Hoffbrand's
Essential Haematology

D1434915

WITHDRAWN
BRITISH MEDICAL ASSOCIATION
FROM LIBRARY

1007304

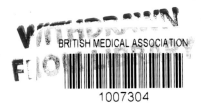

This title is also available as an e-book.

For more details, please see

www.wiley.com/buy/9781119495901

or scan this QR code:

Hoffbrand's Essential Haematology

A. Victor Hoffbrand
MA DM FRCP FRCPath FRCP(Edin) DSc FMedSci
Emeritus Professor of Haematology
University College London
London, UK

David P. Steensma
MD, FACP
Edward P. Evans Chair
Institute Physician, Dana-Farber Cancer Institute
Associate Professor of Medicine, Harvard Medical School
Boston, MA, USA

Eighth Edition

WITHDRAWN FROM LIBRARY

WILEY Blackwell

This edition first published 2020 © 2020 by John Wiley & Sons Ltd

Edition History
1e 1980, Blackwell Publishing; 2e 1984 - Blackwell Publishing; 3e 1993, Blackwell Publishing; 4e 2001, Blackwell Publishing; 5e 2006, Blackwell Publishing; 6e 2011, Wiley-Blackwell; 7e 2015, Wiley-Blackwell

All rights reserved. No part of this publication may be reproduced, stored in a retrieval system, or transmitted, in any form or by any means, electronic, mechanical, photocopying, recording or otherwise, except as permitted by law. Advice on how to obtain permission to reuse material from this title is available at http://www.wiley.com/go/permissions.

The right of A. Victor Hoffbrand and David P. Steensma to be identified as the authors of this work has been asserted in accordance with law.

Registered Offices
John Wiley & Sons, Inc., 111 River Street, Hoboken, NJ 07030, USA
John Wiley & Sons Ltd, The Atrium, Southern Gate, Chichester, West Sussex, PO19 8SQ, UK

Editorial Office
9600 Garsington Road, Oxford, OX4 2DQ, UK

For details of our global editorial offices, customer services, and more information about Wiley products visit us at www.wiley.com.

Wiley also publishes its books in a variety of electronic formats and by print-on-demand. Some content that appears in standard print versions of this book may not be available in other formats.

Limit of Liability/Disclaimer of Warranty
The contents of this work are intended to further general scientific research, understanding, and discussion only and are not intended and should not be relied upon as recommending or promoting scientific method, diagnosis, or treatment by physicians for any particular patient. In view of ongoing research, equipment modifications, changes in governmental regulations, and the constant flow of information relating to the use of medicines, equipment, and devices, the reader is urged to review and evaluate the information provided in the package insert or instructions for each medicine, equipment, or device for, among other things, any changes in the instructions or indication of usage and for added warnings and precautions. While the publisher and authors have used their best efforts in preparing this work, they make no representations or warranties with respect to the accuracy or completeness of the contents of this work and specifically disclaim all warranties, including without limitation any implied warranties of merchantability or fitness for a particular purpose. No warranty may be created or extended by sales representatives, written sales materials or promotional statements for this work. The fact that an organization, website, or product is referred to in this work as a citation and/or potential source of further information does not mean that the publisher and authors endorse the information or services the organization, website, or product may provide or recommendations it may make. This work is sold with the understanding that the publisher is not engaged in rendering professional services. The advice and strategies contained herein may not be suitable for your situation. You should consult with a specialist where appropriate. Further, readers should be aware that websites listed in this work may have changed or disappeared between when this work was written and when it is read. Neither the publisher nor authors shall be liable for any loss of profit or any other commercial damages, including but not limited to special, incidental, consequential, or other damages.

Library of Congress Cataloging-in-Publication Data
Names: Hoffbrand, A. V., author. | Steensma, David P., author.
Title: Hoffbrand's essential haematology / Allan Victor Hoffbrand, David Peter Steensma.
Other titles: Essential haematology
Description: Eighth edition. | Hoboken : Wiley, 2019. | Revision of: Essential haematology / A.V.
Hoffbrand, P.A.H. Moss, J.E. Pettit. 2011.
    6th ed.
Identifiers: LCCN 2019026455 (print) | LCCN 2019026456 (ebook) | ISBN 9781119495901
(paperback) | ISBN 9781119495925 (adobe pdf) | ISBN 9781119495956 (epub)
Subjects: LCSH: Blood—Diseases. | Hematology.
Classification: LCC RC633 .H627 2019 (print) | LCC RC633 (ebook) | DDC 616.1/5—dc23
LC record available at https://lccn.loc.gov/2019026455
LC ebook record available at https://lccn.loc.gov/2019026456

Cover image: © DENNIS KUNKEL MICROSCOPY/science source. Human red blood cells, activated platelets, T lymphocyte (turquoise) and granulocytes (green), coloured scanning electron micrograph (SEM). Magnification: x1000 when shortest axis printed at 25 millimetres.
Cover design by Wiley

Set in 10/12pt Adobe Garamond Pro by Aptara Inc., New Delhi, India
Printed and bound in Singapore by Markono Print Media Pte Ltd

10 9 8 7 6 5 4 3 2 1

Contents

Preface to the Eighth Edition

It is only three years since the 7th edition of this book appeared, but the rapid advances in knowledge of the pathogenesis of blood diseases and in their treatment have necessitated the early publication of this 8th edition. The application of next generation sequencing has revealed the driving mutations underlying many of the neoplastic haematological diseases. Advances in genomic, immunological and immunohistochemical techniques have improved their classification and also enabled highly sensitive tracking of response to therapy. The detection and quantification of minimal residual disease is increasingly recognized as important in planning protocols for treatment of haematological malignancies and for deciding when to end therapy or to intensify it.

The latest (2016) World Health Organization classification of the haematological neoplastic diseases, which relies on much new cytogenetic and molecular genetic information, has been incorporated into the relevant chapters of this new edition. Preclinical clonal abnormalities and their significance in relation to future overt haematological or systemic diseases are being increasingly discovered and are discussed here.

Treatment has also changed substantially. This is partly due to the introduction of many new drugs, often targeted at the signalling pathway, which has been aberrantly activated by a specific mutation. The range of monoclonal antibodies used in therapy, some with conjugated toxins, has also increased. Chimeric antigen receptor (CAR)-T cells are now licensed for treatment of patients with relapsed and refractory B-cell malignancies and are in clinical trials for a wide range of other haematological malignancies. Gene therapy has become a reality for haemophilia and thalassaemia major, and is now also in trials for sickle cell anaemia. Drugs which promote effective erythropoiesis are proving beneficial for alleviating anaemia and transfusion dependence in myelodysplastic syndromes and thalassaemia. The treatment by anticoagulation of venous thrombosis and atrial fibrillation has undergone a major shift from warfarin to the new direct-acting oral anticoagulant drugs for the majority of patients. New text, figures and tables have been added throughout the book to incorporate and illustrate these major advances.

Professor Paul Moss co-authored four previous editions of *Essential Haematology*. We are immensely grateful for his outstanding expert input over many years in keeping its content up to date in a rapidly changing field and maintaining the style of the book. For this 8th edition, David Steensma, from Harvard Medical School and the Dana-Farber Cancer Institute in Boston, has joined as co-author. David is internationally known for his research in the myeloid malignancies and as a writer and teacher within the broader field of haematology.

Jean Connors, also Professor of Haematology at Harvard Medical School and Consultant Haematologist at Brigham and Women's Hospital and the Dana-Farber Cancer Institute Hospital, has substantially helped to update the five chapters dealing with platelets, blood coagulation and their disorders. We are grateful to Jean for her expert knowledge in revising these chapters, where considerable changes in practice have taken place in the last few years. We also thank Dr Keith Gomez of the Royal Free Hospital for his help in updating of the section of the multiple-choice questions relating to Chapters 24-28 which accompany the electronic version of the printed book.

We hope *Essential Haematology* will continue to be used worldwide by medical students and as a primer for those entering haematology as a speciality. The book is also aimed at clinical and non-clinical scientists, nurses and others with a special interest in the blood and its diseases. We thank our publishers Wiley-Blackwell and in particular Jennifer Seward, Nick Morgan and Magenta Styles for their tremendous support in producing this new 8th edition and Jane Fallows for her expert drawing of new figures. We hope *Essential Haematology* will continue internationally to provide a stimulating and comprehensive introduction to one of the most exciting and advanced fields in medicine.

Victor Hoffbrand
David Steensma
2019

Preface to the First Edition

The major changes that have occurred in all fields of medicine over the last decade have been accompanied by an increased understanding of the biochemical, physiological and immunological processes involved in normal blood cell formation and function and the disturbances that may occur in different diseases. At the same time, the range of treatment available for patients with diseases of the blood and blood-forming organs has widened and improved substantially as understanding of the disease processes has increased and new drugs and means of support care have been introduced.

We hope the present book will enable the medical student of the 1980s to grasp the essential features of modern clinical and laboratory haematology and to achieve an understanding of how many of the manifestations of blood diseases can be explained with this new knowledge of the disease processes.

We would like to thank many colleagues and assistants who have helped with the preparation of the book. In particular, Dr H.G. Prentice cared for the patients whose haematological responses are illustrated in Figs 5.3 and 7.8 and Dr J. McLaughlin supplied Fig. 8.6. Dr S. Knowles reviewed critically the final manuscript and made many helpful suggestions. Any remaining errors are, however, our own. We also thank Mr J.B. Irwin and R.W. McPhee who drew many excellent diagrams, Mr Cedric Gilson for expert photomicrography, Mrs T. Charalambos, Mrs B. Elliot, Mrs M. Evans and Miss J. Allaway for typing the manuscript, and Mr Tony Russell of Blackwell Scientific Publications for his invaluable help and patience.

AVH, JEP
1980

How to use your textbook

Features contained within your textbook

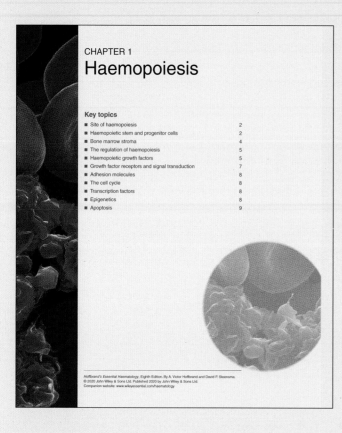

CHAPTER 1

Haemopoiesis

Key topics

Hoffbrand's Essential Haematology, Eighth Edition. By A. Victor Hoffbrand and David P. Steensma.
© 2020 John Wiley & Sons Ltd. Published 2020 by John Wiley & Sons Ltd.
Companion website: www.wileyessential.com/haematology

◀ Every chapter begins
with a list of **Key topics**
of the chapter.

▶ Every chapter ends
with a **Summary** that can
be used for study and
revision purposes.

and may act through regulation of cytochrome c release from mitochondria.

Many of the genetic changes associated with malignant disease lead to a reduced rate of apoptosis and hence prolonged cell survival. The clearest example is the translocation of the *BCL2* gene to the immunoglobulin heavy chain locus in the t(14;18) translocation in follicular lymphoma (see p. 248). Over-expression of the BCL2 protein makes the malignant B cells less susceptible to apoptosis. Apoptosis is the normal fate for most B cells undergoing selection in the lymphoid germinal centres.

Several translocations leading to the generation of fusion proteins, such as t(9;22), t(1;14) and t(15;17), also result in

inhibition of apoptosis (see Chapter 11). In addition, genes encoding proteins that are involved in mediating apoptosis following DNA damage, such as p53 and ATM, are also frequently mutated and therefore inactivated in haemopoietic malignancies.

Necrosis is death of cells and adjacent cells due to ischaemia, chemical trauma or hyperthermia. The cells swell and the plasma membrane loses integrity. There is usually an inflammatory infiltrate in response to spillage of cell contents. Autophagy is the digestion of cell organelles by lysosomes. It may be involved in cell death, but in some situations also in maintaining cell survival by recycling nutrients.

SUMMARY

- Haemopoiesis (blood cell formation) arises from pluripotent stem cells in the bone marrow. Haemopoietic stem cells give rise to mixed and then single lineage progenitor and precursor cells, which, after multiple cell divisions and differentiation, form red cells, granulocytes (neutrophils, eosinophils and basophils), monocytes, platelets, B and T lymphocytes and natural killer cells.
- Haemopoietic tissue occupies about 50% of the marrow space in normal adult marrow. Haemopoiesis in adults is confined to the central skeleton, but in infants and young children haemopoietic tissue extends down the long bones of the arms and legs.
- Stem cells reside in the bone marrow in osteoblastic or endothelial niches formed by stromal cells and circulate in the blood.
- Growth factors attach to specific cell receptors and produce a cascade of phosphorylation events to the cell nucleus. Transcription factors carry the message to those genes that are to be 'switched on', to stimulate

- cell division, differentiation or functional activity or to suppress apoptosis.
- Adhesion molecules are a large family of glycoproteins that mediate the attachment of marrow precursors and mature leucocytes and platelets to extracellular matrix, endothelium and each other.
- Epigenetics refers to changes in DNA and chromatin that affect gene expression other than those that affect DNA sequence. Histone modification and DNA (cytosine) methylation are two important examples relevant to haemopoiesis and haematological malignancies.
- Transcription factors are molecules that bind to DNA and control the transcription of specific genes or gene families.
- Apoptosis is a physiological process of cell death resulting from activation of caspases. The intracellular ratio of pro-apoptotic proteins (e.g. BAX) to anti-apoptotic proteins (e.g. BCL2) determines the cell susceptibility to apoptosis.

 Now visit **www.wileyessential.com/haematology**
to test yourself on this chapter.

▶ Your textbook is full of **photographs, illustrations and tables.**

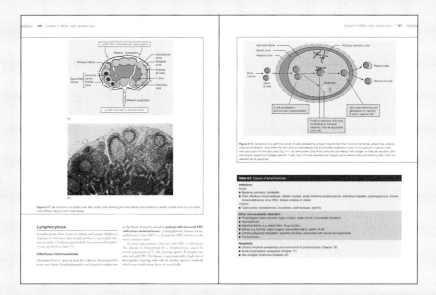

◀ **The website icon**

indicates that you can find accompanying multiple-choice questions and answers on the book's companion website.

5–7 days each week; vitamin C can be given to further increase iron excretion. Most iron is lost in the urine, but up to one-third is also excreted in the stools. Because of the difficult administration, lack of patient adherence is a major problem. It may be given on one or more each days each week in combination with daily deferiprone (or deferasirox) and can be used intravenously in combination with oral deferiprone in patients with severe iron overload at risk of dying from cardiac failure. Side-effects are particularly frequent if high doses are used in children and in adults without heavy iron overload. These include high tone deafness, retinal damage, bone abnormalities and growth retardation. Patients receiving deferoxamine should have auditory and fundoscopic examinations at regular intervals.

All three chelators can be given in children. Deferasirox is most frequently used and a liquid formulation of deferiprone and a sprinkle form of deferasirox are available.

Chelation is typically started in thalassaemia major after 10–15 units have been transfused or the serum ferritin is >800–1000 μg/L. In other conditions such as myelodysplastic

syndromes, there is controversy about when to initiate chelation and hepatic and cardiac T2* MRI may help guide this decision.

Chelation is given to keep the cardiac T2* test at >20 msecs, liver to <7 mg/g dry weight and serum ferritin level at less than 1000–1500 μg/L, when the body iron stores are approximately 5–10 times normal. MRI assesses cardiac and liver iron accurately and should be repeated annually or more frequently if there is definite cardiac or liver damage (Fig. 4.5). Serum ferritin is useful in monitoring changes in iron stores, but as it is an acute phase reactant it may be elevated in the presence of recent infection or physiological stress such as surgery, and this may falsely suggest inadequate chelation.

Serial tests of heart, liver and endocrine function are also needed to monitor therapy.

Life expectancy has improved dramatically for thalassaemia major patients since the introduction of iron chelation. Chelation may even reverse liver, endocrine and cardiac damage in cases where this has developed before chelation is started or is due to inadequate chelation therapy.

SUMMARY

■ Iron overload is caused by excessive absorption of iron from food (genetic haemochromatosis) or by repeated blood transfusions in patients with refractory anaemias. Each unit of blood contains 200–250 mg of iron.
■ Excess iron absorbed from the gastrointestinal tract in genetic haemochromatosis accumulates in the parenchymal cells of the liver, the endocrine organs and, in severe cases, the heart.
■ Genetic haemochromatosis is usually caused by homozygous mutation of the *HFE* gene causing C282Y protein change and a low serum hepcidin level. Rarer forms exist caused by mutations of other genes coding for proteins involved in iron regulation (hemojuvelin, hepcidin, transferrin receptor 2 and ferroportin). Repeated venesections are used to reduce the body iron burden.
■ Transfusional iron overload most frequently occurs in thalassaemia major, but also in other transfusion-dependent refractory anaemias (e.g. some cases of myelodysplastic syndromes, sickle cell anaemia, primary myelofibrosis, red cell aplasia and aplastic anaemia).
■ Transfusional iron overload causes damage to the liver, endocrine organs and heart, with iron accumulation also in macrophages of the reticuloendothelial system.
■ Cardiac failure or arrhythmia caused by cardiac siderosis, best detected by MRI, is the most frequent cause of death from transfusional iron overload.
■ Treatment is with iron chelating drugs: deferiprone and deferasirox, which are active orally, or deferoxamine, given subcutaneously or intravenously.
■ Life expectancy has improved dramatically in thalassaemia major as a result of iron chelation therapy and the use of T2*MRI to accurately measure cardiac and liver iron.

 Now visit www.wileyessential.com/haematology to test yourself on this chapter.

About the companion website

Don't forget to visit the companion website for this book:

www.wileyessential.com/haematology

There you will find invaluable material designed to enhance your learning, including:

- Interactive multiple-choice questions
- Figures and tables from the book

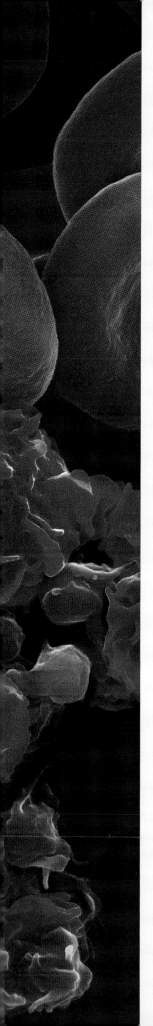

CHAPTER 1
Haemopoiesis

Key topics

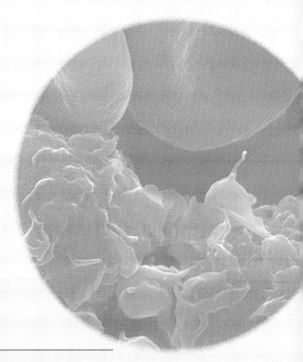

Hoffbrand's Essential Haematology, Eighth Edition. By A. Victor Hoffbrand and David P. Steensma.
© 2020 John Wiley & Sons Ltd. Published 2020 by John Wiley & Sons Ltd.
Companion website: www.wileyessential.com/haematology

This first chapter is concerned with the general aspects of blood cell formation (haemopoiesis). The processes that regulate haemopoiesis and the early stages of formation of red cells (erythropoiesis), granulocytes and monocytes (myelopoiesis) and platelets (thrombopoiesis) are also discussed.

Site of haemopoiesis

In the first few weeks of gestation, the embryonic yolk sac is a transient site of haemopoiesis called 'primitive haemopoiesis'. However, 'definitive haemopoiesis' derives from a population of stem cells first observed on the aorta-gonads-mesonephros (AGM) region of the developing embryo. These common precursors of endothelial and haemopoietic cells are called haemangioblasts and are believed to seed the liver, spleen and bone marrow.

From 6 weeks until 6–7 months of fetal life, the liver and spleen are the major haemopoietic organs and continue to produce blood cells until about 2 weeks after birth (Table 1.1; see Fig. 7.1b). The placenta also contributes to fetal haemopoiesis. The bone marrow is the most important site from 6–7 months of fetal life. During normal childhood and adult life, the marrow is the only source of new blood cells. The developing cells are situated outside the bone marrow sinuses; mature cells are released into the sinus spaces, the marrow microcirculation and so into the general circulation.

In infancy all the bone marrow is haemopoietic, but during childhood and beyond there is progressive fatty replacement of marrow throughout the long bones, so that in adult life haemopoietic marrow is confined to the central skeleton and proximal ends of the femurs and humeri (Table 1.1). Even in these active haemopoietic areas, approximately 50% of the marrow consists of fat in the middle-aged adult (Fig. 1.1). The remaining fatty marrow is capable of reversion to haemopoiesis and in many diseases there is also expansion of haemopoiesis down the long bones. Moreover, in certain disease states the liver and spleen can resume their fetal haemopoietic role ('extramedullary haemopoiesis').

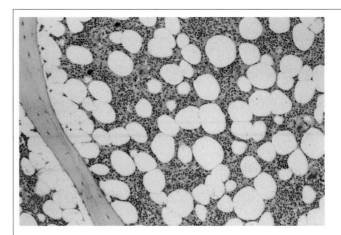

Figure 1.1 Normal bone marrow trephine biopsy (posterior iliac crest). Haematoxylin and eosin stain; approximately 50% of the intertrabecular tissue is haemopoietic tissue and 50% is fat.

Haemopoietic stem and progenitor cells

Haemopoiesis starts with a pluripotential stem cell that can self-renew by asymmetrical cell division, but also gives rise to the separate cell lineages. These cells are able to repopulate a bone marrow from which all stem cells have been eliminated by lethal irradiation or chemotherapy. Self-renewal and repopulating ability define the **haemopoietic stem cell** (HSC). HSCs are rare, perhaps 1 in every 20 million nucleated cells in bone marrow. Newer DNA sequencing techniques suggest that a typical adult has approximately 50 000 HSCs.

HSCs are heterogeneous, with some able to repopulate a bone marrow for more than 16 weeks, called **long-term HSCs**, while others, although able to produce all haemopoietic cell types, engraft only transiently for a few weeks and are called **short–term HSCs**. Although the exact cell surface marker phenotype of the HSC is still unknown, on immunological testing these cells are positive for the marker Cluster of Differentiation 34 (CD34⁺) and negative for CD38⁻ and for cell lineage-defining markers (Lin⁻). Morphologically, HSCs have the appearance of a small or medium-sized lymphocyte (see Fig. 23.3). The cells reside adjacent to osteoblasts or to endothelial cells of sinusoidal vessels in endosteal or vascular 'niches', where they are surrounded by stromal cells, with which they interact in numerous ways. The niches also contain sympathetic nerve endings.

Cell differentiation occurs from the stem cells via committed **haemopoietic progenitors**, which are restricted in their developmental potential (Fig. 1.2). The existence of the separate progenitor cells can be demonstrated by *in vitro* culture techniques. Stem cells and very early progenitors are assayed by culture on bone marrow stroma as long-term culture-initiating cells, whereas late progenitors are generally assayed in semi-solid media. As examples, in the erythroid series progenitors can be identified in special cultures as burst-forming units

Table 1.1 Dominant sites of haemopoiesis at different stages of development.	
Fetus	0–2 months (yolk sac)
	2–7 months (liver, spleen)
	5–9 months (bone marrow)
Infants	Bone marrow (practically all bones); dwindling post-parturition contribution from liver/spleen that ceases in the first few months of life
Adults	Vertebrae, ribs, sternum, skull, sacrum and pelvis, proximal ends of femur

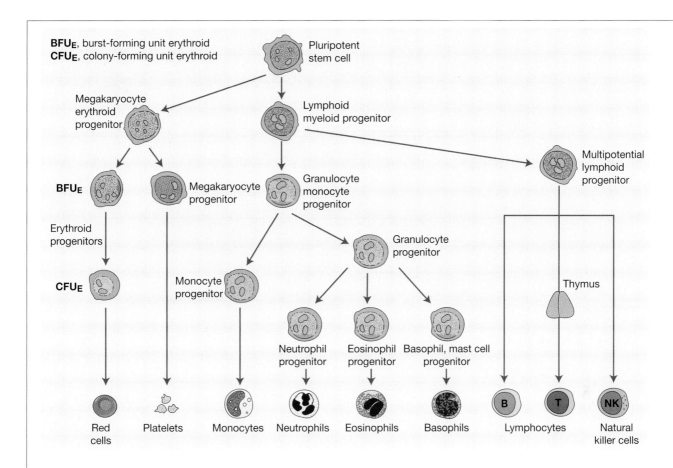

Figure 1.2 Diagrammatic representation of the bone marrow pluripotent stem cells (haemopoietic stem cells, HSC) and the cell lines that arise from them. A megakaryocytic/erythroid progenitor (MkEP) and a mixed lymphoid/myeloid progenitor are formed from the pluripotent stem cells. Each gives rise to more differentiated progenitors. The MkEP divides into erythroid and megakaryocyte progenitors. The mixed lymphoid progenitor gives rise to B and T lymphocytes and to natural killer cells. A granulocyte/monocyte progenitor gives rise to progenitors for monocytes, neutrophils, eosinophils, basophils and mast cells. The erythroid progenitors are also termed BFU-E and CFU-E. BFU-E, burst-forming unit erythroid; CFU-E, colony-forming unit erythroid.

(BFU-E, describing the 'burst' with which they form in culture) and colony-forming units (CFU-E; Fig 1.2); the mixed granulocyte/monocyte progenitor is identified as a colony-forming unit-granulocyte/monocyte (CFU-GM) in culture. Megakaryocytes form from the CFU-Meg.

In the haemopoietic hierarchy, the pluripotent stem cell gives rise to a **mixed erythroid and megakaryocyte progenitor**, which then divides into separate erythroid and megakaryocyte progenitors. The pluripotent stem cell also gives rise to a **mixed lymphoid, granulocyte and monocyte progenitor**, which divides into a progenitor of granulocytes and monocytes and a mixed lymphoid progenitor, from which B- and T-cell lymphocytes and natural killer (NK) cells develop (Fig. 1.2). The spleen, lymph nodes and thymus are secondary sites of lymphocyte production (see Chapter 9).

The stem cell has the capability for **self-renewal** (Fig. 1.3), so that marrow cellularity remains constant in a normal, healthy steady state. There is considerable amplification in the

system: one stem cell is capable of producing about 10^6 mature blood cells after 20 cell divisions (Fig. 1.3). In humans HSCs are capable of about 50 cell divisions (the 'Hayflick limit'), with progressive telomere shortening with each division affecting viability.

Under normal conditions most HSCs are dormant, with at most only a few percent actively in cell cycle on any given day. In humans it has been estimated that any given HSC enters the cell cycle approximately once every 3 months to 3 years. By contrast, progenitor cells are much more numerous and highly proliferative. With ageing, the number of stem cells falls and the relative proportion giving rise to lymphoid rather than myeloid progenitors falls too. Stem cells also accumulate genetic mutations with age, an average of 8 exonic coding mutations by age 60 years (1.3 per decade), and these, either passengers without oncogenic potential or drivers that cause clonal expansion, may be present in neoplasms arising from these stem cells (see Chapter 11).

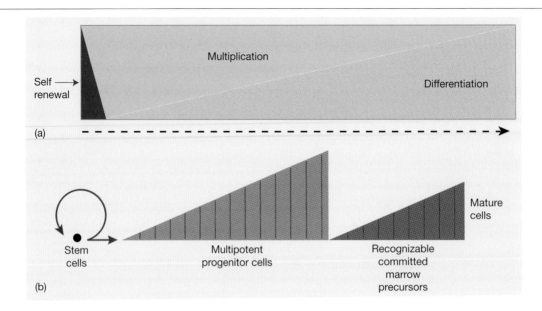

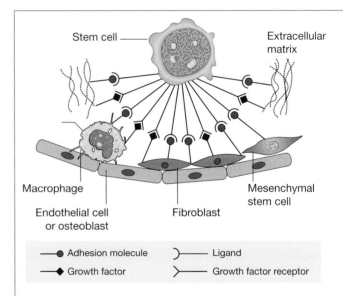

Figure 1.3 **(a)** Bone marrow cells are increasingly differentiated and lose the capacity for self-renewal as they mature. **(b)** A single stem cell gives rise, after multiple cell divisions (shown by vertical lines), to >10^6 mature cells.

The progenitor and precursor cells are capable of responding to haemopoietic growth factors with increased production of one or other cell line when the need arises. The development of the **mature cells** (red cells, granulocytes, monocytes, megakaryocytes and lymphocytes) is considered further in other sections of this book.

Bone marrow stroma

The bone marrow forms a suitable environment for stem cell survival, self-renewal and formation of differentiated progenitor cells. It is composed of various types of stromal cells and a microvascular network (Fig. 1.4). **The stromal cells include mesenchymal stem cells, adipocytes. fibroblasts, osteoblasts, endothelial cells and macrophages**, and they secrete extracellular molecules such as collagen, glycoproteins (fibronectin and thrombospondin) and glycosaminoglycans (hyaluronic acid and chondroitin derivatives) to form an extracellular matrix. In addition, stromal cells secrete several growth factors necessary for stem cell survival.

Mesenchymal stem cells are critical in stromal cell formation. Together with osteoblasts or endothelial cells, they form niches and provide some of the growth factors, adhesion molecules and cytokines which support stem cells, maintaining their viability and reproduction. For example, stem cell factor (SCF) and the protein Jagged1 expressed by stromal cells bind to their respective receptors, KIT (CD117) and NOTCH1, on stem cells. NOTCH1 then becomes a transcription factor involved in the cell cycle.

Stem cells are able to traffic around the body and are found in peripheral blood in low numbers. In order to exit the bone marrow, cells must cross the blood vessel endothelium, and this

Figure 1.4 Haemopoiesis occurs in a suitable microenvironment ('niche') provided by a stromal matrix on which stem cells grow and divide. The niche may be vascular (lined by endothelium) or endosteal (lined by osteoblasts). There are specific recognition and adhesion sites; extracellular glycoproteins and other compounds are involved in the binding.

process of **mobilization** is enhanced by the administration of growth factors such as granulocyte colony-stimulating factor (G-CSF; see p. 100). The reverse process of stem cell **homing** appears to depend on a chemokine gradient in which the stromal-derived factor 1 (SDF-1) which binds to its receptor CXCR4 on HSC is critical.

The regulation of haemopoiesis

Haemopoiesis starts with stem cell division in which one cell replaces the stem cell (*self-renewal*) and the other is committed to differentiation. These early committed progenitors express low levels of transcription factors that may commit them to discrete cell lineages. Which cell lineage is selected for differentiation may depend both on chance and on the external signals received by progenitor cells. Several transcription factors (see p. 8) regulate the survival of stem cells (e.g. SCL, GATA2, NOTCH1), whereas others are involved in differentiation along the major cell lineages. For instance, PU.1 and the CEBP family of transcription factors commit cells to the myeloid lineage, whereas GATA2 and then GATA1 and FOG1 have essential roles in erythropoietic and megakaryocytic differentiation. These transcription factors interact, so that reinforcement of one transcription programme may suppress that of another lineage. The transcription factors induce synthesis of proteins specific to a cell lineage. For example, the erythroid-specific genes for globin and haem synthesis have binding motifs for GATA1.

Haemopoietic growth factors

The haemopoietic growth factors are a group of glycoprotein hormones that regulate the proliferation and differentiation of haemopoietic progenitor cells and the function of mature blood cells. **They may act locally at the site where they are produced by cell–cell contact (e.g. SCF) or circulate in plasma (e.g. G-CSF or erythropoietin, EPO).** They also bind to the extracellular matrix to form niches to which stem and progenitor cells adhere. The growth factors may cause cell proliferation, but can also stimulate differentiation and maturation, prevent apoptosis and affect the function of mature cells (Fig. 1.5).

The growth factors share a number of common properties (Table 1.2) and act at different stages of haemopoiesis (Table 1.3; Fig. 1.6). **Stromal cells are the major source of growth factors except for EPO, 90% of which is synthesized in the kidney, and thrombopoietin (TPO), made largely in the liver.** An important feature of growth factor action is that two or more factors may synergize in stimulating a particular cell to proliferate or differentiate. Moreover, the action of one growth factor on a cell may stimulate production of another growth factor or growth factor receptor.

SCF, TPO and FLT3 ligand act locally on the pluripotential stem cells and on myeloid /lymphoid progenitors (Fig. 1.6). Interleukin-3 (IL-3) has widespread activity on lymphoid/myeloid and megakaryocyte/erythroid progenitors. Granulocyte–macrophage colony-stimulating factor (GM-CSF), G-CSF and macrophage colony-stimulating factor (M-CSF) enhance neutrophil and macrophage/monocyte production, IL-5 eosinophil, KIT mast cell, TPO platelet and EPO red cell production. These lineage-specific growth factors also enhance the effects of SCF, FLT3-L and IL-3 on the survival and differentiation of early haemopoietic

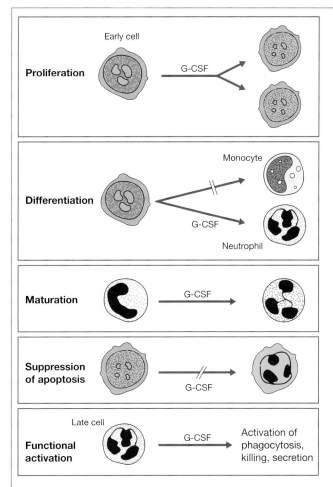

Figure 1.5 Growth factors may stimulate the proliferation of early bone marrow cells, direct differentiation to one or other cell type, stimulate cell maturation, suppress apoptosis or affect the function of mature non-dividing cells, as illustrated here for granulocyte colony-stimulating factor (G-CSF) for an early myeloid progenitor and a neutrophil.

Table 1.2 General characteristics of myeloid and lymphoid growth factors.

Glycoproteins that act at very low concentrations

Act hierarchically

Usually produced by many cell types

Usually affect more than one lineage

Usually active on stem/progenitor cells and on differentiated cells

Usually show synergistic or additive interactions with other growth factors

Often act on the neoplastic equivalent of a normal cell

Multiple actions: proliferation, differentiation, maturation, functional activation, prevention of apoptosis of progenitor cells

Table 1.3 Haemopoietic growth factors (see also Fig. 1.6).

Act on stromal cells
IL-1, TNF

Act on pluripotential stem cells
SCF, TPO, FLT3-L

Act on multipotential lymphoid/myeloid progenitor cells
IL-3, IL-7, SCF, FLT3-L,TPO, GM-CSF

Act on lineage-committed progenitor cells
Granulocyte/monocyte production: IL-3, GM-CSF, G-CSF, M-CSF, IL-5 (eosinophil CSF)
Mast cell production: KIT-ligand
Red cell production: IL-3, EPO
    Platelet production: IL-3, TPO
    Lymphocyte/NK cell production: IL-1, IL-2, IL-4, IL-7, IL-10, other ILs

CSF, colony-stimulating factor; EPO, erythropoietin; FLT3-L, FLT3 ligand; G-CSF, granulocyte colony-stimulating factor; GM-CSF, granulocyte–macrophage colony-stimulating factor; IL, interleukin; M-CSF, macrophage/monocyte colony-stimulating factor; NK, natural killer; SCF, stem cell factor (also known as TAL1); TNF, tumour necrosis factor; TPO, thrombopoietin.

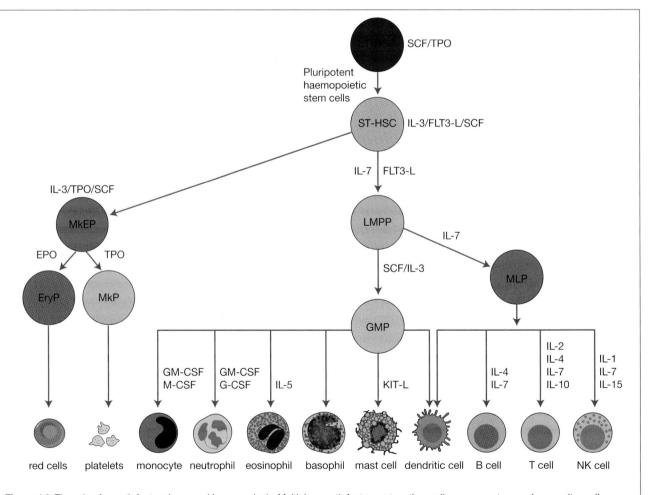

Figure 1.6 The role of growth factors in normal haemopoiesis. Multiple growth factors act on the earlier marrow stem and progenitor cells. EPO, erythropoietin; EryP, erythroid progenitor; FLT3-L, FLT3 ligand; G-CSF, granulocyte colony-stimulating factor; GM-CSF, granulocyte–macrophage colony-stimulating factor; GMP, granulocyte–macrophage progenitor; HSC, haemopoietic stem cells; IL, interleukin; LMPP, lymphoid-primed multipotential progenitor; M-CSF, macrophage/monocyte colony-stimulating factor; MkEP, megakaryocyte–erythroid progenitor; MkP, megakaryocyte progenitor; MLP, multipotential lymphoid progenitor; ST, short-term; LT, long-term; NK, natural killer; PSC, pluripotential stem cell; SCF, stem cell factor; TLR, toll-like receptor; TPO, thrombopoietin. Source: Adapted from A.V. Hoffbrand *et al.* (2019) *Color Atlas of Clinical Hematology: Molecular and Cellular Basis of Disease,* 5th edn. Reproduced with permission of John Wiley & Sons.

cells. Interleukin 7 is involved at all stages of lymphocyte production and various other interleukins and Toll-like receptor ligands (not shown) direct B and T lymphocyte and NK cell production (Fig 1.6).

These factors maintain a pool of haemopoietic stem and progenitor cells on which later-acting factors, EPO, G-CSF, M-CSF, IL-5 and TPO, act to increase production of one or other cell lineage in response to the body's need. Granulocyte and monocyte formation, for example, can be stimulated by infection or inflammation through release of IL-1 and tumour necrosis factor (TNF), which then stimulate stromal cells to produce growth factors in an interacting network (see Fig. 8.4). In contrast, cytokines, such as transforming growth factor-β (TGF-β) and γ-interferon (IFN-γ), can exert a negative effect on haemopoiesis and may have a role in the development of aplastic anaemia (see p. 276).

Growth factor receptors and signal transduction

The biological effects of growth factors are mediated through specific receptors on target cells. Many receptors, such as EPO receptor (EPO-R), GM-CSF-R, are from the **haemopoietin receptor superfamily** which dimerize after binding their ligand.

Dimerization of the receptor leads to activation of a complex series of intracellular signal transduction pathways, of which the three major ones are the JAK/STAT, the mitogen-activated protein (MAP) kinase and the phosphatidylinositol 3 (PI3) kinase pathways (Fig. 1.7; see also Fig. 9.4 and Fig. 15.2). The Janus-associated kinase (JAK) proteins are a family of four tyrosine-specific protein kinases that associate with the intracellular domains of the growth factor receptors (Fig. 1.7). A growth factor molecule binds simultaneously to the extracellular domains of two or three receptor molecules, resulting in their aggregation. Receptor aggregation induces activation of the JAKs, which then phosphorylate members of the signal transducer and activator of transcription (STAT) family of transcription factors. This results in their dimerization and translocation from the cell cytoplasm across the nuclear membrane to the cell nucleus. Within the nucleus STAT dimers activate the transcription of specific genes. A model for the control of gene expression by a transcription factor is shown in Fig. 1.8. The clinical importance of this pathway is revealed for example by the finding of an activating mutation of the *JAK2* gene as the cause of polycythaemia vera and related myeloproliferative neoplasms (see p. 183).

JAK can also activate the MAPK pathway, which is regulated by RAS and controls proliferation. PI3 kinases phosphorylate inositol lipids, which have a wide range of downstream effects, including activation of AKT leading to block of apoptosis and other actions (Fig. 1.7; see Fig. 15.2). Different domains of the intracellular receptor protein may signal for the different processes (e.g. proliferation or suppression of apoptosis) mediated by growth factors.

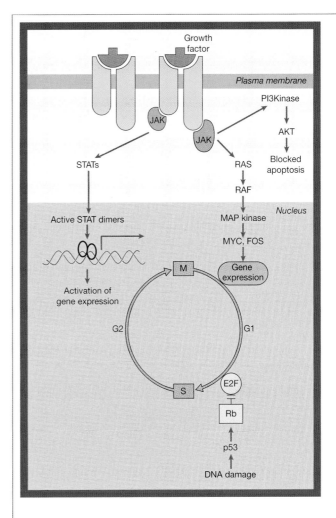

Figure 1.7 Control of haemopoiesis by growth factors. The factors act on cells expressing the corresponding receptors. Binding of a growth factor to its receptor activates the JAK/STAT, MAPK and phosphatidyl-inositol 3-kinase (PI3K) pathways (see Fig. 15.2), which leads to transcriptional activation of specific genes. E2F is a transcription factor needed for cell transition from G1 to S phase. E2F is inhibited by the tumour suppressor gene Rb (retinoblastoma), which can be indirectly activated by p53. The synthesis and degradation of different cyclins stimulate the cell to pass through the different phases of the cell cycle. The growth factors may also suppress apoptosis by activating AKT (protein kinase B).

A second, smaller group of growth factors, including SCF, FLT-3L and M-CSF (Table 1.3), bind to receptors that have an extracellular immunoglobulin-like domain linked via a transmembrane bridge to a cytoplasmic tyrosine kinase domain. Growth factor binding results in dimerization of these receptors and consequent activation of the tyrosine kinase domain. Phosphorylation of tyrosine residues in the receptor itself generates binding sites for signalling proteins which initiate complex cascades of biochemical events, resulting in changes in gene expression, cell proliferation and prevention of apoptosis.

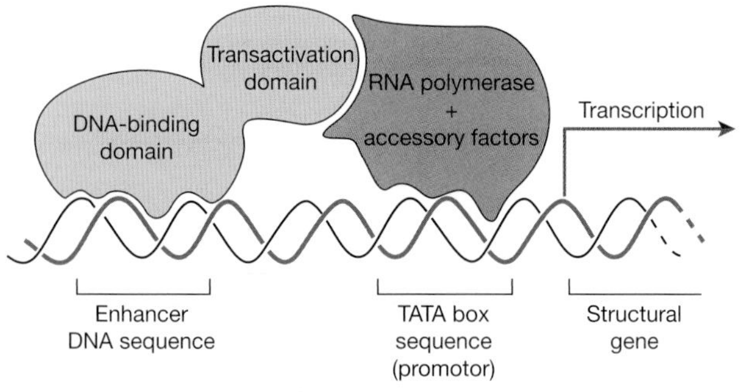

Figure 1.8 Model for control of gene expression by a transcription factor. The DNA-binding domain of a transcription factor binds a specific enhancer sequence adjacent to a structural gene. The transactivation domain then binds a molecule of RNA polymerase, thus augmenting its binding to the TATA box. The RNA polymerase now initiates transcription of the structural gene to form mRNA. Translation of the mRNA by the ribosomes generates the protein encoded by the gene.

Adhesion molecules

A large family of glycoprotein molecules termed adhesion molecules mediate the attachment of marrow precursors, leucocytes and platelets to various components of the extracellular matrix, to endothelium, to other surfaces and to each other. The adhesion molecules on the surface of leucocytes are termed receptors and these interact with proteins termed ligands on the surface of target cells, e.g. endothelium. The adhesion molecules are important in the development and maintenance of inflammatory and immune responses, and in platelet–vessel wall and leucocyte–vessel wall interactions Glycoprotein IIb/IIIa, for example, is an adhesion molecule, also called integrin IIbeta/IIIalpha, involved in platelet adhesion to vessel walls and to each other (Chapter 24).

The pattern of expression of adhesion molecules on tumour cells may determine their mode of spread and tissue localization (e.g. the pattern of metastasis of carcinoma cells to specific visceral organs or bone, or non-Hodgkin lymphoma cells into a follicular or diffuse pattern). The adhesion molecules may also determine whether or not cells circulate in the bloodstream or remain fixed in tissues. They may also partly determine whether or not tumour cells are susceptible to the body's immune defences.

The cell cycle

The cell division cycle, generally known simply as the **cell cycle**, is a complex process that lies at the heart of haemopoiesis. Dysregulation of cell proliferation is also the key to the development of malignant disease. The duration of the cell cycle is variable between different tissues, but the basic principles remain constant. The cycle is divided into the mitotic phase (**M phase**), during which the cell physically divides, and **interphase**, during which the chromosomes are duplicated and cell growth occurs prior to division (Fig. 1.7). The M phase is further partitioned into classical **mitosis**, in which nuclear division is accomplished, and **cytokinesis**, in which cell fission occurs.

Interphase is divided into three main stages: a G_1 **phase**, in which the cell begins to commit to replication, an **S phase**, during which DNA content doubles and the chromosomes replicate, and the G_2 **phase**, in which the cell organelles are copied and cytoplasmic volume is increased. If cells rest prior to division they enter a G_0 state where they can remain for long periods of time. The number of cells at each stage of the cell cycle can be assessed by exposing cells to a chemical or radiolabel that gets incorporated into newly generated DNA or by flow cytometry.

The cell cycle is controlled by two **checkpoints** which act as brakes to coordinate the division process at the end of the G_1 and G_2 phases. Two major classes of molecules control these checkpoints, **cyclin-dependent protein kinases** (Cdk), which phosphorylate downstream protein targets, and **cyclins**, which bind to Cdk and regulate their activity. An example of the importance of these systems is demonstrated by mantle cell lymphoma, which results from the constitutive activation of cyclin D1 as a result of a chromosomal translocation (see p. 249).

Transcription factors

Transcription factors regulate gene expression by controlling the transcription of specific genes or gene families (Fig. 1.8). Typically, they contain at least two domains: a **DNA-binding domain**, such as a leucine zipper or helix–loop–helix motif which binds to a specific DNA sequence, and an **activation domain**, which contributes to assembly of the transcription complex at a gene promoter. Examples of transcription factors involved in haemopoiesis include GATA1, GATA2 and FOG1 in erythropoiesis, PU.1 in granulopoiesis, PAX5 in B lymphocyte and NOTCH in T lymphocyte development. Mutation, deletion or translocation of transcription factors underlies many cases of haematological neoplasms (see Chapter 11).

Epigenetics

Epigenetics refers to changes in DNA and chromatin that affect gene expression other than those that affect DNA sequence (see Fig. 16.1).

Cellular DNA is packaged by wrapping it around histones, a group of specialized nuclear proteins. The complex is tightly compacted as chromatin. In order for the DNA code to be read, transcription factors and other proteins need to physically attach to DNA. Histones act as custodians for this access and so for gene expression. **Histones may be modified by methylation, acetylation and phosphorylation**, which can result in increased or decreased gene expression and so changes in cell phenotype.

Epigenetics also includes changes to DNA itself, such as methylation of DNA bases, which regulates gene expression in normal and tumour tissues. The methylation of cytosine residues to methyl cytosine results in inhibition of gene transcription. The DNA methyltransferase genes *DNMT3A* and *B* are involved in the methylation, and *TET1,2,3* and *IDH1* and *IDH2* in the hydroxylation and breakdown of methylcytosine and restoration of gene expression (see Fig. 16.1). These genes are frequently mutated in the myeloid malignancies, especially myelodysplastic syndromes and acute myeloid leukaemia (see Chapters 13, 15 and 16).

Apoptosis

Apoptosis (programmed cell death) is a regulated process of physiological cell death in which individual cells are triggered to activate intracellular proteins that lead to the death of the cell. Morphologically it is characterized by cell shrinkage, condensation of the nuclear chromatin, fragmentation of the nucleus and cleavage of DNA at internucleosomal sites. It is an important process for maintaining tissue homeostasis in haemopoiesis and lymphocyte development.

Apoptosis results from the action of intracellular cysteine proteases called **caspases**, which are activated following cleavage and lead to endonuclease digestion of DNA and disintegration of the cell skeleton (Fig. 1.9). There are two major pathways by which caspases can be activated. The first is by signalling through membrane proteins such as Fas or TNF receptor via their intracellular death domain. An example of this mechanism is shown by activated cytotoxic T cells expressing Fas ligand, which induces apoptosis in target cells. The second pathway is via the release of cytochrome c from mitochondria. Cytochrome c binds to APAF-1, which then activates caspases. DNA damage induced by irradiation or chemotherapy may act through this pathway.

The protein P53 encoded by the *TP53* gene on chromosome 17 has an important role in sensing DNA damage. It activates apoptosis by raising the cell level of BAX, which then increases cytochrome c release (Fig. 1.9). P53 also shuts down the cell cycle to stop the damaged cell from dividing (Fig. 1.7). The cellular level of P53 is controlled by a second protein, MDM2. Following death, apoptotic cells display molecules that lead to their ingestion by macrophages. Loss of TP53 is a major mechanism by which malignant cells evade controls that would induce cell death.

As well as molecules that mediate apoptosis, there are several intracellular proteins that protect cells from apoptosis. The best-characterized example is BCL2. BCL2 is the prototype of a family of related proteins, some of which are antiapoptotic and some, like BAX, pro-apoptotic. The intracellular ratio of BAX and BCL2 determines the relative susceptibility of cells to apoptosis (e.g. determines the lifespan of platelets)

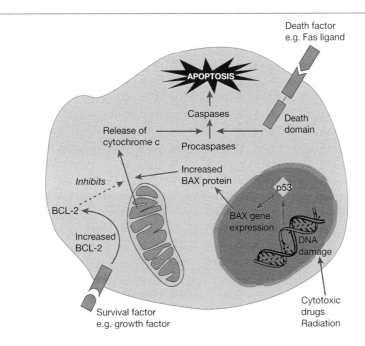

Figure 1.9 Representation of apoptosis. Apoptosis is initiated via two main stimuli: (i) signalling through cell membrane receptors such as FAS or tumour necrosis factor (TNF) receptor; or (ii) release of cytochrome c from mitochondria. Membrane receptors signal apoptosis through an intracellular death domain leading to activation of caspases which digest DNA. Cytochrome c binds to the cytoplasmic protein Apaf-1 leading to activation of caspases. The intracellular ratio of pro-apoptotic (e.g. BAX) or anti-apoptotic (e.g. BCL-2) members of the BCL-2 family may influence mitochondrial cytochrome c release. Growth factors raise the level of BCL-2, inhibiting cytochrome c release, whereas DNA damage, by activating p53, raises the level of BAX, which enhances cytochrome c release.

and may act through regulation of cytochrome c release from mitochondria.

Many of the genetic changes associated with malignant disease lead to a reduced rate of apoptosis and hence prolonged cell survival. The clearest example is the translocation of the *BCL2* gene to the immunoglobulin heavy chain locus in the t(14;18) translocation in follicular lymphoma (see p. 248). Over-expression of the BCL2 protein makes the malignant B cells less susceptible to apoptosis. Apoptosis is the normal fate for most B cells undergoing selection in the lymphoid germinal centres.

Several translocations leading to the generation of fusion proteins, such as t(9;22), t(1;14) and t(15;17), also result in inhibition of apoptosis (see Chapter 11). In addition, genes encoding proteins that are involved in mediating apoptosis following DNA damage, such as p53 and ATM, are also frequently mutated and therefore inactivated in haemopoietic malignancies.

Necrosis is death of cells and adjacent cells due to ischaemia, chemical trauma or hyperthermia. The cells swell and the plasma membrane loses integrity. There is usually an inflammatory infiltrate in response to spillage of cell contents. Autophagy is the digestion of cell organelles by lysosomes. It may be involved in cell death, but in some situations also in maintaining cell survival by recycling nutrients.

SUMMARY

- Haemopoiesis (blood cell formation) arises from pluripotent stem cells in the bone marrow. Haemopoietic stem cells give rise to mixed and then single lineage progenitor and precursor cells which, after multiple cell divisions and differentiation, form red cells, granulocytes (neutrophils, eosinophils and basophils), monocytes, platelets, B and T lymphocytes and natural killer cells.
- Haemopoietic tissue occupies about 50% of the marrow space in normal adult marrow. Haemopoiesis in adults is confined to the central skeleton, but in infants and young children haemopoietic tissue extends down the long bones of the arms and legs.
- Stem cells reside in the bone marrow in osteoblastic or endothelial niches formed by stromal cells and circulate in the blood.
- Growth factors attach to specific cell receptors and produce a cascade of phosphorylation events to the cell nucleus. Transcription factors carry the message to those genes that are to be 'switched on', to stimulate

cell division, differentiation or functional activity or to suppress apoptosis.
- Adhesion molecules are a large family of glycoproteins that mediate the attachment of marrow precursors and mature leucocytes and platelets to extracellular matrix, endothelium and each other.
- Epigenetics refers to changes in DNA and chromatin that affect gene expression other than those that affect DNA sequence. Histone modification and DNA (cytosine) methylation are two important examples relevant to haemopoiesis and haematological malignancies.
- Transcription factors are molecules that bind to DNA and control the transcription of specific genes or gene families.
- Apoptosis is a physiological process of cell death resulting from activation of caspases. The intracellular ratio of pro-apoptotic proteins (e.g. BAX) to anti-apoptotic proteins (e.g. BCL2) determines the cell susceptibility to apoptosis.

 Now visit **www.wileyessential.com/haematology** to test yourself on this chapter.

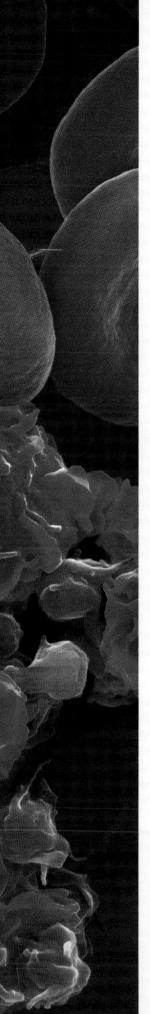

CHAPTER 2
Erythropoiesis and general aspects of anaemia

Key topics

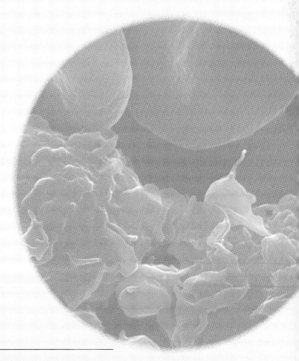

Hoffbrand's Essential Haematology, Eighth Edition. By A. Victor Hoffbrand and David P. Steensma.
© 2020 John Wiley & Sons Ltd. Published 2020 by John Wiley & Sons Ltd.
Companion website: www.wileyessential.com/haematology

Blood cells

All the circulating blood cells derive from pluripotential stem cells in the marrow. They divide into three main types. The most numerous are **red cells**, which are specialized for the carriage of oxygen from the lungs to the tissues and of carbon dioxide in the reverse direction (Table 2.1). They have a 4-month lifespan, whereas the smallest cells, **platelets** involved in haemostasis, circulate for only 10 days. **The white cells are made up of four types of phagocyte: neutrophils, eosinophils, basophils and monocytes**, which protect against bacterial and fungal infections (see Chapter 8); and of **lymphocytes**, which include **B cells**, involved in antibody production, **T cells** (CD4 helper and CD8 suppressor), concerned with the immune response and in protection against viruses and other foreign cells, and natural killer cells, a subset of CD8 T cells (see Chapter 9). White cells have a wide range of lifespan (Table 2.1).

The red cells and platelets are counted and their diameter and other parameters measured by an automated cell counter (Fig. 2.1). The counter also enumerates the different types of white cell by flow cytometry and detects abnormal cells.

We each make approximately 10^{12} new erythrocytes (red cells) each day by the complex and finely regulated process of erythropoiesis. Erythropoiesis passes from the stem cell through the progenitor cells, colony-forming unit (CFU), erythroid and megakaryocyte (CFU_{MkE}), burst-forming unit erythroid (BFU_E) and erythroid CFU (CFU_E; Fig. 1.2) to the first recognizable erythrocyte precursor in the bone marrow, the pronormoblast (Fig. 2.2). This process occurs in an erythroid niche in which about 30 erythroid cells at various stages of development surround a central macrophage.

The pronormoblast is a large cell with dark blue cytoplasm, a central nucleus with nucleoli and slightly clumped chromatin (Fig. 2.2). It gives rise to a series of progressively smaller normoblasts by a number of cell divisions. They also contain progressively more haemoglobin (which stains pink) in the cytoplasm; the cytoplasm stains paler blue as it loses its RNA and protein synthetic apparatus, while nuclear chromatin becomes more condensed (Figs 2.2 and 2.3). The nucleus is finally extruded from the late normoblast within the marrow and a reticulocyte results, which still contains some ribosomal RNA and is still able to synthesize haemoglobin (Fig. 2.4).

Table 2.1 The blood cells.

Cell	Diameter (μm)	Lifespan in blood	Number	Function
Red cells	6–8	120 days	Male: $4.5–6.5 \times 10^{12}$/L Female: $3.9–5.6 \times 10^{12}$/L	Oxygen and carbon dioxide transport
Platelets	0.5–3.0	10 days	$140–400 \times 10^9$/L	Haemostasis
Phagocytes				
Neutrophils	12–15	6–10 h	$1.8–7.5 \times 10^9$/L	Protection from bacteria, fungi
Monocytes	12–20	20-40 h	$0.2–0.8 \times 10^9$/L	Protection from bacteria, fungi
Eosinophils	12–15	Days	$0.04–0.44 \times 10^9$/L	Protection against parasites
Basophils	12–15	Days	$0.01–0.1 \times 10^9$/L	
Lymphocytes B T	7–9 (resting) 12–20 (active)	Weeks or years	$1.5–3.5 \times 10^9$/L	B cells: immunoglobulin synthesis T cells: protection against viruses; immune functions
Natural killer cells NK	10 (resting) 10–20 (active)	Hours or days	0.1–0.4	Protection against virus-infected and neoplastic cells

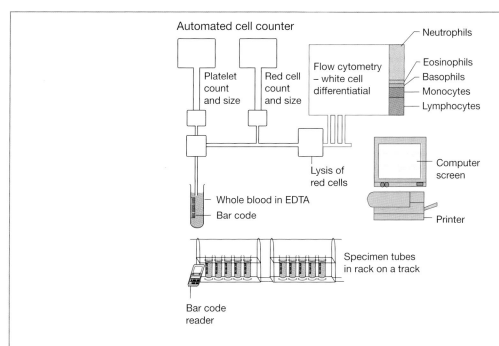

Automated cell counter

Figure 2.1 Automated blood cell counter. Source: A.B. Mehta, A.V. Hoffbrand (2014) *Haematology at a Glance*, 4th edn. Reproduced with permission of John Wiley & Sons.

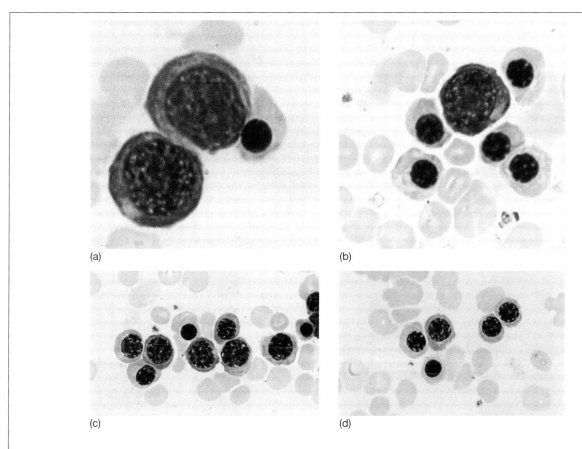

(a)

(b)

(c)

(d)

Figure 2.2 Erythroblasts (normoblasts) at varying stages of development. The earlier cells are larger, with more basophilic cytoplasm and a more open nuclear chromatin pattern. The cytoplasm of the later cells is more eosinophilic as a result of haemoglobin formation.

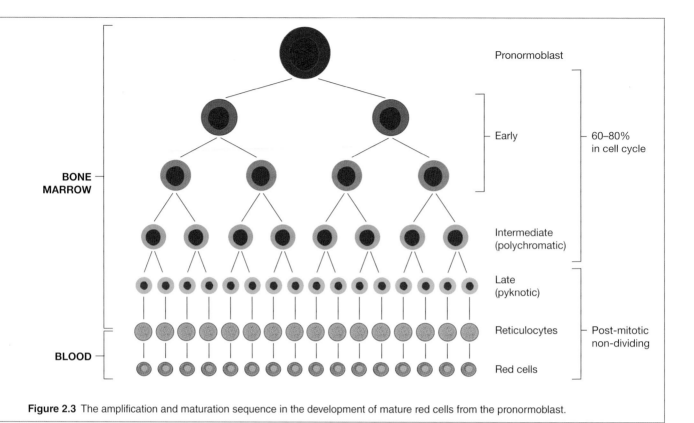

Figure 2.3 The amplification and maturation sequence in the development of mature red cells from the pronormoblast.

This cell is slightly larger than a mature red cell, and circulates in the peripheral blood for 1–2 days before maturing, when RNA is completely lost. A completely pink-staining mature erythrocyte results, which is a non-nucleated biconcave disc (see Fig. 24.3). One pronormoblast usually gives rise to 16 mature red cells (Fig. 2.3). Nucleated red cells (normoblasts) are not present in normal human peripheral blood (Fig. 2.4). They appear in the blood if erythropoiesis is occurring outside the marrow (extramedullary erythropoiesis) and also with some marrow diseases.

Erythropoietin

Erythropoiesis is regulated by the hormone erythropoietin, a heavily glycosylated polypeptide. Normally, 90% of the hormone is produced in the peritubular interstitial cells of the kidney and 10% in the liver and elsewhere. There are no preformed stores and the stimulus to erythropoietin production is the oxygen (O_2) tension in the tissues of the kidney (Fig. 2.5). Hypoxia induces synthesis of hypoxia-inducible factors (HIF-1α and β), which stimulate erythropoietin production and also new vessel formation and transferrin receptor synthesis, and reduce hepcidin synthesis, increasing iron absorption. Von Hippel-Lindau (VHL) protein breaks down HIFs and PHD2 hydroxylates HIF-1α, allowing VHL binding (Fig. 2.5). Mutations in the genes for these proteins may cause polycythaemia (see Chapter 15).

Erythropoietin production therefore increases in anaemia, and also when haemoglobin for some metabolic or structural reason is unable to give up O_2 normally, when atmospheric O_2 is low or when defective cardiac or pulmonary function or damage to the renal circulation affects O_2 delivery to the kidney.

Erythropoietin stimulates erythropoiesis by increasing the number of progenitor cells committed to erythropoiesis.

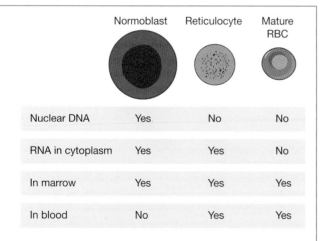

	Normoblast	Reticulocyte	Mature RBC
Nuclear DNA	Yes	No	No
RNA in cytoplasm	Yes	Yes	No
In marrow	Yes	Yes	Yes
In blood	No	Yes	Yes

Figure 2.4 Comparison of the DNA and RNA content, and marrow and peripheral blood distribution, of the erythroblast (normoblast), reticulocyte and mature red blood cell (RBC).

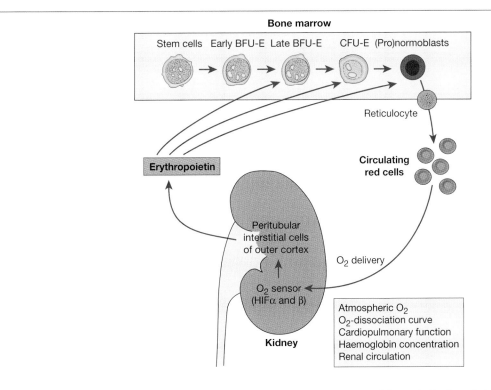

Figure 2.5 The production of erythropoietin by the kidney in response to its oxygen (O_2) supply. Erythropoietin stimulates erythropoiesis and so increases O_2 delivery. BFU_E, erythroid burst-forming unit; CFU_E, erythroid colony-forming unit. Hypoxia induces hypoxia inducible factors (HIFs) α and β, which stimulate erythropoietin production. Von-Hippel–Lindau (VHL) protein breaks down HIFs. PHD2 (prolyl hydroxylase) hydroxylates HIF-1α, allowing VHL binding to HIFs. Mutations in VHL, PHD2 or HIF-1α underlie congenital polycythaemia (see p. 189).

The transcription factor GATA2 is involved in initiating erythroid differentiation from pluripotential stem cells. Subsequently the transcription factors GATA1 and FOG1 are activated by erythropoietin receptor stimulation and are important in enhancing expression of erythroid-specific genes (e.g. globin, haem biosynthetic and red cell membrane proteins) and also enhancing expression of anti-apoptotic genes and of the transferrin receptor (CD71). Late BFU_E and CFU_E, which have erythropoietin receptors, are stimulated to proliferate, differentiate and produce haemoglobin. The proportion of erythroid cells in the marrow increases and, in the chronic state, there is anatomical expansion of erythropoiesis into fatty marrow and sometimes into extramedullary sites. In infants, the marrow cavity may expand into cortical bone, resulting in bone deformities with frontal bossing and protrusion of the maxilla (see p. 85).

Conversely, increased O_2 supply to the tissues (because of an increased red cell mass or because haemoglobin is able to release its O_2 more readily than normal) reduces the erythropoietin drive. Plasma erythropoietin levels can be valuable in clinical diagnosis. They are high in anaemia, unless this is due to renal failure or if a tumour-secreting erythropoietin is present, but low in severe renal disease or polycythaemia vera (Fig. 2.6).

Indications for erythropoietin therapy

Recombinant erythropoietin is needed for treating anaemia resulting from renal disease or from various other causes. It is given subcutaneously either three times weekly, once every 1–2 weeks or every 4 weeks, depending on the indication and on the preparation used (erythropoietin alpha or beta; darbepoetin alpha, a heavily glycosylated longer-acting form; or Micera, the longest-acting preparation). The main indication is end-stage renal disease (with or without dialysis). The patients often also need oral or intravenous iron. Other indications are listed in Table 2.2. The haemoglobin level and quality of life may be improved. A low serum erythropoietin level prior to treatment is valuable in predicting an effective response. Side effects include a rise in blood pressure, thrombosis and local injection site reactions. It has been associated with progression of some tumours which express EPO receptors.

The marrow requires many other precursors for effective erythropoiesis. These include metals such as iron and cobalt, vitamins (especially vitamin B_{12}, folate, vitamin C, vitamin E, vitamin B_6, thiamine and riboflavin) and hormones such as androgens and thyroxine. Deficiency in any of these may be associated with anaemia.

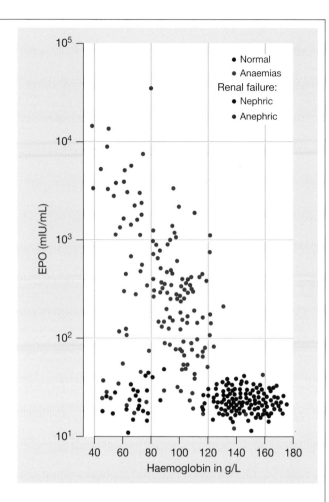

Figure 2.6 The relation between erythropoietin (EPO) in plasma and haemoglobin concentration. Anaemias exclude conditions shown to be associated with impaired production of EPO. Source: Modified from M. Pippard *et al.* (1992) *Br. J. Haematol.* 82: 445. Reproduced with permission of John Wiley & Sons.

Table 2.2 Clinical indications (in selected subjects) for erythropoietin.

Anaemia of chronic renal disease
Myelodysplastic syndrome
Anaemia associated with malignancy and chemotherapy
Anaemia of chronic diseases, e.g. rheumatoid arthritis
Anaemia of prematurity
Perioperative uses

Haemoglobin

Haemoglobin synthesis

The main function of red cells is to carry O_2 to the tissues and to return carbon dioxide (CO_2) from the tissues to the lungs. In order to achieve this gaseous exchange they contain

Table 2.3 Normal haemoglobins in adult blood.

	Hb A	Hb F	Hb A$_2$
Structure	$\alpha_2\beta_2$	$\alpha_2\gamma_2$	$\alpha_2\delta_2$
Normal (%)	96–98	0.5–0.8	1.5–3.2

the specialized protein haemoglobin. Each molecule of normal adult **haemoglobin** A (Hb A, the dominant haemoglobin in blood after the age of 3–6 months) consists of four polypeptide chains, $\alpha_2\beta_2$, each with its own haem group. Normal adult blood also contains small quantities of two other haemoglobins: Hb F and Hb A$_2$. These also contain α chains, but with γ and δ chains, respectively, instead of β (Table 2.3). The synthesis of the various globin chains in the fetus and adult is discussed in more detail in Chapter 7.

Haem synthesis occurs largely in the mitochondria by a series of biochemical reactions, commencing with the condensation of glycine and succinyl coenzyme A under the action of the key rate-limiting enzyme δ-aminolaevulinic acid (ALA) synthase (Fig. 2.7). Pyridoxal phosphate (vitamin B$_6$) is a coenzyme for this reaction. The main sources of succinyl CoA are glutamine and glucose, which are converted to alpha-ketoglutarate, a succinate precursor inside the erythroid cells. Ultimately, protoporphyrin combines with iron in the ferrous

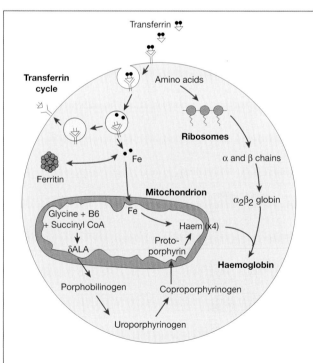

Figure 2.7 Haemoglobin synthesis in the developing red cell. The mitochondria are the main sites of protoporphyrin synthesis, iron (Fe) is supplied from circulating transferrin and globin chains are synthesized on ribosomes. δ-ALA, δ-aminolaevulinic acid; CoA, coenzyme A.

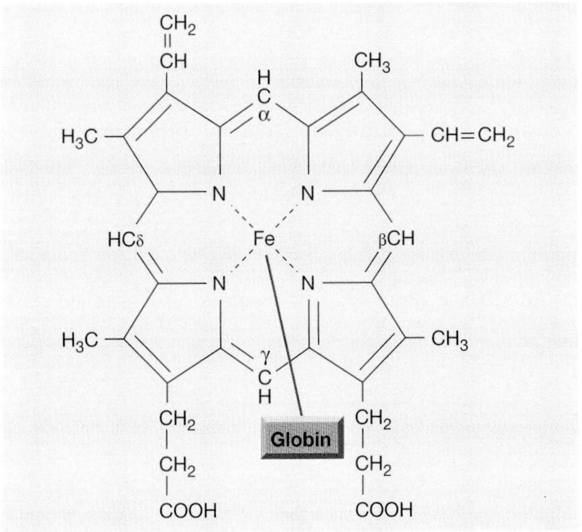

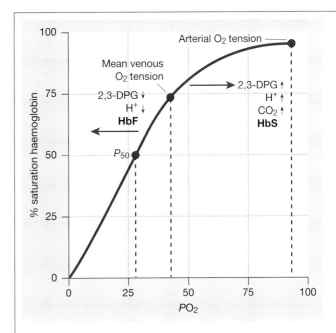

Figure 2.8 The structure of haem.

Figure 2.10 The haemoglobin oxygen (O_2) dissociation curve. 2,3-DPG, 2,3-diphosphoglycerate.

(Fe^{2+}) state to form haem (Fig. 2.8). A tetramer of four globin chains, each with its own haem group in a 'pocket', is then formed to make up a haemoglobin molecule (Fig. 2.9).

Haemoglobin function

The red cells in systemic arterial blood carry O_2 from the lungs to the tissues and return in venous blood with CO_2 to the lungs. As the haemoglobin molecule loads and unloads O_2, the individual globin chains move on each other (Fig. 2.9). The $\alpha_1\beta_1$ and $\alpha_2\beta_2$ contacts stabilize the molecule. When O_2 is unloaded the β chains are pulled apart, permitting entry of the metabolite 2,3-diphosphoglycerate (2,3-DPG), resulting in a lower affinity of the molecule for O_2. This movement is responsible for the sigmoid form of the haemoglobin O_2 dissociation curve (Fig. 2.10). The P_{50} (i.e. the partial pressure of

O_2 at which haemoglobin is half saturated with O_2) of normal blood is 26.6 mmHg. With increased affinity for O_2, the curve shifts to the left (i.e. the P_{50} falls), while with decreased affinity for O_2, the curve shifts to the right (i.e. the P_{50} rises).

Normally, *in vivo*, O_2 exchange operates between 95% saturation (arterial blood) with a mean arterial O_2 tension of 95 mmHg and 70% saturation (venous blood) with a mean venous O_2 tension of 40 mmHg (Fig. 2.10).

The normal position of the curve depends on the concentration of 2,3-DPG, H$^+$ ions and CO_2 in the red cell and on the structure of the haemoglobin molecule. High concentrations of 2,3-DPG, H$^+$ or CO_2, and the presence of sickle haemoglobin (Hb S), shift the curve to the right (oxygen is given up more easily), whereas fetal haemoglobin (Hb F) – which is unable to bind 2,3-DPG – and certain rare abnormal haemoglobins associated with polycythaemia shift the curve to the left, because they give up O_2 less readily than normal.

Methaemoglobinaemia

This is a clinical state in which circulating haemoglobin is present with iron in the oxidized (Fe^{3+}) instead of the usual Fe^{2+} state. It may arise because of a hereditary deficiency of methaemoglobin reductase or inheritance of a structurally abnormal haemoglobin (Hb M). Hb Ms contain an amino acid substitution affecting the haem pocket of the globin chain. Toxic methaemoglobinaemia (and/or sulphaemoglobinaemia) occurs when a drug or other toxic substance oxidizes haemoglobin. In all these states, the patient is likely to show cyanosis.

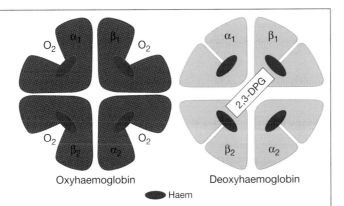

Figure 2.9 The oxygenated and deoxygenated haemoglobin molecule. α, β, globin chains of normal adult haemoglobin (Hb A); 2,3-DPG, 2,3-diphosphoglycerate.

The red cell

In order to carry haemoglobin into close contact with the tissues and for successful gaseous exchange, the red cell, 8 μm in diameter, must be able to pass repeatedly through the microcirculation, whose minimum diameter is 3.5 μm; to maintain haemoglobin in a reduced (ferrous) state; and to maintain osmotic equilibrium despite the high concentration of protein (haemoglobin) in the cell. A single journey round the body takes 20 seconds and its total journey throughout its 120-day lifespan has been estimated to be 480 km (300 miles). To fulfil these functions, the cell is a flexible biconcave disc with an ability to generate energy as adenosine triphosphate (ATP) by the anaerobic glycolytic (Embden–Meyerhof) pathway (Fig. 2.11) and to generate reducing power as nicotinamide adenine dinucleotide (NADH) by this pathway and as reduced nicotinamide adenine dinucleotide phosphate (NADPH) by the hexose monophosphate shunt (see Fig. 6.6).

Red cell metabolism

Embden–Meyerhof pathway

In this series of biochemical reactions, glucose that enters the red cell from plasma by facilitated transfer is metabolized to lactate (Fig. 2.11). For each molecule of glucose used, two molecules of ATP and thus two high-energy phosphate bonds are generated. This ATP provides energy for maintenance of red cell volume, shape and flexibility.

The Embden–Meyerhof pathway also generates NADH, which is needed by the enzyme methaemoglobin reductase to reduce functionally dead methaemoglobin containing ferric iron (produced by oxidation of approximately 3% of haemoglobin each day) to functionally active, reduced haemoglobin containing ferrous ions. The Luebering–Rapoport shunt, or side arm, of this pathway (Fig. 2.11) generates 2,3-DPG, important in the regulation of haemoglobin's oxygen affinity (Fig. 2.9).

Hexose monophosphate (pentose phosphate) shunt

Approximately 10% of glycolysis occurs by this oxidative pathway in which glucose-6-phosphate is converted to 6-phosphogluconate and so to ribulose-5-phosphate (see Fig. 6.6). NADPH is generated and is linked with glutathione, which maintains sulphydril (SH) groups intact in the cell, including those in haemoglobin and the red cell membrane. In one of the most common inherited abnormalities of red cells, glucose-6-phosphate dehydrogenase (G6PD) deficiency, the red cells are extremely susceptible to oxidant stress (see p. 70).

Red cell membrane

The red cell membrane comprises a lipid bilayer, integral membrane proteins and a membrane skeleton (Fig. 2.12). Approximately 50% of the membrane is protein, 20% phospholipids, 20% cholesterol molecules and up to 10% is carbohydrate. Carbohydrates occur only on the external surface, while proteins are either peripheral or integral, penetrating the lipid bilayer. Several red cell proteins have been numbered according to their mobility on polyacrylamide gel electrophoresis (PAGE), e.g. band 3, proteins 4.1, 4.2 (Fig. 2.12).

The membrane skeleton is formed by structural proteins that include α and β spectrin, ankyrin, protein 4.1 and actin. These proteins form a horizontal lattice on the internal side of the red cell membrane and are important in maintaining the biconcave shape. Spectrin is the most abundant and consists of two chains, α and β, wound around each other to form heterodimers, which then self-associate head to head to form tetramers. These tetramers are linked at the tail end to actin and are attached to protein band 4.1. At the head end, the β spectrin chains attach to ankyrin, which connects to band 3, the transmembrane protein that acts as an anion channel ('vertical connections'; Fig. 2.12). Protein 4.2 enhances this interaction.

Defects of the membrane proteins explain some of the abnormalities of shape of the red cell membrane (e.g. hereditary spherocytosis and elliptocytosis; see Chapter 6), while alterations in lipid composition because of congenital or acquired abnormalities in plasma cholesterol or phospholipid may be associated with other membrane abnormalities (see Fig. 2.16).

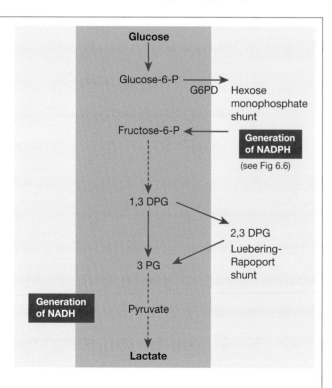

Figure 2.11 The Embden–Meyerhof glycolytic pathway. The Luebering–Rapoport shunt regulates the concentration of 2,3-diphosphoglycerate (2,3-DPG) in the red cell. ATP, adenosine triphosphate; NAD, NADH, nicotinamide adenine dinucleotide; PG, phosphoglycerate.

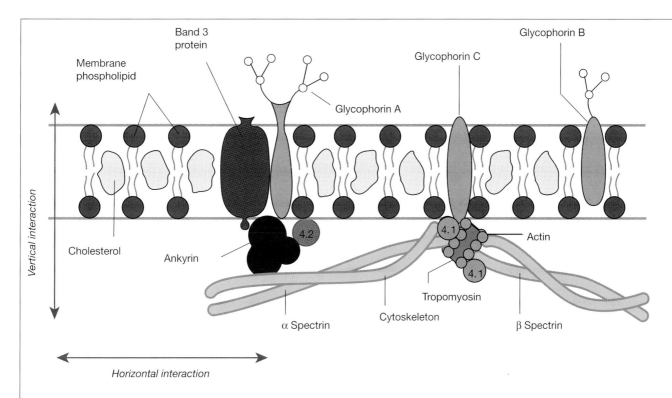

Figure 2.12 The structure of the red cell membrane. Some of the penetrating and integral proteins carry carbohydrate antigens; other antigens are attached directly to the lipid layer.

Anaemia

Anaemia is defined as a reduction in the haemoglobin concentration of the blood below normal for age and sex (Table 2.4). Although normal values can vary between laboratories, typical values would be less than 135 g/L in adult males and less than 115 g/L in adult females (Fig. 2.13). From the age of 2 years to puberty, less than 110 g/L indicates anaemia. As newborn infants have a high haemoglobin level, 140 g/L is taken as the lower limit at birth (Fig. 2.13). Anaemia in pregnancy and neonates is discussed in Chapter 31.

Alterations in total circulating plasma volume as well as in total circulating haemoglobin mass determine the haemoglobin concentration. Reduction in plasma volume (as in dehydration) may mask anaemia or even cause (apparent, pseudo) polycythaemia (see p. 185); conversely, an increase in plasma volume (as with splenomegaly or pregnancy) may cause anaemia even with a normal total circulating red cell and haemoglobin mass.

After acute major blood loss, anaemia is not immediately apparent because the total blood volume is reduced. It takes up to a day for the plasma volume to be replaced and so for the degree of anaemia to become apparent (see p. 385). Regeneration of red cells and haemoglobin mass takes substantially longer. The initial clinical features of major blood loss are therefore a result of reduction in blood volume rather than of anaemia.

Global incidence

The World Health Organization defines anaemia in adults as a haemoglobin less than 130 g/L in males and less than 120 g/L in females. On this basis, anaemia was estimated in 2010 to occur in about 33% of the global population. Prevalence was greater in females than males at all ages and most frequent in children less than 5 years old. Anaemia was most frequent in South Asia, and Central, West and East Sub-Saharan Africa. The main causes are iron deficiency (life-long poor diet combined with menstruation and/or repeated pregnancies, hookworm, schistosomiasis), the anaemia of chronic disorders (see p. 38), sickle cell diseases, thalassaemia and malaria.

Clinical features of anaemia

The major adaptations to anaemia are in the cardiovascular system (with increased stroke volume and tachycardia) and in the haemoglobin O2 dissociation curve. In some patients with quite severe anaemia there may be no symptoms or signs, whereas others with mild anaemia may be severely incapacitated. The presence or absence of clinical features can be considered under four major headings.

1 ***Speed of onset*** Rapidly progressive anaemia causes more symptoms than anaemia of slow onset, because there is less time for adaptation in the cardiovascular system and in the O_2 dissociation curve of haemoglobin.

Table 2.4 Normal values for blood cells and haematinics.

	Males	Females
Haemoglobin (g/L)	135.0–175.0	115.0–155.0
Red cells (erythrocytes) (× 10^{12}/L)	4.5–6.5	3.9–5.6
PCV (haematocrit) (%)	40–52	36–48
Mean cell volume (MCV) (fL)	80–95	
Mean cell haemoglobin (MCH) (pg)	27–34	
Reticulocyte count (× 10^9/L)	50–150	
White cells (leucocytes)		
Total (× 10^9/L)	4.0–11.0	
Neutrophils (× 10^9/L)	1.8–7.5*	
Lymphocytes (× 10^9/L)	1.5–3.5	
Monocytes (× 10^9/L)	0.2–0.8	
Eosinophils (× 10^9/L)	0.04–0.44	
Basophils (× 10^9/L)	0.01–0.1	
Platelets (× 10^9/L)	150–400	
Serum iron (µmol/L)	10–30	
Total iron-binding capacity (µmol/L)	40–75 (2.0–4.0 g/L as transferrin)	
Serum ferritin** (µg/L)	40–340	14–150
Serum vitamin B$_{12}$** (ng/L)	160—925 (20–680 pmol/L)	
Serum folate** (µg/L)	3.0–15.0 (4–30 nmol/L)	
Red cell folate** (µg/L)	160–640 (360–1460 nmol/L)	

*Lower limit 1.5 × 10^9/L in some ethnic groups, e.g. in Middle East and black-skinned people.

**Normal ranges differ between different laboratories. PCV, packed cell volume.

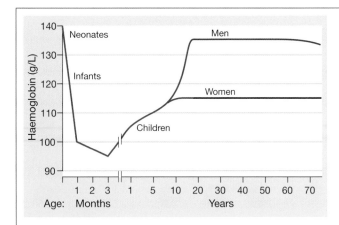

Figure 2.13 The lower limit of normal blood haemoglobin concentration in men, women and children of various ages.

is particularly marked in some anaemias that either raise 2,3-DPG directly, e.g. pyruvate kinase deficiency (p. 72), or that are associated with a low-affinity haemoglobin, e.g. Hb S (see Fig. 2.10).

Symptoms

If the patient does have symptoms these are usually shortness of breath, particularly on exertion, weakness, lethargy, palpitation and headaches. In older subjects, symptoms of cardiac failure, angina pectoris or intermittent claudication or confusion may be present. Visual disturbances because of retinal haemorrhages may complicate very severe anaemia, particularly of rapid onset (Fig. 2.14).

Signs

These may be divided into general and specific. General signs include pallor of mucous membranes or nail beds, which

2 **Severity** Mild anaemia often produces no symptoms or signs, but these are usually present when the haemoglobin is less than 90 g/L. Even severe anaemia (haemoglobin concentration as low as 60 g/L) may produce remarkably few symptoms, when there is very gradual onset in a young subject who is otherwise healthy.

3 **Age** The elderly tolerate anaemia less well than the young because normal cardiovascular compensation is impaired.

4 **Haemoglobin O$_2$ dissociation curve** Anaemia, in general, is associated with a rise in 2,3-DPG in the red cells and a shift in the O$_2$ dissociation curve to the right, so that oxygen is given up more readily to tissues. This adaptation

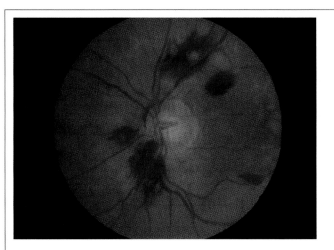

Figure 2.14 Retinal haemorrhages in a patient with severe anaemia (haemoglobin 25 g/L) caused by severe haemorrhage.

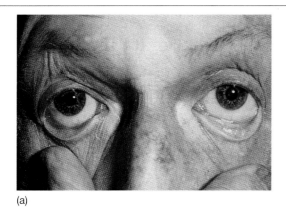
(a)

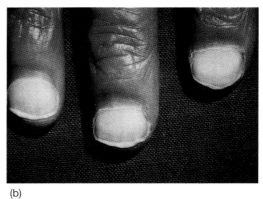
(b)

Figure 2.15 Pallor of the conjunctival mucosa **(a)** and of the nail bed **(b)** in two patients with severe anaemia (haemoglobin 60 g/L).

occurs if the haemoglobin level is less than 90 g/L (Fig. 2.15). Conversely, skin colour is not a reliable sign. A hyperdynamic circulation may be present with tachycardia, a bounding pulse, cardiomegaly and a systolic flow murmur, especially at the apex. Particularly in the elderly, features of congestive heart failure may be present.

Specific signs are associated with particular types of anaemia, e.g. koilonychia (spoon nails) with iron deficiency, jaundice with haemolytic or megaloblastic anaemias, leg ulcers with sickle cell and other haemolytic anaemias, or bone deformities with thalassaemia major.

The association of features of anaemia with excess infections or spontaneous bruising suggests that neutropenia or thrombocytopenia may be present, possibly as a result of bone marrow failure.

Classification and laboratory findings in anaemia

Red cell indices

The most useful classification is that based on red cell indices (Table 2.4). This divides the anaemia into microcytic, normocytic and macrocytic (Table 2.5). As well as suggesting

Table 2.5 Classification of anaemia.

Microcytic, hypochromic	Normocytic, normochromic	Macrocytic
MCV <80 fL	MCV 80–95 fL	MCV >95 fL
MCH <27 pg	MCH ≥27 pg	Megaloblastic: vitamin B_{12} or folate deficiency Non-megaloblastic: alcohol, liver disease, myelodysplasia, aplastic anaemia, etc. (see Table 5.10)
Iron deficiency	Many haemolytic anaemias	
Thalassaemia Anaemia of chronic disease (some cases) Lead poisoning Sideroblastic anaemia (some cases)	Anaemia of chronic disease (some cases)	
	After acute blood loss	
	Renal disease	
	Mixed deficiencies	
	Bone marrow failure (e.g. post-chemotherapy, infiltration by carcinoma, etc.)	

MCH, mean corpuscular haemoglobin; MCV, mean corpuscular volume.

the nature of the primary defect, this classification may also indicate an underlying abnormality before overt anaemia has developed.

In two common physiological situations, the mean corpuscular volume (MCV) may be outside the normal adult range. In the newborn for a few weeks the MCV is high, but in infancy it is low (e.g. 70 fL at 1 year of age) and rises slowly throughout childhood to the normal adult range. In normal pregnancy there is a slight rise in MCV, even in the absence of other causes of macrocytosis (e.g. folate deficiency).

Other laboratory findings

Although the red cell indices will indicate the type of anaemia, further useful information can be obtained from the initial blood sample.

Leucocyte and platelet counts

Measurement of these helps to distinguish 'pure' anaemia from 'pancytopenia' (subnormal levels of red cells, neutrophils and platelets), which suggests a more general marrow defect or destruction of cells (e.g. hypersplenism). In anaemias caused by haemolysis or haemorrhage, the neutrophil and platelet counts are often raised; in infections and leukaemias, the leucocyte count is also often raised and there may be abnormal leucocytes or neutrophil precursors present.

Reticulocyte count

The normal percentage is 0.5–2.5%, and the absolute count $50–150 \times 10^9/L$ (Table 2.4). This should rise in anaemia because of erythropoietin increase, and be higher the more severe the anaemia. This is particularly so when there has been time for erythroid hyperplasia to develop in the marrow as in chronic haemolysis. After an acute major haemorrhage there is an erythropoietin response in 6 hours, and the reticulocyte count rises within 2–3 days, reaches a maximum in 6–10 days and remains raised until the haemoglobin returns to the normal level. If the reticulocyte count is not raised in an anaemic patient, this suggests impaired marrow function or lack of erythropoietin stimulus (Table 2.6).

Blood film

It is important to examine the blood film in all cases of anaemia. Abnormal red cell morphology (Fig. 2.16) or red cell inclusions (Fig. 2.17) may suggest a particular diagnosis. During the blood film examination, white cell abnormalities are sought, platelet number and morphology are assessed and the presence or absence of abnormal cells (e.g. normoblasts, granulocyte precursors or blast cells) is noted.

Bone marrow examination

This is needed when the cause of anaemia or other abnormality of the blood cells cannot be diagnosed from the blood count, film and other blood tests alone. It may be performed by aspiration or trephine biopsy (Fig. 2.18). For bone marrow aspiration a needle is inserted into the marrow cavity and a liquid sample of marrow is sucked into a syringe. This is then spread on a slide for microscopy and stained by the usual Romanowsky technique. The detail of the developing cells can be examined (e.g. normoblastic or megaloblastic) and the proportion of the different cell lines assessed (myeloid:erythroid ratio, the proportion of granulocyte precursors to red cell precursors in the bone marrow, normally 2.5:1 to 12:1). The presence of cells foreign to the marrow (e.g. secondary carcinoma) can also be observed. The cellularity of the marrow can be viewed provided fragments are obtained. An iron stain is performed routinely so that the amount of iron in reticuloendothelial stores (macrophages) and as fine granules ('siderotic' granules) in the developing erythroblasts can be assessed (see Fig. 3.10).

An aspirate sample may also be used for a number of other specialized investigations (Table 2.7).

A trephine biopsy provides a solid core of bone including marrow and is examined as a histological specimen after fixation in formalin, decalcification and sectioning. Usually immunohistology is performed, depending on the diagnosis suspected (see Chapter 11). A trephine biopsy specimen is less valuable than aspiration when individual cell detail is to be examined, but provides a panoramic view of the marrow, from which overall marrow architecture, cellularity and presence of fibrosis or abnormal infiltrates can, with immunohistology if needed, be reliably determined.

Table 2.6 Factors impairing the normal reticulocyte response to anaemia.

Marrow diseases, e.g. hypoplasia, infiltration by carcinoma, lymphoma, myeloma, acute leukaemia, tuberculosis
Deficiency of iron, vitamin B_{12} or folate
Lack of erythropoietin, e.g. renal disease
Reduced tissue O_2 consumption, e.g. myxoedema, protein deficiency
Ineffective erythropoiesis, e.g. thalassaemia major, megaloblastic anaemia, myelodysplasia, myelofibrosis
Chronic inflammatory or malignant disease

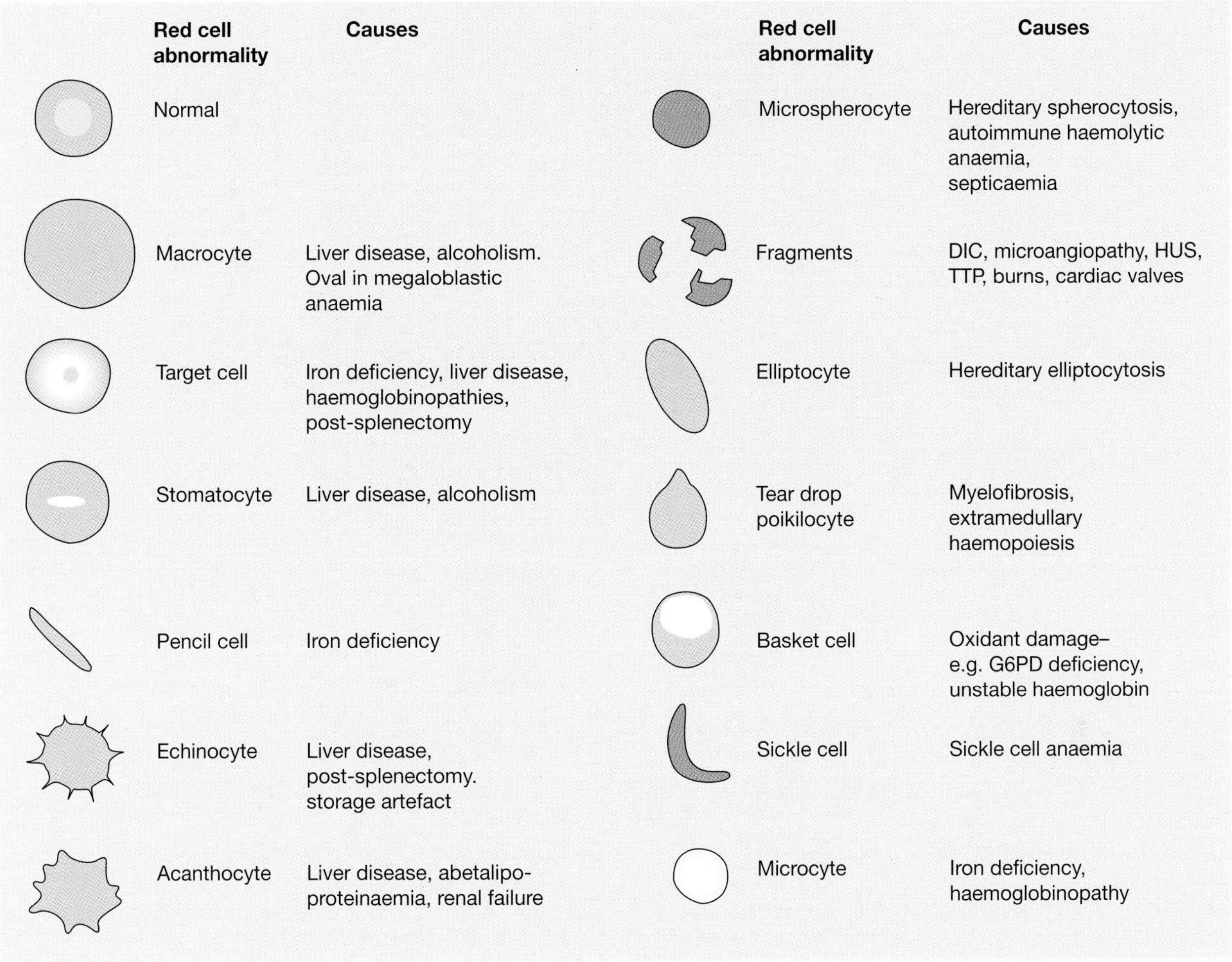

Red cell abnormality	Causes	Red cell abnormality	Causes
Normal		Microspherocyte	Hereditary spherocytosis, autoimmune haemolytic anaemia, septicaemia
Macrocyte	Liver disease, alcoholism. Oval in megaloblastic anaemia	Fragments	DIC, microangiopathy, HUS, TTP, burns, cardiac valves
Target cell	Iron deficiency, liver disease, haemoglobinopathies, post-splenectomy	Elliptocyte	Hereditary elliptocytosis
Stomatocyte	Liver disease, alcoholism	Tear drop poikilocyte	Myelofibrosis, extramedullary haemopoiesis
Pencil cell	Iron deficiency	Basket cell	Oxidant damage– e.g. G6PD deficiency, unstable haemoglobin
Echinocyte	Liver disease, post-splenectomy. storage artefact	Sickle cell	Sickle cell anaemia
Acanthocyte	Liver disease, abetalipo-proteinaemia, renal failure	Microcyte	Iron deficiency, haemoglobinopathy

Figure 2.16 Some of the more frequent variations in size (anisocytosis) and shape (poikilocytosis) that may be found in different anaemias. DIC, disseminated intravascular coagulopathy; G6PD, glucose-6-phosphate dehydrogenase; HUS, haemolytic uraemic syndrome; TTP, thrombotic thrombocytopenic purpura.

Ineffective erythropoiesis

Erythropoiesis is not entirely efficient because approximately 10–15% of developing erythroblasts die within the marrow without producing mature cells. This is termed ineffective erythropoiesis and it is substantially increased in a number of chronic anaemias (Fig. 2.19). The serum unconjugated bilirubin (derived from breaking down haemoglobin) and lactate dehydrogenase (LDH, derived from breaking down cells) are usually raised when ineffective erythropoiesis is marked. The reticulocyte count is low in relation to the degree of anaemia and to the proportion of erythroblasts in the marrow.

Assessment of erythropoiesis

Total erythropoiesis and the amount of erythropoiesis that is effective in producing circulating red cells can be assessed by examining the bone marrow, haemoglobin level and reticulocyte count.

Total erythropoiesis is assessed from the marrow cellularity and the myeloid : erythroid ratio. This ratio falls and may be reversed when total erythropoiesis is selectively increased.

Effective erythropoiesis is assessed by the reticulocyte count. This is raised in proportion to the degree of anaemia when erythropoiesis is effective, but is low when there is ineffective erythropoiesis or an abnormality preventing normal marrow response (Table 2.6).

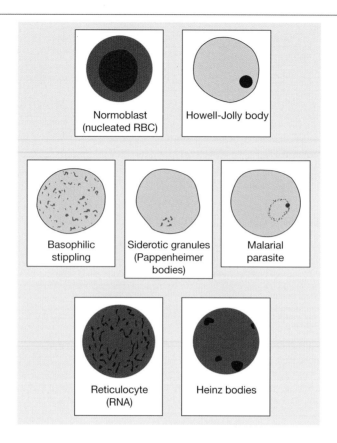

Figure 2.17 Red blood cell (RBC) inclusions which may be seen in the peripheral blood film in various conditions. The reticulocyte RNA and Heinz bodies are only demonstrated by supravital staining (e.g. with new methylene blue). Heinz bodies are oxidized denatured haemoglobin. Siderotic granules (Pappenheimer bodies) contain iron. They are purple on conventional staining, but blue with Perls' stain. The Howell–Jolly body is a DNA remnant. Basophilic stippling is denatured RNA.

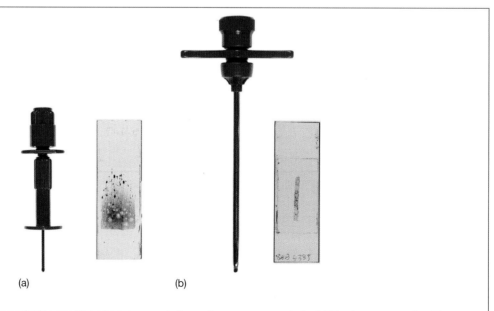

Figure 2.18 (a) The bone marrow aspiration needle and a smear made from a bone marrow aspirate. **(b)** The bone marrow trephine (biopsy) needle and a normal trephine section.

Table 2.7 Indications for bone marrow aspiration and trephine biopsy.

	Aspiration	Trephine
Site	Posterior iliac crest (sternum if obese; tibia in infants)	Posterior iliac crest
Stains	Romanowsky; Perls' reaction (for iron)	Haematoxylin and eosin; reticulin (silver stain)
Result available	1–2 hours	1–7 days (according to decalcification method)
Indications	Investigation of unexplained anaemia, neutropenia, thrombocytopenia, suspicion of leukaemia, myeloproliferative disorders, myelodysplasia, aplastic anaemia, lymphoma, myeloma, amyloid, secondary carcinoma, cases of splenomegaly or pyrexia of undetermined cause	
Special tests	Flow cytometry, cytogenetics and molecular tests such as FISH (see p. 142) and DNA or RNA analysis for gene abnormalities. Consider microbiological culture, cytochemical markers and progenitor cell culture	Immunohistological staining

FISH, fluorescence *in situ* hybridization.

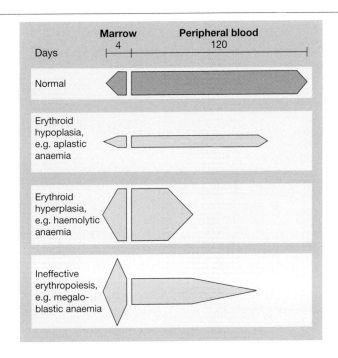

Figure 2.19 The relative proportions of marrow erythroblastic activity, circulating red cell mass and red cell lifespan in normal subjects and in three types of anaemia.

SUMMARY

- Erythropoiesis (red cell production) is regulated by erythropoietin, which is secreted by the kidney in response to hypoxia. Erythropoiesis occurs from mixed progenitor cells through a series of nucleated red cell precursors (normoblasts) to a reticulocyte stage, containing RNA but not DNA.

- Various short- or long-acting preparations of erythropoietin are used clinically to treat anaemia in renal failure and other diseases.

- Haemoglobin is the main protein in red cells. It consists of four polypeptide (globin) chains, in adults dominantly 2α and 2β, each containing an iron atom bound to protoporphyrin to form haem.

- The red cell has two biochemical pathways for metabolizing glucose, the Embden–Meyerhof pathway, which generates ATP, needed for maintenance of red cell shape and flexibility, and NADH, which prevents oxidation of haemoglobin; and the hexose monophosphate pathway, which generates NADPH, important for maintaining glutathione, which keeps haemoglobin and cell proteins in the membrane in the reduced state.

- The red cell membrane consists of a lipid bilayer with a membrane skeleton of penetrating and integral proteins and carbohydrate surface antigens.

- Anaemia is defined as a haemoglobin level in blood below the normal level for age and sex. It is classified according to the size of the red cells into macrocytic, normocytic and microcytic. The reticulocyte count, morphology of the red cells and changes in the white cell and/or platelet count help in the diagnosis of the cause of anaemia.

- The general clinical features of anaemia include shortness of breath on exertion, pallor of mucous membranes and tachycardia.

- Other features relate to particular types of anaemia, e.g. jaundice, leg ulcers.

- Bone marrow examination by aspiration or trephine biopsy may be important in the investigation of anaemia as well as of many other haematological diseases. Special tests, e.g. immunology by flow cytometry or immunohistology, cytogenetics or molecular genetics, can be performed on the cells obtained.

Now visit **www.wileyessential.com/haematology** to test yourself on this chapter.

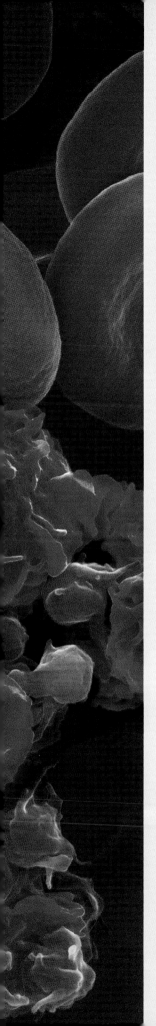

CHAPTER 3
Hypochromic anaemias

Key topics

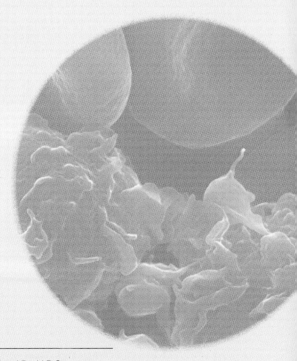

Hoffbrand's Essential Haematology, Eighth Edition. By A. Victor Hoffbrand and David P. Steensma.
© 2020 John Wiley & Sons Ltd. Published 2020 by John Wiley & Sons Ltd.
Companion website: www.wileyessential.com/haematology

Iron is one of the most common elements in the Earth's crust, yet iron deficiency is the most common cause of anaemia, affecting about 500 million people worldwide. It is particularly frequent in low-income populations, such as in sub-Saharan Africa or South Asia, where the diet can be of poor quality and parasites (e.g. hookworm or schistosomiasis), which cause iron loss due to haemorrhage, may be present. Moreover, the body has limited ability to absorb iron. Iron deficiency is the major cause of a microcytic, hypochromic anaemia, in which the two red cell indices, mean corpuscular volume (MCV) and mean corpuscular haemoglobin (MCH), are reduced and the blood film shows small (microcytic) and pale (hypochromic) red cells. This appearance is caused by a defect in haemoglobin synthesis. The major differential diagnosis of a microcytic, hypochromic anaemia is between iron deficiency and the anaemia of chronic disease, which are both dealt with in this chapter, and thalassaemia, which is considered in Chapter 7 (Fig 3.1).

Nutritional and metabolic aspects of iron

Body iron distribution and transport

The transport and storage of iron are largely mediated by three proteins: transferrin, transferrin receptor 1 (TfR1) and ferritin.

Each transferrin molecule can contain up to two atoms of iron. Transferrin delivers iron to tissues that have transferrin receptors, especially erythroblasts in the bone marrow, which incorporate the iron into haemoglobin (Figs 2.7, 3.2). The transferrin is then reutilized. At the end of their life, red cells are broken down in the macrophages of the reticuloendothelial system and the iron is released from haemoglobin, enters the plasma and provides most of the iron attached to transferrin. Only a small proportion of plasma transferrin iron comes from dietary iron, absorbed each day through the duodenum and jejunum. Iron in excess of that needed for haemoglobin synthesis is also released from erythroblasts and erythrocytes to plasma transferrin.

Some iron is stored in the macrophages as **ferritin and haemosiderin**, the amount varying widely according to overall body iron status. Ferritin is a water-soluble protein–iron

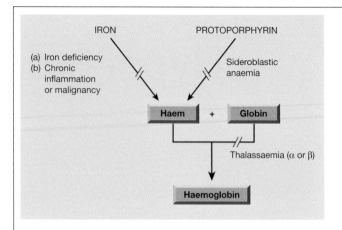

Figure 3.1 The causes of a hypochromic microcytic anaemia. These include lack of iron (iron deficiency) or of iron release from macrophages to serum (anaemia of chronic inflammation or malignancy), failure of protoporphyrin synthesis (sideroblastic anaemia) or of globin synthesis (α- or β-thalassaemia). Lead also inhibits haem and globin synthesis.

complex. It is made up of an outer protein shell, apoferritin, consisting of 22 subunits and an iron–phosphate–hydroxide core. It contains up to 20% of its weight as iron and is not visible by light microscopy. Specialized intracellular carrier proteins transfer iron to ferritin and from ferritin to phagolysosmes for its degradation and release of its iron.

Haemosiderin is an insoluble protein–iron complex of varying composition containing approximately 37% iron by weight. It is derived from partial lysosomal digestion of ferritin molecules and is visible in macrophages and other cells by light microscopy after staining by Perls' (Prussian blue) reaction (see Fig. 3.10). Iron in ferritin and haemosiderin is in the ferric form. It is mobilized after reduction to the ferrous form. A copper-containing enzyme, caeruloplasmin, catalyses oxidation of the iron to the ferric form for binding to plasma transferrin.

Iron is also present in muscle as myoglobin and in most cells of the body in iron-containing enzymes (e.g. cytochromes or catalase; Table 3.1). This tissue iron is less likely to become

Table 3.1 The distribution of body iron.			
Amount of iron in average adult	**Male (g)**	**Female (g)**	**Percentage of total**
Haemoglobin	2.4	1.7	65
Ferritin and haemosiderin	1.0 (0.3–1.5)	0.3 (0–1.0)	30
Myoglobin	0.15	0.12	3.5
Haem enzymes (e.g. cytochromes, catalase, peroxidases, flavoproteins)	0.02	0.015	0.5
Transferrin-bound iron	0.004	0.003	0.1

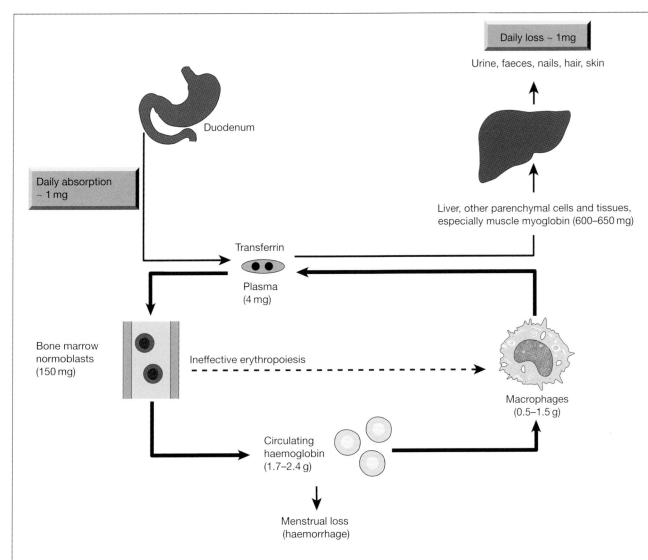

Figure 3.2 Daily iron cycle. Most of the iron in the body is contained in circulating haemoglobin (see Table 3.1) and is reutilized for haemoglobin synthesis after the red cells die. Iron is transferred from macrophages to plasma transferrin and so to bone marrow erythroblasts. Iron absorption is normally just sufficient to make up for iron loss. The dashed line indicates ineffective erythropoiesis.

depleted than haemosiderin, ferritin and haemoglobin in states of iron deficiency, but some reduction of these haem-containing enzymes may occur.

Regulation of ferritin and transferrin receptor 1 synthesis

The levels of ferritin, TfR1, δ-aminolaevulinic acid synthase (ALA-S) and divalent metal transporter 1 (DMT-1) are linked to iron status, so that iron overload causes a rise in tissue ferritin and a fall in TfR1 and DMT-1, whereas in iron deficiency ferritin and ALA-S are low and TfR1 increased. This linkage arises through the binding of an iron regulatory protein (IRP) to iron response elements (IREs) on the ferritin, TfR1, ALA-S and DMT-1 mRNA molecules. Iron deficiency increases the ability of IRP to bind to the IREs, whereas iron overload reduces the binding. The site of IRP binding to IREs, whether upstream (5′) or downstream (3′) from the coding gene, determines whether the amount of mRNA and so protein produced is increased or decreased (Fig. 3.3). Upstream binding reduces translation, whereas downstream binding stabilizes the mRNA, increasing translation and so protein synthesis.

When plasma iron is raised and transferrin is saturated, the amount of iron transferred to parenchymal cells (e.g. those of the liver, endocrine organs and heart) is increased and this is the basis of the pathological changes associated with iron loading conditions. There may also be free iron in plasma (non-transferrin bound iron) which enters and is toxic to different organs (see Chapter 4).

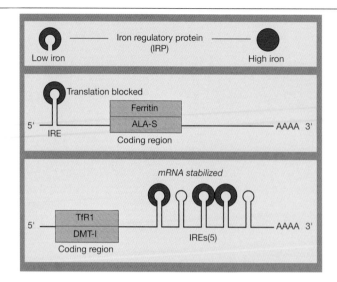

Figure 3.3 Regulation of transferrin receptor 1 (TfR1), divalent metal transporter 1 (DMT-1) and ferritin expression by iron regulatory protein (IRP) sensing of intracellular iron levels. IRPs are able to bind to stem-loop structures called iron response elements (IREs). IRP binding to the IRE within the 3′ untranslated region of TfR1 and DMT-1 leads to stabilization of the mRNA and increased protein synthesis, whereas IRP binding to the IRE within the 5′ untranslated region of ferritin and δ-aminolaevulinic acid synthase (ALA-S) mRNA reduces translation. IRPs can exist in two states: at times of high iron levels the IRP binds iron and exhibits a reduced affinity for the IREs, whereas when iron levels are low the binding of IRPs to IREs is increased. In this way, synthesis of TfR, ALA-S, DMT-1 and ferritin is coordinated to physiological requirements.

Hepcidin

Hepcidin is a polypeptide produced by liver cells. It is the major hormonal regulator of iron homeostasis (Fig. 3.4a). It inhibits iron release from macrophages, from intestinal epithelial cells and from other cells by its interaction with the transmembrane iron exporter, ferroportin. It accelerates degradation of ferroportin protein. Raised hepcidin levels therefore profoundly affect iron metabolism by reducing its absorption and its release from macrophages.

Control of hepcidin expression

The synthesis of hepcidin in the liver is stimulated or inhibited by several factors, including iron status, cytokines circulating in inflammation, erythropoiesis and hypoxia (Fig. 3.4a). Control by iron status is best considered by comparing the control in iron overload when plasma hepcidin levels are high (Fig. 3.4b; except in genetic haemochromatosis, see Chapter 4) with that in iron deficiency when plasma hepcidin levels are low (Fig. 3.4c).

In **iron overload**, diferric transferrin stimulates liver sinusoidal cells to secrete bone morphogenetic proteins (BMPs), especially BMP6 (Fig. 3.4b). The BMPs bind to their receptors (BMPRs) on the hepatic cell membrane. Diferric transferrin also binds to and stabilizes the transferrin receptor 2 (TFR2) on the cell membrane. Binding of BMPs to BMPRs results in the formation of a signalling complex consisting of BMPRs and three proteins, TFR2, hemojuvelin (HJV) and HFE. This complex stimulates hepcidin synthesis via the signalling proteins SMADs, which transfer the message to the cell nucleus. Diferric transferrin also binds to TFR1 to provide the cell with iron.

In **iron deficiency** there is little if any circulating diferric transferrin. This results in reduced synthesis of BMPs by the liver sinusoidal cells (Fig. 3.4c). Also in the absence of binding to diferric transferrin, TFR2 is degraded or shed from the cell membrane and HFE is deviated to bind to the unoccupied TFR1. Iron deficiency also stimulates the protease matriptase 2 (TMPRSS6) to cleave HJV from the cell surface. The result of all these reactions is failure to form the necessary complex to signal for hepcidin synthesis. Finally, iron deficiency stimulates a histone deacetylase which acts on the hepcidin locus to suppress the transcription of hepcidin.

Erythroblasts secrete **erythroferrone** and probably other proteins, which suppress BMP-mediated signalling for hepcidin secretion (Fig. 3.4a). This results in low plasma hepcidin levels in conditions with increased numbers of early erythroblasts in the marrow, e.g. conditions of ineffective erythropoiesis, such as thalassaemia major, so iron absorption is inappropriately increased despite the presence of iron overload due to transfusions. Hypoxia also suppresses hepcidin synthesis, whereas in inflammation interleukin 6 (IL-6) and other cytokines increase hepcidin synthesis (Fig. 3.4a). This results in lowering of plasma iron and helps to protect against infection by depriving bacteria of any non-transferrin-bound iron in plasma.

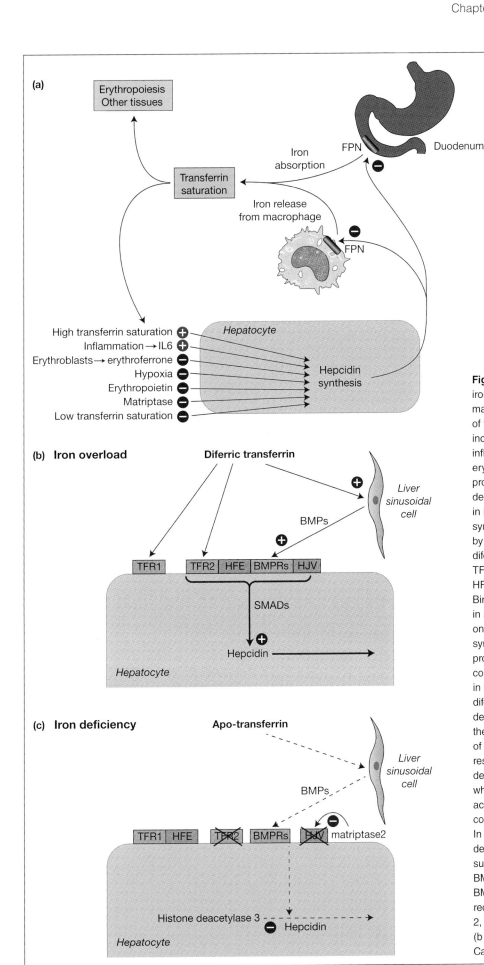

Figure 3.4 (a) Hepcidin reduces iron absorption and release from macrophages by stimulating degradation of ferroportin. Its synthesis is increased by diferric transferrin and by inflammation, but reduced by increased erythropoiesis and hypoxia. **(b)** The proposed mechanism by which the degree of transferrin saturation by iron in iron overload stimulates hepcidin synthesis (see also text). BMP synthesis by liver sinusoidal cells is stimulated by diferric transferrin, which also stabilizes TFR2 and by binding to TFR1 prevents HFE being deviated by attaching to TFR1. Binding of BMPs to BMPRs stimulates, in a complex with HFE, TFR2 and HJV on the hepatic cell membrane, hepcidin synthesis by signalling through SMAD proteins. **(c)** In iron deficiency low concentrations of diferric transferrin result in reduced BMP synthesis. Also lack of diferric iron to bind to TFR2 results in degradation or shedding of TFR2 from the cell membrane. Additionally, failure of diferric transferrin to bind to TFR1 results in HFE binding to TFR1. Iron deficiency also activates matriptase2, which cleaves HJV. The result of all these actions is failure to form the necessary complex to stimulate hepcidin synthesis. In addition in iron deficiency, a histone deacetylase 3 is activated and this suppresses transcription of hepcidin. BMP, bone morphogenetic protein; BMPR, bone morphogenetic protein receptor; HJV, hemojuvelin; TFR1 and 2, transferrin receptor 1 and 2. Source: (b and c) Courtesy of Professor Clara Camaschella.

Table 3.2 Iron absorption.

Factors favouring absorption	Factors reducing absorption
Inorganic iron	Haem iron
Ferrous form (Fe^{2+})	Ferric form (Fe^{3+})
Acids (hydrochloric acid, vitamin C)	Alkalis – antacids, pancreatic secretions
Solubilizing agents (e.g. sugars, amino acids)	Precipitating agents – phytates, phosphates, tea
Reduced serum hepcidin	Increased serum hepcidin
Ineffective erythropoiesis	Decreased erythropoiesis
Pregnancy	Inflammation
Hereditary haemochromatosis	

Dietary iron

Iron is present in food as ferric hydroxides and ferric–protein and haem–protein complexes. Both the iron content and the proportion of iron absorbed differ from food to food; in general meat, in particular liver, is a better source than vegetables, eggs or dairy foods. The average Western diet contains 10–15 mg iron daily, from which only 5–10% is normally absorbed. The proportion can be increased to 20–30% in iron deficiency or pregnancy (Table 3.2), but even in these situations most dietary iron remains unabsorbed.

Iron absorption

Organic dietary iron is partly absorbed as haem and partly broken down in the stomach and duodenum to inorganic iron. Absorption occurs through the duodenum. Haem is absorbed through a receptor on the apical membrane of the duodenal enterocyte. Haem is then broken down to release its iron. Inorganic iron absorption is favoured by factors such as acid and reducing agents that keep iron in the gut lumen in the Fe^{2+} rather than the Fe^{3+} state (Table 3.2). The protein DMT-1 is involved in transfer of iron from the lumen of the gut across the enterocyte microvilli (Fig. 3.5). Ferroportin at the basolateral surface controls the exit of iron from the cell into portal plasma. The amount of iron absorbed is regulated according to the body's needs by changing the levels of DMT-1 and ferroportin. For DMT-1 this occurs by the IRP/IRE binding mechanism (Fig. 3.3) and for ferroportin by hepcidin (Fig. 3.4a). Ferroportin is also present in heart, kidney, brain and placenta, where it is important in exporting iron.

Ferrireductase present at the enterocyte's apical surface converts iron from the Fe^{3+} to Fe^{2+} state and another enzyme, hephaestin (ferrioxidase), converts Fe^{2+} to Fe^{3+} at the basal surface prior to its binding to transferrin.

Iron requirements

The amount of iron required each day to compensate for losses from the body and for growth varies with age and sex; it is highest in pregnancy, and adolescent and menstruating females (Table 3.3). Therefore these groups are particularly likely to develop iron deficiency if there is additional iron loss or prolonged reduced intake.

Table 3.3 Estimated daily iron requirements. Units are mg/day.

	Urine, sweat, faeces	Menses	Pregnancy	Growth	Total
Adult male	0.5–1				0.5–1
Postmenopausal female	0.5–1				0.5–1
Menstruating female*	0.5–1	0.5–1			1–2
Pregnant female*	0.5–1		1–2		1.5–3
Children (average)	0.5			0.6	1.1
Female (age 12–15)*	0.5–1	0.5–1		0.6	1.6–2.6

*These groups are more likely to develop iron deficiency.

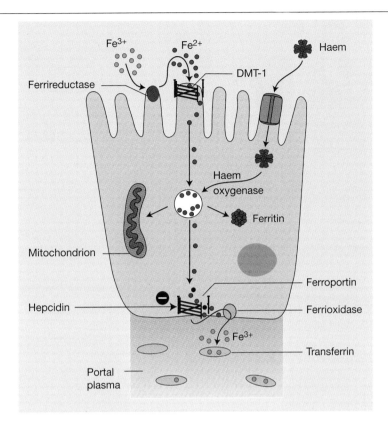

Figure 3.5 The regulation of iron absorption. Dietary ferric (Fe^{3+}) iron is reduced to Fe^{2+} and its entry to the enterocyte is through the divalent cation binder DMT-1. Its export into portal plasma is controlled by ferroportin. It is oxidized before binding to transferrin in plasma. Haem is absorbed after binding to its receptor protein.

Iron deficiency

Clinical features

When iron deficiency is developing, the reticuloendothelial stores (haemosiderin and ferritin) become completely depleted before anaemia occurs (Fig. 3.6). As the condition develops, the patient may show the general symptoms and signs of anaemia (see p. 19) and also a painless glossitis, angular stomatitis, brittle, ridged or spoon nails (koilonychia; Fig. 3.7) and unusual dietary cravings (pica). The cause of the epithelial cell changes is not clear, but may be related to reduction of iron-containing enzymes. Neonatal iron deficiency is associated with cognitive and behavioural abnormalities, while in children it can cause irritability, poor cognitive function and a decline in psychomotor development. There is also evidence that oral or parenteral iron may reduce fatigue in iron-deficient (low serum ferritin) non-anaemic women.

Causes of iron deficiency

In developed countries, chronic blood loss, especially uterine or from the gastrointestinal tract, is the dominant cause of iron deficiency (Table 3.4) and dietary deficiency **is rarely a cause on its own.** Five hundred millilitres of blood contain approximately 250 mg iron and, despite the increased absorption of food iron at an early stage of iron deficiency, negative iron balance is usual in chronic blood loss.

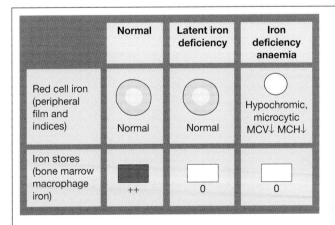

Figure 3.6 The development of iron deficiency anaemia. Reticuloendothelial (macrophage) stores are lost completely before anaemia develops. MCH, mean corpuscular haemoglobin; MCV, mean corpuscular volume.

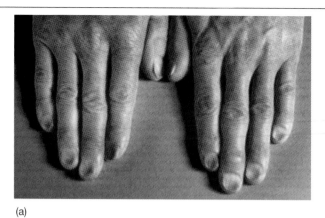

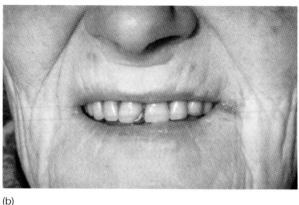

(a)

(b)

Figure 3.7 Iron deficiency anaemia. **(a)** Koilonychia: typical 'spoon' nails. **(b)** Angular cheilosis: fissuring and ulceration of the corner of the mouth.

Increased demands during infancy, adolescence, pregnancy, lactation and in menstruating women account for the high risk of iron deficiency anaemia in these particular clinical groups. Newborn infants have a store of iron derived from delayed clamping of the cord and the breakdown of excess red cells. From 3 to 6 months there is a tendency for a negative iron balance because of growth. From 6 months, supplemented formula milk and mixed feeding, particularly with iron-fortified foods, prevent iron deficiency.

In pregnancy increased iron is needed for an increased maternal red cell mass of approximately 35%, transfer of 300 mg of iron to the fetus and because of blood loss at delivery. Although iron absorption is also increased, iron therapy is often needed if the haemoglobin (Hb) falls below 100 g/L or the mean cell volume (MCV) is below 82 fL in the third trimester.

Menorrhagia (a loss of 80 mL or more of blood at each cycle) is difficult to assess clinically, although the loss of clots, the use of large numbers of pads or tampons or prolonged periods all suggest excessive loss.

It takes about 8 years for a normal adult male to develop iron deficiency anaemia solely as a result of a poor diet or malabsorption resulting in no iron intake at all. In developed countries inadequate intake or malabsorption is only rarely the sole cause of iron deficiency anaemia. Gluten-induced enteropathy,

Table 3.4 Causes of iron deficiency.
Chronic blood loss
Uterine
Gastrointestinal, e.g. peptic ulcer; oesophageal varices; aspirin (or other non-steroidal anti-inflammatory drugs) ingestion; gastrectomy; carcinoma of the stomach, caecum, colon or rectum; hookworm; schistosomiasis; angiodysplasia; inflammatory bowel disease; piles; diverticulosis
Rarely, haematuria, haemoglobinuria, pulmonary haemosiderosis, self-inflicted blood loss
Increased demands (see also Table 3.3)
Prematurity
Growth
Pregnancy
Erythropoietin therapy
Malabsorption
Gluten-induced enteropathy, gastrectomy, autoimmune gastritis
Poor diet
A major factor in many developing countries, but rarely the sole cause in developed countries

partial or total gastrectomy and atrophic gastritis (often auto-immune and with *Helicobacter pylori* infection) may, however, predispose to iron deficiency. In developing countries, iron deficiency may occur as a result of a life-long poor diet, consisting mainly of cereals and vegetables. Hookworm may aggravate iron deficiency, as may repeated pregnancies or growth and menorrhagia in young females.

Laboratory findings

These are summarized and contrasted with those in other hypochromic anaemias in Table 3.7.

Red cell indices and blood film

Even before anaemia occurs, the red cell indices fall, and they fall progressively as the anaemia becomes more severe. The blood film shows hypochromic, microcytic cells with occasional target cells and pencil-shaped poikilocytes (Fig. 3.8). The reticulocyte count is low in relation to the degree of anaemia. When iron deficiency is associated with severe folate or vitamin B_{12} deficiency, a 'dimorphic' film occurs with a dual population of red cells of which one is macrocytic and the other microcytic and hypochromic; the indices may be normal. A dimorphic blood film is also seen in patients with iron deficiency anaemia who have received recent iron therapy and produced a population of new haemoglobinized normal-sized red cells (Fig. 3.9) and when the patient has been transfused. The platelet count is often moderately raised in iron deficiency, particularly when haemorrhage is continuing.

Bone marrow iron

Bone marrow examination is not needed to assess iron stores except in complicated cases. In iron deficiency anaemia there is a complete absence of iron from stores (macrophages) and from developing erythroblasts (Fig. 3.10). The erythroblasts are small and have a ragged cytoplasm.

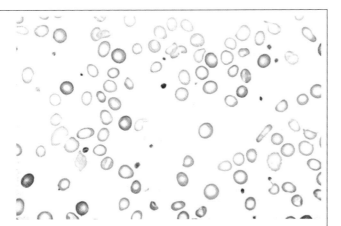

Figure 3.8 The peripheral blood film in severe iron deficiency anaemia. The cells are microcytic and hypochromic with occasional target cells.

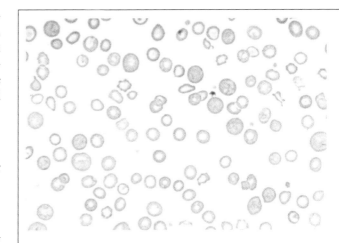

Figure 3.9 Dimorphic blood film in iron deficiency anaemia responding to iron therapy. Two populations of red cells are present: one microcytic and hypochromic, the other normocytic and well haemoglobinized.

Serum iron and total iron-binding capacity

The serum iron falls and total iron-binding capacity (TIBC) rises so that the TIBC is less than 20% saturated (Fig. 3.11). This contrasts both with the anaemia of chronic disorders (see below), when the serum iron and the TIBC are both reduced, and with other hypochromic anaemias where the serum iron is normal or even raised.

Serum ferritin

A small fraction of body ferritin circulates in the serum, the concentration being related to tissue, particularly reticulo-endothelial, iron stores. The normal range in men is higher than in women (Fig. 3.11). In iron deficiency anaemia the serum ferritin is very low, while a raised serum ferritin indicates iron overload or excess release of ferritin from damaged tissues or an acute phase response (e.g. in inflammation). The serum ferritin is normal or raised in the anaemia of chronic disorders.

Investigation of the cause of iron deficiency (Fig. 3.12)

In premenopausal women, menorrhagia and/or repeated pregnancies are the usual causes of the deficiency. If these are not present, other causes must be sought. In some patients with menorrhagia a clotting or platelet abnormality (e.g. von Willebrand disease) is present. In poor countries, the combination of prolonged inadequate intake of iron with expansion of blood volume with growth, and the onset of menstruation and repeated pregnancies in young women, is the major cause of iron deficiency in childhood and adolescence. In men and postmenopausal women, gastrointestinal blood loss is the main cause of iron deficiency and the exact site is sought from the clinical history, physical and rectal examination, by occult

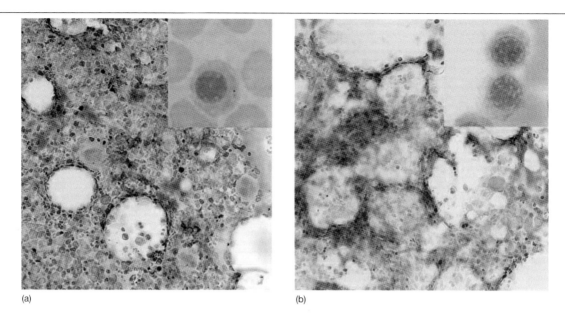

(a)   (b)

Figure 3.10 Bone marrow iron assessed by Perls' stain. **(a)** Normal iron stores indicated by blue staining in the macrophages. Inset: normal siderotic granule in erythroblast. **(b)** Absence of blue staining (absence of haemosiderin) in iron deficiency. Inset: absence of siderotic granules in erythroblasts.

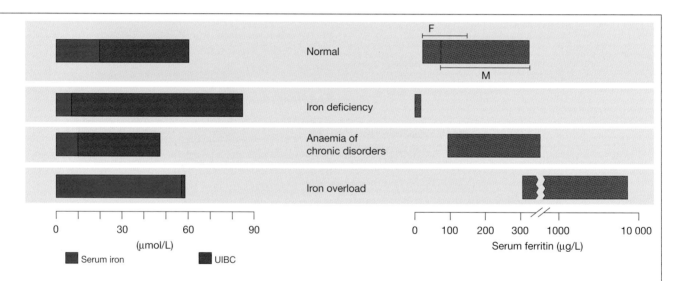

Figure 3.11 The serum iron, unsaturated serum iron-binding capacity (UIBC) and serum ferritin in normal subjects and in those with iron deficiency, anaemia of chronic disorders and iron overload. The total iron-binding capacity (TIBC) is made up of the serum iron and the UIBC. In some laboratories, the transferrin content of serum is measured directly by immunodiffusion, rather than by its ability to bind iron, and is expressed in g/L. Normal serum contains 2–4 g/L transferrin (1 g/L transferrin = 20 μmol/L binding capacity). Normal ranges for serum iron are 10–30 μmol/L; for TIBC, 40–75 μmol/L; for serum ferritin, male, 40–340 μg/L; female, 14–150 μg/L.

blood tests, and by appropriate use of upper and lower gastrointestinal endoscopy and/or radiology, e.g. computed tomography (CT) of the pneumocolon, or virtual colonoscopy using the 3D colon system (Figs 3.12 and 3.13). Tests for parietal cell antibodies, *Helicobacter* infection and serum gastrin level may help to diagnose autoimmune gastritis. In difficult cases a camera in a capsule can be swallowed which relays pictures of the gastrointestinal tract electronically. Tests for transglutaminase antibodies and duodenal biopsy to look for gluten-induced enteropathy can be valuable. Hookworm and schistosomiasis ova are sought in stools of subjects from areas where these infestations occur, and serology for schistosomiasis can be performed. Rarely, a coeliac axis angiogram is needed to demonstrate angiodysplasia.

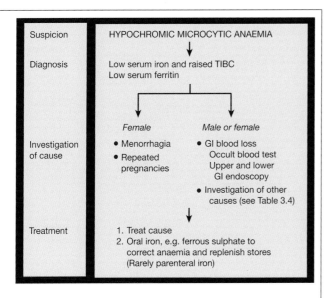

Figure 3.12 Investigation and management of iron deficiency anaemia. GI, gastrointestinal; TIBC, total iron-binding capacity.

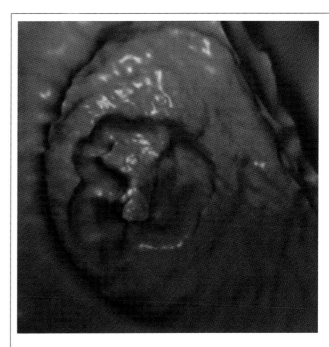

Figure 3.13 Virtual colonoscopy to show carcinoma of colon causing colonic obstruction and iron deficiency.

If gastrointestinal blood loss is excluded, loss of iron in the urine as haematuria or haemosiderinuria (resulting from chronic intravascular haemolysis) is considered. A normal chest X-ray excludes the rare condition of pulmonary haemosiderosis. Rarely, patients bleed themselves, producing iron deficiency.

Treatment

The underlying cause is treated as far as possible. In addition, iron is given to correct the anaemia and replenish iron stores.

Oral iron

The best preparation is ferrous sulphate, which is cheap, contains 67 mg iron in each 200 mg tablet and is usually given on an empty stomach. Once daily rather than three times daily doses are now advocated based on the rise in plasma hepcidin levels (which block further iron absorption) within hours after a single dose of iron is ingested. Ferrous fumarate is equally cheap and effective. If side-effects occur (e.g. nausea, abdominal pain, constipation or diarrhoea), these can be reduced by giving iron with food or by using a preparation with a lower iron content, e.g. ferrous gluconate, which contains less iron (37 mg) per 300 mg tablet. An elixir is available for children. Slow-release preparations should not be used.

Oral iron therapy should be given for long enough both to correct the anaemia and to replenish body iron stores, which usually means for at least 6 months. The haemoglobin should rise at the rate of approximately 20 g/L every 3 weeks. Failure of response to oral iron has several possible causes (Table 3.5), which should all be considered before parenteral iron is used. Iron fortification of the diet in infants in Africa reduces the incidence of anaemia, but increases susceptibility to malaria.

Parenteral iron

Many different preparations are available with varying licensing in different countries (Table 3.6). The dose may be calculated according to body weight and degree of anaemia, but it is more usual in order not to waste costly drugs to give 1000 mg

Table 3.5 Failure of response to oral iron.
Continuing haemorrhage
Failure to take tablets
Wrong diagnosis – especially thalassaemia trait, sideroblastic anaemia, IRIDA
Mixed deficiency – associated folate or vitamin B_{12} deficiency
Another cause for anaemia (e.g. malignancy, inflammation)
Malabsorption – coeliac disease, atrophic gastritis, *Helicobacter* infection
Use of slow-release preparation
IRIDA, non-refractory iron deficiency anaemia.

Table 3.6 Intravenous iron preparations.

Trade name	Cosmofer (Europe) INFeD (USA)	Ferinject (Europe) Injectafer (USA)	Feraheme	Monofer (Europe only)	Ferrlecit	Venofer (Europe only)
Carbohydrate	Low molecular weight dextran	Carboxymaltose	Ferumoxytol	Isomaltoside	Ferric gluconate in sucrose solution	Sucrose
Vial	50 mg/uL	50 mg/uL	30 mg/uL	100 mg/uL	5 ml (12.5 mg/uL)	20 mg/uL
Total dose	Yes	Yes	Yes	Yes	No	No
Test dose required	Yes	No	No	No	No	No
Infusion time	1 hour	15 min	15 min	15 min	60 min	15 min
Slow intravenous injection	Yes	Yes	No	Yes	Yes	Yes

as a single dose to moderately anaemic patients and 1500 mg divided into two doses, given at least 48 hours apart, to those more severely anaemic or of large body mass. All the preparations contain ferric (usually ferric hydroxide) iron. Iron dextran can be given in small doses by slow intravenous injection or by infusion as a total dose in one day. Ferric carboxymaltose and ferric isomaltoside may be given as a total dose in one day by intravenous infusion or by slow intravenous injections. Ferumoxytol is given only by intravenous infusion. Ferric hydroxide–sucrose, which releases iron from its sugar more rapidly than the other preparations, is administered by slow intravenous injection or infusion, to a maximum of 200 mg iron in each dose. Rarely there may be hypersensitivity or anaphylactoid reactions to parenteral iron, especially in those with a previous reaction, multiple drug allergies and severe atopy. If the reaction is severe, it is treated with intravenous hydrocortisone and possibly adrenaline.

Parenteral iron is given when there are high iron requirements, as in gastrointestinal bleeding, severe menorrhagia, middle or late pregnancy, chronic haemodialysis and chronic renal failure with erythropoietin therapy, post-operative after major surgery. It is avoided in the first trimester. It is also given when oral iron is ineffective (e.g. iron malabsorption resulting from gluten-induced enteropathy, atrophic gastritis, bariatric surgery), if IRIDA (see below) is present, or when oral iron causes intolerable side-effects) or is impractical (e.g. active inflammatory bowel disease). The haematological response to parenteral iron is no faster than to adequate dosage of oral iron, but the stores are replenished faster. Intravenous iron has also been found to increase functional capacity and quality of life in some patients with congestive heart failure, even in the absence of anaemia (see p. 365) and it has been found effective in restless leg syndrome.

Anaemia of chronic disorders

One of the most common anaemias occurs in patients with a variety of chronic inflammatory and malignant diseases (Table 3.7). With iron deficiency it accounts for about two-thirds of the world's anaemias. The characteristic features are:

1 Normochromic, normocytic or mildly hypochromic (MCV rarely <75 fL) indices and red cell morphology.
2 Mild and non-progressive anaemia (haemoglobin rarely <90 g/L) – the severity being related to the severity of the underlying disease.
3 Both the serum iron and TIBC are reduced.
4 The serum ferritin is normal or raised.
5 Bone marrow storage (reticuloendothelial) iron is normal, but erythroblast iron is reduced (Table 3.8).

Table 3.7 Causes of the anaemia of chronic disorders.

Chronic inflammatory diseases

Infections (e.g. pulmonary abscess, tuberculosis, osteomyelitis, pneumonia, bacterial endocarditis)

Non-infectious (e.g. rheumatoid arthritis, systemic lupus erythematosus and other connective tissue diseases, sarcoidosis, inflammatory bowel disease)
Congestive heart failure
Chronic pulmonary disease
Chronic renal disease
Obesity

Malignant diseases

Carcinoma, lymphoma, sarcoma

Table 3.8 Laboratory diagnosis of a hypochromic anaemia.

	Iron deficiency	Chronic inflammation or malignancy	Thalassaemia trait (α or β)	Sideroblastic anaemia	IRIDA
MCV/ MCH	Reduced in relation to severity of anaemia	Normal or mild reduction	Reduced; very low for degree of anaemia	Usually low in congenital type but MCV usually raised in acquired type	Reduced in relation to severity of anaemia
Serum iron	Reduced	Reduced	Normal	Raised	Reduced
TIBC	Raised	Reduced	Normal	Normal	Reduced
Serum ferritin	Reduced	Normal or raised	Normal	Raised	Raised
Bone marrow iron stores	Absent	Present	Present	Present	Present
Erythroblast iron	Absent	Absent	Present	Ring forms	Absent
Haemoglobin electrophoresis	Normal	Normal	Hb A$_2$ raised in β form	Normal	

Hb, haemoglobin; IRIDA, non-refractory iron deficiency anaemia; MCH, mean corpuscular haemoglobin; MCV, mean corpuscular volume; TIBC, total iron-binding capacity.

Table 3.9 Classification of sideroblastic anaemia.

Hereditary

X chromosome-linked ALA-S mutation or rarely with spinocerebellar degeneration and ataxia

Usually occurs in males, transmitted by females; also occurs rarely in females

Other rare autosomal types involving mitochondrial proteins or thiamine phosphorylation (see text)

Acquired

Primary

Myelodysplasia (refractory anaemia with ring sideroblasts; see p. 197). N.B. Ring sideroblast formation (<15% of erythroblasts) may also occur in the bone marrow in:
other malignant diseases of the marrow (e.g. other types of myelodysplasia, myelofibrosis, myeloid leukaemia, myeloma)
drugs, e.g. antituberculous (isoniazid, cycloserine), alcohol, lead
other benign conditions (e.g. haemolytic anaemia, megaloblastic anaemia, rheumatoid arthritis)

ALA-S, δ-aminolaevulinic acid synthase.

The pathogenesis of this anaemia appears to be related to decreased release of iron from macrophages to plasma, because of raised serum hepcidin levels stimulated by IL-6 and IL-1 and an inadequate erythropoietin response to anaemia caused by the effects of cytokines such as IL-1 and tumour necrosis factor, as well as direct inhibition of erythropoiesis by these cytokines and interferon-gamma. Erythrocyte lifespan is reduced due to activation of macrophages and to deposition of antibody and complement on erythrocytes. In addition, interferon-γ binds to thrombopoietin and forms a heterodimer, inhibiting thrombopoietin binding to its receptor on marrow cells.

The anaemia is corrected by successful treatment of the underlying disease and does not respond to iron therapy. Erythropoietin injections improve the anaemia in some cases. In many conditions this anaemia is complicated by anaemia resulting from other causes (e.g. iron, vitamin B$_{12}$ or folate deficiency, renal failure, bone marrow failure, hypersplenism, endocrine abnormality or leucoerythroblastic anaemia) and these are discussed in Chapter 29.

Iron refractory iron deficiency anaemia (IRIDA)

Rare autosomal recessive cases of hypochromic microcytic anaemia have been described caused by inherited mutations of matriptase 2, which allow uninhibited hepcidin secretion, or even more rarely of *DMT-1* genes (Figs 3.4 and 3.5). The serum iron is low with <5% saturation of the iron binding capacity (Table 3.8). There may be a haematological response to intravenous but usually not to oral iron.

Sideroblastic anaemia

This is a refractory anaemia defined by the presence of many pathological ring sideroblasts in the bone marrow (Fig. 3.14). These are abnormal erythroblasts containing numerous iron granules arranged in a ring or collar around the nucleus, instead of the one or two randomly distributed iron granules seen when normal erythroblasts are stained for iron. There is also usually erythroid hyperplasia with ineffective erythropoiesis. Sideroblastic anaemia is diagnosed when 15% or more of marrow erythroblasts are ring sideroblasts. They can be found at lower numbers in a variety of other haematological conditions.

Sideroblastic anaemia is classified into different types (Table 3.8) and the common link is a defect in haem synthesis. In the **hereditary forms** the anaemia is usually characterized by a markedly hypochromic and microcytic blood picture. The most common mutations are in the *ALA-S* gene, which is on the X chromosome. Pyridoxal-6-phosphate is a coenzyme for ALA-S. Other rare types include an X-linked disease with spinocerebellar degeneration and ataxia, mitochondrial defects (e.g. Pearson's syndrome, when there is also pancreatic insufficiency), thiamine-responsive and other autosomal defects. The much more common form is **refractory anaemia with ring sideroblasts**, which is a subtype of myelodysplasia (see Chapter 16). Acquired reversible forms may be due to alcohol, lead and drugs, e.g. isoniazid.

In some patients, particularly with the hereditary type, there is a response to pyridoxine therapy. Folate deficiency may occur and folic acid therapy may also be tried. Other treatments, e.g. erythropoietin, may be tried in the myelodysplasia form (see Chapter 16). In many severe cases, however, repeated blood transfusions are the only method of maintaining a satisfactory haemoglobin concentration, and transfusional iron overload requiring iron chelation therapy becomes a major problem.

Lead poisoning

Lead inhibits both haem and globin synthesis at a number of points. In addition, it interferes with the breakdown of RNA by inhibiting the enzyme pyrimidine 5′ nucleotidase, causing accumulation of denatured RNA in red cells, the RNA giving an appearance called basophilic stippling on the ordinary (Romanowsky) stain (see Fig. 2.17). The anaemia may be hypochromic or predominantly haemolytic, and the bone marrow may show ring sideroblasts. Free erythrocyte protoporphyrin is raised.

Differential diagnosis of hypochromic anaemia

Table 3.8 lists the laboratory investigations that may be necessary. The clinical history is particularly important, as the source of the haemorrhage leading to iron deficiency or the presence of a chronic disease may be revealed. The ethnic group and the family history may suggest a possible diagnosis of thalassaemia or other genetic defect of haemoglobin. Physical examination may also be helpful in determining a site of haemorrhage, features of a chronic inflammatory or malignant disease, koilonychia or, in some haemoglobinopathies, an enlarged spleen or bony deformities.

In thalassaemia trait the red cells tend to be very small, often with an MCV of 70 fL or less, even when anaemia is mild or absent; the red cell count is usually over 5.5×10^{12}/L. Conversely, in iron deficiency anaemia the indices fall progressively with the degree of anaemia and when anaemia is mild the indices are normal or only just reduced below normal (e.g. MCV 75–80 fL). In the anaemia of chronic disorders the indices are also not markedly low, an MCV in the range 75–82 fL being usual.

It is usual to perform a serum iron and TIBC measurement, or alternatively serum ferritin estimation, to confirm a diagnosis of iron deficiency. Haemoglobin high-performance liquid chromatography (HPLC) or electrophoresis with an

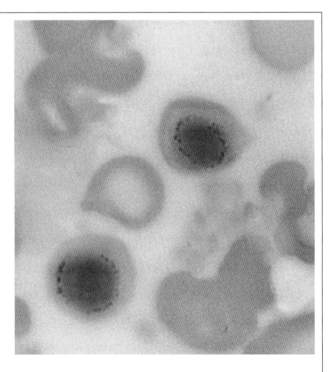

Figure 3.14 Ring sideroblasts with a perinuclear ring of iron granules in sideroblastic anaemia.

estimation of Hb A$_2$ and Hb F is carried out in all patients suspected of thalassaemia or other genetic defect of haemoglobin, because of the family history, ethnic group, red cell indices and blood film. Iron deficiency or the anaemia of chronic disorders may also occur in these subjects. β-Thalassaemia trait is characterized by a raised Hb A$_2$ above 3.5%, but in α-thalassaemia trait there is no abnormality on simple haemoglobin studies, so the diagnosis is usually made by exclusion of all other causes of hypochromic red cells and by the presence of a red cell count $>5.5 \times 10^{12}$/L. DNA studies can be used to confirm the diagnosis.

Bone marrow examination is essential if a diagnosis of sideroblastic anaemia is suspected, but is not usually needed in diagnosis of the other hypochromic anaemias.

SUMMARY

- Iron is present in the body in haemoglobin, myoglobin, haemosiderin and ferritin, and in iron-containing enzymes. Transferrin is the main transport protein in blood.
- Hepcidin is the main regulator of iron absorption and iron release from macrophages and other cells.
- Iron metabolism is regulated according to iron status by intracellular iron regulatory proteins and by control of hepcidin synthesis. Hepcidin synthesis is also affected by erythropoiesis and by inflammation.
- Iron deficiency is the most common cause of anaemia throughout the world. The serum ferritin, serum iron and saturation of the iron-binding capacity are reduced.
- In Western countries, it is usually caused by haemorrhage from the gastrointestinal or the female genital tract. Dietary intake is important, particularly in developing countries, where hookworm and schistosomiasis are also important causes of blood loss.
- The red cells are hypochromic and microcytic. It is treated by oral or parenteral iron to correct the anaemia and to restore body stores of iron, and by treating, as far as possible, the underlying cause.
- Other frequent causes of a hypochromic, microcytic anaemia are the anaemia of chronic disorders, which occurs in patients with chronic inflammatory or malignant diseases, and α- or β-thalassaemia. Less frequent causes include sideroblastic anaemia (some cases), iron refractory iron deficiency anaemia and lead poisoning.
- Sideroblastic anaemias are characterised by ring sideroblasts in the marrow. The most frequent is a subtype of myelodysplasia.

Now visit **www.wileyessential.com/haematology** to test yourself on this chapter.

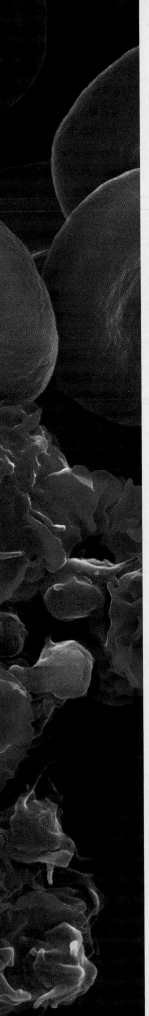

CHAPTER 4
Iron overload

Key topics

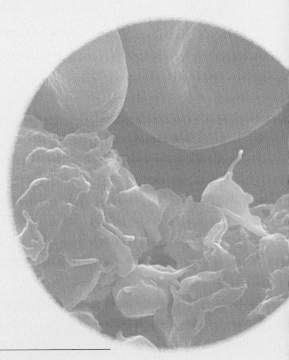

Hoffbrand's Essential Haematology, Eighth Edition. By A. Victor Hoffbrand and David P. Steensma.
© 2020 John Wiley & Sons Ltd. Published 2020 by John Wiley & Sons Ltd.
Companion website: www.wileyessential.com/haematology

There is no physiological mechanism for eliminating excess iron from the body, so iron absorption by the small intestine is normally carefully regulated to avoid accumulation of excess iron. Iron overload (haemosiderosis) occurs in genetic disorders associated with inappropriately increased iron absorption (haemochromatosis), or in patients with severe chronic anaemias, especially those who receive regular blood transfusions. Excessive iron deposition in tissues may result in serious damage to organs, particularly the heart, liver and endocrine organs. The causes of iron overload are listed in Table 4.1 and of genetic haemochromatosis in Table 4.2.

Assessment of iron status and organ function

The tests that can be performed to assess iron overload and the degree of damage caused by iron are listed in Table 4.3. The serum ferritin is easy to obtain and is thus the most widely

Table 4.1 The causes of iron overload.

Increased iron absorption	Hereditary (primary) haemochromatosis
	Ineffective erythropoiesis, e.g. thalassaemia intermedia or myelodysplastic syndromes
	Chronic liver disease
Increased iron intake	African siderosis (dietary and genetic components)
Repeated red cell transfusions	Transfusion siderosis

Table 4.2 Genetic causes of haemochromatosis and of hyperferritinaemia.

Type	Inheritance	Clinical condition	Gene defect
1	AR	Classical hereditary haemochromatosis	HFE
2	AR	Juvenile haemochromatosis	Hemojuvelin (*HJV*) Hepcidin (*HAMP*)
3	AR	Hereditary haemochromatosis	Transferrin receptor 2 (*TFR2*)
4	AD	Marked increase in RE iron, less hepatic iron (see text)	Ferroportin 1 (*SLC40A1*)
5	AD	Hereditary hyperferritinaemia–cataract syndrome (no iron deposition)	Ferritin heavy chain (*FTH1*)

AD, autosomal dominant; AR, autosomal recessive; RE, reticuloendothelial.

Table 4.3 Assessment of iron overload.

Assessment of iron stores

Serum ferritin

Serum iron and percentage saturation of transferrin (iron-binding capacity)

Serum non-transferrin-bound iron (NTBI)

Bone marrow biopsy (Perls' stain) for iron within reticuloendothelial stores

Liver biopsy (parenchymal and reticuloendothelial stores)

Liver CT scan or MRI (T_2^* or Ferriscan technique)

Cardiac MRI (gated T_2^* technique)

Pancreas and pituitary MRI (not yet widely available)

Assessment of tissue damage caused by iron overload

Cardiac	Clinical; chest X-ray; ECG; 24-h monitor; echocardiography or radionuclide (MUGA) scan to assess left and right ventricular ejection fraction at rest and with stress
Liver	Liver function tests, alphafetoprotein; liver biopsy; CT scan or MRI, fibroscan
Endocrine	Clinical examination (including for growth and sexual development); glucose tolerance test; pituitary gonadotrophin release tests; thyroid, parathyroid, gonadal, adrenal function and growth hormone assays; radiology for bone age; isotopic bone density study
Musculoskeletal	Hand X-rays with assessment of metacarpophalangeal joints

CT, computed tomography; ECG, electrocardiography; MRI, magnetic resonance imaging; MUGA, multiple gated acquisition.

used to assess iron overload and for monitoring its treatment, although inflammation can increase serum ferritin levels even in the absence of iron overload. The percentage saturation of transferrin (which is a measure of iron-binding capacity) is also valuable. Serum non-transferrin-bound (NTBI) iron, also known as labile plasma iron, is a toxic form of iron that occurs in severe transfusional iron overload. Clinical tests for NTBI are not widely available.

Liver biopsy with staining for iron (Fig. 4.1) and chemical analysis of iron content is useful for assessment of both parenchymal iron (within hepatic cells) and reticuloendothelial iron (within Kupffer cells). Liver biopsy also allows estimation

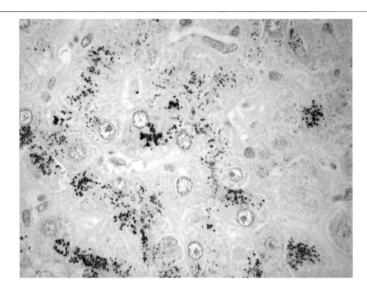

Figure 4.1 Liver biopsy in genetic haemochromatosis. Iron loading of hepatic parenchymal cells (Perls' stain). Source: Courtesy of Professor A.P. Dhillon.

of the degree of fibrosis. Fibroscan (transient elastography) is a non-invasive ultrasound method of assessing liver fibrosis of any cause, including iron overload. Magnetic resonance imaging (MRI) using the T2* technique is the best non-invasive guide to liver and cardiac iron. A commercial Ferriscan MRI technique is widely used for measuring liver iron. Serum alpha fetoprotein and liver ultrasound are used for serial screening for hepatocellular carcinoma in patients with known iron overload, typically on an annual basis.

Hereditary (genetic, primary) haemochromatosis

Hereditary or genetic haemochromatosis is a group of diseases in which there is from birth excessive absorption of iron from the gastrointestinal tract leading to iron overload of the parenchymal cells, dominantly of the liver (Fig. 4.1) and at later stages the endocrine organs and the heart. In contrast to transfusional iron overload, the macrophages are not iron overloaded.

Most patients are homozygous for a missense mutation in the *HFE* gene, which leads to insertion of a tyrosine residue rather than cysteine in the mature protein (C282Y). This allele has the highest prevalence (approximately 1 in 10) within populations of Northern European origin. However, gene penetrance is low; only a small proportion of this ethnic group who are homozygous for the mutation (about 1 in 300) present with clinical features of the disease. Affected individuals usually show a serum ferritin greater than 1000 μg/L. A second mutation resulting in a histidine to aspartic acid substitution H63D is found with the C282Y mutation in approximately 5% of patients with genetic haemochromatosis, but homozygotes for the H63D mutation usually do not have the

disease. HFE H63D has a broader global distribution than C282Y.

HFE is involved in regulating hepcidin synthesis and therefore hereditary haemochromatosis caused by *HFE* mutation is due to low serum hepcidin levels (see Fig. 3.4). Low serum hepcidin levels lead to high levels of ferroportin and therefore increased iron absorption and increased release of iron from macrophages. Iron overload develops over decades and damages parenchymal cells, such that patients may present in adult life with hepatic disease (fibrosis, cirrhosis, hepatocellular carcinoma), endocrine disturbances (diabetes mellitus, hypothyroidism or impotence) or melanin skin pigmentation (Fig. 4.2). In some severe cases

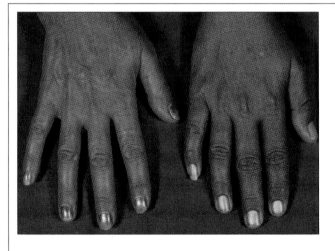

Figure 4.2 Melanin skin pigmentation. The right hand is of a teenager with iron overload caused by thalassaemia major. The left hand is of her mother, who has normal iron status.

there is cardiac failure or arrhythmia. Homozygosity for the *HFE* mutation also underlies an arthropathy due to calcium pyrophosphate deposition and not related to the degree of iron overload. The most commonly affected joints include the second and third metacarpophalangeals.

Other non-HFE genetic factors as well as dietary iron intake, alcohol consumption, pregnancies, menstrual blood loss, other blood loss (e.g. gastrointestinal bleeding) or blood donation affect the phenotype and time of presentation of the disease. Regular blood donors on average present several years later than individuals with hereditary haemochromatosis who never donate blood.

The initial clinical presentation is often with non-specific symptoms such as fatigue, loss of libido or arthralgias. Diagnosis is suspected in the presence of increased levels of serum iron, serum transferrin saturation and ferritin. The diagnosis is confirmed by testing for the *HFE* mutation, but a negative result does not exclude the diagnosis, since mutations of other genes may cause a similar disease phenotype (see Table 4.2 and below). Liver biopsy is useful to quantify the degree of iron overload and assess liver damage, but is associated with risks, including bleeding. MRI can also be used to measure liver and cardiac iron non-invasively.

Treatment is with regular venesection, initially at 1–2-week intervals, with each unit of blood removing 200–250 mg of iron. Organ function may improve and liver fibrosis resolve, but the arthropathy does not respond to iron removal and response of the endocrinopathy is variable. There are differences of opinion as to whether patients without evidence of organ dysfunction due to iron overload should be treated, but usually this is done when the serum ferritin is raised to over 1000 µg/L. Venesection is monitored by serum ferritin and the aim is to restore this to normal, usually to <100 µg/L, and then keep it there with further less frequent venesections, e.g. a few times per year. Some patients elect to become blood donors, but some blood banks and regulatory agencies do not allow blood donation from patients with haemochromatosis. Patients with abnormal liver tests are excluded from donating blood due to the inability to exclude viral causes of hepatic enzyme elevation.

Rarer forms of genetic haemochromatosis are caused by mutations in genes for other iron regulatory proteins, including hemojuvelin, transferrin receptor 2 and hepcidin. All of these (types II and III disease; Table 4.2) are associated, like homozygous HFE disease, with low levels of hepcidin in serum. They often present as severe iron overload with cardiomyopathy in children, adolescents or young adults. Hypogonadism is another particular feature of these forms of haemochromatosis, whereas arthropathy is absent. Genetic iron overload in Asian populations is usually due to these mutations rather than mutation of *HFE*.

On the other hand, ferroportin gene mutations (type IV disease) usually cause reticuloendothelial but not parenchymal cell iron overload. They may rarely cause parenchymal overload if the mutations in the ferroportin gene are at the hepcidin binding site. Mutations of the ferritin light chain gene (type V disease) cause a raised monoclonal serum ferritin with cataracts resulting from ferritin deposition in the eye, but no other tissue iron overload.

African iron overload

This occurs in sub-Saharan Africa through a combination of increased iron absorption due to a genetic defect, possibly in the ferroportin gene, and consumption of beverages, especially beer, with a high iron content due to the use of iron brewing or cooking pots.

Thalassaemia intermedia (non-transfusion-dependent thalassaemia)

Moderately severe forms of thalassaemia may lead to increased iron levels even in patients who do not need regular blood transfusions (see Chapter 7). This is due to increased absorption and may lead to increased levels of iron in the liver. The heart is spared from this iron loading. Blood transfusions at times of increased anaemia, e.g. with intercurrent infections, may increase the iron burden. Iron chelation is indicated if the liver iron concentration is above 5 mg/g dry weight, when serum ferritin reaches 800 µg/L or when the iron leads to organ damage (see also Chapter 7).

Transfusional iron overload

This develops in patients with chronic severe anaemia not due to haemorrhage who need to have regular blood transfusions. Each 500 mL of transfused blood contains approximately 250 mg iron and iron overload is inevitable unless iron chelation therapy is given (Table 4.4). To make matters worse, iron absorption from food is *increased* in β-thalassaemia major and many other anaemias secondary to ineffective erythropoiesis because of inappropriately low serum hepcidin levels. This is due to release from early erythroblasts of erythroferrone and other proteins that inhibit hepcidin synthesis (see Fig. 3.4). Non-transferrin-bound iron may appear in plasma when transferrin is >70% saturated and cause widespread iron deposition in parenchymal tissues.

Cardiac damage due to iron is a dominant problem in transfusional iron overload. As for hereditary haemochromatosis, iron also damages the liver (Fig. 4.3) and the endocrine organs, including the hypothalamus and pituitary, with failure of growth, delayed or absent puberty, diabetes mellitus, hypothyroidism and hypoparathyroidism. Skin pigmentation as a result of excess melanin and haemosiderin gives a slate grey appearance even at an early stage of iron overload.

In the absence of intensive iron chelation, death occurs in the second or third decade of life in thalassaemia major, usually from congestive heart failure or cardiac arrhythmias. **T_2^* MRI is a valuable measure of cardiac and liver iron loading (Fig. 4.4)**. It can detect increased cardiac iron and predict for cardiac failure or arrhythmia before sensitive tests detect

Table 4.4 Causes of anaemia that may lead to transfusional iron overload.

Congenital	Acquired
β-Thalassaemia major	Myelodysplastic syndromes
β-Thalassaemia/Hb E disease	Red cell aplasia
Congenital dyserythropoietic anaemias	Acute leukaemias
Sickle cell anaemia (some cases)	Aplastic anaemia
Red cell aplasia (Diamond–Blackfan)	Primary myelofibrosis
Congenital sideroblastic anaemia	
Dyserythropoietic anaemia	

Hb, haemoglobin.

impaired cardiac function. The shorter the relaxation time, the greater the cardiac iron burden and the greater risk of subsequent cardiac failure or arrhythmia (Fig. 4.5). Serum ferritin and liver iron correlate poorly with cardiac iron (Figs 4.4 and 4.5). Moreover, serum ferritin is raised in viral hepatitis and other inflammatory disorders and should therefore be interpreted in conjunction with more accurate tests of iron status, such as T_2^* MRI or liver biopsy.

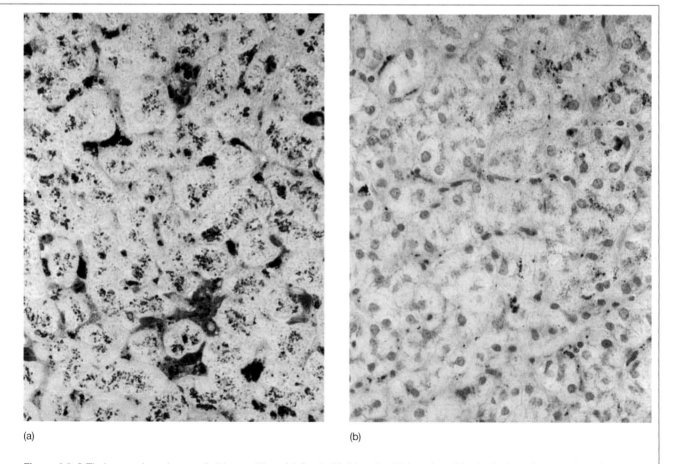

(a) (b)

Figure 4.3 β-Thalassaemia major: needle biopsy of liver. **(a)** Grade IV siderosis with iron deposition in the hepatic parenchymal cells, bile duct epithelium, macrophages and fibroblasts (Perls' stain). **(b)** Reduction of iron excess in liver after intensive chelation therapy.

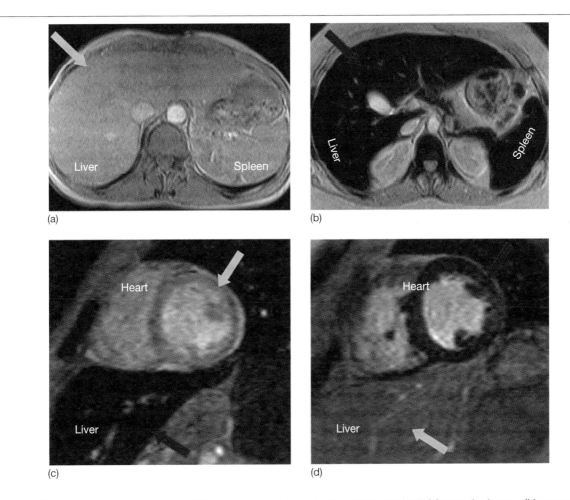

Figure 4.4 T$_2$* magnetic resonance images (MRIs) showing tissue appearance in iron overload: **(a)** normal volunteer, **(b)** severe iron overload. Green arrow, normal appearance; red arrow, iron overload. Lack of correlation: liver and cardiac iron in two cases of thalassaemia major, **(c)** and **(d)**.

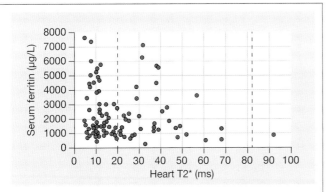

Figure 4.5 Comparison of T2* magnetic resonance imaging **(MRI)** measurement of cardiac iron and serum ferritin in thalassaemia major patients. There are substantial numbers of patients with very high serum ferritin (>3000 μg/L) but normal heart iron (T2* >20 msecs) and, conversely, patients with serum ferritin levels <1000 μg/L with severe cardiac iron loading (T2* <10 msecs). Source: L.J. Anderson *et al.* (2001) *Eur. Heart J.* 22: 2171–79.

Iron chelation therapy

Iron chelation therapy is used to treat transfusional iron overload and three effective drugs are available: orally administered deferasirox and deferiprone, and parenterally administered deferoxamine. Thalassaemia major is the most frequent indication worldwide, but chelation is also used for iron overloaded, heavily transfused patients with the other anaemias listed in Table 4.4.

Deferasirox is given orally once daily and leads to iron loss in the faeces. Skin rashes and transient changes in liver enzymes and rise in serum creatinine are the main side-effects. Its licensing for young children and lack of major side-effects have resulted in its widespread use, but high cost means that the other drugs may be preferred in some countries. Defer-asirox is the least effective of the three drugs for eliminating cardiac iron (Fig. 4.6).

Deferiprone is also an oral chelator and causes predominantly urinary iron excretion. It is usually given in three doses daily. It may be used alone or, if this is inadequate, in combination with deferoxamine infused on one or more days a week, since the drugs have an additive or even synergetic effect on iron excretion. Alone it is the most effective of the three drugs at removing cardiac iron and improving left and right heart function (Fig. 4.6). Side-effects include an arthropathy, agranulocytosis (in about 1%), neutropenia, gastrointestinal disturbance and, rarely in patients with diabetes, zinc deficiency. Monitoring of the blood count weekly for the first year and fortnightly in the second is recommended for all patients receiving deferiprone. Combination therapy with the two orally active chelators, if either alone is not sufficiently effective, has been effective without unexpected toxicity in several trials, but is not yet licensed in any country.

The third drug, **deferoxamine**, was the first of the three drugs to be used in clinical practice. It is not active orally and is usually given by subcutaneous infusion over 8–12 hours for

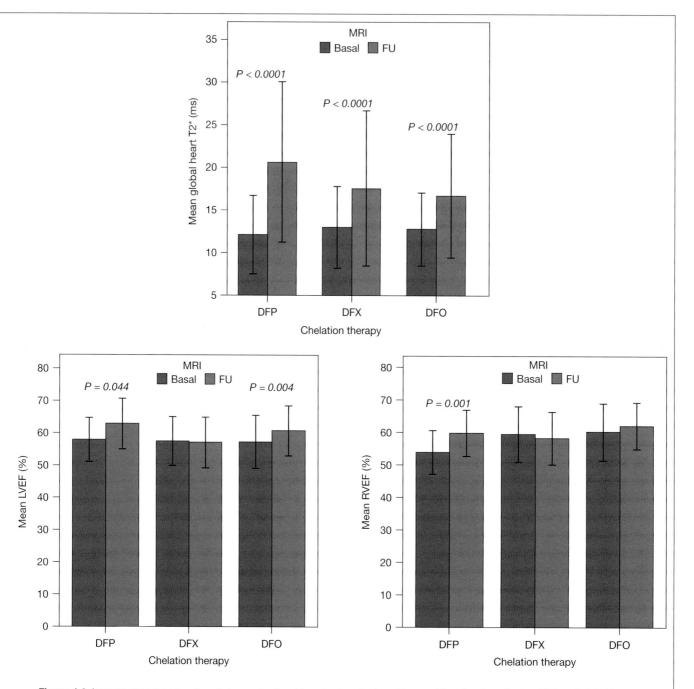

Figure 4.6 Intra-treatment comparison between final and basal values for heart iron and function in patients with basal global heart T2* value <20 ms. DFO, desferrioxamine; DFP, deferiprone; DFX, deferasirox; FU, follow-up; LVEF, left ventricular ejection fraction; MRI, magnetic resonance imaging; RVEF, right ventricular ejection fraction. Source: A. Pepe *et al.* (2018) *Br. J. Haematol.* 180(6): 879–88.

5–7 days each week; vitamin C can be given to further increase iron excretion. Most iron is lost in the urine, but up to one-third is also excreted in the stools. Because of the difficult administration, lack of patient adherence is a major problem. It may be given on one or more each days each week in combination with daily deferiprone (or deferasirox) and can be used intravenously in combination with oral deferiprone in patients with severe iron overload at risk of dying from cardiac failure. Side-effects are particularly frequent if high doses are used in children and in adults without heavy iron overload. These include high tone deafness, retinal damage, bone abnormalities and growth retardation. Patients receiving deferoxamine should have auditory and fundoscopic examinations at regular intervals.

All three chelators can be given in children. Deferasirox is most frequently used and a liquid formulation of deferiprone and a sprinkle form of deferasirox are available.

Chelation is typically started in thalassaemia major after 10–15 units have been transfused or the serum ferritin is >800–1000 µg/L. In other conditions such as myelodysplastic syndromes, there is controversy about when to initiate chelation and hepatic and cardiac T2* MRI may help guide this decision.

Chelation is given to keep the cardiac T2* test at >20 msecs, liver to <7 mg/g dry weight and serum ferritin level at less than 1000–1500 µg/L, when the body iron stores are approximately 5–10 times normal. MRI assesses cardiac and liver iron accurately and should be repeated annually or more frequently if there is definite cardiac or liver damage (Fig. 4.5). Serum ferritin is useful in monitoring changes in iron stores, but as it is an acute phase reactant it may be elevated in the presence of recent infection or physiological stress such as surgery, and this may falsely suggest inadequate chelation.

Serial tests of heart, liver and endocrine function are also needed to monitor therapy.

Life expectancy has improved dramatically for thalassaemia major patients since the introduction of iron chelation. Chelation may even reverse liver, endocrine and cardiac damage in cases where this has developed before chelation is started or is due to inadequate chelation therapy.

SUMMARY

- Iron overload is caused by excessive absorption of iron from food (genetic haemochromatosis) or by repeated blood transfusions in patients with refractory anaemias. Each unit of blood contains 200–250 mg of iron.
- Excess iron absorbed from the gastrointestinal tract in genetic haemochromatosis accumulates in the parenchymal cells of the liver, the endocrine organs and, in severe cases, the heart.
- Genetic haemochromatosis is usually caused by homozygous mutation of the *HFE* gene causing C282Y protein change and a low serum hepcidin level. Rarer forms exist caused by mutations of other genes coding for proteins involved in iron regulation (hemojuvelin, hepcidin, transferrin receptor 2 and ferroportin). Repeated venesections are used to reduce the body iron burden.
- Transfusional iron overload most frequently occurs in thalassaemia major, but also in other transfusion-dependent refractory anaemias (e.g. some cases of myelodysplastic syndromes, sickle cell anaemia, primary myelofibrosis, red cell aplasia and aplastic anaemia).
- Transfusional iron overload causes damage to the liver, endocrine organs and heart, with iron accumulation also in macrophages of the reticuloendothelial system.
- Cardiac failure or arrhythmia caused by cardiac siderosis, best detected by MRI, is the most frequent cause of death from transfusional iron overload.
- Treatment is with iron chelating drugs: deferiprone and deferasirox, which are active orally, or deferoxamine, given subcutaneously or intravenously.
- Life expectancy has improved dramatically in thalassaemia major as a result of iron chelation therapy and the use of T2*MRI to accurately measure cardiac and liver iron.

Now visit **www.wileyessential.com/haematology** to test yourself on this chapter.

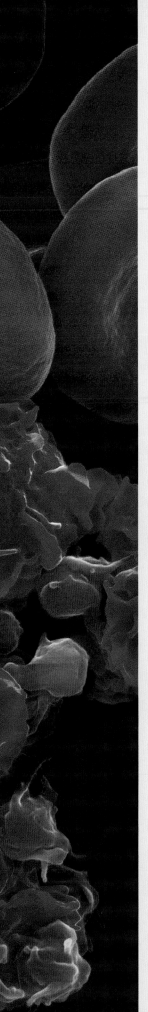

CHAPTER 5
Megaloblastic anaemias and other macrocytic anaemias

Key topics

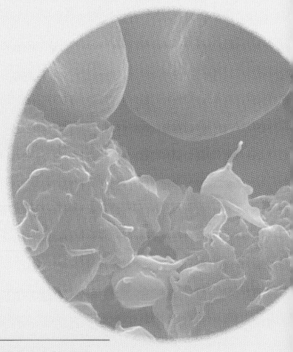

Hoffbrand's Essential Haematology, Eighth Edition. By A. Victor Hoffbrand and David P. Steensma.
© 2020 John Wiley & Sons Ltd. Published 2020 by John Wiley & Sons Ltd.
Companion website: www.wileyessential.com/haematology

Introduction to macrocytic anaemia

In macrocytic anaemia, the red cells are abnormally large (mean corpuscular volume, MCV >98 fL). There are several causes (see Table 2.5), but they can be broadly subdivided into megaloblastic and non-megaloblastic (Table 5.10), based on the appearance of developing erythroblasts in the bone marrow. An elevated MCV may also be an artefact reported by an automated cell counter if red cell agglutination or a paraprotein is present.

Megaloblastic anaemias

This is a group of anaemias in which the erythroblasts in the bone marrow show a characteristic abnormality: maturation of the nucleus is delayed relative to that of the cytoplasm. The underlying defect accounting for the asynchronous maturation of the nucleus is defective DNA synthesis; this is usually caused by deficiency of vitamin B_{12} or folate. Less commonly, abnormalities of the metabolism of these vitamins (including abnormalities induced by drugs) or inherited lesions in DNA synthesis may cause an identical haematological appearance (Table 5.1). Morphologically, this asynchrony is manifest by a persistently open, loosely organized chromatin in the erythropoietic cell nucleus, while the cytoplasm exhibits staining changes of haemoglobinization typical of a later stage of maturation.

Vitamin B_{12} (B_{12}, cobalamin)

Vitamin B_{12} is synthesized in nature by microorganisms; animals acquire it by eating food of animal origin, by internal production from intestinal bacteria (not in humans) or by eating bacterially contaminated foods. The vitamin consists of a small group of compounds, the cobalamins, which have the same basic structure, with a cobalt atom at the centre of a corrin ring (Fig. 5.1). The reactive centre of the molecule

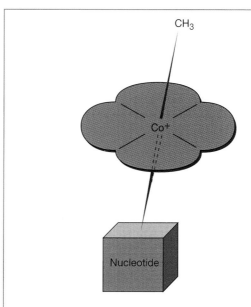

Figure 5.1 The structure of methylcobalamin (methyl B_{12}), the main form of vitamin B_{12} in human plasma. Other forms include deoxyadenosylcobalamin (ado B_{12}), the main form in human tissues; and hydroxocobalamin (hydroxo B_{12}) and cyanocobalamin, the main forms used in treatment of deficiency and in multivitamin supplements.

is attached to either a cyano group (-CN, cyanocobalamin), a hydroxyl group (-OH, hydroxocobalamin), a methyl group (-CH^3, methylcobalamin) or 5-deoxyadenosyl (adenosylcobalamin). The vitamin is found in foods of animal origin such as liver, meat, fish and dairy produce, but does not occur in fruit, cereals or vegetables, except in small amounts due to contamination by insect parts in harvesting or by micro-organisms in a natural environment (Table 5.2).

Absorption

A normal diet contains a large excess of B_{12} compared with daily needs (Table 5.2). B_{12} is released from protein binding in food by pepsin in the stomach. It is then mainly combined with the glycoprotein, **intrinsic factor (IF)**. IF is synthesized by the gastric parietal cells. The IF–B_{12} complex subsequently binds in the ileum to a specific surface receptor for IF, **cubam**, a complex of cubilin and amnionless proteins. Amnionless directs endocytosis of the cubilin IF–B_{12} complex into the ileal cell so that B_{12} is absorbed and IF destroyed (Fig. 5.2). The maximum amount of B_{12} that can be absorbed from a single oral dose (either in the form of food or a supplement) via the IF–cubam mechanism is about 1–2 μg.

Some dietary B_{12}, after release from food, first binds to a glycoprotein haptocorrin (also known as R-factor, R-protein, or transcobalamin I), which is present in saliva and gastric juice. Release of dietary B_{12} from haptocorrin for binding to IF depends largely on proteases from the pancreas.

Table 5.1 Causes of megaloblastic anaemia.

Vitamin B_{12} deficiency (causes are listed in Table 5.3)

Folate deficiency (causes are listed in Table 5.5)

Combined folate and B_{12} deficiency

Abnormalities of vitamin B_{12} or folate metabolism (e.g. transcobalamin deficiency, nitrous oxide, antifolate drugs such as methotrexate, phenytoin or trimethoprim)

Inherited defects of DNA synthesis or methionine synthase

Congenital enzyme deficiencies (e.g. orotic aciduria, which impairs pyrimidine synthesis)

Acquired enzyme deficiencies (e.g. due to hydroxyurea, purine synthesis antagonists such as 6-mercaptopurine, pyrimidine antagonists such as cytosine arabinoside)

Table 5.2 Vitamin B$_{12}$ and folate: nutritional aspects.

	Vitamin B$_{12}$	Folate
Typical daily dietary intake	7–30 µg	200–250 µg
Food sources	Animal products only	Many foods, especially liver, greens and yeast
Effect of cooking	Little effect	Easily destroyed
Minimal adult daily requirement	2 µg	100–200 µg
Body stores when replete	2–3 mg (sufficient for 2–4 years)	10–12 mg (sufficient for 4 months)
Absorption Site Mechanism Limit	Ileum Bound to intrinsic factor, absorbed by cubam 2–3 µg/day	Duodenum and jejunum Conversion to methyltetrahydrofolate 50–80% of dietary content
Enterohepatic circulation	5–10 µg/day	90 µg/day
Transport in plasma	Most bound to haptocorrin; TC essential for cell uptake	Weakly bound to albumin
Major intracellular physiological forms	Methyl- and deoxyadenosylcobalamin	Reduced polyglutamate derivatives
Usual therapeutic form	Hydroxocobalamin or cyanocobalamin	Folic (pteroylglutamic) acid

TC, transcobalamin II; haptocorrin = transcobalamin 1.

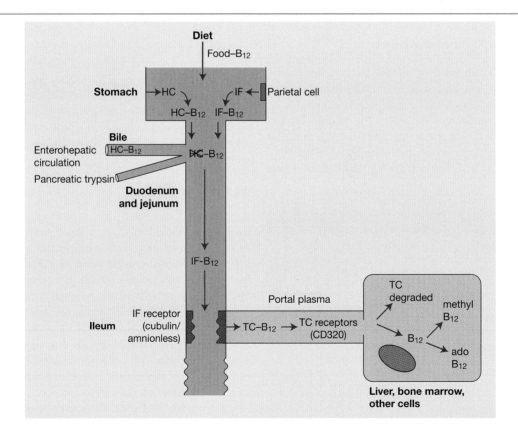

Figure 5.2 The absorption of dietary vitamin B$_{12}$ after combination with intrinsic factor (IF), through the ileum. TC, transcobalamin; IF, intrinsic factor; HC, haptocorrin; ado B$_{12}$, see text.

Transport of vitamin B₁₂: the transcobalamins

Vitamin B_{12} is absorbed from the ileal cell into portal blood, where it becomes attached to the plasma-binding protein transcobalamin (TC, also called transcobalamin II), which delivers B_{12} to the bone marrow and other tissues. Although TC is the essential plasma protein for transferring B_{12} into the cells of the body, the amount of B_{12} on TC is normally very low (<50 ng/L).

Congenital TC deficiency due to germline mutations in the *TCN2* gene causes megaloblastic anaemia because of failure of B_{12} to enter marrow (and other cells) from plasma, but the serum B_{12} level in TC deficiency is normal. This is because most B_{12} in plasma is bound to haptocorrin. In addition to haptocorrin synthesis in saliva, gastric juice and milk, this glycoprotein is synthesized by granulocytes and macrophages. In myeloproliferative neoplasms where granulocyte production may be greatly increased, the haptocorrin and B_{12} levels in serum both rise considerably. This also occurs in some liver diseases. B_{12} bound to haptocorrin in the blood does not transfer to marrow; it appears to be functionally 'dead'.

Biochemical function

Vitamin B_{12} is a coenzyme for two biochemical reactions. First, as methyl B_{12} it is a cofactor for methionine synthase, the enzyme responsible for methylation of homocysteine to methionine using methyltetrahydrofolate (methylTHF) as methyl donor (Fig. 5.3). Second, as deoxyadenosyl B_{12} (ado B_{12}) it assists in conversion of methylmalonyl coenzyme A (CoA) to succinyl CoA, a key intermediate in the citric acid cycle (Fig. 5.3).

Folate

Folic (pteroylglutamic) acid is the parent compound of a large group of compounds, the folates, that are derived from it (Fig. 5.4).

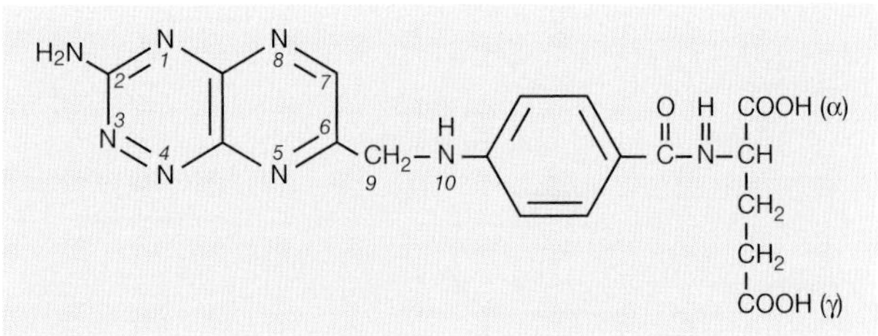

Figure 5.4 The structure of folic (pteroylglutamic) acid. Dietary folates may contain (i) additional hydrogen atoms at positions 7 and 8 (dihydrofolate) or 5, 6, 7 and 8 (tetrahydrofolate); (ii) a formyl group at N_5 or N_{10}, a methyl group at N_5 or other 1-carbon groups; and (iii) additional glutamate moiety attached to the γ-carboxyl group of the glutamate moiety.

Absorption, transport and function

Dietary folates are a complex mixture of variously reduced and polyglutamated folates. They are all converted to one compound, methylTHF, a reduced monoglutamate form which circulates in plasma (Fig. 5.5a). After entering cells, this is converted, after de-methylation to THF, to folate polyglutamate forms by addition of usually four, five or six glutamate moieties (Fig. 5.6). Folic (pteroylglutamic) acid itself is a poor substrate for reduction by dihydrofolate reductase and, while converted to methylTHF at doses of 200–400 μg, larger doses of folic acid enter portal plasma unchanged and are then reduced in the liver or excreted in the urine (Fig 5.5b).

Folates are needed in a variety of biochemical reactions in the body involving single carbon unit transfer, in amino acid interconversions (e.g. homocysteine conversion to methionine; Figs 5.3, 5.6) and serine to glycine, or in synthesis of purine precursors of DNA.

Biochemical basis for megaloblastic anaemia (Fig. 5.6)

DNA is formed by polymerization of the four deoxyribonucleoside monophosphates derived from their triphosphates. Folate deficiency is thought to cause megaloblastic anaemia by limiting synthesis of thymidine monophosphate (dTMP), a rate-limiting step in DNA synthesis. This reaction needs 5,10-methylene THF polyglutamate as coenzyme. Consequent starvation of the precursor dTTP leads to prolongation of the S phase during mitosis, failure to form new double-stranded DNA and apoptotic cell death.

The role of B_{12} in DNA synthesis is indirect. B_{12} is needed in the conversion of methylTHF, which enters marrow and other cells from plasma, to THF. In this reaction, homocysteine is converted to methionine. THF (but not methylTHF) is the substrate for folate polyglutamate synthesis. The folate polyglutamates are the intracellular folate coenzymes. B_{12} deficiency therefore indirectly reduces the supply of the critical

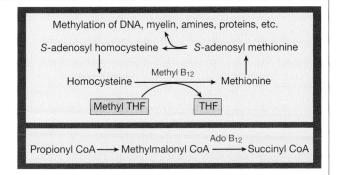

Figure 5.3 The biochemical reactions of vitamin B_{12} in humans. Ado B_{12}, deoxyadenosylcobalamin; CoA, coenzyme A; THF, tetrahydrofolate.

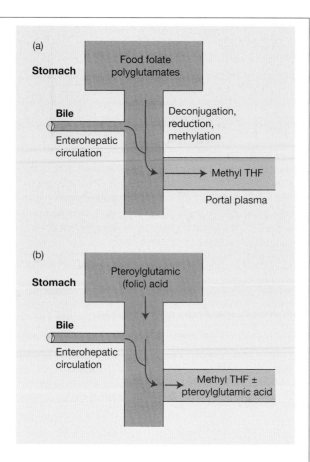

Figure 5.5 **(a)** The absorption of dietary folates; **(b)** The absorption of pteroylglutamic acid. At doses up to 400 μg, most pteroylglutamic (folic) acid is converted to methyltetrahydrofolate (methylTHF). At higher doses, unchanged pteroylglutamic acid enters portal plasma.

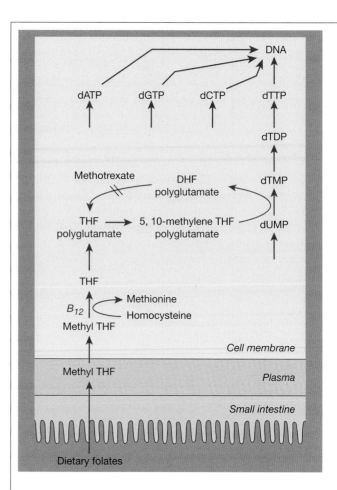

Figure 5.6 The biochemical basis of megaloblastic anaemia caused by vitamin B$_{12}$ or folate deficiency. Folate is required in one of its coenzyme forms, 5,10-methylene tetrahydrofolate (methylTHF) polyglutamate, in the synthesis of thymidine monophosphate from its precursor deoxyuridine monophosphate. Vitamin B$_{12}$ is needed to convert methylTHF, which enters the cells from plasma, to THF, from which polyglutamate forms of folate are synthesized. Dietary folates are all converted to methylTHF (a monoglutamate) by the small intestine. A, adenine; C, cytosine; d, deoxyribose; DHF, dihydrofolate; DP, diphosphate; G, guanine; MP, monophosphate; T, thymine; TP, triphosphate; U, uracil.

folate coenzyme 5,10-methylene THF polyglutamate, needed for synthesis of thymidine monophosphate (dTMP) (Fig. 5.6). Other congenital or acquired causes of megaloblastic anaemia (e.g. antimetabolite drug therapy) inhibit purine or pyrimidine synthesis at one or another step. The result is a reduced supply of one or other of the four precursors needed for DNA synthesis.

Folate reduction

During the synthesis of dTMP, the folate polyglutamate coenzyme becomes oxidized from the THF to the dihydrofolate (DHF) state (Fig. 5.6). Regeneration of active THF coenzymes requires the enzyme DHF reductase. As already mentioned, the enzyme reduces dietary folate during their absorption. Inhibitors of this enzyme (e.g. methotrexate) inhibit folate biochemical reactions, and so DNA synthesis (Fig. 5.6). Methotrexate is a useful drug, mainly in the treatment of malignant (e.g. acute

lymphoblastic leukaemia; see p. 215) or inflammatory disease (e.g. rheumatoid arthritis, psoriasis) with excessive cell turnover. The weaker antagonist, pyrimethamine, is used primarily against malaria. Trimethoprim, active against bacterial DHF reductase but only very weakly against the human enzyme, is used alone or in combination with a sulphonamide, as cotrimoxazole, an antibiotic. Toxicity caused by methotrexate or pyrimethamine may be reversed by giving the reduced folate, folinic acid (5-formyl THF). In the protocols used, this reversal does not eliminate the effectiveness of methotrexate when used in anti-cancer chemotherapy.

Causes of severe vitamin B$_{12}$ deficiency

In developed countries, severe deficiency is usually caused by (Addisonian, autoantibody-mediated) pernicious anaemia (Table 5.3). Less commonly, severe deficiency may be caused by lack of B$_{12}$ in the diet (as in veganism without dietary supplementation), gastrectomy or small intestinal lesions. In vegetarians and people subsisting on a poor-quality diet low in B$_{12}$-rich foods, an intact entero-hepatic circulation usually but not invariably helps to protect them from severe B$_{12}$ deficiency, although they often develop mild B$_{12}$ deficiency. The deficiency takes at least 2 years to develop (i.e. the time needed for body stores to deplete at the rate of 1–2 µg/day) when there is severe malabsorption of B$_{12}$ from the diet. There is no syndrome of B$_{12}$ deficiency as a result of increased utilization or loss of the vitamin. Nitrous oxide, however, may rapidly inactivate body B$_{12}$ (see p. 52).

Causes of mild vitamin B$_{12}$ deficiency

The most frequent cause worldwide of mild B$_{12}$ deficiency is an inadequate diet. Other causes of mild B$_{12}$ deficiency are malabsorption of B$_{12}$ due to atrophic gastritis (particularly in the elderly), therapy with proton pump inhibitors, chronic pancreatitis, gluten-induced enteropathy, HIV infection, and prolonged treatment with metformin or cholestyramine. In the Zollinger–Ellison syndrome, the pH in the duodenum falls so low that pancreatic enzymes that normally release B$_{12}$ from haptocorrin are inactivated. These malabsorption conditions do not usually lead to B$_{12}$ deficiency sufficient to cause anaemia or neuropathy. In pregnancy, serum B$_{12}$ levels fall in some women to below the normal range, but spontaneously return to normal after delivery (see Chapter 31).

Pernicious anaemia

Pernicious anaemia (PA) is caused by autoimmune attack on the gastric mucosa, leading to atrophy of the stomach.

Table 5.3 Causes of severe vitamin B$_{12}$ deficiency.

Nutritional
Especially strict vegans

Malabsorption
Gastric causes
Pernicious anaemia
Congenital lack or abnormality of intrinsic factor
Total or partial gastrectomy

Intestinal causes
Intestinal stagnant loop syndrome – jejunal diverticulosis, blind-loop, stricture, etc.
Chronic tropical sprue
Ileal resection and Crohn's disease
Congenital selective malabsorption with proteinuria (autosomal recessive megaloblastic anaemia)
Fish tapeworm

Table 5.4 Pernicious anaemia: associations.

Female	Vitiligo
Blue eyes	Myxoedema
Early greying	Hashimoto's disease
Northern European	Thyrotoxicosis
Familial	Addison's disease
Blood group A	Hypoparathyroidism
Type I diabetes
Hypogammaglobulinaemia
Carcinoma of the stomach

The wall of the stomach becomes thin, with a plasma cell and lymphoid infiltrate of the lamina propria. Intestinal metaplasia may occur. Destruction of parietal cells results in achlorhydria and secretion of IF is absent or almost absent. Serum gastrin levels are raised. *Helicobater pylori* infection may initiate an autoimmune gastritis, which presents in younger subjects as iron deficiency and in the elderly as PA.

More females than males are affected (1.6 : 1), with a peak occurrence at 60 years, and there may be associated autoimmune disease, particularly thyroid diseases (Table 5.4). The disease is found in all races, but is most common in Northern Europeans and tends to occur in families. There is also an increased incidence of carcinoma of the stomach (approximately 2–3% of all cases of pernicious anaemia).

Antibodies

Ninety per cent of patients with PA show parietal cell antibody in the serum directed against the gastric proton pump H$^+$/K$^+$-ATPase. The antibody, however, is not specific for PA. PA is distinguished from simple atrophic or autoimmune gastritis by the presence of antibodies to IF. **Fifty to seventy per cent of PA patients show in serum an antibody to IF which inhibits IF binding to B$_{12}$.** An antibody blocking IF attachment to its ileal binding site is less frequent. IF antibodies also occur in PA in gastric juice, where they block any remaining IF binding B$_{12}$. IF antibodies are specific for PA, but as they occur in the serum of only half of patients, their absence from serum does not exclude the diagnosis. The more common parietal cell antibody is less specific, as it occurs quite commonly in older subjects (e.g. 16% of normal women over 60 years) even without PA.

Other causes of severe vitamin B$_{12}$ deficiency

Congenital lack or abnormality of IF due to mutations of its gene usually presents at approximately 2 years of age, when stores of B$_{12}$ that were derived from the mother *in utero* have been used up. Specific malabsorption of B$_{12}$ is due to genetic mutation of the IF–B$_{12}$ receptor proteins, cubilin or amnionless. It usually presents in infancy or childhood and is associated

Table 5.5 Causes of folate deficiency.

Nutritional
Especially old age, institutions, poverty, famine, special diets, goat's milk anaemia, etc.

Malabsorption
Tropical sprue, gluten-induced enteropathy (adult or child). Possible contributory factor to folate deficiency in some patients with partial gastrectomy, extensive jejunal resection or Crohn's disease

Excess utilization

Physiological
Pregnancy and lactation, prematurity

Pathological
Haematological diseases: haemolytic anaemias, myelofibrosis
Malignant disease: carcinoma, lymphoma, myeloma
Inflammatory diseases: Crohn's disease, tuberculosis, rheumatoid arthritis, psoriasis, exfoliative dermatitis, malaria

Excess urinary folate loss
Active liver disease, congestive heart failure

Drugs
Anticonvulsants, sulfasalazine

Mixed
Liver disease, alcoholism, intensive care

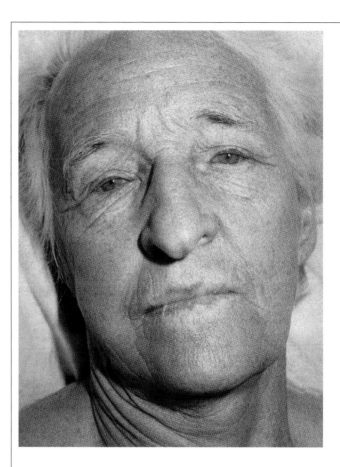

Figure 5.7 Megaloblastic anaemia: pallor and mild icterus in a patient with a haemoglobin count of 70.0 g/L and a mean corpuscular volume of 132 fL.

with proteinuria in 90% of cases. Infants born to and breast fed by B_{12}-deficient mothers may also develop symptomatic B_{12} deficiency

Folate deficiency

This is most often a result of a poor dietary intake of folate alone or in combination with a condition of increased folate utilization or malabsorption (Table 5.5). Excess cell turnover of any sort, including pregnancy, is the main cause of an increased need for folate, because the folate molecule becomes degraded when DNA synthesis, and so thymidine monophosphate synthesis, is increased. The mechanism by which anticonvulsants and barbiturates cause the deficiency is still controversial.

Clinical features of megaloblastic anaemia

The onset is usually insidious, with gradually progressive symptoms and signs of anaemia (see Chapter 2). The patient may be mildly jaundiced (lemon yellow; Fig. 5.7) because of the excess breakdown of haemoglobin resulting from increased ineffective erythropoiesis in the bone marrow. Glossitis (a beefy-red sore tongue; Fig. 5.8), angular cheilosis (Fig. 5.9) and mild symptoms of malabsorption with loss of weight may

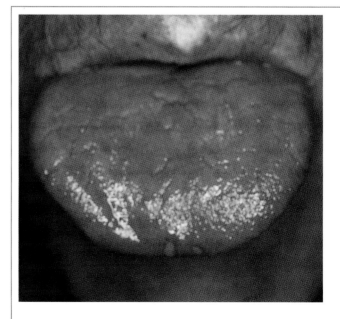

Figure 5.8 Megaloblastic anaemia: glossitis – the tongue is beefy-red and painful.

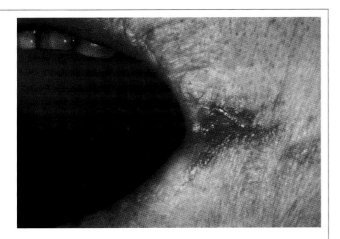

Figure 5.9 Megaloblastic anaemia: angular cheilosis (stomatitis).

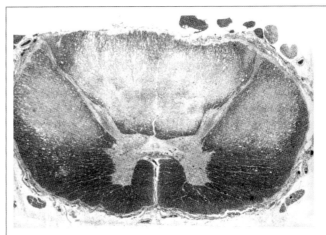

Figure 5.10 Cross-section of the spinal cord in a patient who died with subacute combined degeneration of the cord (Weigert–Pal stain). There is demyelination of the dorsal and dorsolateral columns.

be present because of the epithelial abnormality. Purpura as a result of thrombocytopenia and widespread melanin pigmentation (the cause of which is unclear) are less frequent presenting features (Table 5.6). Many asymptomatic patients are diagnosed when a blood count performed for another reason reveals macrocytosis.

Vitamin B$_{12}$ neuropathy (subacute combined degeneration of the cord)

Severe B$_{12}$ deficiency can cause a progressive neuropathy affecting the peripheral sensory nerves and posterior and lateral columns (Fig. 5.10). The neuropathy is symmetrical and affects the lower more than the upper limbs. The patient notices tingling in the feet, difficulty in walking and may fall over in the dark due to loss of positional sense. Rarely, optic atrophy or severe psychiatric symptoms are present. Anaemia may be severe, mild or even absent, but the blood film and bone marrow appearances are abnormal. The duration and severity of the neurological defects predict the outcome. The peripheral neuropathy is usually reversible with B$_{12}$ therapy, but spinal cord recovery is usually incomplete, especially if

the neuropathy has been present for more than a few weeks or months. Prolonged deficiency in infants impairs motor function, which also may be irreversible.

The cause of the neuropathy is likely to be related to the accumulation of *S*-adenosyl homocysteine and reduced levels of *S*-adenosyl methionine in nervous tissue, resulting in defective methylation of myelin and other substrates.

Neural tube defect

Folate (or B$_{12}$ deficiency) in the mother predisposes to neural tube defect (NTD; anencephaly, spina bifida or encephalocoele) in the fetus (Fig. 5.11). The lower the maternal serum or red cell folate or serum B$_{12}$ levels, the higher the incidence of NTDs. Moreover, supplementation of the diet with folic acid at the time of conception and in early pregnancy reduces the incidence of NTD by up to 75%. The exact mechanism is uncertain, but is thought to be related to the build-up of homocysteine and *S*-adenosyl homocysteine in the fetus, which may impair methylation of various proteins and lipids. A common polymorphism (677C → T) in the enzyme 5,10-methylene tetrahydrofolate reductase (5,10-MTHFR), which reduces 5,10-MTHF to methylTHF, results in higher serum homocysteine and lower serum and red cell folate levels compared with controls. The incidence of the mutation is higher in the parents and fetuses with NTD than in controls.

Other tissue abnormalities

Sterility is frequent in either sex with severe B$_{12}$ or folate deficiency. Macrocytosis, excess apoptosis and other morphological abnormalities of cervical, buccal, bladder and other epithelia occur. Widespread reversible melanin pigmentation may also occur. B$_{12}$ deficiency is associated with reduced osteoblastic activity.

Table 5.6 Effects of vitamin B$_{12}$ or folate deficiency.

Megaloblastic anaemia
Macrocytosis of epithelial cell surfaces
Neuropathy (for B$_{12}$ deficiency only)
Sterility
Rarely, reversible melanin skin pigmentation
Decreased osteoblast activity
Neural tube defects in the fetus are related to folate or B$_{12}$ deficiency

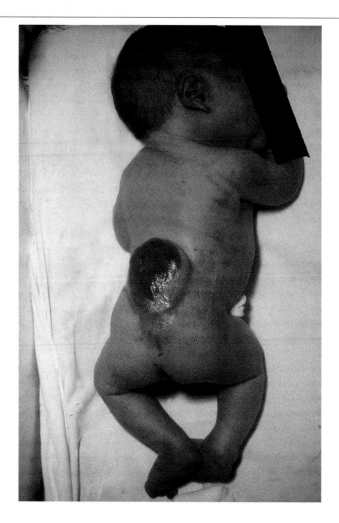

Figure 5.11 A baby with neural tube defect (spina bifida). Source: Courtesy of Professor C.J. Schorah.

Raised serum homocysteine levels and low serum or red cell folate and the polymorphism in the MTHFR enzyme (see above) have been associated with an increased incidence of cardiovascular diseases, including myocardial infarct, peripheral vascular diseases, stroke and venous thrombosis (see p. 342). Folic acid prophylaxis, however, has not reduced the incidence of the arterial diseases or cardiovascular events, except for stroke in hypertensive subjects, where a reduction of 15% has been shown in large-scale controlled studies in China.

Various associations have been found between folate status and malignant diseases, but meta-analysis of subjects randomized in trials to take folic acid or placebo for 2 years or more does not show any difference in cancer incidence between those taking folic acid and the controls.

Laboratory findings

The anaemia is macrocytic (MCV >98 fL by definition and often as high as 120–140 fL in severe cases) and the macrocytes are typically oval (Fig. 5.12). In severe cases megaloblasts

may appear in the peripheral blood due to extramedullary haemopoiesis. If iron deficiency is also present the MCV may be normal, but the red cell distribution width (RDW) in such

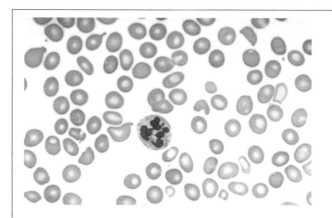

Figure 5.12 Megaloblastic anaemia: peripheral blood film showing oval macrocytes.

cases will be very wide and the blood film dimorphic, with distinct populations of large and small cells.. The reticulocyte count is low and the total white cell and platelet counts may be reduced, especially in severely anaemic patients with pancytopenia. **A proportion of the neutrophils show hypersegmented nuclei (with six or more lobes)**. The bone marrow is usually hypercellular and the erythroblasts are large and show an open, fine, lacy primitive chromatin pattern, but normal cytoplasmic haemoglobinization (Fig. 5.13). Giant and abnormally shaped metamyelocytes are characteristic.

The serum unconjugated bilirubin and lactate dehydrogenase are raised as a result of marrow cell breakdown.

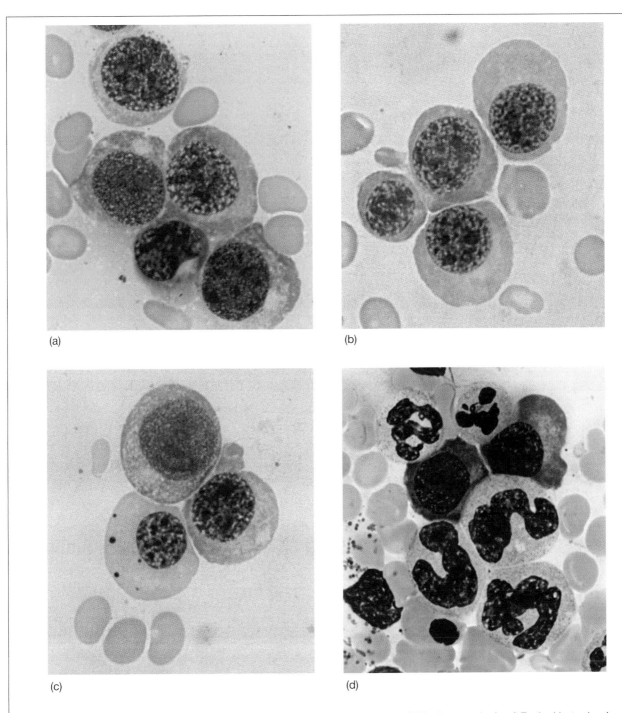

(a)

(b)

(c)

(d)

Figure 5.13 Megaloblastic changes in the bone marrow in a patient with severe megaloblastic anaemia. **(a–c)** Erythroblasts showing fine, open stippled (primitive) appearance of the nuclear chromatin even in late cells (pale cytoplasm with some haemoglobin formation). **(d)** Abnormal giant metamyelocytes and band forms.

Diagnosis of vitamin B_{12} or folate deficiency

It is usual to assay serum B_{12} and folate and in many laboratories also red blood cell folate (Table 5.7). The serum B_{12} is low in megaloblastic anaemia or neuropathy caused by B_{12} deficiency. In B_{12} deficiency, the serum folate tends to rise but the red cell folate falls. In the absence of B_{12} deficiency, however, the red cell folate may be a more accurate guide to tissue folate status than the serum folate. Serum and red cell folate are both low in megaloblastic anaemia caused by folate deficiency. Serum folate in contrast to red cell folate is more labile, and even one or two nutritious meals in a hospitalized patient admitted with severe deficiency may normalize serum folate. However, red cell folate will remain low for some time.

Measurement of serum or urine methylmalonic acid is a test for B_{12} deficiency and measurement of homocysteine is a test for folate or B_{12} deficiency. These are not specific, however, and it is difficult to establish normal levels in different age groups. These tests are also not widely available.

Tests for cause of vitamin B_{12} or folate deficiency

Useful tests are listed in Table 5.8. These are mainly concerned with assessing gastric function and testing for antibodies to gastric antigens. In all cases of pernicious anaemia, endoscopy studies should be performed at diagnosis to confirm the presence of gastric atrophy and exclude carcinoma of the stomach.

For folate deficiency, the dietary history is most important, although it is difficult to estimate folate intake accurately. Unsuspected gluten-induced enteropathy or other underlying conditions should also be considered (Table 5.5).

Treatment

Most cases only need therapy with the appropriate vitamin (Table 5.9). If large doses of folic acid (e.g. 5 mg/day) are given in B_{12} deficiency they cause a haematological response, but will allow a neuropathy to appear or progress. Folic acid should therefore not be given alone unless B_{12} deficiency has been excluded. In severely anaemic patients who need treatment urgently, it may be safer to initiate treatment with

Table 5.8 Tests for cause of vitamin B_{12} or folate deficiency.

Vitamin B_{12}	Folate
Diet history	Diet history
Serum gastrin	Tests for intestinal malabsorption
IF, parietal cell antibodies	Anti-transglutaminase and endomysial antibodies
Endoscopy	Duodenal biopsy Underlying disease

IF, intrinsic factor.

both vitamins after blood has been taken for B_{12} and folate assay. Patients with megaloblastic anaemia or neuropathy due to B_{12} deficiency should be treated initially with injections of B_{12}.

Either parenteral or oral B_{12} therapy may be used for subsequent life-long maintenance. Large oral doses are needed daily, however, to achieve sufficient B_{12} absorption in PA and compliance with long-term therapy may be a problem. Oral therapy is more appropriate for those with mild degrees of B_{12} deficiency, e.g. with malabsorption of food B_{12}. For folate deficiency, an oral dose of 5 mg daily is indicated, with parenteral therapy reserved for those receiving parenteral nutrition. It is usual to continue for 4 months and then to decide whether or not to continue this long term (Table 5.9). In the elderly, the presence of heart failure should be corrected with diuretics. Blood transfusion should be avoided if possible, as it may cause circulatory overload.

Response to therapy

The patient usually begins to feel better after 24–48 hours of correct vitamin therapy, with increased appetite and well-being. The haemoglobin should rise by 20–30 g/L each fortnight. The white cell and platelet counts become normal in 7–10 days (Fig. 5.14) and the marrow is normoblastic in about 48 hours, although giant metamyelocytes persist for up to 12 days.

Table 5.7 Laboratory tests for vitamin B_{12} and folate deficiency.

Test	Normal values*		Result in	
			Vitamin B_{12} deficiency	Folate deficiency
Serum vitamin B_{12}	160–925 ng/L	120–680 pmol/L	Low	Normal or borderline low
Serum folate	3.0–15.0 µg/L	4–30 nmol/L	Normal or raised	Low
Red cell folate	160–640 µg/L	360–1460 nmol/L	Normal or low	Low

*Normal values differ with different commercial kits.

Table 5.9 Treatment of megaloblastic anaemia.

	Vitamin B$_{12}$ deficiency	Folate deficiency
Compound	Hydroxocobalamin*	Folic acid
Route	Intramuscular**	Oral
Dose	1000 µg	5 mg
Initial dose	6 × 1000 µg over 2–3 weeks	Daily for 4 months
Maintenance	1000 µg every 3 months*; usually life-long or daily large (500–1000 µg) oral doses of B$_{12}$	Depends on underlying disease; life-long therapy may be needed in chronic inherited haemolytic anaemias, myelofibrosis, renal dialysis
Prophylactic	Total gastrectomy Ileal resection Daily oral B$_{12}$ for vegans and in developing countries during pregnancy and lactation	Pregnancy, severe haemolytic anaemias, dialysis, prematurity In over 80 countries the diet (grain or flour) is fortified with folic acid to reduce the incidence of NTD

*In the USA cyanocobalamin is commonly used and maintenance B$_{12}$ injections are given monthly.
**Some authors recommend daily oral or sublingual therapy of vitamin B$_{12}$ deficiency (see text).

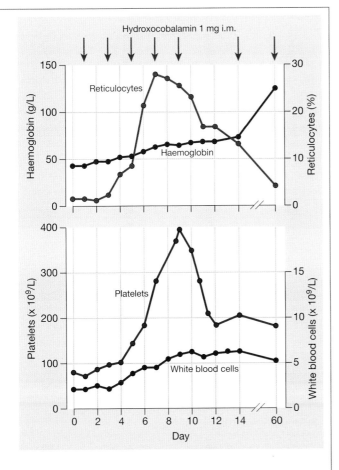

Figure 5.14 Typical haematological response to vitamin B$_{12}$ (hydroxocobalamin) therapy in pernicious anaemia.

Prophylactic therapy

Vitamin B$_{12}$ is given 3-monthly to patients who are total vegetarians or have ileal resection. Oral supplements and consumption of dairy products or of foods fortified with B$_{12}$ are recommended for vegetarians and those living because of poverty on a diet low in B$_{12}$-rich foods. In developing countries oral B$_{12}$ supplements are recommended for all pregnant and lactating women.

Folic acid is given in pregnancy at a typical dosage of 400 µg/day and all women of child-bearing age are recommended to have an intake of at least 400 µg/day (by increased intake of folate-rich or folate-supplemented foods or as folic acid) to prevent a first occurrence of an NTD fetus.

Food fortification with folic acid (e.g. in flour or grain) is practised in over 80 countries (including North America since 1998) to reduce the incidence of NTD. Folic acid supplementation of foods has not been approved in Europe.

Folic acid is also given to patients undergoing chronic dialysis, with severe chronic haemolytic anaemias, e.g. sickle cell anaemia, and to premature babies.

Other megaloblastic anaemias

The most frequent (see Table 5.1) causes are drugs inhibiting DNA synthesis, e.g. hyroxycarbamide (hydroxyurea) or cytosine arabinoside, or drugs inhibiting dihydrofolate reductase, e.g. methotrexate of pyrimethamine. Myelodysplastic syndromes are also a relatively frequent cause in the elderly. Congenital deficiencies involved in DNA synthesis, e.g. orotic aciduria, are extremely rare.

Abnormalities of vitamin B$_{12}$ or folate metabolism

These include rare congenital deficiencies of enzymes concerned in B$_{12}$ or folate intracellular trafficking or metabolism, or of the serum transport protein for B$_{12}$, TC. Nitrous oxide (N$_2$O) anaesthesia causes rapid inactivation of body B$_{12}$ by oxidizing the reduced cobalt atom of methyl B$_{12}$. Megaloblastic marrow changes occur with several days of N$_2$O administration and can cause pancytopenia. Chronic exposure (as in dentists and anaesthetists) has been associated with neurological damage resembling B$_{12}$ deficiency neuropathy. Antifolate drugs, particularly those which inhibit DHF reductase (e.g. methotrexate and pyrimethamine), may also cause megaloblastic change.

Other macrocytic anaemias

There are many non-megaloblastic causes of macrocytic anaemia (Table 5.10). The exact mechanism creating large red cells in each of these conditions is not clear, although increased lipid deposition on the red cell membrane or alterations of erythroblast maturation time in the marrow may be implicated. Alcohol is the most frequent cause of a raised MCV in the absence of anaemia. Reticulocytes are bigger than mature red cells, so haemolytic anaemia is an important cause of macrocytic anaemia. Antimetabolite drugs such as hydroxycarbamide (see Table 12.1) cause macrocytosis and the marrow may show megaloblastic changes. The other underlying conditions listed in Table 5.10 are usually easily diagnosed provided that they are considered and the appropriate investigations to exclude B$_{12}$ or folate deficiency are carried out.

Differential diagnosis of macrocytic anaemias

The clinical history and physical examination may suggest B$_{12}$ or folate deficiency as the cause. Diet, drugs, alcohol intake, family history, history suggestive of malabsorption, presence of autoimmune diseases or other associations with pernicious

Table 5.10 Causes of macrocytosis other than megaloblastic anaemia.

Alcohol
Liver disease
Myxoedema
Myelodysplastic syndromes
Antimetabolite drugs, e.g. hydroxycarbamide
Aplastic anaemia
Pregnancy
Smoking
Reticulocytosis
Myeloma and paraproteinaemia
RBC agglutination (artifactual)

anaemia (Table 5.4), previous gastrointestinal disease or operations are all important. The presence of jaundice, glossitis or symmetrical neuropathy is also an important indication of megaloblastic anaemia.

The laboratory features of particular importance are the shape of macrocytes (oval in megaloblastic anaemia), the presence of hypersegmented neutrophils, leucopenia and thrombocytopenia in megaloblastic anaemia, and the bone marrow appearance. Assay of serum B$_{12}$ and folate is essential. Exclusion of alcoholism (particularly if the patient is not anaemic), liver and thyroid function tests, and bone marrow examination for myelodysplasia, aplasia or myeloma are important in the investigation of macrocytosis not caused by B$_{12}$ or folate deficiency.

SUMMARY

- Macrocytic anaemias show an increased size of circulating red cells (MCV >98 fL). The bone marrow (erythropoiesis) may be megaloblastic or normoblastic. B$_{12}$ or folate deficiency causes megaloblastic anaemia, in which the bone marrow erythroblasts have a typical abnormal appearance with delayed maturation of the nucleus compared to the degree of cytoplasmic haemoglobinization.
- Folates take part in biochemical reactions in DNA synthesis. B$_{12}$ has an indirect role in DNA synthesis by its involvement in folate metabolism.
- B$_{12}$ deficiency may also cause a neuropathy due to damage to the spinal cord and peripheral nerves.

- Severe B$_{12}$ deficiency is usually caused by B$_{12}$ malabsorption due to pernicious anaemia in which there is autoimmune gastritis, resulting in failure of synthesis of intrinsic factor, a glycoprotein made in the stomach which facilitates B$_{12}$ absorption by the ileum.
- Other gastrointestinal diseases as well as a vegan diet may cause B$_{12}$ deficiency.
- Folate deficiency may be caused by a poor diet, malabsorption (e.g. gluten-induced enteropathy) or excess cell turnover (e.g. pregnancy, haemolytic anaemias, malignancy).
- Treatment of B$_{12}$ deficiency is usually with injections of hydroxocobalamin and that of folate deficiency is with oral folic (pteroylglutamic) acid.

- Rare causes of megaloblastic anaemia include inborn errors of B_{12} or folate transport or metabolism, and defects of DNA synthesis not related to B_{12} or folate.
- Causes of macrocytic red cells with or without anaemia and usually with normoblastic erythropoiesis include alcohol, liver disease, hypothyroidism, myelodysplasia, paraproteinaemia, cytotoxic drugs, aplastic anaemia, pregnancy and the neonatal period. In the non-anaemic patient, alcohol is the most frequent cause.

 Now visit **www.wileyessential.com/haematology** to test yourself on this chapter.

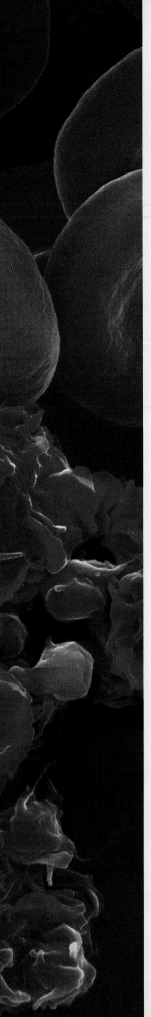

CHAPTER 6
Haemolytic anaemias

Key topics

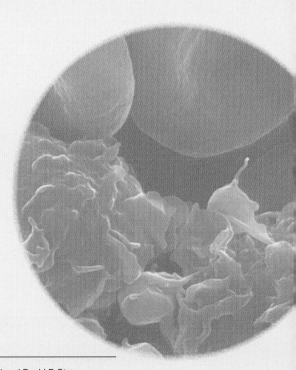

Hoffbrand's Essential Haematology, Eighth Edition. By A. Victor Hoffbrand and David P. Steensma.
© 2020 John Wiley & Sons Ltd. Published 2020 by John Wiley & Sons Ltd.
Companion website: www.wileyessential.com/haematology

Normal red cell destruction

Normal (physiological) red cell destruction occurs after a mean lifespan of 120 days, when aged cells are removed extravascularly by the macrophages of the reticuloendothelial (RE) system, especially in the marrow but also in the liver and spleen. As red cells have no nucleus and therefore cannot synthesize new RNA and proteins, cell metabolism gradually deteriorates as enzymes are degraded, and the cells also become stiffer and less deformable in the microcirculation as structural proteins are degraded. Eventually senescent red cells become non-viable.

The breakdown of haem from haemoglobin liberates iron from macrophages for recirculation via plasma transferrin, which is mainly used by marrow erythroblasts. Protoporphyrin, the organic ring into which ferrous iron is embedded to form haem, is broken down in the macrophages to biliverdin and then to bilirubin. Bilirubin, which is lipid soluble, circulates to the liver, where it is conjugated to glucuronides to make it water soluble and facilitate excretion. Conjugated bilirubin is excreted into the gut via bile and converted to stercobilinogen and stercobilin, which are brown in colour and excreted in faeces (Fig. 6.1). Stercobilinogen and stercobilin are partly reabsorbed after reduction by bacterial action in the intestines to urobilinogen and urobilin (also known as urochrome and responsible for the yellow colour of urine) and are then excreted in urine. Globin chains are broken down to individual amino acids, which are reutilized for general protein synthesis in the body.

Haptoglobins are proteins in normal plasma which bind haemoglobin if either intravascular or significant extravascular haemolysis is present. The haemoglobin–haptoglobin complex is removed by the RE system. Intravascular haemolysis (i.e. the breakdown of red cells within blood vessels) plays little or no part in normal red cell destruction, but is important in some pathological states, discussed later.

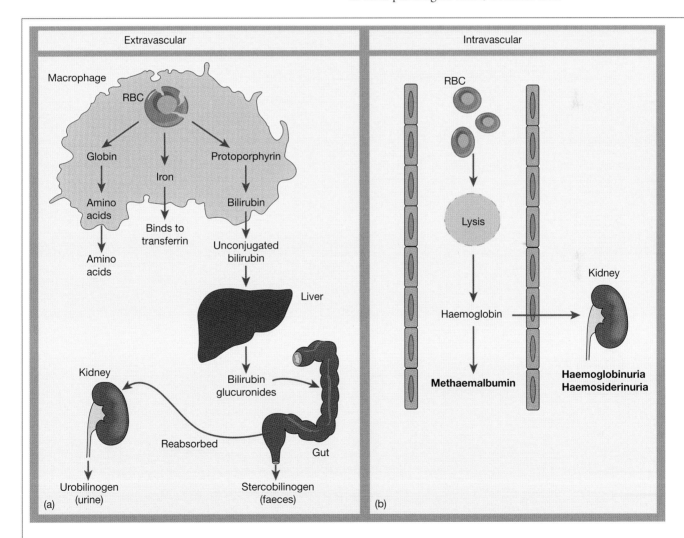

Figure 6.1 **(a)** Normal red blood cell (RBC) breakdown. This takes place extravascularly in the macrophages of the reticuloendothelial system. **(b)** Intravascular haemolysis within the blood vessel occurs in some pathological disorders, and is associated with haemoglobinaemia, haemoglobinuria and haemosiderinuria.

Introduction to haemolytic anaemias

Haemolytic anaemias are defined as anaemias that result from an increase in the rate of red cell destruction. Because of erythropoietic hyperplasia and anatomical extension of bone marrow, red cell destruction may increase several-fold before the patient becomes anaemic – this is called compensated haemolytic disease. The normal adult marrow, after full expansion, is able to produce red cells at 6–8 times the normal rate. This expanded production leads to a marked reticulocytosis. Therefore, anaemia due to haemolysis may not be seen until the red cell lifespan drops to less than 30 days.

Classification

Table 6.1 is a simplified classification of the haemolytic anaemias. **Hereditary haemolytic anaemias are typically the result of 'intrinsic' red cell defects, whereas acquired haemolytic anaemias are usually the result of an 'extracorpuscular' or 'environmental' change**. Paroxysmal nocturnal haemoglobinuria (PNH) is an exception because, although it is an acquired disorder, the PNH red cells have an intrinsic defect. PNH is associated with marrow hypoplasia and is therefore discussed in Chapter 22. Clonal disorders such as myelodysplastic syndromes may also be associated with acquired intrinsic red cell defects.

Clinical features

The patient may show pallor of the mucous membranes, mild fluctuating jaundice and splenomegaly. There is no bilirubin in urine, but the urine may turn dark on standing because of excess urobilinogen, which is colourless but oxidizes in light to highly coloured urobilin. Pigment (bilirubin) gallstones may complicate the condition (Fig. 6.2).

Some patients with haemolysis develop disease-specific complications. For instance, patients with sickle cell disease, hereditary spherocytosis, or rarely other haemolytic anaemias may develop ulcers around the ankle (see Fig. 7.19), while those with thalassaemia major who do not receive regular transfusions develop bone deformities (Figs 7.9, 7.10). Patients with cold-reactive autoantibodies may exhibit discoloration in peripheral (acral) regions of the body such as the earlobes or fingertips, and patients with PNH may develop thrombosis.

Aplastic crises may occur, usually precipitated by infection with parvovirus, which 'switches off' erythropoiesis. These crises are characterized by a sudden increase in anaemia and drop in reticulocyte count (see Fig. 22.7). Rarely, folate deficiency may cause an aplastic crisis in which the bone marrow becomes megaloblastic.

Laboratory findings

The laboratory findings are conveniently divided into three groups.

1 **Features of increased red cell breakdown:**
   (a) serum bilirubin raised, unconjugated and bound to albumin;
   (b) urine urobilinogen increased;
   (c) serum haptoglobins absent because the haptoglobins become saturated with haemoglobin and the complex is removed by RE cells.

Table 6.1 Classification of haemolytic anaemias.

Hereditary	Acquired
Membrane defects Hereditary spherocytosis, hereditary elliptocytosis *Metabolic disorders* G6PD deficiency, pyruvate kinase deficiency	*Autoimmune* Warm antibody type (see Table 6.5) Cold antibody type
Haemoglobinopathies and thalassaemias Hb SS, Hb SC, Hb CC, unstable haemoglobins, thalassaemia major and others; see Chapter 7	*Alloimmune* Haemolytic transfusion reactions (acute or delayed) Haemolytic disease of the newborn Allografts, especially in marrow transplantation Drug-associated *Red cell fragmentation syndromes* (see Table 6.6) Microangiopathy, e.g. disseminated intravascular coagulation March haemoglobinuria *Infections:* malaria, clostridia, tick-borne illnesses such as babesiosis *Chemical or physical agents:* especially drugs, industrial/domestic substances (e.g. naphthalene in moth balls), severe burns *Secondary:* severe liver and renal disease *Paroxysmal nocturnal haemoglobinuria* (see Chapter 22)

G6PD, glucose-6-phosphate dehydrogenase; Hb, haemoglobin.

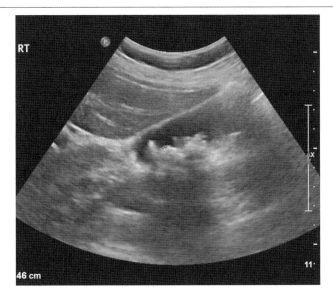

Figure 6.2 Ultrasound of multiple small pigment gallstones typical of those associated with hereditary spherocytosis. Source: Courtesy of Dr P. Wylie.

2 Features of increased red cell production:
 (a) reticulocytosis;
 (b) bone marrow erythroid hyperplasia – the normal marrow myeloid : erythroid ratio of 2 : 1 to 12 : 1 is reduced to 1 : 1 or reversed.

3 Damaged red cells, visualized by:
 (a) routine blood film morphology (e.g. microspherocytes, elliptocytes, fragments);
 (b) flow cytometry after eosin-maleimide (EMA) staining;
 (c) specific enzyme, protein or DNA tests.

Intravascular and extravascular haemolysis

There are two mechanisms whereby red cells are destroyed in haemolytic anaemia. There may be excessive removal of red cells by cells of the RE system (**extravascular haemolysis**) or they may be broken down directly in the circulation (**intravascular haemolysis**) (Fig. 6.1; Table 6.2). Whichever mechanism dominates will depend on the pathology involved.

In intravascular haemolysis, free haemoglobin is released which rapidly saturates plasma haptoglobins and the excess free haemoglobin is filtered by the glomerulus. If the rate of haemolysis saturates the renal tubular reabsorptive capacity, free haemoglobin enters urine (Fig. 6.3). Iron released from haemoglobin in the renal tubules is seen as haemosiderin in

Table 6.2 Causes of intravascular haemolysis.
Mismatched blood transfusion (usually ABO)
G6PD deficiency with oxidant stress
Red cell fragmentation syndromes
Some severe autoimmune haemolytic anaemias
Some drug- and infection-induced haemolytic anaemias
Paroxysmal nocturnal haemoglobinuria
March haemoglobinuria
Unstable haemoglobin

G6PD, glucose-6-phosphate dehydrogenase

a urinary deposit. Methaemalbumin is also formed from the process of intravascular haemolysis.

The main laboratory features of intravascular haemolysis therefore are (Fig. 6.3):

1 Haemoglobinaemia and haemoglobinuria.
2 Haemosiderinuria.
3 Methaemalbuminaemia (detected spectrophotometrically).

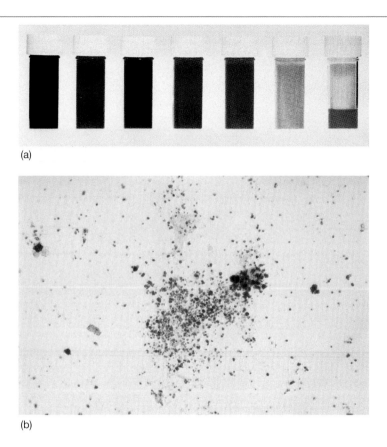

(a)

(b)

Figure 6.3 (a) Progressive urine samples in an acute episode of intravascular haemolysis showing haemoglobinuria of decreasing severity. **(b)** Prussian blue-positive deposits of haemosiderin in a urine spun deposit (Perls' stain).

Hereditary haemolytic anaemias

Membrane defects

Hereditary spherocytosis

Hereditary spherocytosis (HS) is the most common hereditary haemolytic anaemia in Northern Europeans.

Pathogenesis

HS is usually caused by defects in the proteins involved in the vertical interactions between the membrane skeleton and the lipid bilayer of the red cell (Table 6.3; see Fig. 2.12). The marrow produces red cells of normal biconcave shape, but these lose membrane and become increasingly spherical (loss of surface area relative to volume) as they circulate through the spleen and the rest of the RE system. The loss of membrane may be caused by the release of parts of the lipid bilayer that are not supported by the skeleton. Ultimately, the spherocytes are unable to pass through the microcirculation, especially in the spleen, and die prematurely.

Clinical features

The inheritance is usually autosomal dominant with variable expression; rarely, it may be autosomal recessive. In about 25% of cases the mutation is new (spontaneous) and there is no family history. The anaemia can present at any age from infancy to old age. Jaundice is typically fluctuating and is particularly marked if the haemolytic anaemia is associated with Gilbert's disease (a defect of hepatic conjugation of bilirubin);

Table 6.3 Molecular basis of hereditary spherocytosis and elliptocytosis.

Hereditary spherocytosis

- Ankyrin deficiency or abnormalities (most common cause – about 50% of patients)
- α- or β-spectrin deficiency or abnormalities
- Band 3 abnormalities
- Pallidin (protein 4.2) abnormalities

Hereditary elliptocytosis

- α- or β-spectrin mutants leading to defective spectrin dimer formation
- α- or β-spectrin mutants leading to defective spectrin–ankyrin associations
- Protein 4.1 deficiency or abnormality
- South-East Asian ovalocytosis band 3 deletion

splenomegaly occurs in most patients. Pigment gallstones are frequent (Fig. 6.2); aplastic crises, usually precipitated by parvovirus infection, may cause a sudden increase in the severity of anaemia (see Fig. 22.7).

Haematological findings

Anaemia is usual but not invariable; its severity tends to be similar in members of the same family. Reticulocytes are usually 5–20%. The blood film shows microspherocytes (Fig. 6.4a), which are densely staining with smaller diameters than normal red cells.

Investigation and treatment

A rapid flow cytometric analysis of EMA bound to erythrocytes is used as a test for HS and membrane protein deficiency (Fig. 6.5). Identification of the exact molecular defect is not needed for management, but electrophoresis of membrane proteins is carried out in difficult cases. EMA is a dye that binds specifically to band 3 of the red blood cell cytoskeleton and measures the content of erythrocyte structural proteins, which is altered in HS. The EMA test has replaced the osmotic fragility test, which showed the red cells to be excessively fragile compared to normal red cells in dilute saline solutions. The

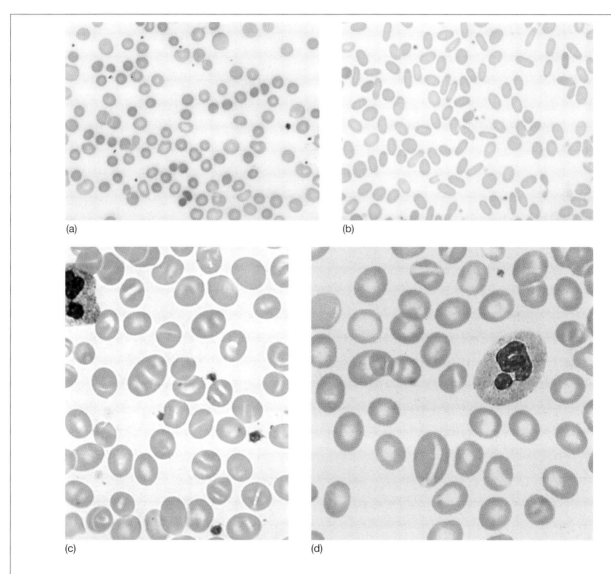

(a)

(b)

(c)

(d)

Figure 6.4 **(a)** Blood film in hereditary spherocytosis. The spherocytes are deeply staining and of small diameter. Larger polychromatic cells are reticulocytes (confirmed by supravital staining). **(b)** Blood film in hereditary elliptocytosis. **(c)** Hereditary stomatocytosis: peripheral blood film showing many cells with the characteristic loosely folded appearance of the membrane. **(d)** Southeast Asian ovalocytosis.
Source: A.V. Hoffbrand *et al.* (2019) *Color Atlas of Clinical Hematology: Molecular and Cellular Basis of Disease,* 5th edn. Reproduced with permission of John Wiley & Sons.

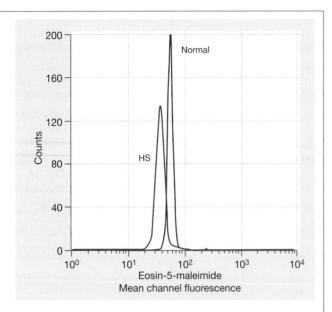

Figure 6.5 Eosin-5-maleimide staining in hereditary spherocytosis (HS) showing reduced mean channel fluorescence due to membrane band 3 protein deficiency. Source: Courtesy of Mr G. Ellis.

direct antiglobulin (Coombs') test is normal in HS, excluding an autoimmune cause of spherocytosis and haemolysis.

The principal form of treatment is splenectomy, preferably laparoscopic, although this should not be performed unless clinically indicated by symptomatic anaemia or gallstones, leg ulcers or growth retardation, because of the risk of post-splenectomy sepsis, particularly in early childhood (see p. 131). Cholecystectomy should be performed with splenectomy if symptomatic gallstones are present. Unless there is additional pathology, splenectomy in HS should always produce a rise in the haemoglobin level to normal, even though microspherocytes formed in the rest of the RE system will remain. Folic acid is given in severe cases to prevent folate deficiency.

Hereditary elliptocytosis

Hereditary elliptocytosis (HE) has similar clinical and laboratory features to HS, except for the appearance of the blood film (Fig. 6.4b), but HE is usually a clinically milder disorder. HE is predominantly discovered by chance on a blood film and there may be no evidence of haemolysis. Occasional patients require splenectomy. The basic defect is a failure of spectrin heterodimers. A number of genetic mutations affecting horizontal interactions of red cell skeletal proteins have been detected (Table 6.3).

Patients with homozygous or doubly heterozygous elliptocytosis present with a severe haemolytic anaemia termed hereditary pyropoikilocytosis; this is most common in patients of African descent. In severe cases, splenectomy can be performed and results in clinical improvement. Folic acid supplementation is also appropriate.

Hereditary stomatocytosis

This is a group of rare red cell membrane defects including xerocytosis and overhydrated stomatocytosis, in which the red cells have mouth-like slits in a stained blood film (Fig 6.4c). The cells leak cations and anaemia is variable. Stomatocytosis may also occur as an artifact if blood films are prepared improperly.

South-East Asian ovalocytosis

This is common in Melanesia, Malaysia, Indonesia and the Philippines and is caused by a 9-amino acid deletion at the junction of the cytoplasmic and transmembrane domains of the band 3 protein. The cells are rigid and resist invasion by malarial parasites. The blood film shows ovalocytes and stomatocytes (Fig 6.4d). Most cases are not anaemic and are asymptomatic. Treatment is rarely required.

Defective red cell metabolism

Glucose-6-phosphate dehydrogenase deficiency

Glucose-6-phosphate dehydrogenase (G6PD) functions to reduce nicotinamide adenine dinucleotide phosphate (NADP) to NADPH. The reaction catalysed by G6PD is the only source of NADPH, which is needed for the production of reduced glutathione; a deficiency renders the red cell susceptible to oxidant stress (Fig. 6.6).

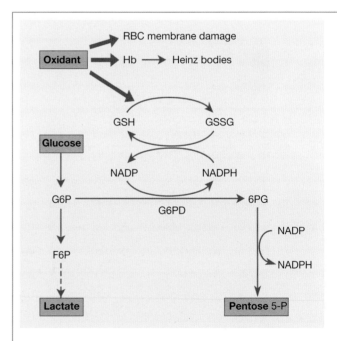

Figure 6.6 Haemoglobin and red blood cell (RBC) membranes are usually protected from oxidant stress by reduced glutathione (GSH). In G6PD deficiency, NADPH and GSH synthesis is impaired. F6P, fructose-6-phosphate; G6P, glucose-6-phosphate; G6PD, glucose-6-phosphate dehydrogenase; 6-PG, 6-phosphogluconate; GSSG, glutathione (oxidized form); NADP, NADPH, nicotinamide adenine dinucleotide phosphate.

Epidemiology

There is a wide variety of normal genetic variants of the enzyme G6PD, the most common isoform being type B (designated G6PD-Mediterranean and most commonly seen in the Middle East) and type A (designated G6PD-A(-)) in Africans, found in about 10% of African-Americans. In addition, more than 400 variants caused by point mutations or deletions that alter the activity of the G6PD enzyme have been characterized, and worldwide over 400 million people are G6PD deficient (Fig. 6.7).

The inheritance is sex-linked, affecting males, and carried by females who show approximately half the normal red cell G6PD values. The female heterozygotes have an advantage of resistance to *Falciparum* malaria. The degree of deficiency varies with ethnic group and G6PD genotype, often being mild (10–60% of normal activity) in black African people, more severe in Middle Eastern and South-East Asian people, and most severe in Mediterranean people (e.g. with G6PD Mediterranean, <10% of normal activity). The degree of enzyme activity and the clinical severity of the syndrome do not always correlate. Severe deficiency occurs occasionally in Northern European people.

Clinical features

G6PD deficiency is usually asymptomatic, with a normal blood count between attacks of haemolysis. The main clinical syndromes that occur with levels between 2% and 60% of normal are as follows:

1 **Acute haemolytic anaemia in response to oxidant stress**, e.g. drugs, fava beans or infections (Table 6.4). Fava beans (*Vica fava*) contain an oxidant chemical, divicine. The acute haemolytic anaemia is caused by rapidly developing intravascular haemolysis with haemoglobinuria (Fig. 6.3a). Depending on the G6PD genotype, the anaemia may be self-limiting, as new young red cells are made with near normal enzyme levels, or may be life-threatening.

2 **Neonatal jaundice**, usually without haemolysis.

3 **Rarely, a congenital non-spherocytic haemolytic anaemia**. This chronic anaemia may result from different types of severe enzyme deficiency (levels <2% of normal).

Diagnosis

Between acute crises (except in the rare cases of congenital non-spherocytic haemolytic anaemia) the blood count is normal. The enzyme deficiency is detected by one of a number of screening tests or by direct enzyme assay on red cells.

During a crisis the blood film may show contracted and fragmented cells, 'bite' cells and 'blister' cells (Fig. 6.8), which have had Heinz bodies removed by the spleen. Heinz bodies (oxidized, denatured and insoluble haemoglobin that precipitates in the red cell) may be seen in the reticulocyte preparation, particularly if the spleen is absent (Fig 2.17). There are also features of intravascular haemolysis.

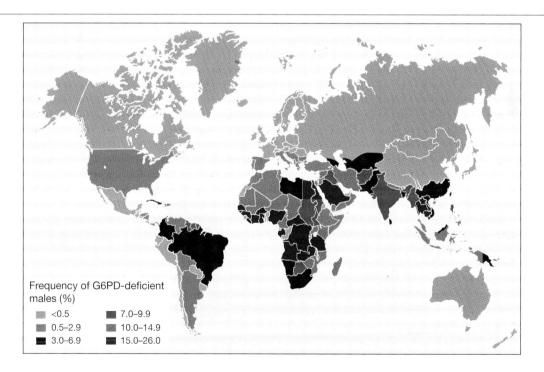

Frequency of G6PD-deficient males (%)

- <0.5
- 0.5–2.9
- 3.0–6.9
- 7.0–9.9
- 10.0–14.9
- 15.0–26.0

Figure 6.7 Global distribution of *G6PD* gene variants causing glucose-6-phosphate dehydrogenase (G6PD) deficiency. Shaded areas indicate the prevalence of G6PD deficiency. The distribution is similar to that of malaria; in countries where endogenous G6PD deficiency is not found, the distribution reflects immigration patterns. Source: Adapted from L. Luzzatto, R. Notaro (2001) *Science* 293: 442.

Table 6.4 Agents that may cause haemolytic anaemia in glucose-6-phosphate dehydrogenase (G6PD) deficiency.

Infections and other acute illnesses (e.g. diabetic ketoacidosis)

Drugs
- Antimalarials (e.g. primaquine, pamaquine, chloroquine, Fansidar, Maloprim, quinine)
- Sulphonamides and sulphones (e.g. co-trimoxazole, sulfanilamide, dapsone, sufasalazine)
- Other antibacterial agents (e.g. quinolones, nitrofurans, nalidixic acid, chloramphenicol)
- Analgesics (e.g. aspirin); moderate doses are safe
- Antihelminths (e.g. β-naphthol, stibophen)
- Miscellaneous (e.g. vitamin K analogues, rasburicase, glibenclamide, naphthalene (mothballs), probenecid)

Fava beans

Chemical oxidants

N.B. Many common drugs have been reported to precipitate haemolysis in G6PD deficiency in some patients (e.g. aspirin, quinine and penicillin), but not at conventional dosage.

Because of the higher enzyme level in young red cells in some G6PD genotypes, red cell enzyme assay may give a 'false' normal level in the phase of acute haemolysis with a reticulocyte response. Subsequent assay after the acute phase reveals the low G6PD level when the red cell population is of normal age distribution.

Treatment

The offending drug is stopped, any underlying infection is treated, a high urine output is maintained with fluid

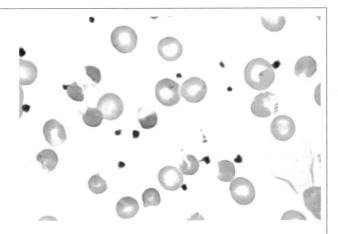

Figure 6.8 Blood film in glucose-6-phosphate dehydrogenase (G6PD) deficiency with acute haemolysis after an oxidant stress. Some of the cells show loss of cytoplasm with separation of remaining haemoglobin from the cell membrane ('blister' cells). There are also numerous contracted and deeply staining cells. Supravital staining (as for reticulocytes) showed the presence of Heinz bodies (see Fig. 2.17).

supplementation and blood transfusion undertaken where necessary for severe anaemia. G6PD-deficient babies are prone to neonatal jaundice and in severe cases phototherapy and exchange transfusion may be needed. The jaundice is usually not caused by excess haemolysis, but by deficiency of G6PD affecting neonatal liver function.

Glutathione deficiency and other syndromes

Other defects in the pentose phosphate pathway leading to similar syndromes to G6PD deficiency have been described – particularly glutathione deficiency.

Glycolytic (Embden–Meyerhof) pathway defects

These are all uncommon and lead to a congenital non-spherocytic haemolytic anaemia. In some there are defects of other systems (e.g. a myopathy). The most frequently encountered is pyruvate kinase deficiency (see Fig. 2.11).

Pyruvate kinase deficiency

This is inherited as an autosomal recessive condition, the affected patients being homozygous or doubly heterozygous. Over 100 different mutations have been described. The red cells become rigid as a result of reduced adenosine triphosphate (ATP) formation. The severity of the anaemia varies widely (haemoglobin 40–100 g/L) and causes relatively mild symptoms because of a shift to the right in the oxygen (O_2) dissociation curve caused by a rise in intracellular 2,3-diphosphoglycerate (2,3-DPG). Clinically, jaundice is usual and gallstones are frequent. Frontal bossing and leg ulcers (see Chapter 7) may be present. Perinatal complications including hydrops, prematurity, neonatal jaundice and anaemia are common.

The blood film shows poikilocytosis and distorted 'prickle' cells, particularly post-splenectomy. Direct enzyme assay is needed to make the diagnosis. Splenectomy may alleviate the anaemia but does not cure it and is indicated in those patients who need frequent transfusions. Iron loading occurs due to low serum hepcidin levels consequent on increased and ineffective erythropoiesis as well as from blood transfusions. A small-molecule activator of pyruvate kinase, AG-348, is highly effective and is in late-stage clinical trials.

Hereditary disorders of haemoglobin synthesis

Several of these cause clinical haemolysis. They are discussed in Chapter 7.

Acquired haemolytic anaemias

Immune haemolytic anaemias

Autoimmune haemolytic anaemias

Autoimmune haemolytic anaemias (AIHAs) are caused by antibody production by the body against its own red cells. They are characterized by a positive direct antiglobulin test (DAT), also known as the Coombs' test (see Fig. 30.5), and

Table 6.5 Immune haemolytic anaemias: classification.

Warm type	Cold type
Autoimmune	*Primary* ■ Cold agglutinin disease
Primary	*Secondary* ■ Infections – *Mycoplasma* pneumonia, infectious mononucleosis ■ Malignancy – lymphoma, CLL, solid organ ■ Post-allogeneic stem cell transplantation
Secondary ■ SLE, other immune dysregulation diseases –ulcerative colitis, primary biliary cirrhosis, post-allogeneic stem cell transplantation ■ Malignancy – CLL, lymphomas, solid organ ■ Drugs (e.g. fludarabine, cephalosporins, penicillin, methyldopa, Rh(D) immune globulin) ■ Infection (e.g. HIV, hepatitis, cytomegalovirus)	*Paroxysmal cold haemoglobinuria* (rare, sometimes associated with infections, e.g. adenovirus, influenza, syphilis)
Alloimmune	
Induced by red cell antigens	
■ Haemolytic transfusion reactions ■ Haemolytic disease of the newborn ■ Post-allogeneic stem cell grafts	
Drug induced	
■ Drug–red cell membrane complex ■ Immune complex	

CLL, chronic lymphocytic leukaemia; SLE, systemic lupus erythematosus.

divided into 'warm' and 'cold' types (Table 6.5) according to whether the antibody reacts more strongly with red cells at 37°C or 4°C.

Warm autoimmune haemolytic anaemias

In warm AIHA, red cells are coated with immunoglobulin (Ig), usually immunoglobulin G (IgG) alone or together with complement, and are therefore taken up by RE macrophages which have receptors for the Ig Fc fragment. Part of the coated membrane is lost, so the cell becomes progressively more spherical to maintain the same volume and is ultimately prematurely destroyed, predominantly in the spleen. When the cells are coated with IgG and complement (C3d, the degraded fragment of C3) or complement alone, red cell destruction occurs more generally in the RE system.

Clinical features

The disease may occur at any age, in either sex, and presents as a haemolytic anaemia of varying severity. The spleen is often enlarged. The disease tends to remit and relapse. It may occur alone or in association with other diseases, particularly lymphoid malignancies infection and auto-immune disorders (Table 6.5). When associated with idiopathic thrombocytopenic purpura (ITP), a similar condition affecting platelets (p. 316), it is called Evans' syndrome. When secondary to systemic lupus erythematosus, the cells typically are coated with

immunoglobulin and complement. In all 'idiopathic' cases, an underlying lymphoproliferative disease should be considered, and computed tomography (CT) scan of the chest, abdomen and pelvis performed.

Laboratory findings

The haematological and biochemical findings are typical of an extravascular haemolytic anaemia with spherocytosis prominent in the peripheral blood (Fig. 6.9a). The DAT is positive as a result of IgG, IgG and complement or IgA on the cells and, in some cases, the autoantibody shows specificity within the Rh system. The antibodies both on the cell surface and free in serum are best detected at 37°C. Rare cases are DAT negative, e.g. if the surface antibody titre is too low to be detected by the assay. On the other hand, about 5% of patients in hospital show a weakly positive DAT test, usually due to complement only on the surface of red cells, without any evidence of haemolysis.

Treatment

1 **Remove the underlying cause** if one is present (e.g. drug). If an underlying disease is present, e.g. chronic lymphocytic leukaemia or lymphoma, it may be necessary to treat the underlying condition to adequately control the haemolysis.
2 **Corticosteroids**. Prednisolone is the usual first-line treatment; 1 mg/kg/day is a typical starting dose in adults and should then be tapered down. Those with predominantly

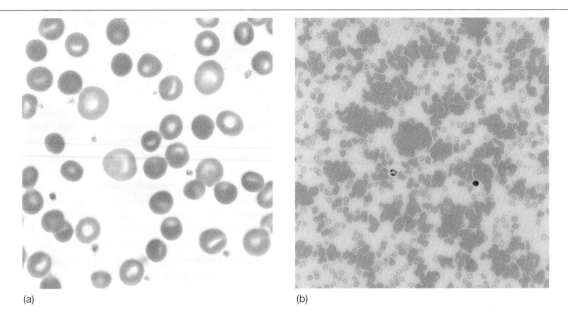

Figure 6.9 **(a)** Blood film in warm autoimmune haemolytic anaemia. Numerous microspherocytes are present and larger polychromatic cells (reticulocytes). **(b)** Blood film in cold autoimmune haemolytic anaemia. Marked red cell agglutination is present in films made at room temperature. The background is caused by the raised plasma protein concentration.

IgG on red cells do best, whereas those with complement often respond poorly, to both corticosteroids and splenectomy. While high-dose dexamethasone has been effective in ITP, it is less well tested and not established in AIHA. Antacid therapy with e.g. a proton pump inhibitor should be given. If steroid therapy is prolonged for over 3 months, especially for those over 40 years, prophylaxis against fractures is considered with vitamin D and calcium supplements and possibly with oral bisphosphonate.

3 **Monoclonal antibody.** Anti-CD20 (rituximab) has produced prolonged remissions in a proportion of cases and may be used with steroids as first-line therapy.
4 **Splenectomy** may be of value in those who fail to respond well or fail to maintain a satisfactory haemoglobin level on an acceptably small (e.g. <15 mg daily) steroid dosage or rituximab maintenance.
5 **Immunosuppression** may be tried after the above measures have failed or even before splenectomy. Azathioprine, bortezomib, cyclophosphamide, chlorambucil, ciclosporin and mycophenolate mofetil have been tried with varying success. Anti-CD52 (alemtuzumab) may be tried third line or later.
6 **Folic acid** is essential in severe and chronic cases.
7 **Blood transfusion** may be needed if anaemia is severe and causing symptoms. The blood should be the least incompatible and, if the specificity of the autoantibody is known, donor blood is chosen that lacks the relevant antigen(s).

The patients also readily make alloantibodies against donor red cells, so donor red cells phenotypically matched as far possible to the recipient are used. It may be challenging for the blood bank to match blood cells and this may take some time.
8 **High-dose immunoglobulin** has been used but with less success than in ITP (p. 317).
9 **Venous thrombosis prophylaxis** is usually indicated.

Cold autoimmune haemolytic anaemias

In these syndromes the IgM autoantibody attaches to red cells, mainly in the peripheral circulation where the blood temperature is cooled (Table 6.5). The autoantibody may be **monoclonal**, as in primary cold haemagglutinin syndrome or associated with lymphoproliferative disorders, or may be a transient **polyclonal** response following infections such as infectious mononucleosis or *Mycoplasma* pneumonia. The IgM antibodies, which bind to red cells optimally at 4°C, are highly efficient at fixing complement such that intravascular and extravascular haemolysis can occur. The clinical severity reflects the thermal amplitude of the specific antibody in a given patient; antibodies that continue to bind at higher temperatures are more dangerous than those that only bind at colder temperatures. Only complement factors can be detected on red cells in laboratory tests, as the IgM antibody is eluted off as cells flow through warmer parts of the circulation.

The cold agglutinin titre is usually high, typically >1:512; low-titre cold agglutinins are widespread and of no clinical significance. In nearly all these cold AIHA syndromes the antibody is directed against the 'I' antigen on the red cell surface. In infectious mononucleosis it is anti-i. Underlying lymphoma should be excluded in all 'idiopathic' cases.

Primary cold agglutinin disease

In this disease the patient has a chronic haemolytic anaemia aggravated by the cold and often associated with intravascular haemolysis. Mild jaundice and splenomegaly may be present. The patient may develop acrocyanosis (purplish skin discoloration) at the tip of the nose, ears, fingers and toes caused by the agglutination of red cells in small vessels.

Laboratory findings are similar to those of warm AIHA, except that spherocytosis is less marked, red cells agglutinate in the cold (Fig. 6.9b) and the DAT reveals complement (C3d) only on the red cell surface. In most patients, nodules of a monoclonal population of B lymphocytes are present in the bone marrow. Their morphology and immunophenotype differ from those in lymphoplasmacytic lymphoma, also associated with an IgM paraprotein; the MYD88 mutation characteristic of that disease is absent. Cold agglutinin disease is indolent, but may transform to an aggressive lymphoma.

Treatment consists of keeping the patient warm. Plasmapheresis may be needed initially to treat hyperviscosity. Rituximab is the best first-line therapy. Rituximab plus fludarabine or bendamustine is equally effective. Bortezomib-based therapy is also used. Alkylating drugs, e.g. chlorambucil or cyclophosphamide, are given as second-line therapy. Inhibition of complement C5 with eculizumab may also be effective (see p. 278), but is extremely expensive. Sutimlimab, which inhibits complement C1, also looks promising in early clinical trials. Splenectomy is not indicated unless massive splenomegaly is present. Corticosteroids are of less value than in warm antibody AIHA.

Paroxysmal cold haemoglobinuria is a rare syndrome of acute intravascular haemolysis after exposure to the cold. It is caused by the Donath–Landsteiner antibody, an IgG antibody with specificity for the P blood group antigens, which binds to red cells in the cold but causes lysis with complement in warm conditions. Viral infections are predisposing causes and the condition is usually self-limiting. In the past this condition was associated with advanced syphilis.

Alloimmune haemolytic anaemias

In these anaemias, antibody produced by one individual reacts with red cells of another. Three important situations are transfusion of ABO-incompatible blood and Rh disease of the newborn (which are considered in Chapters 30 and 31) and after allogeneic transplantation. The increased use of allogeneic transplantation for renal, hepatic, cardiac and bone marrow diseases has led to the recognition of alloimmune haemolytic anaemia, resulting from the destruction of red cells of the recipient by antibodies produced by donor lymphocytes. This occurs before the blood group of the recipient becomes that of the donor.

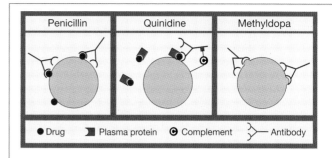

Figure 6.10 Three different mechanisms of drug-induced immune haemolytic anaemia. In each case the coated (opsonized) cells are destroyed in the reticuloendothelial system.

Drug-induced immune haemolytic anaemias

Drugs may cause immune haemolytic anaemias via three mechanisms (Fig. 6.10):

1 Antibody directed against a drug–red cell membrane complex (e.g. penicillin, ampicillin); this only occurs with massive doses of the antibiotic.
2 Deposition of complement via a drug–protein (antigen)– antibody complex onto the red cell surface (e.g. quinidine, rifampicin).
3 A true autoimmune haemolytic anaemia in which the role of the drug is unclear (e.g., fludarabine).

In each case, the haemolytic anaemia gradually disappears when the drug is discontinued.

Red cell fragmentation syndromes

These arise through physical damage to red cells either on abnormal surfaces (e.g. artificial heart valves or arterial grafts), arteriovenous malformations or as a **microangiopathic haemolytic anaemia**. This is caused by red cells passing through abnormal small vessels. The abnormality may be caused by deposition of fibrin strands, often associated with disseminated intravascular coagulation (DIC), or platelet adherence, as in thrombotic thrombocytopenic purpura (TTP; p. 319), or vasculitis (e.g. polyarteritis nodosa) (Table 6.6). The peripheral blood contains many deeply staining red cell fragments (Fig. 6.11). When DIC underlies the haemolysis, clotting abnormalities (p. 334) and a low platelet count are also present. TTP is discussed in detail on p. 319.

March haemoglobinuria

This is caused by damage to red cells between the small bones of the feet, usually during prolonged marching or running. The blood film does not show fragments.

Infections

Infections can cause haemolysis in a variety of ways. They may precipitate an acute haemolytic crisis in G6PD deficiency or cause microangiopathic haemolytic anaemia (e.g. with meningococcal

Table 6.6 Red cell fragmentation syndromes.

Cardiac haemolysis	Prosthetic heart valves
	Patches, grafts
	Perivalvular leaks
Arteriovenous malformations	Kasabach–Merritt syndrome, giant haemangiomas and others
Microangiopathic	TTP-HUS
	Disseminated intravascular coagulation
	Malignant disease
	Vasculitis (e.g. polyarteritis nodosa)
	Malignant hypertension
	Pre-eclampsia/HELLP syndrome
	Renal vascular disorders
	Ciclosporin
	Homograft rejection

HELLP, haemolysis with elevated liver function tests and low platelets; HUS, haemolytic uraemic syndrome; TTP, thrombotic thrombocytopenic purpura.

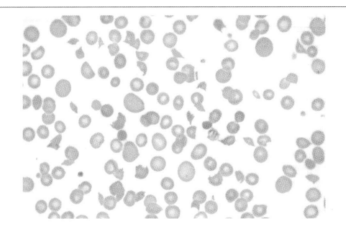

Figure 6.11 Blood film in microangiopathic haemolytic anaemia (in this patient Gram-negative septicaemia). Numerous contracted and deeply staining cells and cell fragments are present.

or pneumococcal septicaemia). Malaria causes haemolysis by extravascular destruction of parasitized red cells as well as by direct intravascular lysis. Blackwater fever is an acute intravascular haemolysis accompanied by acute renal failure caused by *Falciparum* malaria. *Clostridium perfringens* septicaemia can cause intravascular haemolysis with marked microspherocytosis. Tick-borne illnesses such as babesiosis can also enter red cells and cause haemolysis, which is usually not as severe as in malaria.

Chemical and physical agents

Certain drugs (e.g. dapsone and sulfasalazine) in high doses cause oxidative intravascular haemolysis with Heinz body formation in normal subjects. In Wilson disease, an acute haemolytic anaemia can occur as a result of high levels of copper in the blood. Chemical poisoning (e.g. with lead, chlorate or arsine) can cause severe haemolysis. Severe burns damage red cells, causing acanthocytosis or spherocytosis.

Secondary haemolytic anaemias

In many systemic disorders, such as inflammatory bowel disease or rheumatological syndromes, red cell survival is modestly shortened. This may contribute to anaemia (see Chapter 29).

- Haemolytic anaemia is caused by shortening of the red cell life. The red cells may break down in the reticuloendothelial system (extravascular) or in the circulation (intravascular).
- Haemolytic anaemia may be caused by inherited red cell defects, which are usually intrinsic to the red cell, or to acquired causes, which are usually caused by an abnormality of the red cell environment.
- Features of extravascular haemolysis include jaundice, gallstones and splenomegaly with raised reticulocytes, unconjugated serum bilirubin and absent haptoglobins. In intravascular haemolysis (e.g. caused by ABO mismatched blood transfusion), there is haemoglobinaemia, methaemalbuminaemia, haemoglobinuria and haemosiderinuria.
- Genetic defects include those of the red cell membrane (e.g. hereditary spherocytosis or elliptocytosis), enzyme deficiencies (e.g. glucose-6-phosphate dehydrogenase or pyruvate kinase deficiency) or haemoglobin defects (e.g. sickle cell disease, see Chapter 7).
- Acquired causes of haemolytic anaemia include warm or cold, auto- or alloantibodies to red cells, red cell fragmentation syndromes, infections, toxins and paroxysmal nocturnal haemoglobinuria (see Chapter 22).

Now visit **www.wileyessential.com/haematology** to test yourself on this chapter.

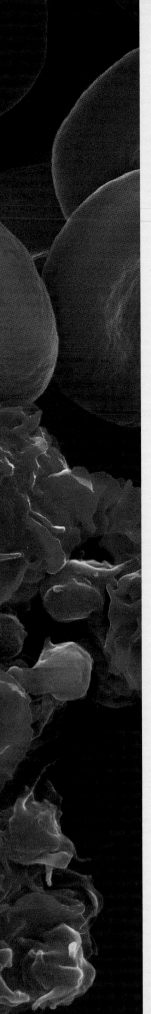

CHAPTER 7

Genetic disorders of haemoglobin

Key topics

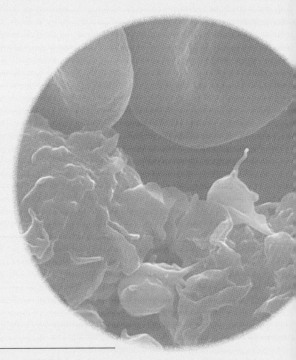

Hoffbrand's Essential Haematology, Eighth Edition. By A. Victor Hoffbrand and David P. Steensma.
© 2020 John Wiley & Sons Ltd. Published 2020 by John Wiley & Sons Ltd.
Companion website: www.wileyessential.com/haematology

This chapter discusses inherited diseases caused by reduced or abnormal synthesis of globin, the protein component of the haemoglobin molecule. Mutations in globin genes are the most prevalent monogenic disorders worldwide and affect approximately 7% of the world's population. Synthesis of normal haemoglobin in the fetus and adult is described first.

Haemoglobin synthesis during human development

Normal adult blood contains three types of haemoglobin (Hb; see Table 2.3). The major component is Hb A, with the molecular structure $\alpha_2\beta_2$ (i.e. two α chains and two β chains forming a tetramer). The minor haemoglobins in adult blood contain γ-globin ($\alpha_2\gamma_2$ in fetal Hb, also known as Hb F) or δ-globin ($\alpha_2\delta_2$ in Hb A$_2$) chains instead of β chains. Hb A$_2$ normally represents 1.5–3.5% of total adult haemoglobin and Hb F about 0.5%.

In the embryo and fetus, Hb Gower 1 (the primary embryonic haemoglobin despite its relative instability) and Hb F dominate at different stages. Minor haemoglobins detectable at early stages of gestation include Hb Portland and Hb Gower 2 (Fig. 7.1). These haemoglobins include ζ- and ε- instead of α- and β-globins.

Molecular aspects of haemoglobin synthesis

The genes for the globin chains and their regulatory elements occur in two clusters: ε, γ, δ and β (the 'β-globin cluster')

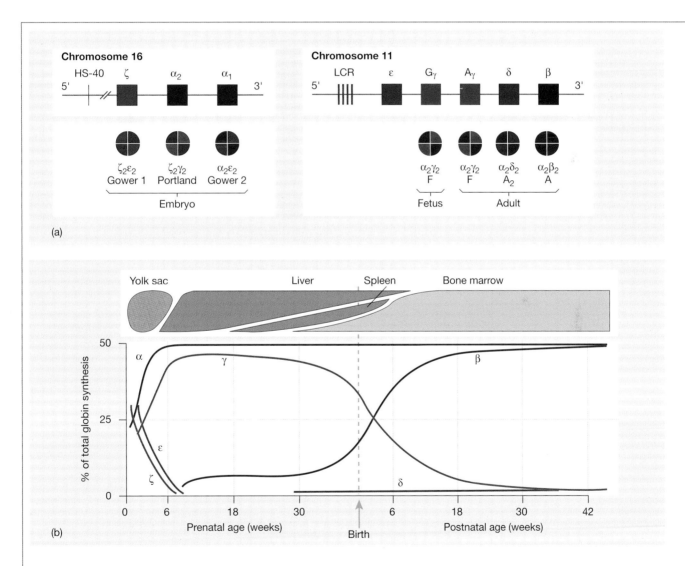

Figure 7.1 (a) The globin gene clusters on chromosomes 16p and 11q. In embryonic, fetal and adult life, different genes are activated or suppressed. The different globin chains are synthesized independently and then combine with each other to produce the different haemoglobins. The γ gene may have two sequences, which code for either a glutamic acid or alanine residue at position 136 (Gγ or Aγ, respectively). LCR, locus control region; HS-40, see text for description. **(b)** Synthesis of individual globin chains in prenatal and postnatal life.

located on chromosome 11q, and ζ and α (the 'α-globin cluster') on chromosome 16p. Several inactive globin pseudogenes are also part of these globin gene clusters. Two types of γ-globin occur, Gγ and Aγ, which are interchangeable and differ by having either a glycine or an alanine amino acid at position 136 in the polypeptide chain. The α-globin gene is duplicated, and both α genes (α_1 and α_2) on each chromosome 16 are active. Thus, in health there are four α-globin genes and two β-globin genes (Fig. 7.1), yet the cell regulates expression of these genes such that α-globin and β-globin protein synthesis is balanced.

All the globin genes have three exons (coding regions) and two introns (non-coding regions whose DNA is not represented in the finished protein). An initial globin RNA is transcribed from both introns and exons, and from this transcript the RNA derived from introns is removed by splicing (Fig. 7.2). Introns almost always begin with a G-T dinucleotide and end with an A-G dinucleotide, and the introns in the globin genes are typical in this regard. The pre-mRNA splicing machinery recognizes these sequences as well as neighbouring conserved sequences and excises the introns from the newly formed transcript. The newly formed mature mRNA resulting from transcription is polyadenylated at the 3′ end (Fig. 7.2) and this stabilizes it. Thalassaemia may arise from mutations or deletions of any of these sequences.

A number of other conserved regulatory sequences are important in globin synthesis, and mutations at these sites may also give rise to thalassaemia by reducing synthesis of one of the globin chains. These regulatory sequences influence gene transcription, ensure its fidelity, specify sites for the initiation and termination of transcription, and ensure the stability of newly synthesized mRNA.

Promoters are found 5′ of the gene (see Fig. 1.8). Enhancers occur either 5′ or 3′ to the gene and are important in the tissue-specific regulation of globin gene expression and in regulation of the synthesis of the various globin chains during fetal and postnatal life. The locus control region (LCR) is a genetic regulatory element situated upstream of the β-globin cluster, which controls genetic activity by opening up the chromatin to allow several key transcription factors to bind. A similar region, called HS-40 because it is approximately 40 kilobases 5′ to the gene cluster, and due to the open nature of its chromatin is hypersensitive (HS) to DNA cleavage by endonuclease enzymes that are used experimentally, regulates α-globin synthesis. In addition, mutations in transcription factors such as GATA1 that bind to these regulatory sequences but are encoded on other chromosomes can cause altered globin synthesis and a clinical syndrome if mutated.

Switch from fetal to adult haemoglobin

The globin genes are arranged on chromosomes 11 and 16 in the order in which they are expressed in development (Fig. 7.1). Embryonic haemoglobins are usually only expressed in yolk sac erythroblasts. **The β-globin gene is expressed at a low level in early fetal life, but the main switch to adult haemoglobin occurs 3–6 months after birth, when synthesis of the γ chain is largely replaced by β chains**. This explains why clinical defects in β-globin synthesis may not be detected at birth but are usually manifest by the end of the first year of life.

BCL11A is a major transcriptional regulator of this switch. Other nuclear transcriptional factors are involved. The cytosine methylation state of the gene (expressed genes are associated with hypomethylated cytosine bases in the promoter regions, while non-expressed are associated with hypermethylated cytosines), as well as the state of the chromosome packaging (i.e. status of histone proteins) and DNA enhancer sequences all play a part in determining whether a particular gene will be transcribed.

Haemoglobin abnormalities

These result from the following:
1 **Synthesis of an abnormal haemoglobin with an altered amino acid sequence.**
2 **Reduced rate of synthesis of normal α- or β-globin chains (the α- and β-thalassaemias, Fig. 7.3), leading to a globin deficit and imbalance.**

Table 7.1 shows some of the abnormal haemoglobins that arise from synthesis of an α- or β-globin chain with an amino acid substitution. Clinically most important is sickle cell disease, resulting most commonly from homozygous Hb S, described further below. Hb C, D and E are also common and, like Hb S, result from DNA sequence variants leading to amino acid

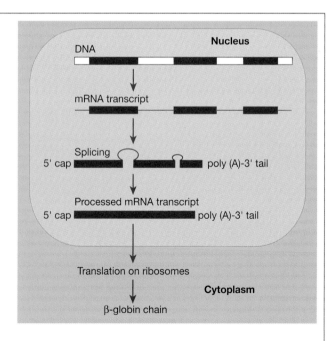

Figure 7.2 The expression of a human β-globin gene from transcription, excision of introns, splicing of exons and translation to ribosomes. The primary transcript is 'capped' at the 5′ end and a poly-A tail is then added.

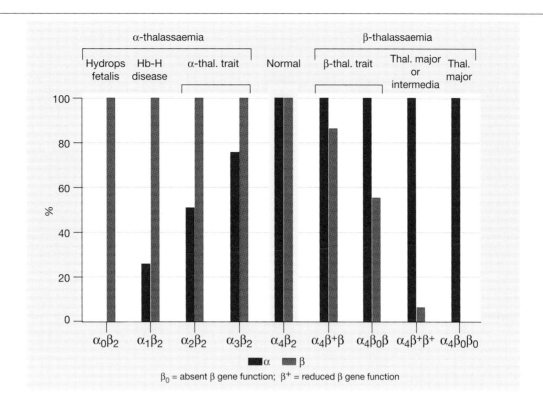

β₀ = absent β gene function; β⁺ = reduced β gene function

Figure 7.3 The ratio of $\alpha\!:\!\beta$-globin chain synthesis (y axis) depending on the number of functioning α and β chain genes (x axis). Source: A.B. Mehta, A.V. Hoffbrand (2014) *Haematology at a Glance*, 4th edn. Reproduced with permission of John Wiley & Sons.

Table 7.1 The clinical syndromes produced by haemoglobin abnormalities.

Syndrome	Abnormality
Haemolysis	Crystalline haemoglobins (Hb S, C, D, E, etc.)
	Unstable haemoglobins (e.g. Hb Köln, Hb Zurich) resulting in 'Heinz body' congenital haemolytic anaemias
Thalassaemia	α- or β-thalassaemia, resulting from reduced and imbalanced globin synthesis
Familial polycythaemia (erythrocytosis)	Altered oxygen affinity (e.g. Hb Chesapeake, Hb Montefiore)
Methaemoglobinaemia	Failure of reduction (various types of Hb M)

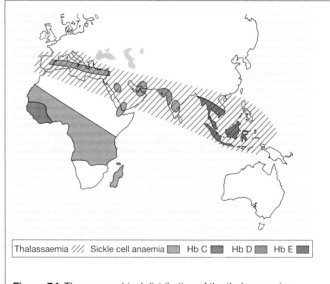

Figure 7.4 The geographical distribution of the thalassaemias and the more common, inherited, structural haemoglobin abnormalities.

changes in the β chain and altered physicochemical properties. Hb C is found most commonly in persons of sub-Saharan African origin, while Hb D is detected frequently in western China and South Asia, and Hb E in South-East Asia (Fig. 7.4).

Unstable haemoglobins are rare and cause a chronic haemolytic anaemia of varying severity with intravascular haemolysis (see Table 6.2). Heinz bodies represent denatured haemoglobin resulting from the instability and can be detected in blood films with use of special stains. Abnormal haemoglobins may also cause (familial) polycythaemia or erythrocytosis (Chapter 15) or congenital methaemoglobinaemia (Chapter 2). Many amino acid substitutions in haemoglobin are of no clinical consequence.

The genetic defects of haemoglobin are the most common genetic disorders worldwide. They occur primarily in tropical and sub-tropical areas (Fig. 7.4) and most appear to have been selected because the carrier state affords some protection against malaria.

Thalassaemias

These are a heterogeneous group of genetic disorders that result from a reduced rate of synthesis of α- or β-globin chains (Fig. 7.3; Table 7.2). β-Thalassaemia is more common in the Mediterranean region, while α-thalassaemia is more common in South and South-East Asia (Fig. 7.4).

Clinically the three main syndromes are transfusion-dependent **thalassaemia major**, non-transfusion-dependent thalassaemia **(thalassaemia intermedia)** with a moderate degree of anaemia due to a variety of genetic defects (see Table 7.3) and **thalassaemia minor**, usually due to a carrier state for α- or β-thalassaemia and characterized by erythrocyte microcytosis and mild or no anaemia.

α-Thalassaemia syndromes

These are caused by α-globin gene deletions or less frequently mutations (Table 7.2). The clinical severity is related to the number of the four α-globin genes missing or inactive. Loss of all four genes completely suppresses α chain synthesis (Fig. 7.5) and because the α chain is essential in fetal as well as in adult haemoglobin, this is incompatible with life and leads to death *in utero* (**hydrops fetalis**; Fig. 7.6). Deletion of three α genes leads to a moderately severe (haemoglobin 70–110 g/L) microcytic, hypochromic anaemia (Fig. 7.7) with splenomegaly. This is known as **Hb H disease** because haemoglobin H (a tetramer of self-associating β-globin chains, β_4) can be detected in red cells of these patients by electrophoresis or in reticulocyte preparations (Fig. 7.7). In fetal and early infant life, before β-globin chains are produced at high levels, **Hb Barts** (γ_4) occurs.

The α- thalassaemia traits are caused by loss of one or two genes and are usually not associated with anaemia. The mean corpuscular volume (MCV) and mean corpuscular haemoglobin (MCH) are low and the red cell count is over 5.5×10^{12}/L. Haemoglobin electrophoresis is usually normal and DNA analysis is needed to be certain of the diagnosis. Uncommon non-deletional forms of α-thalassaemia are

---

Table 7.2 Classification of thalassaemia*

Clinical syndromes

Hydrops fetalis
- Four-gene-deletion α-thalassaemia

Thalassaemia major
- Transfusion dependent; resulting from homozygous β^0-thalassaemia or other combinations of β-thalassaemia trait

Thalassaemia minor
- β^0-thalassaemia trait
- β^+-thalassaemia trait
- α^0-thalassaemia trait
- α^+ thalassaemia trait

Thalassaemia intermedia (non-transfusion-dependent thalassaemia)
- Many potential genetic mechanisms; see Table 7.3

Genetic type	Haplotype	Heterozygous thalassaemia trait (minor)*	Homozygous
α-*Thalassaemias*[†]			
α^0	– –/	MCV, MCH low	Hydrops fetalis
α^+	–α/	MCV, MCH minimally reduced	As heterozygous α^0-thalassaemia
			Compound heterozygote $\alpha^0\alpha^+$ (– –/–α) is haemoglobin H disease
β-*Thalassaemias*			
β^0		MCV, MCH low (Hb A_2 >3.5%)	Thalassaemia major (Hb F 98%, Hb A_2 2%)
β^+		MCV, MCH low (Hb A_2 >3.5%)	Thalassaemia major or intermedia (Hb F 70–80%, Hb A 10–20%, Hb A_2 variable)

*See text for the less common diseases: δβ-thalassaemia, Hb Lepore and dominant β-thalassaemia trait. α^0 = 2 α genes deleted or mutated, α^+ = one α gene deleted or mutated.
MCV, mean corpuscular (or cell) volume; MCH, mean cell haemoglobin.

Table 7.3 Non-transfusion-dependent thalassaemia (thalassaemia intermedia) – a clinical syndrome resulting from many genotypes.

With homozygous β-thalassaemia

   Homozygous or compound heterozygotes with mild (β+) thalassaemia

   Coinheritance of α-thalassaemia

   Enhanced ability to make fetal haemoglobin (γ chain production)

With heterozygous β-thalassaemia

   Coinheritance of additional α-globin genes (ααα/αα or ααα/ααα) increasing globin imbalance

   Dominant β-thalassaemia trait

δβ-thalassaemia and hereditary persistence of fetal haemoglobin

   Homozygous δβ-thalassaemia

   Heterozygous δβ-thalassaemia/β-thalassaemia

   Homozygous Hb Lepore (some cases)

Haemoglobin E/β-thalassaemia compound heterozygote
(some cases)

Haemoglobin H disease

caused by point mutations producing dysfunction of the genes, or rarely by mutations affecting termination of translation, which give rise to an elongated but unstable chain (e.g. Hb Constant Spring).

Two rare forms of α-thalassaemia are associated with developmental neurological abnormalities. They are caused by small germline chromosomal deletions resulting in a loss of a group of genes on chromosome 16, including the α-globin cluster (ATR-16 syndrome), or by mutation of a gene on chromosome X (*ATRX*) that controls the transcription of the globin and other genes; the latter only affects males. α-Thalassaemia has also been described in myelodysplastic syndromes due to an acquired mutation in the *ATRX* gene.

β-Thalassaemia syndromes

β-*Thalassaemia major*

This condition occurs on average in one in four offspring if both parents are carriers of the β-thalassaemia trait. Either no β chain (β⁰) or small amounts (β⁺) are synthesized (Fig. 7.3). Excess unpaired α chains precipitate in erythroblasts and in mature red cells, causing severe ineffective erythropoiesis and chronic haemolysis that are typical of this disease. The greater the α chain excess, the more severe the anaemia. Production of γ-chains helps to 'mop up' some excess α chains

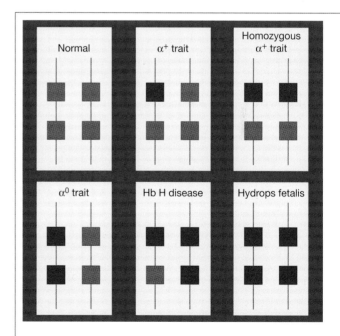

Figure 7.5 The genetics of α-thalassaemia. Each α gene may be deleted or (less frequently) dysfunctional. The orange boxes represent normal genes, and the blue boxes represent gene deletions or dysfunctional genes.

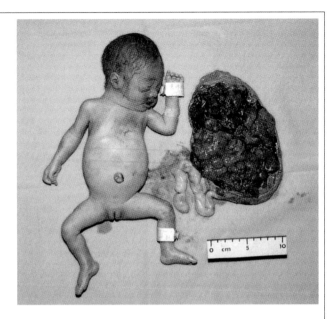

Figure 7.6 α-Thalassaemia: hydrops fetalis, the result of the deletion of all four α-globin genes (homozygous α⁰-thalassaemia). The main haemoglobin present is Hb Barts (γ₄). The condition is incompatible with life beyond the fetal stage. Source: Courtesy of Professor D. Todd.

and to ameliorate the condition. Over 400 different genetic defects have been detected (Fig. 7.8).

Unlike α-thalassaemia, the majority of genetic lesions in β-thalassaemia are point mutations rather than gene deletions. These mutations may be within the gene complex itself or in promoter or enhancer regions. Certain mutations are particularly frequent in some ethnic communities and this may simplify antenatal diagnosis aimed at detecting the mutations in fetal DNA.

Thalassaemia major is often a result of inheritance of two different mutations, each affecting β-globin synthesis (compound heterozygotes). In some cases, deletion of the β gene, δ and β genes or even δ, β and γ genes occurs. In others, unequal chromosome crossing-over has produced δβ fusion genes (so called Lepore syndrome, named after the Italian-American family in which this was first diagnosed; p. 89).

Clinical features

1 **Severe anaemia** becomes apparent at 3–6 months after birth when the switch from γ to β chain production should take place. Typically the infant presents in the first year with failure to thrive, pallor and a swollen abdomen.

2 **Enlargement of the liver and spleen** occurs as a result of excessive red cell destruction, extramedullary haemopoiesis and later because of iron overload. The large spleen increases

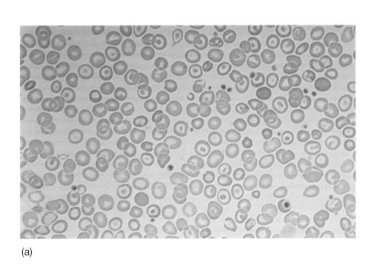

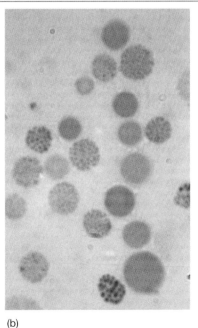

(a)   (b)

Figure 7.7 (a) α-Thalassaemia: Hb H disease (three α-globin gene deletion). The blood film shows marked hypochromic, microcytic cells with target cells and poikilocytosis. **(b)** α-Thalassaemia: Hb H disease. Supravital staining with brilliant cresyl blue or methylene blue reveals multiple fine, deeply stained deposits ('golf ball' cells) caused by precipitation of aggregates of β-globin chains. Hb H can also be detected as a fast-moving band on haemoglobin electrophoresis (see Fig. 7.12).

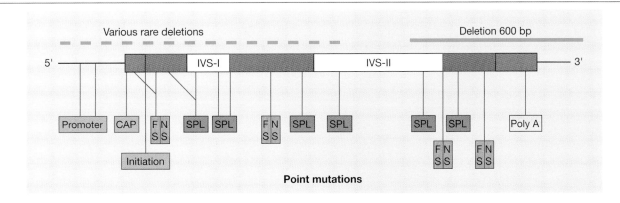

Figure 7.8 Examples of mutations that produce β-thalassaemia. These include single base changes, small deletions and insertions of one or two bases affecting introns, exons or the flanking regions of the β-globin gene. FS, 'frameshifts': deletion of nucleotide(s) that places the reading frame out of phase downstream of the lesion; NS, 'non-sense': premature chain termination as a result of a new translational stop codon (e.g. UAA); SPL, 'splicing': inactivation of splicing or new splice sites generated (aberrant splicing) in exons or introns; promoter, CAP, initiation: reduction of transcription or translation as a result of lesion in promoter, CAP or initiation regions; Poly A, mutations on the polyadenylation addition signal resulting in failure of poly A addition and an unstable mRNA.

blood requirements by increasing red cell destruction and pooling, and by causing expansion of the plasma volume.

3 **Expansion of bones** caused by intense marrow hyperplasia leads to a thalassaemic facies (Fig. 7.9) and to thinning of the cortex of many bones, with a tendency to fractures and bossing of the skull with a 'hair-on-end' appearance on X-ray (Fig. 7.10). This is seen less commonly in the modern era, since it is prevented by transfusion.

4 **Thalassaemia major is the disease that most frequently underlies transfusional iron overload.** Regular transfusions are usually commenced in the first year of life and, unless the disease is cured by stem cell transplantation or improved by gene therapy, are continued for life. Also, iron absorption is increased because of low serum hepcidin levels due to release of proteins such as erythroferrone from the increased numbers of early red cell precursors in the marrow. In children, failure of growth and delayed puberty are frequent, and without iron chelation, death from cardiac damage usually occurs in teenagers. The clinical features of iron overload are further discussed in Chapter 4.

5 **Infections** occur frequently. In infancy, without adequate transfusion, anaemia predisposes to bacterial infections. Pneumococcal, *Haemophilus* and meningococcal infections are likely if splenectomy has been carried out. *Yersinia enterocolitica* occurs, particularly in iron-loaded patients being treated with deferoxamine; it may cause severe gastroenteritis. Iron overload itself also predisposes to certain bacterial infections, e.g. *Klebsiella* or *Yersinia*, and to fungal infection. Transfusion of viruses by blood transfusion is now uncommon. As a result of reduction of deaths from cardiac iron overload by improved chelation therapy, infections now account for an increasing proportion of deaths in thalassaemia major.

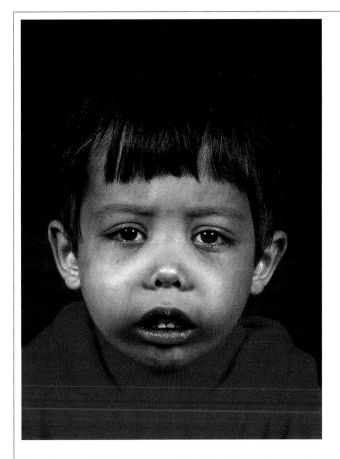

Figure 7.9 The facial appearance of a child with β-thalassaemia major. The skull is bossed with prominent frontal and parietal bones; the maxilla is also enlarged. This is a result of chronic anaemia and compensatory expansion (hyperplasia) of the marrow, and can be prevented by transfusion.

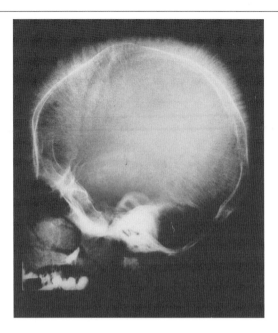

Figure 7.10 Skull X-ray in β-thalassaemia major without chronic transfusion support. There is a 'hair-on-end' appearance as a result of expansion of the bone marrow into cortical bone.

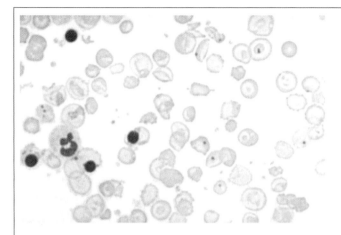

Figure 7.11 Blood film in β-thalassaemia major post-splenectomy. There are hypochromic cells, target cells and many nucleated red cells (normoblasts). Howell–Jolly bodies are seen in the same red cells.

6 **Liver disease** in thalassaemia major is most frequently a result of hepatitis C, but hepatitis B is also common where the virus is endemic. Human immunodeficiency virus (HIV) has been transmitted to some patients by blood transfusion. Iron overload may also cause liver damage.

7 **Hepatocellular carcinoma** incidence is increased in those with iron overload, resulting in hepatic fibrosis/cirrhosis and with chronic hepatitis B or C. Ultrasound and measurement of serum alpha fetoprotein every 6–12 months are advisable in such patients.

8 **Osteoporosis** may occur even in well-transfused patients. It is more common in diabetic patients with endocrine abnormalities, including those resulting from iron-related injury to the pituitary gland.

Laboratory diagnosis

1 There is a severe hypochromic, microcytic anaemia with normoblasts, target cells and basophilic stippling in the blood film (Fig. 7.11).

2 High-performance liquid chromatography (HPLC) is now usually used as the first-line method to diagnose haemoglobin disorders (Fig. 7.12a). HPLC or haemoglobin electrophoresis (Fig. 7.12b) reveals the absence or almost complete absence of Hb A, with almost all the circulating haemoglobin being Hb F. The Hb A$_2$ percentage is normal, low or slightly raised. DNA analysis is used to identify the defect on each allele, important in antenatal diagnosis.

3 The assessment of the degree of iron overload and of the consequent organ damage is described in Chapter 4.

Treatment

1 **Regular blood transfusions** are needed to maintain the haemoglobin over 100 g/L at all times. This usually requires 2–3 units every 3–4 weeks. Fresh blood, filtered to remove white cells, gives the best red cell survival with the fewest reactions. The patients should be genotyped at the start of the transfusion programme in case red cell antibodies against transfused red cells develop. Transfusions prevent complications, including skeletal deformation.

2 As a result of chronic transfusions, **thalassaemia major is the dominant disease worldwide for which iron chelation is essential**. The three available drugs, deferiprone, deferoxamine and deferasirox, have considerably improved quality of life and life expectancy for thalassemia patients. They are described in Chapter 4.

3 Regular **folic acid** (e.g. 5 mg weekly or 0.4–1 mg daily) is given due to the ongoing haemolysis with risk for folate deficiency, especially if the diet is poor.

4 **Splenectomy** may be needed to reduce blood transfusion requirements. If possible, this should be delayed until the patient is over 6 years old because of the high risk of dangerous infections post-splenectomy. The vaccinations and antibiotics to be given are described in Chapter 10.

5 **Endocrine therapy** is given either as replacement because of end-organ failure or to stimulate the pituitary if puberty is delayed. Diabetes will require insulin therapy. Patients with osteoporosis may need additional therapy with increased calcium and vitamin D, together with a bisphosphonate and appropriate endocrine therapy.

6 **Immunization** against hepatitis B should be carried out in all non-immune patients. Treatment for transfusion-transmitted hepatitis C is given if viral genomes are detected in plasma.

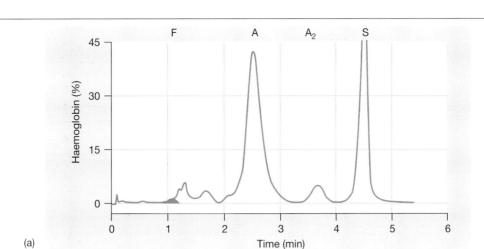

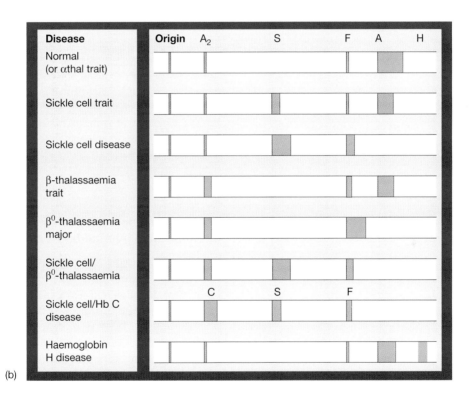

Figure 7.12 (a) High-performance liquid chromatography. The different haemoglobins elute at different times from the column and their concentrations are read automatically. In this example, the patient is a carrier of sickle cell disease. **(b)** Haemoglobin electrophoretic patterns in normal adult human blood and in subjects with sickle cell (Hb S) trait or disease, β-thalassaemia trait, β-thalassaemia major, Hb S/β-thalassaemia or Hb S/Hb C disease and Hb H disease.

7 **Allogeneic stem cell transplantation** offers the prospect of permanent cure. The success rate (long-term thalassaemia major-free survival) is over 80% in well-chelated younger patients without liver fibrosis or hepatomegaly. A human leucocyte antigen-matching sibling (or rarely other family member or matching unrelated volunteer) acts as donor. Failure is mainly a result of recurrence of thalassaemia, death (e.g. from infection) or severe chronic graft-versus-host disease.

8 Trials of **gene therapy** for treating the thalassaemia major phenotype are in progress. These aim to introduce a normal β-globin gene or to enhance Hb F production to reduce haemolysis using an autologous stem cell transplantation technique. Patient stem cells are harvested from bone

marrow or peripheral blood, and a lentiviral vector is used to introduce a gene construct *in vitro* into these stem cells. The construct is designed to enhance normal β-globin synthesis, or else to improve fetal haemoglobin synthesis by editing the *BC11A* gene, which normally suppresses γ-globin chain synthesis or its enhancers or promoters. In some of these techniques the CRISPR/Cas9 technique for gene editing is employed (Fig. 7.13). The 'corrected' stem cells are then reinfused into the patient, who has been treated with myeloablative conditioning, e.g with busulphan. In early

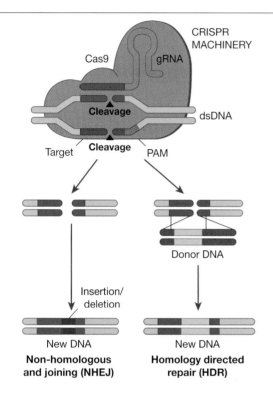

Figure 7.13 CRISPR/Cas9 gene editing. CRISPR, pronounced 'crisper', is commonly used in biotechnology as a shorthand term for CRISPR/Cas9 gene editing. CRISPR (clusters of regularly interspaced short palindromic repeats) is a specialized region of DNA consisting of nucleotide repeats and 'spacers', DNA elements that are interspersed among these repeated sequences and that in bacteria usually represent integrated viral genetic elements, and for which cells have evolved protective machinery to excise and repair DNA. In CRISPR/Cas9 gene editing, a short RNA template is created that matches a target sequence in the genome DNA. This guide RNA directs the CRISPR machinery to the target DNA. Associated Cas9 nuclease then site-specifically cleaves double-stranded DNA, activating the endogenous double-strand break DNA repair machinery, which includes homology-directed repair and non-homologous end joining. In the absence of a homologous repair template, non-homologous end joining can result in insertions and deletions (indels), disrupting the target sequence. Alternatively, precise mutations and knock-ins can be made by providing a homologous repair template with the new sequence of interest and exploiting the homology directed repair pathway. Source: New England Bio Labs Inc.

clinical trials, this approach has reduced or eliminated the need for long-term red cell transfusions in most patients treated.

9 The drug **luspatercept** is also proving beneficial in early clinical trials in thalassaemia major, as well as in thalassaemia intermedia and myelodysplastic syndromes. This 'ligand trap; (synthetic IgG1 antibody–activin II receptor fusion protein) inhibits growth differentiation factor 11 (GDF11), an inhibitor of erythropoiesis, binding to activin II receptors on erythroblasts, and so promote increased effective erythropoiesis, since GDF11 binding to the receptor blocks late-stage erythropoiesis.

β-Thalassaemia trait (minor)

This is a common, usually symptomless abnormality characterized like α-thalassaemia trait by a hypochromic, microcytic blood picture (MCV and MCH low) but high red cell count ($>5.5 \times 10^{12}$/L) and mild anaemia (haemoglobin 100–120 g/L). It is usually more severe than α-thalassaemia trait. A raised level of Hb A_2 ($>3.5\%$) confirms the diagnosis. Since iron deficiency lowers the Hb A_2 level, a falsely normal result may be found in the presence of concomitant iron deficiency.

The diagnosis of β-thalassaemia trait allows the possibility of prenatal counselling, which is legally mandated in some areas of the world with a high incidence of thalassaemia major, such as Cyprus. If the partner also has β-thalassaemia trait, there is a 25% risk of a child with thalassaemia major.

Non-transfusion-dependent thalassaemia (thalassaemia intermedia): a clinical syndrome

This is thalassaemia of moderate severity (haemoglobin 70–100 g/L) without the need for regular transfusions (Table 7.3), although transfusion may occasionally be required, for example during an acute illness with temporary suppression of erythropoiesis. **Thalassaemia intermedia is a *clinical* syndrome caused by a variety of genetic defects**, such as homozygous β-thalassaemia with production of more Hb F than usual, e.g. due to mutations of the *BCL11A* gene, or with milder defects in β chain synthesis. Additionally, the syndrome may result from β-thalassaemia trait alone of unusual severity ('dominant' β-thalassaemia trait), or by β-thalassaemia trait in association with another mild globin abnormality such as Hb Lepore.

The coexistence of α-thalassaemia trait improves the haemoglobin level in homozygous β-thalassaemia by reducing the degree of α:β chain imbalance and thus of α chain precipitation and ineffective erythropoiesis, and may result in an intermedia syndrome rather than thalassaemia major. Conversely, patients with β-thalassaemia trait who also have excess (five or six) α genes tend to be more anaemic than usual for the trait due to the greater chain imbalance.

The patient with thalassaemia intermedia may show liver fibrosis and cirrhosis, endocrine abnormalities, bone deformity and extramedullary erythropoiesis (Fig. 7.14), leg ulcers,

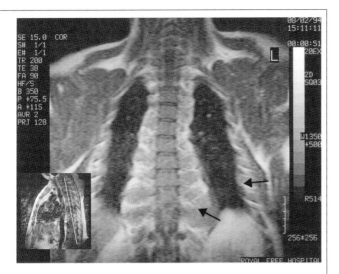

Figure 7.14 β-Thalassaemia intermedia: magnetic resonance imaging (MRI) scan showing masses of extramedullary haemopoietic tissue arising from the ribs and in the paravertebral region without encroachment of the spinal cord.

gallstones, osteoporosis, pulmonary hypertension and venous thrombosis. Iron overload is caused by increased iron absorption (due to low erythroferrone levels caused by ineffective erythropoiesis, see Chapter 3) and occasional transfusions, e.g. during pregnancy or infections or given to reduce bone deformity. Iron chelation, usually with oral drugs, may be needed to treat this, e.g. if the serum ferritin is greater than 800 μg/L or liver iron is greater than 5 mg/g dry weight. Splenectomy may be required to avoid the need for transfusions. Luspatercept (see above) enhances effective erythropoiesis and can reduce the level of anaemia, the extent of organ damage and iron overload.

Hb H disease (three-gene-deletion α-thalassaemia) is a type of thalassaemia intermedia without iron overload or extramedullary haemopoiesis.

δβ-Thalassaemia

This involves failure of production of both β and δ chains. Hb F production is increased to 5–20% in the heterozygous state, which resembles thalassaemia minor haematologically. In the homozygous state, only Hb F is present and haematologically the picture is one of thalassaemia intermedia.

Haemoglobin Lepore

This is an abnormal haemoglobin caused by unequal crossing-over of the β and δ genes to produce a polypeptide chain consisting of the δ chain at its amino end and the β chain at its carboxyl end. The δβ-fusion chain is synthesized inefficiently and normal δ and β chain production is abolished. The Hb Lepore homozygotes show thalassaemia intermedia and the heterozygotes thalassaemia trait.

Hereditary persistence of fetal haemoglobin

Hereditary persistence of fetal haemoglobin (HPFH) is a heterogeneous group of genetic conditions caused by deletions or cross-overs affecting the production of β and γ chains or, in non-deletion forms, by point mutations upstream from the γ-globin genes or in the *BCL11A* gene (p. 80).

Association of β-thalassaemia trait with other genetic disorders of haemoglobin

The combination of β-thalassaemia trait with Hb E trait usually causes a transfusion-dependent thalassaemia major syndrome, but some cases are intermediate. β-Thalassaemia trait co-inherited with Hb S trait produces the clinical picture of sickle cell disease rather than of thalassaemia. β-Thalassaemia trait with Hb D trait causes a hypochromic, microcytic anaemia of varying severity.

Sickle cell disease

Sickle cell disease is a group of haemoglobin disorders resulting from the inheritance of the sickle β-globin gene (Hb S). The sickle β-globin abnormality is caused by substitution of valine for glutamic acid in position 6 in the β chain (Fig. 7.15). Homozygous sickle cell anaemia (Hb SS) is the most common severe syndrome, while the doubly heterozygote conditions of Hb S/C and Hb S/β-thalassaemia also cause sickling disease that varies in severity.

Hb S (Hb $\alpha_2\beta_2^S$) is insoluble and forms crystals when exposed to low oxygen tension (Fig. 7.16). Deoxygenated sickle haemoglobin polymerizes into long fibres, each consisting of seven intertwined double strands with cross-linking (Fig. 7.16). The red cells containing this denatured fibrous haemoglobin experience membrane damage and form sickle shapes, and may block different areas of the microcirculation or large vessels, causing infarcts of various organs. The carrier state is widespread (Fig. 7.4) and is found in up to 30% of West African people, maintained at this level because of the protection against malaria that is afforded by the carrier state.

		pro	glu	glu
Normal β-chain	Amino acid	pro	glu	glu
	Base composition	CCT	G A G	GAG
Sickle β-chain	Base composition	CCT	G T G	GAG
	Amino acid	pro	val	glu

Figure 7.15 Molecular pathology of sickle cell anaemia. There is a single base change in the DNA coding for the amino acid in the sixth position in the β-globin chain (adenine is replaced by thymine). This leads to an amino acid change from glutamic acid to valine. A, adenine; C, cytosine; G, guanine; glu, glutamic acid; pro, proline; T, thymine; val, valine.

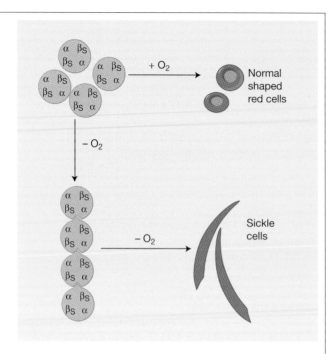

Figure 7.16 The formation of the sickle polymer. Source: Adapted from H.F. Bunn, J.C. Aster (2011) *Hematologic Pathophysiology*. New York: McGraw Hill.

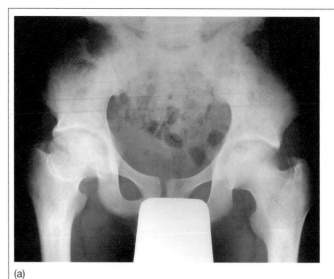

(a)

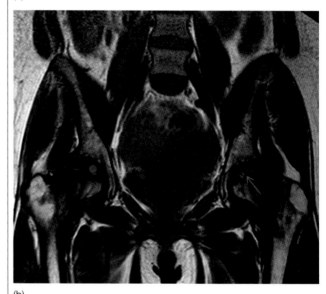

(b)

Figure 7.17 Sickle cell anaemia. **(a)** Radiograph of the pelvis of a young man of West Indian origin which shows avascular necrosis with flattening of the femoral heads, more marked on the right, coarsening of the bone architecture and cystic areas in the right femoral neck caused by previous infarcts. **(b)** Coronal hip magnetic resonance image (MRI) revealing established osteonecrosis of femoral heads bilaterally (yellow arrow) with crescent sclerotic margin (blue dot) as a consequence of sickle cell. Source: Courtesy of Dr A. Malhotra.

Homozygous disease

Clinical features

Clinical features are of a severe haemolytic anaemia punctuated by crises. The symptoms of anaemia are often mild in relation to the severity of the anaemia because Hb S gives up oxygen (O_2) to tissues relatively easily compared with Hb A (see Fig. 2.10). The clinical expression of Hb SS is very variable, some patients having an almost normal life, free of crises, but others develop severe crises even as infants and may die in early childhood or as young adults. Crises may be vaso-occlusive (painful or visceral), aplastic or haemolytic. There may be serious damage to many organs. The co-inheritance of α-thalassaemia or raised Hb F production with Hb SS results in a milder clinical course.

Vaso-occlusive crises

Painful

These are the most frequent type of crisis in sickle cell disease. They may be sporadic and unpredictable or precipitated by infection, acidosis, dehydration or deoxygenation (e.g. altitude, operations, obstetric delivery, stasis of the circulation, exposure to cold, violent exercise). Infarcts causing severe pain occur in the bones (hips, shoulders and vertebrae are commonly affected). Avascular necrosis of bones, especially of the femoral head, causes long term problems (Fig. 7.17). The 'hand–foot' syndrome (painful dactylitis caused by infarcts of the small bones) is frequently the first presentation of the disease, typically before age 5, and may lead to digits of varying lengths (Fig. 7.18).

Visceral

These are caused by sickling within organs causing infarction and sequestration of blood, often with a severe exacerbation of anaemia. The **acute sickle chest syndrome** is the most common cause of death in both children and adults. It

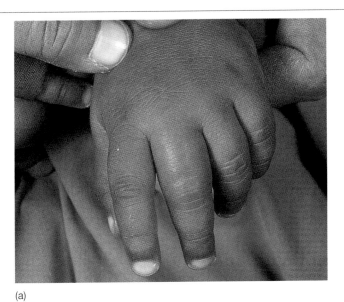

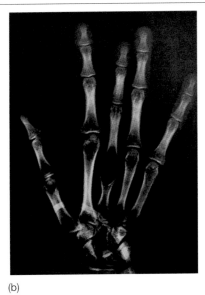

(a)

(b)

Figure 7.18 Sickle cell anaemia: **(a)** painful swollen fingers (dactylitis) in a child and **(b)** the hand of an 18-year-old Nigerian boy with the 'hand–foot' syndrome. There is marked shortening of the right middle finger because of dactylitis in childhood affecting the growth of the epiphysis.

presents with dyspnoea, falling arterial PO_2, chest pain and pulmonary infiltrates on chest X-ray. Treatment is with analgesia, oxygen, exchange transfusion and ventilatory support if necessary. Hepatic and girdle sequestration crises may lead to severe illness requiring exchange transfusions.

Splenic sequestration is typically seen in infants and presents with an enlarging spleen, falling haemoglobin and abdominal pain. Treatment is with transfusion. Attacks tend to be recurrent and splenectomy is often needed.

Aplastic crises

These occur as a result of infection with parvovirus or from folate deficiency and are characterized by a sudden fall in haemoglobin and reticulocytes, usually requiring transfusion (see Fig. 22.7).

Haemolytic crises

These are characterized by an increased rate of haemolysis and fall in haemoglobin but rise in reticulocytes and usually accompany a painful crisis.

Other organ damage

The most serious is of the brain (a stroke occurs in 7% of all patients) or spinal cord. Up to a third of children have had a silent cerebral infarct by the age of 6 years (Fig. 7.19). Transcranial Doppler ultrasonography detects abnormal blood flow

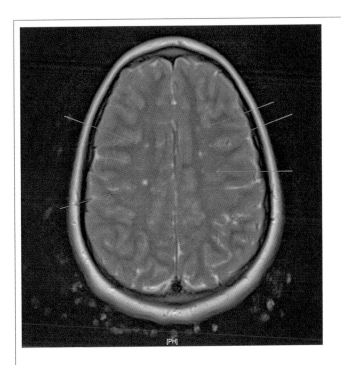

Figure 7.19 T2-weighted magnetic resonance image (MRI) of a 9-year-old girl with sickle cell anaemia, showing five hyperintensities in the deep white matter (arrows), which are silent cerebral infarcts. Source: Courtesy of Dr David Rees, Kings College Hospital.

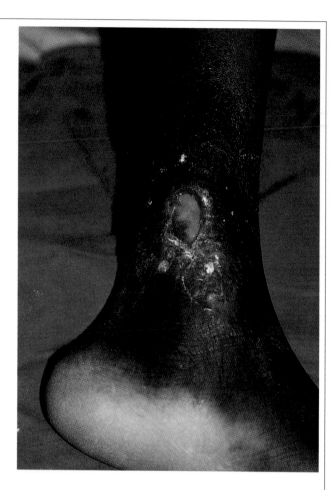

Figure 7.20 Sickle cell anaemia: medial aspect of the ankle of a 15-year-old Nigerian boy showing necrosis and ulceration.

indicative of arterial stenosis. This may be associated with cognitive impairment and predicts for strokes in children. This can be largely prevented by regular blood transfusions and trials of hyroxycarbamide therapy suggest it is also beneficial.

Ulcers of the lower legs are common, as a result of vascular stasis and local ischaemia (Fig. 7.20). The spleen is enlarged in infancy and early childhood, but later is often reduced in size as a result of infarcts (**autosplenectomy**). **Pulmonary hypertension** detected by Doppler echocardiography and an increased tricuspid regurgitant velocity is common and increases the risk of death. **Left ventricular failure** due to myocardial fibrosis is a frequent problem. A **proliferative retinopathy and priapism** are other clinical complications. **Chronic damage to the liver** may occur through microinfarcts. **Pigment (bilirubin) gallstones** are frequent.

The kidneys are vulnerable to infarctions of the medulla with papillary necrosis. There may be acute deterioration in renal function. Failure to concentrate urine aggravates the tendency to dehydration and crisis, and nocturnal enuresis may develop. **Chronic renal insufficiency** is a common complication in adulthood. Infections are frequent partly due to

hyposplenism, and iron overload from repeated transfusions may increase the risk. Pneumonia, urinary tract infections and Gram-negative septicaemia are common. Osteomyelitis may also occur, usually from *Salmonella* species. There is an increased incidence of venous thrombosis and this tends to recur, so long-term anticoagulation may be needed.

Laboratory findings

1 The haemoglobin is usually 60–90 g/L – low in comparison to mild or no symptoms of anaemia.
2 Sickle cells and target cells occur in the blood (Fig. 7.21). Features of splenic atrophy (e.g. Howell–Jolly bodies) may also be present.
3 Screening tests for sickling are positive when the blood is deoxygenated (e.g. with dithionate and disodium phosphate, $Na_2 HPO_4$).
4 HPLC or haemoglobin electrophoresis (Fig. 7.12): in Hb SS, no Hb A is detected. The amount of Hb F is variable and is usually 5–15%; larger amounts are usually associated with a milder disorder.

Treatment

General

1 Prophylactic – avoid those factors known to precipitate crises, especially dehydration, anoxia (e.g. high altitudes), infections, stasis of the circulation and cooling of the skin surface.
2 Folic acid (e.g. 5 mg once weekly).
3 Good general nutrition and hygiene.
4 Pneumococcal, *Haemophilus* and meningococcal vaccination and regular oral penicillin are effective at reducing the infection rate with these organisms. Oral penicillin should start at diagnosis and continue at least until puberty. Hepatitis B vaccination is also given, as transfusions may be needed and malarial prophylaxis is required in countries where malaria is prevalent.

Special situations

1 **Acute crisis**:
  (a) Treat by rest, warmth, rehydration by oral fluids and/or intravenous normal saline (3 L in 24 h) and antibiotics if infection is present.
  (b) Analgesia at the appropriate level should be given. Suitable drugs are paracetamol, a non-steroidal anti-inflammatory agent and opiates, depending on the severity of pain.
  (c) Blood transfusion is given if there is very severe anaemia with symptoms or with impending critical organ complications. Exchange transfusion may be needed, particularly if there is neurological damage or repeated painful crises. This is aimed at achieving an Hb S percentage of less than 30% and, after a stroke, is continued for at least one year with subsequent hydroxycarbamide. For hepatic or splenic sequestration and for aplastic crisis, blood transfusion is essential and may be life-saving.

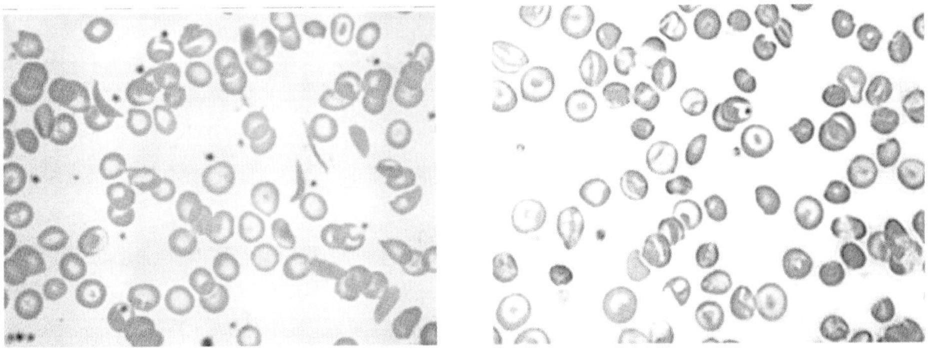

(a)   (b)

Figure 7.21 (a) Sickle cell anaemia: peripheral blood film showing deeply staining sickle cells, target cells and polychromasia. **(b)** Homozygous Hb C disease: peripheral blood film showing many target cells, deeply staining rhomboidal and spherocytic cells.

(d) Crizanlizumab, an antibody directed against P-selectin that is involved in adhesion of sickle cells to blood vessel walls, has been shown to reduce the time to resolution of a painful crisis.

2 **Pregnancy and surgery** Particular care is needed in pregnancy and surgery. There is debate about whether or not all patients need transfusions to reduce Hb S levels during pregnancy or before delivery or for minor operations. Routine transfusions throughout pregnancy are definitely recommended for those with a poor obstetric history, a multiple pregnancy or a history of frequent crises. Careful anaesthetic and recovery techniques must be used to avoid hypoxaemia or acidosis. Preoperative transfusions are indicated before medium-risk, e.g. abdominal or orthopaedic, or high-risk surgery, e.g brain or cardiovascular procedures.

3 **Blood transfusions** Their use in acute crises has been described above. The choice between simple transfusion and exchange transfusion (usually performed with a cell separator as a single procedure) depends on clinical judgement in each case, depending on the indication, avoidance of hyperviscosity and iron overload and on venous access and availability of a cell separator. Transfusions are sometimes given repeatedly as prophylaxis to patients having frequent crises or who have had major organ damage (e.g. of the brain) or show abnormal transcranial Doppler studies. The aim is to suppress Hb S production over a period of several months or even years, with a target haemoglobin S of <30%. Alloimmunization against donated blood is also a common problem. Delayed haemolytic transfusion reactions in which both the transfused and the patient's own red cells are destroyed are particularly dangerous. Recommended treatment is with eculizumab, an inhibitor of C5 convertase in the complement pathway (see p. 277). High doses of steroids or gamma globulin may also be helpful.

4 **Hydroxycarbamide (hydroxyurea)** This increases Hb F levels and improves the clinical course of children or adults. It is now recommended for all infants and children over the age of 9 months with sickle cell disease. In adults it is given to those with severe or moderately severe disease, e.g. who are having three or more painful crises each year. It should not be used during pregnancy. It can be used in primary prevention of stroke or to replace blood transfusions when they have been given for a year to prevent recurrence of stroke. In sub-Saharan Africa, it reduces malarial infections in childhood among Hb SS patients. Careful monitoring is needed to avoid severe neutropenia; there is no evidence that its prolonged administration over many years to children or adults predisposes to any form of neoplastic disease. Research into other drugs (e.g. butyrates) to enhance Hb F synthesis or to increase the solubility of Hb S is taking place.

5 **Iron overload** This is best assessed by the total number of units transfused and by liver iron estimated by magnetic resonance imaging (MRI). Sickle cell patients tend not to adhere to burdensome subcutaneous deferoxamine infusions, so if iron chelation is needed, oral iron chelating drugs are preferred.

6 **L-glutamine** L-glutamine is a precursor of glutathione which protects cells from oxidative damage. Supplementation with L-glutamine in some studies has reduced the frequency and severity of painful crises. A powdered form of the amino acid was approved for treatment of sickle cell anaemia by the US Food and Drug Administration in 2017. It should not be used in pregnancy or lactation or in those with severe renal or liver disease.

7 **Allogeneic stem cell transplantation** Allogeneic transplant can cure sickle cell anaemia, with 80% disease free after the procedure. The mortality rate is less than 10% if patients are carefully selected. Transplantation is only indicated in the severest of cases whose quality of life or life expectancy is substantially impaired.

8 Gene therapy Clinical trials are in progress using an autologous marrow stem cell transplant procedure, as described above for thalassaemia major. Initial trials are aimed at increasing Hb F production in harvested stem cells before they are reinfused. They have produced promising results.

Sickle cell trait

This is a benign condition with no anaemia and normal appearance of red cells in a blood film. Haematuria is the most common symptom and is thought to be caused by minor infarcts of the renal papillae. There is also an increased risk of exertional rhabdomyolysis, chronic kidney disease, venous thrombosis including pulmonary embolus, and splenic infarction. Hb S varies from 25% to 45% of the total haemoglobin (Fig. 7.12). Care must be taken with anaesthesia, pregnancy and at high altitudes.

Combination of haemoglobin S with other genetic defects of haemoglobin

The most common of these are Hb S/β-thalassaemia and sickle cell/C disease. In Hb S/β-thalassaemia, the MCV and MCH are lower than in homozygous Hb SS. The clinical picture is of sickle cell anaemia; splenomegaly is usual. Patients with Hb SC disease have a particular tendency to thrombosis and pulmonary embolism, especially in pregnancy. In general, when compared with Hb SS disease, they have a higher incidence of retinal abnormalities, milder anaemia, splenomegaly and generally a longer life expectancy. Diagnosis is made by haemoglobin electrophoresis or HPLC, particularly with family studies.

Haemoglobin C disease

This genetic defect of haemoglobin is frequent in West Africa and is caused by substitution of lysine for glutamic acid in the β-globin chain at the same point as the substitution in Hb S. Hb C tends to form rhomboidal crystals and in the homozygous state there is a mild haemolytic anaemia with marked target cell formation, cells with rhomboidal shape and microspherocytes (Fig. 7.21b). The spleen is enlarged. The carriers show a few target cells only. When Hb C is co-inherited with Hb S, the resulting sickling disease tends to be milder, with fewer crises and longer preservation of splenic function.

Haemoglobin D disease

This is a group of variants all with the same electrophoretic mobility. Heterozygotes show no haematological abnormality, while homozygotes have a mild haemolytic anaemia. When Hb D is co-inherited with Hb S, the resulting sickling disease may be especially severe.

Haemoglobin E disease

This is the most common haemoglobin variant in South-East Asia. In the homozygous state, there is a mild microcytic, hypochromic anaemia. Haemoglobin E/β⁰-thalassaemia, however, resembles homozygous β⁰-thalassaemia both clinically and haematologically.

Prenatal diagnosis of genetic haemoglobin disorders

It is important to give genetic counselling to couples at risk of having a child with a major haemoglobin defect. If a pregnant woman is found to have a haemoglobin abnormality, her partner should be tested to determine whether he also carries a defect. When both partners show an abnormality and there is a risk of a serious defect in the offspring, particularly β-thalassaemia major, it is important to offer antenatal diagnosis. Several techniques are available, the choice depending on the stage of pregnancy and the potential nature of the defect.

DNA diagnosis

The majority of samples are obtained by chorionic villus biopsy, although amniotic fluid cells are sometimes used. Techniques to sample maternal blood for fetal cells or fetal DNA are being developed. Fetal blood may be sampled directly in mid-trimester. The DNA is then analysed after amplification by the polymerase chain reaction (PCR). It may be performed by using primer pairs that only amplify individual alleles ('allele-specific priming') or by using consensus primers that amplify all the alleles, followed by restriction digestion to detect a particular allele. This is best illustrated by Hb S, in which the bacterially derived enzyme Dde I detects the A-T change (Fig. 7.22).

Pre-implantation genetic diagnosis which avoids the need for pregnancy termination involves performing conventional *in vitro* fertilization, followed by removing one or two cells from the blastomeres on day 3. PCR is used to detect thalassaemia mutations so that unaffected blastomeres can be selected for implantation. HLA typing can also be used to select a blastomere HLA matching a previous thalassaemia major child, so that the new baby could potentially act as a donor for stem cell transplantation into its older sibling. Ethical considerations are important in deciding to use these applications.

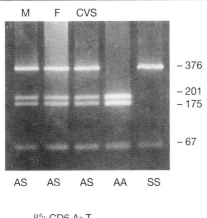

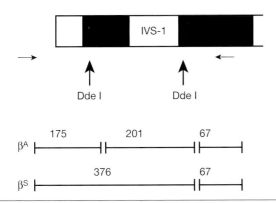

β5: CD6 A>T

Figure 7.22 Sickle cell anaemia: antenatal diagnosis by Dde I-polymerase chain reaction (PCR) analysis. The DNA is amplified by two primers that span the sickle cell gene mutation site and produce a product of 473 base pairs (bp) in size. The product is digested with the restriction enzyme Dde I and the resulting fragments analysed by agarose gel electrophoresis. The replacement of an adenine base in the normal β-globin gene by thymine results in Hb S and removes a normal restriction site for Dde I, producing a larger 376 bp fragment than the normal 175 and 201 bp fragments in the digested amplified product. In this case, the CVS DNA shows both the normal fragments and the larger sickle cell product and so is AS. The gel shows DNA from the mother (M), father (F), fetal DNA from a chorionic villus sample (CVS), a normal DNA control (AA) and a homozygous sickle cell DNA control (SS). Source: Courtesy of Dr. J. Old.

SUMMARY

- Genetic disorders of haemoglobin fall into two main groups:
  1 The thalassaemias in which synthesis of the α- or β-globin chain is reduced.
  2 Structural disorders such as sickle cell anaemia in which an abnormal haemoglobin is produced.
- The α- or β-thalassaemias occur clinically as minor forms with microcytic hypochromic red cells and a raised red cell count with or without anaemia.
- Total absence of function of all four α-globin genes causes hydrops fetalis.
- Total absence of function of both β-globin genes causes β-thalassaemia major, a transfusion-dependent anaemia associated with iron overload with liver, endocrine and cardiac damage. Iron chelation therapy has greatly improved life expectancy
- Thalassaemia intermedia is a clinical term for a group of disorders showing mild to moderate anaemia and is usually caused by variants of β-thalassaemia.

- The most frequent structural defect of haemoglobin is the sickle mutation in the β-globin chain causing, in the homozygous form, a severe haemolytic anaemia, associated with vaso-occlusive crises. These may be painful, affecting bone, or affect soft tissues (e.g. chest, spleen or central nervous system). Crises may also be haemolytic or aplastic.
- Management of sickle cell anaemia involves prevention and treatment of infections and, for acute crises, pain relief and hydration. Blood transfusions are given to prevent organ, especially brain, damage and hydroxycarbamide is valuable in reducing the frequency and severity of acute crises.
- Antenatal diagnosis using PCR technology to amplify chorionic villous DNA is used to detect severe genetic defects of haemoglobin production, with termination of the pregnancy if appropriate.
- Gene therapy for both thalassaemia major and sickle cell anaemia is proving beneficial in early clinical trials.

Now visit **www.wileyessential.com/haematology** to test yourself on this chapter.

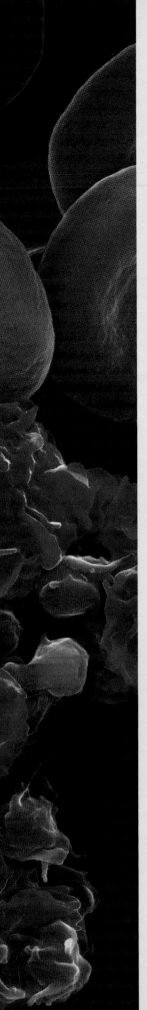

CHAPTER 8
The white cells, part 1: granulocytes, monocytes and their benign disorders

Key topics

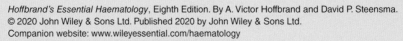

Hoffbrand's Essential Haematology, Eighth Edition. By A. Victor Hoffbrand and David P. Steensma.
© 2020 John Wiley & Sons Ltd. Published 2020 by John Wiley & Sons Ltd.
Companion website: www.wileyessential.com/haematology

The white blood cells (leucocytes) may be divided into two broad groups: the **phagocytes** and the **lymphocytes**. Phagocytes comprise cells of the **innate** immune system, which can act very quickly after an infection, whereas lymphocytes mediate the **adaptive immune response**, which can develop immunological memory, for example after vaccination. Certain lymphocyte subtypes such as natural killer (NK) cells lack memory capacity and are also considered part of the innate immune system.

Phagocytes can themselves be subdivided into granulocytes (which include neutrophils, eosinophils and basophils) and monocytes. Their normal development and function, and benign disorders of white blood cells, are dealt with in this chapter (Table 8.1; Fig. 8.1). Lymphocytes are considered in Chapter 9.

The function of phagocytes and lymphocytes in protecting the body against infection is closely connected with two soluble protein systems of the body: immunoglobulins and complement. These proteins, which may also be involved in blood cell destruction in a number of diseases, are discussed together with the lymphocytes in Chapter 9.

Granulocytes

Neutrophil (polymorph)

This cell has a characteristic dense nucleus consisting of between two and five lobes, and a pale cytoplasm with an irregular outline containing many fine pink–blue (azurophilic) or

Table 8.1 White cells: normal blood counts.			
Adults	**Blood count**	**Children**	**Blood count**
Total leucocytes	$4.0–11.0 \times 10^9$/L*		*Total leucocytes*
Neutrophils	$1.8–7.5 \times 10^9$/L*	Neonates	$10.0–25.0 \times 10^9$/L
Eosinophils	$0.04–0.4 \times 10^9$/L	1 year	$6.0–18.0 \times 10^9$/L
Monocytes	$0.2–0.8 \times 10^9$/L	4–7 years	$6.0–15.0 \times 10^9$/L
Basophils	$0.01–0.1 \times 10^9$/L	8–12 years	$4.5–13.5 \times 10^9$/L
Lymphocytes	$1.5–3.5 \times 10^9$/L		

* Normal subjects of African and Middle Eastern descent may have lower counts. In normal pregnancy the upper limits are total leucocytes 14.5×10^9/L, neutrophils 11×10^9/L. Minor variations in the 'normal' range may be present from laboratory to laboratory.

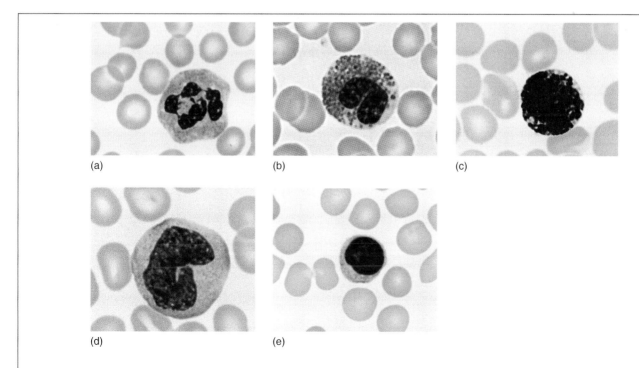

(a) (b) (c)

(d) (e)

Figure 8.1 White blood cells (leucocytes): **(a)** neutrophil (polymorph); **(b)** eosinophil; **(c)** basophil; **(d)** monocyte; **(e)** lymphocyte.

grey–blue granules (Fig. 8.1a). The granules are divided into primary, which appear at the promyelocyte stage, and secondary (specific), which appear at the myelocyte stage and predominate in the mature neutrophil (see Fig. 8.7). Both types of granule are lysosomal in origin: the primary contains myeloperoxidase and other acid hydrolases; the secondary contains lactoferrin, lysozyme and other enzymes. The lifespan of neutrophils in the blood is only 6–10 hours.

Neutrophil precursors

These do not normally appear in normal peripheral blood but are present in the marrow (Fig. 8.2). The earliest recognizable precursor is the **myeloblast**, a cell of variable size which has a large nucleus with fine chromatin and usually two to five nucleoli (Fig. 8.2b). The cytoplasm is basophilic and no granules are present. The normal bone marrow contains up to 5% of myeloblasts.

Myeloblasts give rise to promyelocytes, which are slightly larger cells which retain nucleoli but have developed primary granules in the cytoplasm (Fig. 8.2a). These cells then give rise to myelocytes, which have specific or secondary granules. The nuclear chromatin is now more condensed and nucleoli are not visible. Separate myelocytes of the neutrophil, eosinophil and basophil series can be identified. The myelocytes give rise to **metamyelocytes**, non-dividing cells, which have an indented or horseshoe-shaped nucleus and a cytoplasm filled with primary and secondary granules.

Neutrophil forms between the metamyelocyte and fully mature neutrophil are termed '**band**', 'stab' or 'juvenile'. These cells may occur in normal peripheral blood. They do not contain the clear, fine filamentous distinction between nuclear lobes that is seen in mature neutrophils.

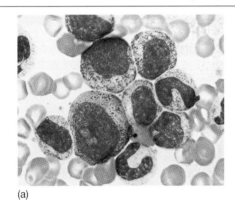

(a)

Figure 8.2 (a) Granulopoiesis. A promyelocyte, myelocytes, and metamyelocytes. Source: A.V. Hoffbrand *et al.* (2019) *Color Atlas of Clinical Hematology: Molecular and Cellular Basis of Disease*, 5th edn. Reproduced by permission of John Wiley & Sons. **(b)** The formation of the neutrophil and monocyte phagocytes. Eosinophils and basophils are also formed in the marrow in a process similar to that for neutrophils.

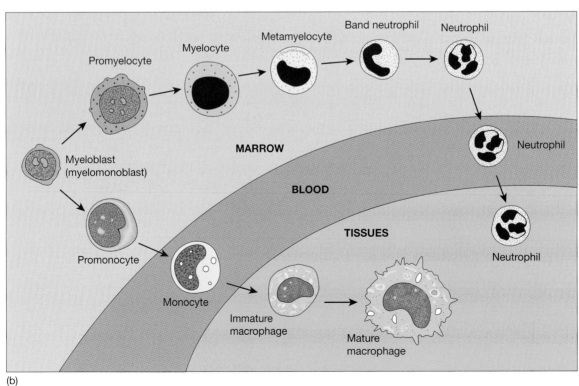

(b)

Monocytes

These are usually larger than other peripheral blood leucocytes and possess a large central oval or indented nucleus with clumped chromatin (Fig. 8.1d). The abundant cytoplasm stains blue and contains many fine vacuoles, giving a ground-glass appearance. Cytoplasmic granules are also often present. The monocyte precursors in the marrow (monoblasts and promonocytes) are difficult to distinguish from myeloblasts and monocytes.

Eosinophils

These cells are similar to neutrophils, except that the cytoplasmic granules are coarser and more deeply red staining and there are rarely more than three nuclear lobes (Fig. 8.1b). Eosinophil myelocytes can be recognized, but earlier stages are indistinguishable from neutrophil precursors. The blood transit time for eosinophils is longer than for neutrophils. They enter inflammatory exudates and have a special role in allergic responses, defence against parasites and removal of fibrin formed during inflammation. Thus they play a role in local immunity and tissue repair.

Basophils

These are only occasionally seen in normal peripheral blood. They have many dark cytoplasmic granules which overlie the nucleus and contain heparin and histamine (Fig. 8.1c). In the tissues they become mast cells. They have immunoglobulin E (IgE) attachment sites and their degranulation is associated with histamine release.

Granulopoiesis

Granulocytes and monocytes are formed in the bone marrow from a common precursor cell (see Fig. 1.2). In the granulopoietic series progenitor cells, myeloblasts, promyelocytes and myelocytes form a proliferative or mitotic pool of cells, while the metamyelocytes, band and segmented granulocytes make up a post-mitotic maturation compartment (Fig. 8.3).

Large numbers of band and segmented neutrophils (10–15 times more than in the blood) are held in the normal marrow as a 'reserve pool'. **The bone marrow normally contains more myeloid cells than erythroid cells in the ratio of 2:1 to 12:1, the largest proportion being neutrophils and metamyelocytes.** Following their release from the marrow, granulocytes spend only 6–10 hours in the circulation before entering tissues, where they perform their phagocytic function. They spend on average 4–5 days in the tissues before they are destroyed during defensive action or as the result of senescence. In the bloodstream there are two pools usually of about equal size: the circulating pool (included in the blood count) and a marginating pool (not included in the blood count).

Control of granulopoiesis: myeloid growth factors

The granulocyte series arises from bone marrow progenitor cells, which are increasingly specialized. Many growth factors are involved in this maturation process including interleukin-1 (IL-1), IL-3, IL-5 (for eosinophils), IL-6, IL-11, granulocyte–macrophage colony-stimulating factor (GM-CSF), granulocyte CSF (G-CSF) and monocyte CSF (M-CSF) (see Fig. 1.6). The growth factors stimulate proliferation and differentiation and also affect the function of the mature cells on which they act (e.g. phagocytosis, superoxide generation and cytotoxicity in the case of neutrophils; see Fig. 1.5). They also inhibit apoptosis.

Increased granulocyte and monocyte production in response to an infection is induced by increased production of growth factors from stromal cells and T lymphocytes, stimulated by endotoxin, and cytokines such as IL-1 or tumour necrosis factor (TNF) (Fig. 8.4).

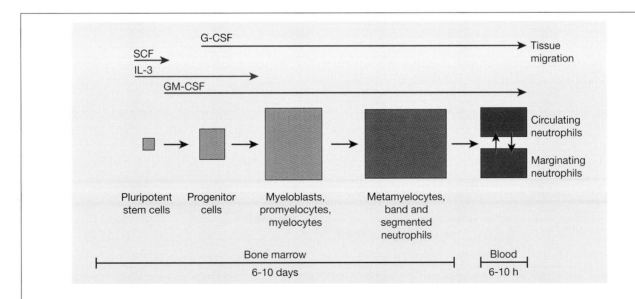

Figure 8.3 Neutrophil kinetics. CSF, colony-stimulating factor; G, granulocyte; IL, interleukin; M, monocyte; SCF, stem cell factor.

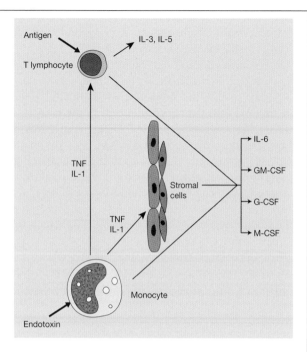

Figure 8.4 Regulation of haemopoiesis; pathways of stimulation of leucopoiesis by endotoxin, for example from infection. It is likely that endothelial and fibroblast cells release basal quantities of granulocyte–macrophage colony-stimulating factor (GM-CSF) and granulocyte colony-stimulating factor (G-CSF) in the normal resting state and that this is enhanced substantially by tumour necrosis factor (TNF) and interleukin-1 (IL-1).

Clinical applications of G-CSF

Clinical administration of G-CSF intravenously or subcutaneously produces a rise in neutrophils. Short-acting G-CSF is given daily. Filgrastim was the original recombinant G-CSF, but numerous bioequivalent forms are now used. A longer-acting PEGylated G-CSF, pegfilgrastim, can be given once in 7–14 days. Indications are:

- **Post-chemotherapy, radiotherapy or stem cell transplantation (SCT)** In these situations, G-CSF accelerates granulocytic recovery and shortens the period of neutropenia (Fig. 8.5). This may translate into a reduction of length of time in hospital, antibiotic usage and frequency of infection, but periods of extreme neutropenia after intensive chemotherapy cannot be prevented. The injections may also allow repeated courses of chemotherapy, e.g. for lymphoma, to be given on schedule rather than being delayed because of prolonged neutropenia, particularly a problem in older patients.
- **Myelodysplastic syndromes and aplastic anaemia** G-CSF has been given alone or in conjunction with erythropoiesis-stimulating agents in an attempt to improve bone marrow function and the neutrophil count.
- **Severe benign neutropenia** Both congenital and acquired neutropenia, including cyclical and drug-induced neutropenia, often respond well to G-CSF.
- **Peripheral blood stem cell mobilization** G-CSF is used to increase the number of circulating multipotent progenitors from donors or the patient, improving the harvest of sufficient peripheral blood stem cells for allogeneic or autologous transplantation.

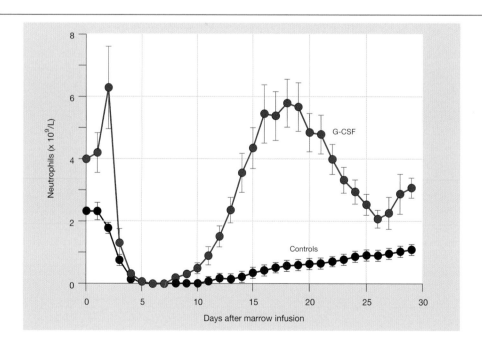

Figure 8.5 Typical effect of granulocyte colony-stimulating factor (G-CSF) on recovery of neutrophils following autologous bone marrow transplantation.

Monocytes

Monocytes spend only a short time in the marrow and, after circulating for 20–40 hours, leave the blood to enter the tissues, where they mature and carry out their principal functions. Their extravascular lifespan after their transformation to **macrophages (histiocytes)** may be as long as several months or even years. In tissues the macrophages become self-replicating without replenishment from the blood. They assume specific functions in different tissues (e.g. skin, gut, liver; Fig. 8.6). One particularly important lineage is that of **dendritic cells**, which are involved in antigen presentation to T cells (see Chapter 9). GM-CSF and M-CSF are involved in their production and activation.

Disorders of neutrophil and monocyte function

The normal function of neutrophils and monocytes may be divided into three phases. Defects resulting in clinical syndromes can occur in each of these phases.

Chemotaxis (cell mobilization and migration)

The phagocyte is attracted to bacteria or the site of inflammation by chemotactic substances released from damaged tissues, by complement components and by the interaction of leucocyte adhesion molecules with ligands on the damaged tissues. The leucocyte adhesion molecules also mediate recruitment and interaction with other immune cells. They are also variously expressed on endothelial cells and platelets (see Chapter 1).

Phagocytosis

The foreign material (e.g. bacteria, fungi) or dead or damaged cells of the host are phagocytosed (Fig. 8.7). Recognition of a foreign particle is aided by opsonization with immunoglobulin or complement, because both neutrophils and monocytes have Fc and C3b receptors (see Chapter 9).

Macrophages have a central role in antigen presentation: processing and presenting foreign antigens on human leucocyte antigen (HLA) molecules to the immune system. They also secrete a large number of growth factors and chemokines, which regulate inflammation and immune responses.

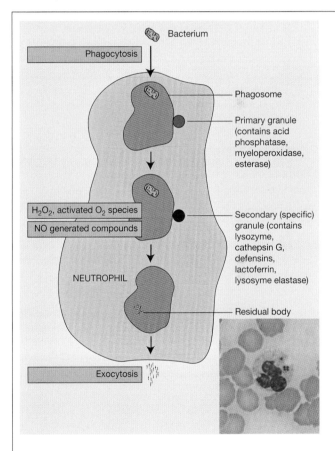

Figure 8.7 Phagocytosis and bacterial destruction. On entering the neutrophil, the bacterium is surrounded by an invaginated surface membrane and fuses with a primary lysosome to form a phagosome. Enzymes from the lysosome attack the bacterium. Secondary granules also fuse with the phagosomes, and new enzymes from these granules including lactoferrin attack the organism. Various types of activated oxygen, generated by glucose metabolism, also help to kill bacteria. Undigested residual bacterial products are excreted by exocytosis. Inset: Neutrophil ingesting meningococci. Source (inset): A.V. Hoffbrand *et al.* (2019) *Color Atlas of Clinical Hematology: Molecular and Cellular Basis of Disease*, 5th edn. Reproduced by permission of John Wiley & Sons.

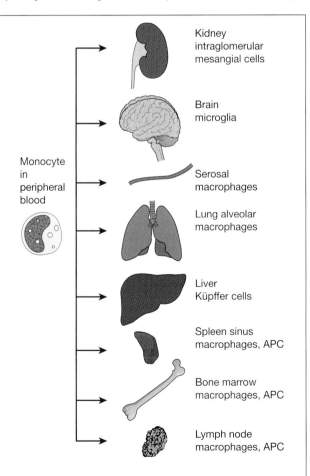

Figure 8.6 Reticuloendothelial system: distribution of macrophages.

Chemokines are chemotactic cytokines which may be produced constitutively and control lymphocyte traffic under physiological conditions; inflammatory chemokines are induced or up-regulated by inflammatory stimuli. They bind to and activate cells via chemokine receptors and play an important part in recruiting appropriate cells to the sites of inflammation.

Killing and digestion

These occur by **oxygen-dependent** and **oxygen-independent** pathways. In the oxygen-dependent reactions, superoxide (O_2^-), hydrogen peroxide (H_2O_2) and other activated oxygen (O_2) species, are generated from O_2 and reduced nicotinamide adenine dinucleotide phosphate (NADPH). In neutrophils, H_2O_2 reacts with myeloperoxidase and intracellular halide to kill bacteria; activated oxygen may also be involved. Nitric oxide (NO), generated through NO synthase from L-arginine, is an oxygen-independent mechanism by which phagocytes also kill microbes.

The other non-oxidative microbicidal mechanisms involve microbicidal proteins. These may act alone (e.g. cathepsin G) or in conjunction with H_2O_2 (e.g. lysozyme, elastase). They may also act with a fall in pH within phagocytic vacuoles into which lysosomal enzymes are released. Lactoferrin, an iron-binding protein, is bacteriostatic by depriving bacteria of iron and generating free radicals (Fig. 8.7).

Defects of phagocytic cell function

Chemotaxis

These defects occur in rare congenital abnormalities (e.g. 'lazy leucocyte' syndrome) and in more common acquired abnormalities, either of the environment, e.g. corticosteroid therapy, or of the leucocytes themselves, e.g. in acute or chronic myeloid leukaemia, myelodysplasia and the myeloproliferative syndromes.

Phagocytosis

These defects usually arise because of a lack of opsonization, which may be caused by congenital or acquired causes of hypogammaglobulinaemia or lack of complement components.

Killing

This abnormality is clearly illustrated by the rare X-linked or autosomal recessive chronic granulomatous disease that results from abnormal leucocyte oxidative metabolism. There is an abnormality affecting different elements of the respiratory burst oxidase or its activating mechanism. The patients have recurring infections, usually bacterial but sometimes fungal, which present in infancy or early childhood.

Other rare congenital abnormalities may result in defects of bacterial killing (e.g. myeloperoxidase deficiency and the Chédiak–Higashi syndrome; see below). Acute or chronic myeloid leukaemia and myelodysplastic syndromes may also be associated with defective killing of ingested microorganisms.

Benign disorders

A number of hereditary conditions may give rise to changes in granulocyte morphology (Fig. 8.8).

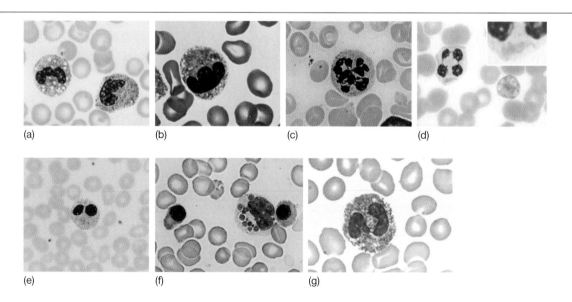

Figure 8.8 Abnormal white blood cells. **(a)** Neutrophil leucocytosis: toxic changes shown by the presence of red–purple granules in the band form neutrophils. **(b)** Neutrophil leucocytosis: a Döhle body can be seen in the cytoplasm of the neutrophil. **(c)** Megaloblastic anaemia: hypersegmented oversized neutrophil in peripheral blood. **(d)** May–Hegglin anomaly: the neutrophils contain basophilic inclusions 2–5 mm in diameter; there is an associated mild thrombocytopenia with giant platelets. **(e)** Pelger–Huët anomaly: coarse clumping of the chromatin in pince nez configuration. **(f)** Chédiak–Higashi syndrome: bizarre giant granules in the cytoplasm of a monocyte. **(g)** Alder anomaly: coarse violet granules in the cytoplasm of a neutrophil.

Pelger–Huët anomaly

In this uncommon symptomless condition, bilobed neutrophils are found in the peripheral blood. Occasional unsegmented neutrophils are also seen. Inheritance is autosomal dominant, usually due to mutations in the gene encoding the lamin B receptor (LBR), which is important for cholesterol synthesis. It is most common in Northern Europeans. In myelodysplastic syndromes, cells resembling Pelger–Huët neutrophils are often seen on a blood film; these are called **pseudo-Pelger–Huët cells** because they lack the LBR mutations characteristic of the inherited condition.

May–Hegglin anomaly

In this rare condition the neutrophils contain basophilic inclusions of RNA (resembling Döhle bodies) in the cytoplasm. There is an associated mild thrombocytopenia with giant platelets. Inheritance is autosomal dominant and usually due to mutations in the *MYH9* gene, which encodes a myosin heavy chain.

Other rare disorders

In contrast to these two benign anomalies, other rare congenital leucocyte disorders may be associated with severe disease. The Chédiak–Higashi syndrome is inherited in an autosomal recessive manner, and there are giant granules in the neutrophils, eosinophils, monocytes and lymphocytes, accompanied by neutropenia, thrombocytopenia and marked hepatosplenomegaly. It is due to mutations in the *CHS1 (LYST)* gene, which encodes a lysosomal trafficking regulator. Abnormal leucocyte granulation or vacuolation is also seen in patients with rare mucopolysaccharide disorders (e.g. Hurler's syndrome).

Common morphological abnormalities

Figure 8.8 also shows some of the more common abnormalities of neutrophil morphology that can be seen in peripheral blood. Hypersegmented forms occur in megaloblastic anaemia, Döhle bodies and toxic changes in infection. A 'drumstick' (Barr body) appears on the nucleus of a proportion of the neutrophils in normal females and is caused by the presence of two X chromosomes (not illustrated).

Causes of neutrophil leucocytosis

An increase in circulating neutrophils to levels greater than 7.5×10^9/L is one of the most frequently observed blood count changes. The causes of neutrophil leucocytosis are given in Table 8.2. Neutrophil leucocytosis is sometimes accompanied by fever as a result of the release of leucocyte pyrogens. Other characteristic features of reactive neutrophilia may include (a) a 'shift to the left' in the peripheral blood differential white cell count, an increase in the number of band forms and the occasional presence of more primitive cells such as metamyelocytes and myelocytes; and (b) the presence of cytoplasmic toxic granulation and Döhle bodies (Fig. 8.8a, b).

Table 8.2 Causes of neutrophil leucocytosis.
Bacterial infections (especially pyogenic bacterial, localized or generalized)
Inflammation and tissue necrosis (e.g. myositis, vasculitis, cardiac infarct, trauma)
Metabolic disorders (e.g. uraemia, eclampsia, acidosis, gout)
Pregnancy
Neoplasms of all types (e.g. carcinoma, lymphoma, melanoma)
Acute haemorrhage or haemolysis
Drugs (e.g. corticosteroid therapy, which inhibits margination; lithium, tetracycline)
Chronic myeloid leukaemia, myeloproliferative neoplasms (polycythaemia vera, myelofibrosis, essential thrombocythaemia)
Treatment with G-CSF (granulocyte colony-stimulating factor)
Rare inherited disorders
Asplenia

The leukaemoid reaction

The leukaemoid reaction is a reactive and excessive leucocytosis usually characterized by the presence of immature cells (e.g. myeloblasts, promyelocytes and myelocytes) in the peripheral blood. Associated disorders include severe or chronic infections, severe haemolysis or metastatic cancer. Leukaemoid reactions are often particularly marked in children.

Leucoerythroblastic reaction

This is characterized by the presence of erythroblast and granulocyte precursors in the blood (Fig. 8.9). It is due to metastatic infiltration of the marrow or certain benign or neoplastic blood disorders (Table 8.3).

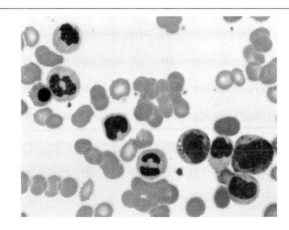

Figure 8.9 Leucoerythroblastic blood film. This shows an erythroblast, promyelocyte, myelocyte and metamyelocytes in a patient with metastatic breast carcinoma in the bone marrow.

Table 8.3 Causes of leucoerythroblastic blood film.

Metastatic neoplasm in the marrow

Primary myelofibrosis

Acute and chronic myeloid leukaemias

Myeloma, lymphoma

Miliary tuberculosis

Severe megaloblastic anaemia

Severe haemolysis

Osteopetrosis

Secondary marrow fibrosis, e.g. due to rheumatological syndromes

Table 8.4 Causes of neutropenia.

Selective neutropenia
Congenital

Acquired
Drug-induced
    Anti-inflammatory drugs (aminopyrene, gold, levamisole, penicillamine)
    Antibacterial drugs (cephalosporins, co-trimoxazole, meropenem)
    Metronidazole, penicillins, sulfasalazine, tobramycin, vancomycin
    Anticonvulsants (carbamazepine, valproate)
    Antithyroids (carbimazole, methimazole)
    Hypoglycaemics (tolbutamide)
    Phenothiazines (chlorpromazine, thioridazine)
    Psychotropics and antidepressants (clozapine, olanzapine, imipramine)
    Miscellaneous (deferiprone, furosemide, mepacrine, rituximab, ticlopidine)

Benign (racial or familial)

Cyclical
Idiopathic and clonal neutropenia of uncertain significance (see Chapter 16)
Autoimmune
Associated with chronic autoimmune diseases, e.g. systemic lupus erythematosus, Sjogren's syndrome
Rheumatoid arthritis (Felty syndrome)
Hypersensitivity and anaphylaxis
Large granular lymphocytic leukaemia (see p. 227)
Infections
Viral (e.g. hepatitis, influenza, HIV)
Fulminant bacterial infection (e.g. typhoid, military tuberculosis)

Part of general pancytopenia (see Table 22.1)

HIV, human immunodeficiency virus.

Neutropenia

The lower limit of the normal neutrophil count is 1.8×10^9/L, except in people of African and Middle Eastern descent where values around 1.5×10^9/L are normal. This has been called 'benign ethnic neutropenia'. Lower normal values are also found from 2–3 weeks after birth for the first few months of life (Table 31.1). When the absolute neutrophil level falls below 0.5×10^9/L, the patient is likely to have recurrent infections, and when the count falls to less than 0.2×10^9/L the risks are very serious, particularly if there is also a functional defect. Neutropenia may be selective (Table 8.4) or part of a general pancytopenia (see Chapter 22). It may also be acute or chronic (lasting >3 months).

Benign ethnic neutropenia

Up to 98% of people of West African origin carry a polymorphism in the Duffy antigen chemokine receptor (*DARC*) gene which leads to loss of DARC expression on red cells. This has been selected during evolution because the malaria parasite *Plasmodium vivax* uses DARC as a receptor to enter the red cell. DARC is a chemokine receptor and the loss of its expression on white cells is associated with a lowering of the median neutrophil count by around 0.5×10^9/L. A similar effect is seen in some populations in the Middle East. The reduction in the neutrophil count may result from increased neutrophil margination, which can also occur in other ethnic groups, but there are no significant clinical consequences.

Congenital neutropenia

Severe congenital neutropenia (previously called Kostmann syndrome) usually presents in the first year of life with life-threatening infections. Most cases are dominantly inherited, caused by mutations of the gene *ELANE2*, coding for neutrophil elastase. Other types are autosomal recessive, and mutations of more than 10 genes have been described. In some cases the neutropenia occurs as part of other syndromes with

non-haematological manifestations, e.g. Wiskott–Aldrich, Shwachman–Diamond (p. 275) or Chédiak–Higashi (p. 103). G-CSF produces a clinical response in most patients. Some of the forms predispose to myelodysplastic syndromes or acute myeloid leukaemia.

Drug-induced neutropenia

A large number of drugs have been implicated (Table 8.4), which may induce neutropenia either by direct toxicity or immune-mediated damage, the drug acting as a hapten. For many drugs the mechanism remains obscure.

Cyclical neutropenia

This is a rare syndrome with 2–4-week periodicity. Severe but temporary neutropenia occurs. Monocytes tend to rise as the neutrophils fall. Germline mutation of *ELANE2*, the gene for neutrophil elastase, underlies some cases.

Idiopathic and clonal neutropenia of uncertain significance

In these conditions there is neutropenia without morphological features in the blood or marrow cells of myelodysplastic syndromes or another haematological neoplasm. They are defined and discussed under the general descriptions of idiopathic and clonal cytopenias in Chapter 16.

In the idiopathic form (benign chronic neutropenia) no clonal genetic mutations are detected. This is the most common type of chronic neutropenia in both children and adults. It is more common in females and thought to be brought about in some cases by immune cells causing inhibition of myelopoiesis in the bone marrow. If an immune aetiology can be confirmed, e.g. by detection of antineutrophil antibodies, a definite diagnosis of autoimmune neutropenia is made (see below). In the clonal form, clonal genetic mutations are found in the blood and bone marrow cells similar to those found in clonal haemopoiesis of indeterminate prognosis (CHIP; see p. 203).

Autoimmune neutropenia

In some cases of chronic neutropenia an autoimmune mechanism can be demonstrated. The antibody may be directed against one of the neutrophil-specific antigens. The detection of neutrophil antibodies requires difficult laboratory procedures and test characteristics (sensitivity and specificity) are poor, so the tests are not performed routinely.

Clinical features

Severe neutropenia is particularly associated with infections of the mouth and throat. Painful and often intractable ulceration may occur at these sites (Fig. 8.10), on the skin or at the anus. Septicaemia rapidly supervenes. Organisms carried as commensals by normal individuals, such as *Staphylococcus epidermidis* or Gram-negative organisms in the bowel, may become pathogens. Other features of infections associated with severe neutropenia are described in Chapter 12.

Diagnosis

Bone marrow examination is useful in determining the severity of damage in granulopoiesis (i.e. whether there is reduction in early precursors or whether there is reduction only of circulating and marrow neutrophils, with late precursors remaining in the marrow). Marrow aspiration and trephine biopsy may also provide evidence of leukaemia, myelodysplasia or other infiltration.

Management

The treatment of patients with acute severe neutropenia is described on p. 150. In many patients with drug-induced neutropenia, spontaneous recovery occurs within 1–2 weeks after stopping the drug. Patients with chronic neutropenia have recurrent infections which are mainly bacterial in origin, although fungal and viral infections (especially herpes) also

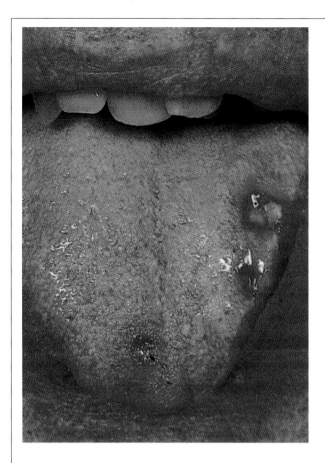

Figure 8.10 Ulceration of the tongue in severe neutropenia.

occur. **Early recognition and vigorous treatment with antibiotics, antifungal or antiviral agents, as appropriate, are essential**. Prophylactic antifungal agents, e.g. fluconazole, are often given and antibacterial agents, e.g. ciprofloxacin, may reduce the risk, but resistance is of concern (see Chapter 12). G-CSF or its PEGylated form is effective at raising the neutrophil count in a variety of benign chronic neutropenic states. Corticosteroid therapy or splenectomy has been associated with good results in some patients with autoimmune neutropenia. Corticosteroids impair neutrophil function and should not be used indiscriminately in patients with neutropenia. Rituximab (anti-CD20) may also be effective, although it may itself be a cause of neutropenia. Haemopoietic stem cell transplantation may be indicated if clonal evolution to myelodysplasia occurs.

Causes of monocytosis, eosinophil and basophil leucocytosis

Monocytosis

A rise in blood monocyte count above 0.8×10^9/L is infrequent. The conditions causing monocytosis are listed in Table 8.5.

Table 8.5 Causes of monocytosis.

Chronic bacterial infections: tuberculosis, brucellosis, bacterial endocarditis, typhoid
Connective tissue diseases: SLE, temporal arteritis, rheumatoid arthritis
Protozoan infections
Chronic neutropenia
Hodgkin lymphoma, AML and other malignancies
Chronic myelomonocytic leukaemia (CMML)

AML, acute myeloid leukaemia; SLE, systemic lupus erythematosus.

Table 8.6 Causes of eosinophilia.

Allergic diseases, especially hypersensitivity of the atopic type (e.g. bronchial asthma, hay fever and food sensitivity)
Parasitic diseases (e.g. amoebiasis, hookworm, ascariasis, tapeworm infestation, filariasis, schistosomiasis, strongyloidiasis and trichinosis)
Recovery from acute infection
Certain skin diseases (e.g. psoriasis, pemphigus and dermatitis herpetiformis, urticaria and angioedema, atopic dermatitis) and skin parasites (e.g. scabies. myiasis)
Drug sensitivity
Polyarteritis nodosa, vasculitis, serum sickness Autoimmune (e.g. inflammatory bowel disease, sarcoidosis)
Graft-versus-host disease
Hodgkin lymphoma and some other lymphoid tumours, especially clonal T-cell disorders, adenocarcinoma
Metastatic malignancy with tumour necrosis
Hypereosinophilic syndrome (idiopathic)
Pulmonary syndromes Eosinophilic pneumonia, transient pulmonary infiltrates (Loeffler's syndrome), allergic granulomatosis (Churg–Strauss syndrome), tropical pulmonary eosinophilia
Chronic eosinophilic leukaemia
Other myeloproliferative neoplasms, including systemic mastocytosis

Eosinophilic leucocytosis (eosinophilia)

The causes of an increase in blood eosinophils (Fig. 8.11) above 0.4×10^9/L are listed in Table 8.6. **It is most frequently due to allergic diseases, parasites, skin diseases or drugs**. If a cause such as asthma or severe atopy is not obvious, a diligent search for precipitants must be undertaken, including testing for *Strongyloides* and stool ova and parasites. Sometimes no underlying cause is found, and no clonal marker can be detected. If the eosinophil count is elevated (above 1.5×10^9/L) for over 6 months and associated with tissue damage for which no other cause can be detected, then the **hypereosinophilic syndrome (HES)** is diagnosed. In the HES, the heart valves, central nervous system (CNS), skin and lungs may be affected. Treatment is usually first with high-dose corticosteroids and second-line with cytotoxic drugs, e.g. imatinib, hydroxycarbamide, methotrexate or immunosuppressants, ciclosporine or alpha-interferon. In 25% of cases a clonal T-cell population is driving the eosinophilia.

Loeffler syndrome is a transient reactive form affecting the lungs and the Churg–Strauss syndrome consists of a vasculitis with eosinophilic granulomas affecting the respiratory tract.

In other cases of chronic eosinophilia, often with similar clinical features to idiopathic cases, a clonal cytogenetic or molecular abnormality is present such as a mutation or rearrangement in *PDGFRA* or *B* or *KIT*, and chronic eosinophilic leukaemia is diagnosed (see p. 194). These cases sometimes respond to tyrosine kinase inhibitors such as imatinib or midostaurin.

Basophil leucocytosis (basophilia)

An increase in blood basophils above 0.1×10^9/L is uncommon. The usual cause is a myeloproliferative disorder such as chronic myeloid leukaemia or polycythaemia vera. Reactive basophil increases are sometimes seen in myxoedema, during smallpox or chickenpox infection and in ulcerative colitis.

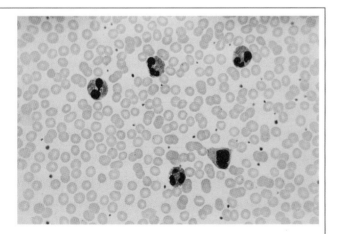

Figure 8.11 Eosinophilia.

Histiocytic and dendritic cell disorders

Histiocytes are myeloid-derived tissue macrophages. The disorders are listed in Table 8.7.

Dendritic cells

These are specialized antigen-presenting cells found mainly in the skin, lymph nodes, spleen and thymus. They comprise:

1 Myeloid-derived cells, including Langerhans' cells, which are present in skin and mucosae and are characterized by the presence of tennis racquet-shaped Birbeck granules, seen in electron-microscopy sections in neutrophils, eosinophils, macrophages and lymphocytes.

2 A lymphocyte-derived subset (Fig. 1.6).

The primary role of dendritic cells is antigen presentation to T and B lymphocytes (p. 119).

Langerhans' cell histiocytosis

Langerhans' cell histiocytosis (LCH) includes diseases previously called histiocytosis X, and falls into three clinical groups: **Letterer–Siwe (multisystem) disease**, **Hand–Schüller–Christian disease** (a triad of bone lesions, polyuria due to posterior pituitary involvement and exophthalmos) and **eosinophilic granuloma** (one or more bone lesions). The disease may be single organ or multisystem. There is a clonal proliferation of myeloid-derived cells resembling antigen-presenting cells of the skin. Mutations of the *BRAF* or *MAP2K1* genes may be present.

The multisystem disease affects children in the first 3 years of life with hepatosplenomegaly, lymphadenopathy and eczematous skin symptoms. Localized lesions may occur, especially in the skull, ribs and long bones, the posterior pituitary causing diabetes insipidus, the CNS, gastrointestinal tract and lungs. The lesions include CD1a-positive Langerhans' cells

(characterized by the presence of Birbeck granules), eosinophils, lymphocytes, neutrophils and macrophages. Cladrabine and cytosine arabinoside have been used in therapy and may improve survival.

Haemophagocytic lymphohistiocytosis

Haemophagocytic lymphohistiocytosis (HLH, haemophagocytic syndrome) is a rare, recessively inherited or more frequently acquired disease, defined by overwhelming activation of macrophages and T lymphocytes. HLH is usually precipitated by a viral (especially Epstein–Barr), bacterial or fungal infection or occurring in association with autoimmune diseases or neoplasms, most commonly non-Hodgkin lymphoma.

In the familial form, various genes involved in regulation of macrophage function or regulation, such as perforin and *UNC13D*, have been shown to be mutated. More damaging mutations may result in presentation in childhood and 'milder' variants may only present in adulthood when a trigger such as a neoplasm develops.

Patients present with fever and pancytopenia, often with splenomegaly and liver dysfunction. **There are increased numbers of histiocytes in the bone marrow which ingest red cells, white cells and platelets (Fig. 8.12)**. Clinical features often also include lymphadenopathy, hepatic and splenic enlargement, coagulopathy and CNS signs. Common laboratory anomalies include very elevated serum ferritin and C-reactive protein, reduced albumin and fibrinogen, low or absent NK cell activity, and elevated CD25 level (soluble IL-2 receptor).

Treatment is of the underlying infection or neoplasm, if known, with support care, and with antimacrophage and immunomodulatory drugs. Chemotherapy with daunorubicin, etoposide, corticosteroids, ciclosporin, ruxolitinib, rituximab (anti-CD20) or antithymocyte globulin may be tried. An antibody to interferon-γ appears effective in some paediatric cases. The condition is often fatal.

Sinus histiocytosis with massive lymphadenopathy

This is also known as the Rosai–Dorfman syndrome. There is painless, chronic cervical lymphadenopathy. There may be fever and weight loss. The histology is typical with sheets of foamy macrophages. The condition usually subsides over months or years. Mutations in *KRAS* and *MAPZK1* have been detected in some cases.

Malignant diseases of histiocytic or dendritic cells include sarcomas, chronic myelomonocytic leukaemia (see Chapter 16) and a rare neoplasm called blastic plasmacytoid dendritic cell neoplasm (see Chapter 13).

Lysosomal storage diseases

Gaucher, Tay–Sachs and Niemann–Pick diseases all result from hereditary deficiency of the enzymes required for glycolipid breakdown.

Table 8.7 Classification of the histiocytic and dendritic cell disorders.

Benign

Dendritic cell related
Langerhans' cell histiocytosis
Solitary dendritic cell histiocytoma

Histiocyte related
Haemophagocytic lymphohistiocytosis primary (familial), secondary (infection, drug, tumour)
Sinus histiocytosis with massive lymphadenopathy (Rosai–Dorfman syndrome)

Malignant
Dendritic and histiocytic sarcomas (localized or disseminated)
Acute myeloid leukaemia, monocytic and myelomonocytic (p. 161)
Chronic myelomonocytic leukaemia (p. 204)

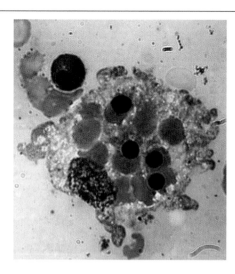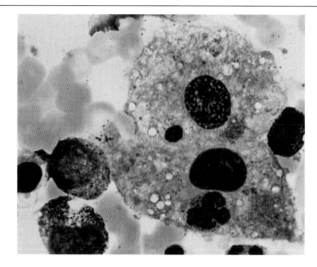

Figure 8.12 Haemophagocytic lymphohistiocytosis: bone marrow aspirates showing histiocytes that have ingested red cells, erythroblasts and neutrophils.

Gaucher disease

Gaucher disease is an uncommon autosomal recessive disorder characterized by an accumulation of glucosylceramide in the lysosomes of reticuloendothelial cells as a result of deficiency of glucocerebrosidase (Fig. 8.13).

Three types occur: a chronic adult type (type I), an acute infantile neuronopathic type (type II) and a subacute neuronopathic type with onset in childhood or adolescence (type III). It is caused by a variety of mutations in the glucocerebrosidase gene, one type of which (a single base pair substitution in codon 444) is particularly common in Ashkenazi Jews and explains the high incidence of Type 1 disease in this group. In type I the outstanding physical sign is splenomegaly. Moderate liver enlargement and pingueculae (conjunctival deposits) are other characteristics. Often the presenting symptom is easy bruising. This is due to thrombocytopenia

with abnormal platelet function and coagulation defects. In many cases, bone deposits cause bone pain and pathological fractures. Osteoporosis is also frequent. Expansion of the lower end of the femur may produce the 'Erlenmeyer flask deformity' (Fig. 8.14).

The clinical manifestations are caused by the accumulation of glucocerebroside-laden macrophages in the spleen, liver and bone marrow (Fig. 8.15). Gaucher disease at all ages is commonly associated with marked anaemia, leucopenia and thrombocytopenia, occurring singly or in combination. Gaucher cells are not inert lipid storage containers but are metabolically active, secreting proteins that cause secondary pathology, e.g. pulmonary hypertension, alveolar fibrosis and cholesterol gallstones. Polyclonal hypergammaglobulinaemia or monoclonal gammopathy is frequent due to activation of B lymphocytes by NK cells, themselves activated by macrophages laden with glycolipids. There is an increased risk of myeloma. Carriers of a Gaucher mutation also have an increased incidence and earlier onset of Parkinson's disease.

Diagnosis is made by assay of white cell glucocerebrosidase and DNA analysis. Lysosomal enyzmes, chitotriosidase and acid phosphatase are raised and useful in monitoring therapy. Serum levels of pulmonary activation regulated cytokine (Parc), angiotensin-converting enzyme (ACE) and ferritin are also elevated.

Enzyme replacement therapy with glucocerebrosidase as imiglucerase (Cerezyme), velaglucerase or taliglucerase, made by recombinant technology and given intravenously once every 2 weeks, is effective in treating the disease with shrinkage of spleen, rise in blood count and improved bone structure (Fig. 8.15). Oral drugs, miglustat or eliglustat, are useful alone in mild forms or in combination with the intravenous enzyme. They inhibit glucosylceramide synthase (Fig. 8.14) and so reduce the amount

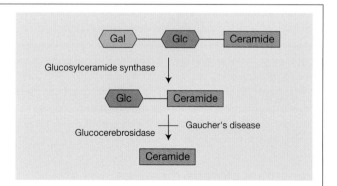

Figure 8.13 Gaucher disease results from a deficiency of glucocerebrosidase. Gal, galactose; Glc, glucose.

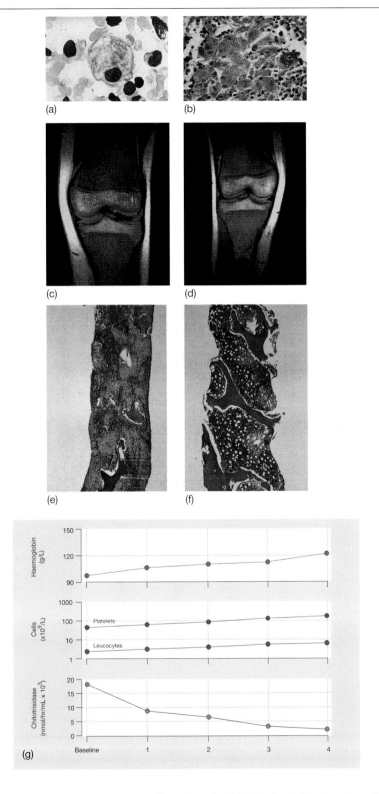

Figure 8.14 Gaucher disease: **(a)** bone marrow aspirate – a Gaucher cell with 'fibrillar' cytoplasmic pattern; **(b)** spleen histology – pale clusters of Gaucher cells in the reticuloendothelial cord; **(c)** magnetic resonance imaging (MRI) scan of the left knee of a patient before treatment showing Erlenmeyer flask deformity with expansion of the marrow and thinning of the cortical bone; **(d)** following a year of glucocerebrosidase therapy with subsequent remodelling of bone; and bone marrow trephine biopsy before **(e)** and after **(f)** 2 years of glucocerebrosidase therapy. **(g)** Improvement in blood counts and chitotriosidase levels with glucocerebrosidase therapy. Source: (g) A.B. Mehta, D.A. Hughes. In A.V. Hoffbrand *et al.* (eds) (2016) *Postgraduate Haematology*, 7th edn. Reproduced with permission of John Wiley & Sons.

of substrate being produced in lysosomes. The use of enzyme replacement has virtually eliminated the need for splenectomy, but it cannot reverse established osteonecrosis, bone deformation, or hepatic, splenic or marrow fibrosis. Enzyme replacement has no impact, however, on CNS disease types II and III. Stem cell transplantation has been carried out successfully in severely affected patients, usually with type II or III disease.

Niemann–Pick disease

Niemann–Pick disease shows certain clinical and pathological similarities to Gaucher disease. It is caused by a sphingomyelinase deficiency. The majority of patients are infants who die in the first few years of life, although occasional patients survive to adult life. Massive hepatosplenomegaly occurs and there is usually lung and nervous system involvement, with retarded physical and mental development. A 'cherry-red' spot is commonly seen in the retina of affected infants. Pancytopenia is a regular feature and in marrow aspirates 'foam cells' of similar size to Gaucher cells are seen. Chemical analysis of the tissues reveals that the disorder is caused by an accumulation of sphingomyelin and cholesterol.

SUMMARY

- Granulocytes include neutrophils (polymorphs), eosinophils and basophils. They are made in the bone marrow under the control of a variety of growth factors and have a short lifespan in the bloodstream before entering tissues.
- Phagocytes (neutrophils and monocytes) are the body's main defence against bacterial infection. Neutrophil leucocytosis occurs in bacterial infection and in other types of inflammation.
- Neutropenia, if severe, predisposes to infections. It may be caused by bone marrow failure, chemotherapy or radiotherapy drugs, or may be selective caused by immune, drug or other mechanisms or occur congenitally. G-CSF may be given to raise the neutrophil count.
- Eosinophilia is most frequently caused by allergic diseases, including skin diseases, parasitic infections or drugs. It can also be caused by a clonal increase in eosinophils, termed chronic eosinophilic leukaemia, or by an idiopathic condition, the hypereosinophilic

  syndrome, which is associated with damage to the lungs, heart, skin or other tissues.
- Defects of function of neutrophils and monocytes may affect their chemotaxis, phagocytosis or killing.
- Histiocytes are tissue macrophages derived from circulation monocytes. They may form clonal diseases called Langerhans' cell histiocytosis, which affect single or multiple organs.
- The haemophagocytic syndrome (HLH) involves destruction of red cells, granulocytes and platelets by tissue macrophages.
- Lysosomal storage diseases are caused by inherited defects in the enzymes responsible for breakdown of glycolipids. Gaucher disease, the most common of them to affect haemopoiesis, is caused by glucocerebrosidase deficiency and is associated with accumulation of glycolipids in the reticuloendothelial system, with splenomegaly, pancytopenia and bone lesions causing the main clinical manifestations. Treatment is with enzyme replacement or substrate reduction therapy.

Now visit **www.wileyessential.com/haematology** to test yourself on this chapter.

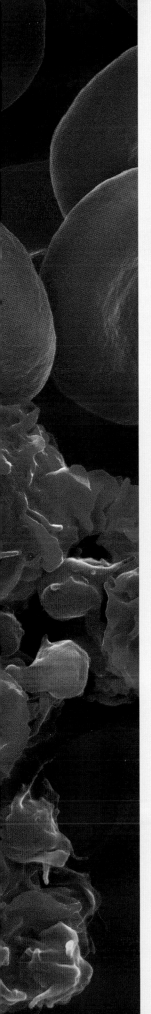

CHAPTER 9

The white cells, part 2: lymphocytes and their benign disorders

Key topics

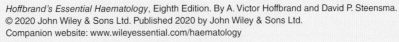

Hoffbrand's Essential Haematology, Eighth Edition. By A. Victor Hoffbrand and David P. Steensma.
© 2020 John Wiley & Sons Ltd. Published 2020 by John Wiley & Sons Ltd.
Companion website: www.wileyessential.com/haematology

Lymphocytes are the immunologically competent cells that assist phagocytes in defence of the body against infection and other foreign invasion, including protection from neoplastic cells (Fig. 9.1). Two unique features characteristic of this component of the immune system are the ability to generate antigenic specificity and the phenomenon of immunological memory. A complete description of the functions of lymphocytes is beyond the scope of this book, but information essential to an understanding of the diseases of the lymphoid system, and of the role of lymphocytes in other haematological diseases, is included here.

Lymphocytes

In postnatal life, the bone marrow and thymus are the primary lymphoid organs in which lymphocytes develop (Fig. 9.2). The secondary lymphoid organs in which specific immune responses are generated are the lymph nodes, spleen and lymphoid tissues of the alimentary and respiratory tracts. In the bone marrow lymphocytes derive from haemopoietic stem cells through a common myeloid lymphoid progenitor.

B and T lymphocytes

The immune response depends upon two types of lymphocytes, B and T cells (Table 9.1), which both derive from the haemopoietic stem cell through myeloid-lymphoid and then lymphoid progenitor cells. Interleukins 4 and 7 are involved (See Fig. 1.6). B cells are named after the avian organ (bursa) in which they were first identified, and T cells are named after the thymus.

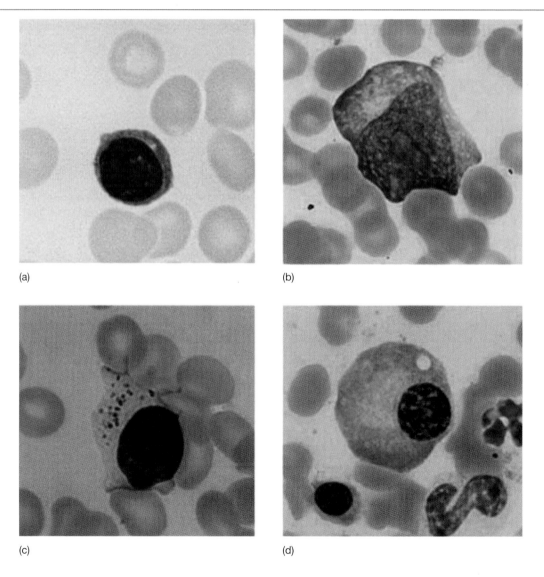

(a)

(b)

(c)

(d)

Figure 9.1 Lymphocytes: **(a)** small lymphocyte; **(b)** activated lymphocyte; **(c)** large granular lymphocyte; **(d)** plasma cell.

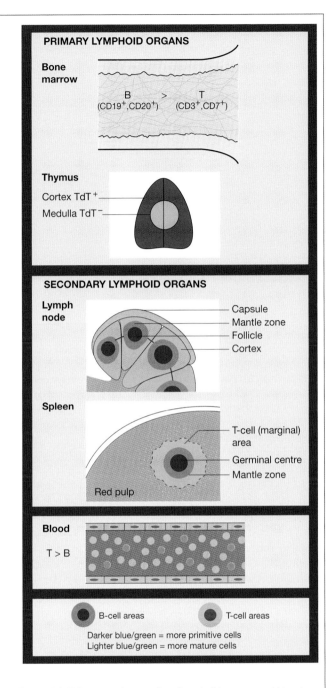

Figure 9.2 Primary and secondary lymphoid organs and blood.

Table 9.1 Functional aspects of T and B cells.

	T cells	B cells
Origin	Thymus	Bone marrow
Tissue distribution	Parafollicular areas of cortex in nodes, periarteriolar in spleen	Germinal centres of lymph nodes, spleen, gut, respiratory tract; also subcapsular and medullary cords of lymph nodes
Blood	80% of lymphocytes; CD4 > CD8	20% of lymphocytes
Membrane receptors	TCR for antigen	BCR (= immunoglobulin) for antigen
Function	CD8⁺: CMI against intracellular organisms CD4⁺: T-cell help for antibody production and generation of CMI	Humoral immunity by generation of antibodies
Characteristic surface markers	CD1 CD2 CD3 CD4 or 8 CD5 CD6 CD7 HLA class I HLA class II when activated	CD19 CD20 CD22 CD9 (pre-B cells) CD10 (precursor B cells) CD79 a and b HLA class I and II
Genes rearranged	TCR α, β, γ, δ	IgH, Igk, Igl

BCR, B-cell receptor; C, complement; CMI, cell-mediated immunity; Ig, immunoglobulin; TCR, T-cell receptor.

B cells mature in the bone marrow and circulate in the peripheral blood until they undergo recognition of antigen. The **B-cell receptor (BCR)** is membrane-bound immunoglobulin (Fig. 9.3) and binds to a specific antigen. This leads to activation of phosphoinositide 3-kinase (PI3K), which produces a second messenger phosphatidylinositol (3,4,5)-trisphosphate (PIP3; Fig. 9.4), and also of Bruton tyrosine kinase (BTK), which phosphorylates further downstream enzymes. The overall effect is to induce expression of AKT, which is an anti-apoptotic pro-survival kinase. Effective drugs for treating the B cell neoplasms, chronic lymphocytic leukaemia and non-Hodgkin lymphoma, inhibit BTK (ibrutinib, acalabrutinib) and PI3K (idelalisib, duvelisib, copanlisib; see Chapter 18). The B-cell receptor itself is secreted as free soluble immunoglobulin (Fig. 9.5). **The B cell can mature into a memory B cell or plasma cell**. Plasma cells home to the bone marrow and have a characteristic morphology with an eccentric round nucleus, a 'clock-face' chromatin pattern, and strongly basophilic cytoplasm (Fig. 9.1d). They express intracellular but not surface immunoglobulin and produce large amounts of antibody.

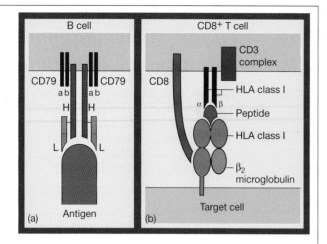

Figure 9.3 Antigen receptors on lymphocytes and their interaction with antigen. **(a)** The B-cell antigen receptor is membrane-bound immunoglobulin (see Fig. 9.4). The antigen-binding immunoglobulin molecule is associated with the CD79 heterodimer, which acts as a signal transduction unit. **(b)** The T-cell receptor consists of a number of components that together constitute the CD3 complex. Two antigen-binding chains (α, β) are associated with several proteins (γ, δ, ε, ζ) that mediate signal transduction. Antigen is recognized in the form of short peptides held on the surface of human leucocyte antigen (HLA) molecules. CD8⁺ T cells interact with peptide on a class I HLA molecule and the CD8 heterodimer interacts with the α_3 domain of the class I protein.

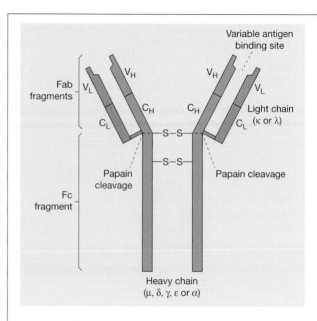

Figure 9.5 Basic structure of an immunoglobulin (Ig) molecule. Each molecule is made up of two light (k or l; blue areas) and two heavy (purple) chains, and each chain is made up of variable (V) and constant (C) portions, the V portions including the antigen-binding site. The heavy chain (m, δ, γ, ε or α) varies according to the immunoglobulin class. IgA molecules form dimers, while IgM forms a ring of five molecules. Papain cleaves the molecules into an Fc fragment and two Fab fragments.

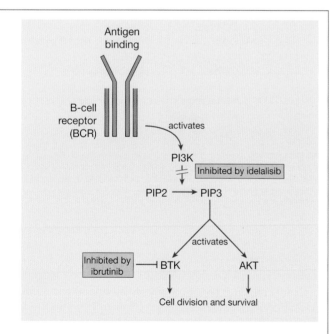

Figure 9.4 Signalling from the B-cell receptor after antigen binding occurs through phosphoinositide-3-kinase (PI3K), which produces a second messenger phosphtidyl triphosphate (PIP3), which activates Bruton tyrosine kinase (BTK) and AKT. Idelalisib inhibits PI3K and ibrutinib inhibits BTK.

T cells develop from cells that have migrated to the thymus, where they differentiate into mature T cells during passage from the cortex to the medulla. During this process, self-reactive T cells are deleted (negative selection), whereas T cells with some specificity for host human leucocyte antigen (HLA) molecules are selected (positive selection). The mature helper cells express CD4 and cytotoxic cells express CD8 (Table 9.1). The cells also express one of two T-cell antigen receptor heterodimers, $\alpha\beta$ (>90%) or $\gamma\delta$ (<10%). They recognize antigen only when it is presented at a cell surface (see below).

Engineering of T cells, including chimeric antigen receptor T cells

The immunological capacity of T cells is being harnessed for different types of therapeutic uses:

1 T lymphocytes can be harvested from patients, manipulated *in vitro* and reinfused as an anti-cancer therapy (Fig 9.6). **Chimeric antigen receptor T cells (CAR-T cells)** are T lymphocytes that have been genetically engineered to express a construct that includes both an antigen-specific receptor and various co-stimulatory molecules (Figure 9.6a) The effectiveness largely depends on which co-stimulatory molecules are chosen. The most promising CAR-T cells have been developed against CD19, an antigen expressed on B-ALL and most B cell lymphomas. Other CAR-T cells

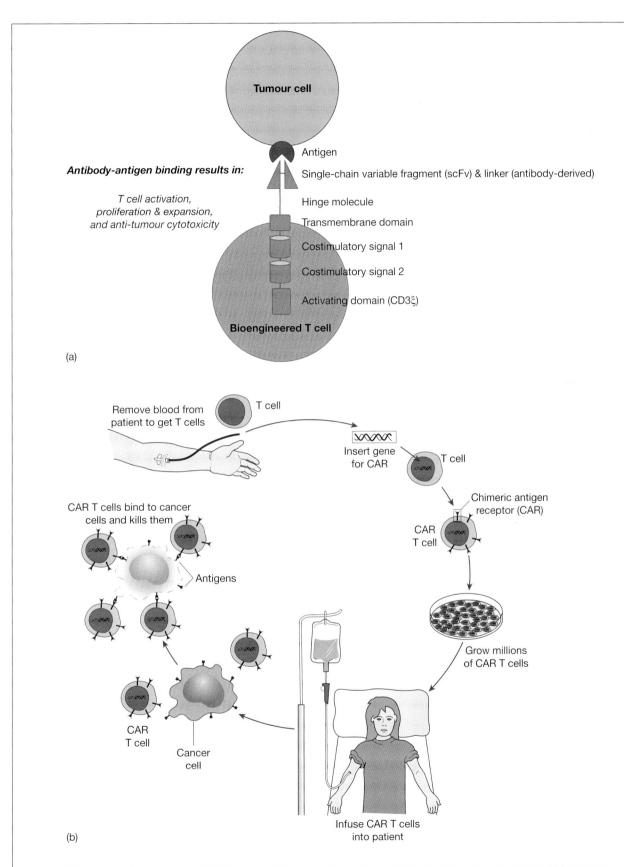

Figure 9.6 Chimeric antigen receptor (CAR)-T cells. **(a)** These T cells are engineered to express a gene construct with immune co-stimulatory and activating signals, and a T-cell receptor with antigen specificity relevant to the tumour target (e.g. CD19 in B-cell lymphoid neoplasms). **(b)** T lymphocytes are harvested from the patient, genetically engineered *in vitro*, expanded and reinfused, aimed at killing neoplastic cells. Source: https://visualsonline.cancer.gov/details.cfm?imageid=11776, reproduced with permission of Terese Winslow.

are being developed against antigens expressed on multiple myeloma cells, e.g. B cell maturation antigen (BCMA) and myeloid-associated antigens, e.g. CD33 and CD123, that are expressed in acute myeloid leukaemia.

2 T cells with particular antigen specificity can be harvested from a healthy donor and infused into a patient to control an infection. This is also being done for difficult post-allogeneic stem cell transplant viral infections, such as cytomegalovirus and Epstein–Barr virus (EBV). Similar procedures have been introduced for treating post-transplantation EBV positive lymphoid malignancies.

Natural killer cells

Natural killer (NK) cells are cytotoxic lymphocytes that lack the T-cell receptor (TCR) and are considered part of the innate rather than the adaptive immune system. They are large cells with cytoplasmic granules (see Fig. 9.1c) and typically express surface molecules CD16 (Fc receptor), CD56 and CD57.

NK cells are designed to kill target cells that have a low level of expression of HLA class I molecules, such as may occur during viral infection or on a malignant cell. NK cells do this by displaying a number of receptors for HLA molecules on their surface. When HLA is expressed on the target cell, these deliver an inhibitory signal into the NK cell. When HLA molecules are absent on the target cell, this inhibitory signal is lost and the NK cell can then kill its target.

In addition, NK cells display antibody-dependent cell-mediated cytotoxicity (ADCC). In this, antibody binds to antigen on the surface of the target cell and then NK cells bind to the Fc portion of the bound antibody and kill the target cell.

Lymphocyte circulation

Lymphocytes in the peripheral blood migrate through **post-capillary venules** into the substance of the lymph nodes or into the spleen or bone marrow. T cells home to the perifollicular zones of the cortical areas of lymph nodes (paracortical areas; Fig. 9.2) and to the periarteriolar sheaths surrounding the central arterioles of the spleen. B cells selectively accumulate in follicles of the lymph nodes and spleen. Lymphocytes

return to the peripheral blood via the efferent lymphatic stream and the thoracic duct.

Immunoglobulins

These are a group of proteins produced by plasma cells and B lymphocytes that bind to antigen. They are divided into five subclasses or isotypes: immunoglobulin G (IgG), IgA, IgM, IgD and IgE. IgG, the most common, contributes approximately 80% of normal serum immunoglobulin and is further subdivided into four subclasses: IgG_1, IgG_2, IgG_3 and IgG_4. IgA is subdivided into two types. IgM is usually produced first in response to antigen, IgG subsequently and for a more prolonged period. The same cell can switch from IgM to IgG, or to IgA or IgE synthesis. IgA is the main immunoglobulin in secretions, particularly of the gastrointestinal tract. IgD and I_gE (involved in delayed hypersensitivity reactions) are minor fractions. Some important biochemical and biological properties of the three main immunoglobulin subclasses are summarized in Table 9.2.

The immunoglobulins are all made up of the same basic structure (Fig. 9.5), consisting of **two heavy chains** which are called gamma (γ) in IgG, alpha (α) in IgA, mu (m) in IgM, delta (δ) in IgD and epsilon (ϵ) in IgE, and **two light chains** – kappa (k) or lambda (λ) – which are common to all five immunoglobulins. The heavy and light chains each have highly variable regions, which give the immunoglobulin specificity, and constant regions, in which there is virtual complete correspondence in amino acid sequence in all antibodies of a given isotype (e.g. IgA, IgG) or isotype subclass (e.g. IgG_1, IgG_2). IgG antibody can be broken into a constant Fc fragment and two highly variable Fab fragments. IgM molecules are much larger because they consist of five subunits.

The main role of immunoglobulins is defence of the body against foreign organisms. They also have a vital role in the pathogenesis of a number of haematological disorders. For example, secretion of a specific immunoglobulin from a monoclonal population of lymphocytes or plasma cells causes **paraproteinaemia** (see p. 256). Bence–Jones protein found in the urine in some cases of myeloma consists of a monoclonal

Table 9.2 Some properties of the three main classes of immunoglobulin (Ig).

	IgG	IgA	IgM
Molecular weight	140000	140000	900000
Normal serum level (g/L)	6.0–16.0	1.5–4.5	0.5–1.5
Present in	Serum and extracellular fluid	Serum and other body fluids (e.g. of bronchi and gut)	Serum only
Complement fixation	Usual	Yes (alternative pathway)	Usual and very efficient
Placental transfer	Yes	No	No
Heavy chain	(γ_{1-4})	α (α_1 or α_2)	μ

secretion of light chains or light-chain fragments (either k or λ). Immunoglobulins may bind to blood cells in a variety of immune disorders and cause their agglutination (e.g. in cold agglutinin disease; p. 75) or destruction following direct complement lysis or after elimination by the reticuloendothelial (RE) system, as in autoimmune haemolytic anaemia and immune thrombocytopenia.

Antigen–receptor gene rearrangements

Immunoglobulin gene rearrangements

The immunoglobulin heavy-chain and κ and λ light-chain genes occur on chromosomes 14, 2 and 22, respectively. **In the germline state, the heavy-chain gene consists of separate segments for variable (V), diversity (D), joining (J) and constant (C) regions. Each of the V, D and J regions contains a number (*n*) of different gene segments (Fig. 9.7).** In cells not committed to immunoglobulin synthesis, these gene segments remain in their separate germline state. During early differentiation of B cells there is rearrangement of heavy-chain genes so that one of the V heavy-chain segments combines with one of the D segments, which has itself already combined with one of the J segments. Thus, they form a transcriptionally active gene for the heavy chain. The protein coding segments of the C region mRNA are joined to the V region after splicing out intervening RNA. The class of immunoglobulin that is secreted depends on which of the nine (4γ, 2α, 1μ, 1δ and 1ε) constant regions is used. Diversity is introduced by the variability of which V segment joins with which D and with which J segment. In the arbitrary example shown in Fig. 9.7, V_2 joins with D_1 and J_2. Additional diversity is generated by the enzyme terminal deoxynucleotidyl transferase (TdT), which inserts a variable number of new bases into the DNA of the D region at the time of gene rearrangement. Further mutation of the V region genes occurs in the germinal centres of secondary lymphoid tissues (called somatic mutation; see below).

Similar rearrangements occur during generation of the light-chain gene (Fig. 9.8). Enzymes called **recombinases** are needed both in B and T cells to join up the adjacent pieces of DNA after excision of intervening sequences. These recognize certain heptamer- and nonamer-conserved sequences flanking the various gene segments. Mistakes in recombinase activity play an important part in the chromosome translocations of B- or T-cell malignancy.

T-cell receptor gene rearrangements

The vast majority of T cells contain a TCR composed of a heterodimer of α and β chains. In a minority of T cells, the TCR is composed of γ and δ chains. The α, β, γ and δ genes of the TCRs each include V, D, J and C regions. During T-cell ontogeny, rearrangements of these gene segments occur in a similar fashion to those for immunoglobulin genes, thus creating T cells expressing a wide variety (10^8 or more) of TCR structures (Figs 9.3, 9.9). TdT is involved in creating additional diversity and the same recombinase enzymes used in B cells are involved in joining up TCR gene segments.

Complement

The complement system includes a series of plasma proteins constituting an amplification enzyme system which is capable of lysis of bacteria (or of blood cells) or can 'opsonize' (coat) bacteria or cells so that they are phagocytosed. The complement sequence consists of nine major

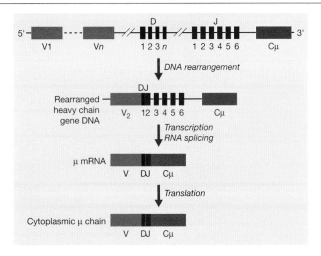

Figure 9.7 Rearrangement of a heavy-chain immunoglobulin gene. One of the V segments is brought into contact with a D, a J and a C (in this case Cm) segment, forming an active transcriptional gene from which the corresponding mRNA is produced. The DJ rearrangement precedes VDJ joining. The class of immunoglobulin depends on which of the nine constant regions (1m, 1δ, 4γ, 2α, 1ε) is used.

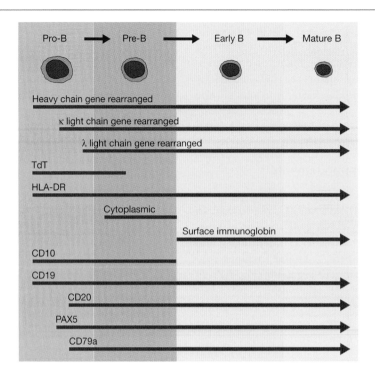

Figure 9.8 The sequence of immunoglobulin gene rearrangement, antigen and immunoglobulin expression during early B-cell development. Intracytoplasmic CD22 is not depicted, but is also a feature of very early B cells. HLA, human leucocyte antigen; TdT, terminal deoxynucleotidyl transferase.

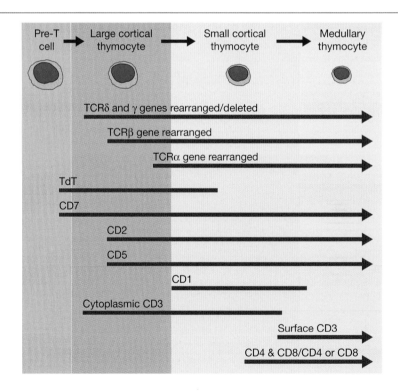

Figure 9.9 The sequence of events during early T-cell development. The earliest events appear to be the expression of surface CD7, intranuclear terminal deoxynucleotidyl transferase (TdT) and intracytoplasmic CD3, followed by T-cell receptor (TCR) gene rearrangement. Early medullary thymocytes express both CD4 and CD8, but they then lose one or other of these structures.

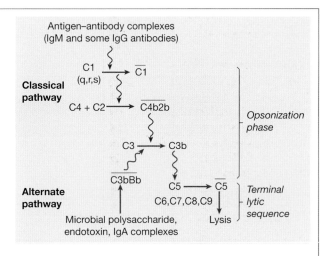

Figure 9.10 The complement (C) sequence. The activated factors are denoted by a bar over the number. Both pathways generate a C3 convertase. In the classic pathway, the convertase is the major (b) component of C4 and C2 (C4b2b). In the alternate pathway, it is the combination of C3b and the major fragment (b) of factor B (C3bBb).

components – C1, C2, etc. – which are activated in turn and form a cascade, resembling the coagulation sequence (Fig. 9.10). The most abundant and pivotal protein is C3, which is present in plasma at a level of approximately 1.2 g/L. The early (opsonizing) stages leading to coating of the cells with C3b can occur by two different pathways:

1 The **classical pathway**, usually activated by IgG or IgM coating of cells; or

2 The **alternate pathway**, which is more rapid and activated by IgA, endotoxin (from Gram-negative bacteria) and other factors (Fig. 9.10).

Macrophages and neutrophils have C3b receptors and they phagocytose C3b-coated cells. C3b is degraded to C3d, detected in the direct antiglobulin test using an anti-complement agent (p. 379). If the complement sequence goes to completion (C9), there is generation of an active phospholipase that punches holes in the cell membrane (e.g. of the red cell or bacterium), causing direct lysis. The complement pathway also generates the biologically active fragments C3a and C5a, which act directly on phagocytes to stimulate the respiratory burst (p. 102). Both may trigger anaphylaxis by release of mediators from tissue mast cells and basophils, which cause vasodilatation and increased permeability.

The immune response

One of the most striking features of the immune system is its capacity to produce a highly *specific* response. For both T and B cells this specificity is achieved by the presence of a particular receptor on the lymphocyte surface (Fig. 9.3). Naïve (or virgin) B and T lymphocytes which leave the bone marrow and

thymus are resting cells that are not in cell division. They recirculate in the lymphatic system. Specialized macrophages called dendritic cells (DCs; p. 107) process antigens before presenting them to B and T lymphocytes – they are therefore known as **antigen-presenting cells** (APCs). The immune system contains many different lymphocytes. Each of these lymphocytes has a receptor that shows differences in structure from that of any other lymphocyte. Consequently, each lymphocyte will bind to only a restricted number of antigens. T and B cells undergo clonal expansion if they meet an APC that is presenting an antigen that can trigger their antigen receptor molecules. At this stage, lymphocytes may develop into effector cells (such as plasma cells or cytotoxic T cells) or memory cells.

DC precursors constitutively migrate at low levels from blood into tissues, but their rate of migration is increased at the site of inflammation. Immature DCs are efficient at macropinocytosis, which allows them to capture antigens from the environment.

T cells are unable to bind antigen free in solution and require it to be presented on APCs in the form of peptides held on the surface of HLA molecules (Fig. 9.3b). T cells recognize the antigen only when it is presented with 'self' HLA molecules and so are known as **HLA-restricted**. The CD4 molecule on helper cells recognizes class II (HLA-DP, -DQ and -DR) molecules, whereas the CD8 molecule recognizes class I (HLA-A, -B and -C) molecules (see Fig. 23.5). The antigen recognition site of the TCR is joined to several other subunits in the CD3 complex, which together mediate signal transduction. Depending on their cytokine production, CD4⁺ T cells can be broadly subdivided into T helper type 1 (Th1) and Th2 cells. Th1 cells produce mainly IL-2, TNF-β and γ-interferon (IFN-γ), and are important in boosting cell-mediated immunity (and granuloma formation), whereas Th2 cells produce IL-4 and IL-10 and are mainly responsible for providing help for antibody production.

Antigen-specific immune responses are generated in **secondary lymphoid organs** and commence when antigen is carried into a lymph node (Fig. 9.11) on dendritic cells. B cells recognize antigen through their surface immunoglobulin and, although most antibody responses require help from antigen-specific T cells, some antigens such as polysaccharides can lead to T-cell-independent B cell antibody production. In the follicle, germinal centres arise as a result of continuing response to antigenic stimulation (Fig. 9.12). These consist of follicular dendritic cells (FDCs), which are loaded with antigen, B cells and activated T cells which have migrated up from the T zone. Proliferating B cells move to the dark zone of the germinal centre as **centroblasts**, where they undergo somatic mutation of their immunoglobulin variable-region genes (Fig. 9.12). Their progeny are known as **centrocytes** and these must be selected for survival by antigen on FDCs, otherwise they undergo apoptosis. If selected they become memory B cells or plasma cells (Fig. 9.12). Plasma cells migrate to the bone marrow and other sites in the RE system and produce high-affinity antibody.

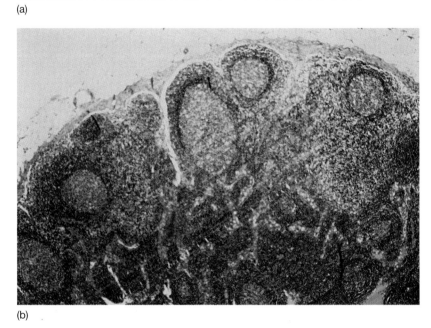

(a)

(b)

Figure 9.11 (a) Structure of a lymph node. **(b)** Lymph node showing germinal follicles surrounded by a darker mantle zone rim and lighter, more diffuse marginal and T-zone areas.

Lymphocytosis

Lymphocytosis often occurs in infants and young children in response to infections that would produce a neutrophil reaction in adults. Conditions particularly associated with lymphocytosis are listed in Table 9.3.

Infectious mononucleosis

Glandular fever is a general term for a disease characterized by fever, sore throat, lymphadenopathy and atypical lymphocytes in the blood. It may be caused by **primary infection with EBV (infectious mononucleosis)**, cytomegalovirus, human immunodeficiency virus (HIV) or *Toxoplasma*. EBV infection is the most common cause.

In most cases primary infection with EBV is subclinical. The disease is characterized by a lymphocytosis caused by clonal expansions of T cells reacting against B lymphocytes infected with EBV. The disease is associated with a high titre of heterophile ('reacting with cells of another species') antibody which reacts with sheep, horse or ox red cells.

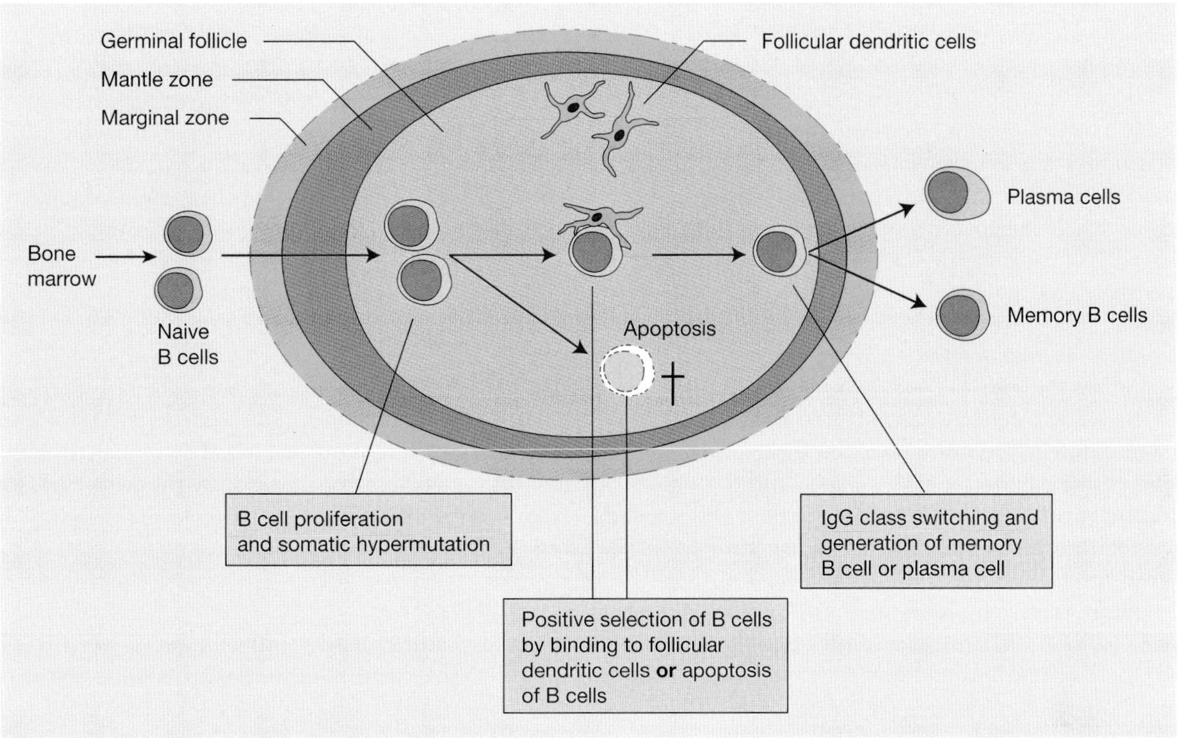

Figure 9.12 Generation of a germinal centre. B cells activated by antigen migrate from the T zone to the follicle, where they undergo massive proliferation. Cells enter the dark zone as centroblasts and accumulate mutations in their immunoglobulin V genes. Cells then pass back into the light zone (Fig. 9.11) as centrocytes. Only those cells that can interact with antigen on follicular dendritic cells and receive signals from antigen-specific T cells (Fig. 9.10) are selected and migrate out as plasma cells and memory cells. Cells not selected die by apoptosis.

Table 9.3 Causes of lymphocytosis.

Infections
Acute
- Bacterial: pertussis, bordetella
- Viral: infectious mononucleosis, rubella, mumps, acute infectious lymphocytosis, infectious hepatitis, cytomegalovirus, human immunodeficiency virus (HIV), herpes simplex or zoster
Chronic
- Tuberculosis, toxoplasmosis, brucellosis, leishmaniasis, syphilis

Other non-neoplastic disorders
- Physiological stress (trauma, major surgery, septic shock, myocardial infarction)
- Hyposplenism
- Hypersensitivity, e.g. insect bites, drug reaction
- Stress, e.g. trauma, major surgery, myocardial infarct, septic shock
- Chronic polyclonal (idiopathic; cigarette smoking, associated with cancer but polyclonal)
- Thyrotoxicosis

Neoplastic
- Chronic lymphoid leukaemias and monoclonal B lymphocytosis (Chapter 18)
- Acute lymphoblastic leukaemia (Chapter 17)
- Non-Hodgkin lymphoma (Chapter 20)

Clinical features

The majority of patients are between the ages of 15 and 40 years. A prodromal period of a few days occurs with lethargy, malaise, headaches, stiff neck and a dry cough. In established disease the following features may be found:

1. Bilateral cervical lymphadenopathy is present in 75% of cases. Symmetrical generalized lymphadenopathy occurs in 50% of cases. The nodes are discrete and may be tender.
2. Over half of patients have a sore throat with inflamed oral and pharyngeal surfaces. Follicular tonsillitis is frequently seen.
3. Fever may be mild or severe.
4. A morbilliform rash, severe headache and eye signs (e.g. photophobia, conjunctivitis and periorbital oedema) are not uncommon. The rash may follow therapy with amoxicillin or ampicillin.
5. Palpable splenomegaly occurs in over half of patients and hepatomegaly in approximately 15%. Approximately 5% of patients are jaundiced.
6. Peripheral neuropathy, severe anaemia (caused by autoimmune haemolysis) or purpura (caused by thrombocytopenia) are less frequent complications.

Diagnosis

Pleomorphic atypical lymphocytosis A moderate rise in white cell count (e.g. $10–20 \times 10^9/L$) with an absolute lymphocytosis is usual, and some patients have even higher counts. Large numbers of atypical lymphocytes are seen in the peripheral blood film (Fig. 9.13). These T cells are variable in appearance, but most have nuclear and cytoplasmic features similar to those seen during reactive lymphocyte transformation. The greatest number of atypical lymphocytes are usually found between the seventh and tenth days of the illness.

Heterophile antibodies

Heterophile antibodies against sheep or horse red cells may be found in the serum at high titres. Slide screening tests, such as the **monospot test**, use formalinized horse red cells to test for the IgM antibodies which agglutinate the cells. Highest titres occur during the second and third weeks and the antibody persists in most patients for six weeks.

EBV antibody

A rise in the titre of IgM antibody against the EBV capsid antigen (VCA) may be demonstrated during the first 2–3

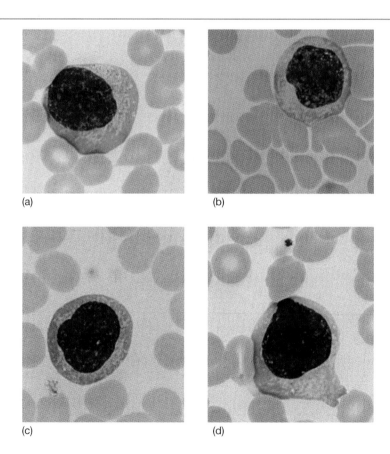

(a)　　　　　　　　(b)

(c)　　　　　　　　(d)

Figure 9.13 (a–d) Infectious mononucleosis: representative 'reactive' T lymphocytes in the peripheral blood film of a 21-year-old man (see also Fig. 9.1b).

weeks. Specific IgG antibody to the EBV nuclear antigen (EBNA) and IgG VCA antibodies develop later and persist for life. A polymerase chain reaction (PCR) assay is also available.

Haematological abnormalities

Haematological abnormalities other than the atypical lymphocytosis are frequent. Occasional patients develop an autoimmune haemolytic anaemia. The IgM autoantibody is typically of the 'cold'-reactive type and usually shows 'i' blood group specificity. Thrombocytopenia is frequent and an autoimmune thrombocytopenic purpura occurs in a smaller number of patients.

Differential diagnosis

The differential diagnosis of infectious mononucleosis includes cytomegalovirus, HIV or toxoplasmosis infection; acute leukaemia; influenza; rubella; bacterial tonsillitis; and infectious hepatitis.

Treatment

In the great majority of patients only symptomatic treatment is required. Corticosteroids are sometimes given to those with severe systemic symptoms. Patients characteristically develop an erythematous rash if given ampicillin therapy. Most patients recover fully 4–6 weeks after initial symptoms. However, convalescence may be slow and associated with severe malaise and lethargy.

Lymphopenia

Lymphopenia may occur in severe bone marrow failure, with corticosteroid and other immunosuppressive therapy, in Hodgkin lymphoma and with widespread irradiation. It also occurs during treatment with the monoclonal antibody alemtuzumab (anti-CD52) and in a variety of immunodeficiency syndromes, the most important of which is HIV infection (see p. 367).

Immunodeficiency

A large number of inherited or acquired deficits in any of the components of the immune system can cause an impaired immune response with increased susceptibility to infection (Table 9.4). If the principal lack is T cells (as in AIDS), this leads not only to bacterial infections, but also to viral, protozoal, fungal and mycobacterial infections. In some cases, however, lack of specific subsets of T cells which control B-cell maturation may lead to a secondary lack of B-cell function, as in many cases of common variable immunodeficiency, which may develop in children or adults of either sex. In others, a primary defect of B cells or of APCs is present. X-linked agammaglobulinaemia is due to an inherited defect of the enzyme Bruton tyrosine kinase (see p. 114) and is characterized by failure of B-cell development; pyogenic bacterial infections dominate the clinical course. Immunoglobulin replacement therapy can be given by monthly courses of intravenous immunoglobulin.

Table 9.4 Classification of immunodeficiencies.

Primary	*Examples:*
B cell (antibody deficiency)	X-linked agammaglobulinaemia, acquired common variable hypogammaglobulinaemia, selective IgA, IgM or IgG subclass deficiencies Thymic aplasia (DiGeorge's syndrome)
T cell Mixed B and T cell	Severe combined immune deficiency (as a result of ADA or PNP or MHC class II deficiency or other causes) Multisystem disorders: ataxia-telangiectasia; Wiskott–Aldrich and polyendocrinopathy syndromes
Secondary	*Examples:*
B cell (antibody deficiency)	Myeloma, nephrotic syndrome, protein-losing enteropathy
T cell	AIDS
T and B cell	Hodgkin lymphoma Non-Hodgkin lymphoma Drugs: steroids, ciclosporin, azathioprine, fludarabine, etc. Radiation therapy Chronic lymphocytic leukaemia Post-stem cell transplantation AntiCD52 (alemtuzumab), other chemotherapy Post-transfusion

ADA, adenosine deaminase; AIDS, acquired immune deficiency syndrome; Ig, immunoglobulin; MHC, major histocompatibility complex; PNP, purine nucleoside phosphorylase.

Rare syndromes include aplasia of the thymus, severe combined (T and B) immunodeficiency as a result of adenosine deaminase deficiency, and selective deficiencies of IgA or IgM. Acquired immune deficiency occurs after cytotoxic chemotherapy or radiotherapy and is particularly pronounced after allogeneic stem cell transplantation, where dysregulation of the immune system persists for 1 year or more. Immunodeficiency is also frequently associated with lymphoid and plasma cell neoplasms such as chronic lymphocytic leukaemia and myeloma. Transfusions can cause a temporary immunodeficiency.

Differential diagnosis of lymphadenopathy

The principal causes of lymphadenopathy are listed in Fig. 9.14. The clinical history and examination give essential information. **The age of the patient, length of history, associated symptoms of possible infectious or malignant disease, whether the nodes are painful or tender, consistency of the nodes and whether there is generalized or local lymphadenopathy are all important.** The size of the liver and spleen are assessed. In the case of local node enlargement, it is important to look for inflammatory or malignant disease in the associated lymphatic drainage area.

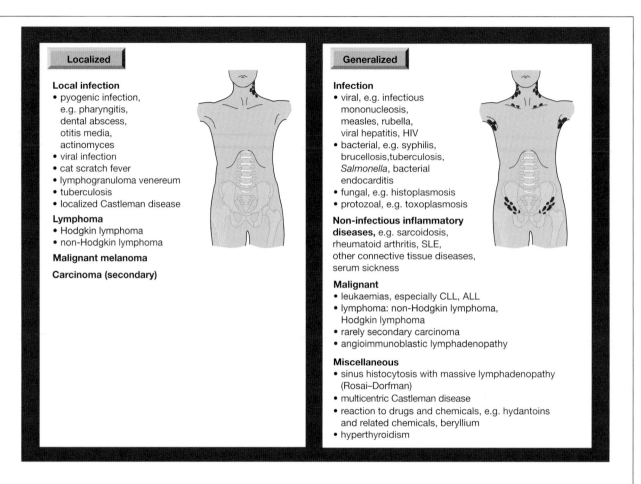

Figure 9.14 Causes of lymphadenopathy. ALL, acute lymphoblastic leukaemia; CLL, chronic lymphocytic leukaemia; SLE, systemic lupus erythematosus. Malignancies are listed in red.

Further investigations will depend on the initial clinical diagnosis, but it is usual to include a full blood count, blood film and erythrocyte sedimentation rate (ESR). Chest X-ray, monospot test or other EBV assay, cytomegalovirus and *Toxoplasma* titres or PCR, and anti-HIV and Mantoux tests are frequently needed. In many cases, it will be essential to make a histological diagnosis by node biopsy, usually core biopsy (e.g. with a Trucut® needle), in which a core of node is removed under radiological control. Fine needle aspirates give less material, destroy the architecture and so are less reliable in diagnosis. **Computed tomography (CT) scanning is valuable in determining the presence and extent of deep node enlargement. Appearances that suggest a 'normal' node include:**

1 **Short axis diameter <1 cm.**
2 **Normal architecture (elongated, fatty hilum, not round or indistinct).**
3 **Normal enhancement (no necrosis or hypervascularity).**
4 **Normal number of nodes (no increase defined as a cluster of ≥3 nodes in a single nodal station or ≥2 nodes in ≥2 node regions.**

In cases of deep node enlargement, where enlarged superficial nodes are not available for biopsy, bone marrow or liver biopsy, CT- or ultrasound-guided Trucut deep node biopsy is needed in an attempt to reach a histological diagnosis. Biopsy of the spleen is not performed, as it may cause splenic rupture requiring splenectomy. Follow-up CT scan after 3-6 months is recommended if nodes are suspicious and biopsy has been performed and there is no underlying disorder. FDG-PET (fluorodeoxyglucose-positron emission tomography) scanning is not recommended, as it is non-specific, more expensive and less effective. It may be negative in some low-grade lymphomas and positive in inflammatory and autoimmune disorders.

SUMMARY

- Lymphocytes are immunologically competent white cells that are involved in antibody production (B cells) and with the body's defence against viral infection or other foreign invasion (T cells).
- They arise from haemopoietic stem cells in the marrow, T cells being subsequently processed in the thymus.
- B cells secrete antibodies specific for individual antigens.
- T lymphocytes are further subdivided into helper (CD4$^+$) and cytotoxic (CD8$^+$) cells. They recognize peptides on HLA antigens.
- Natural killer cells are cytotoxic CD8+ cells that kill target cells with low expression of HLA molecules.
- The immune response occurs in the germinal centre of lymph nodes and involves B-cell and T-cell proliferation, somatic mutation, selection of cells by recognition of antigen on antigen-presenting cells and formation of plasma cells (which secrete immunoglobulin) or memory B cells.
- Immunoglobulins include five subclasses or isotypes, IgG, IgA, IgM, IgD and IgG, all made up of two heavy chains and two light chains (κ or λ).
- Complement is a cascade of plasma proteins that can either lyse cells or coat (opsonize) them so they are phagocytosed.
- Lymphocytosis is usually caused by acute or chronic infections or by lymphoid leukaemias or lymphomas.
- Lymphadenopathy may be localized (because of local infection or malignancy) or generalized because of infection, non-infectious inflammatory diseases, malignancy or drugs.

Now visit **www.wileyessential.com/haematology** to test yourself on this chapter.

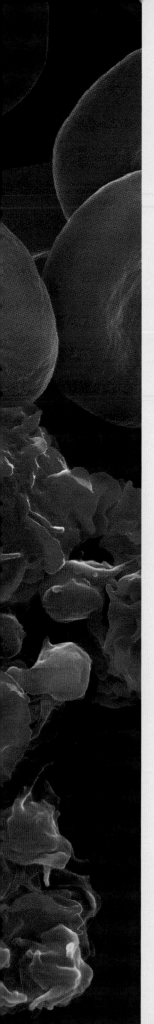

CHAPTER 10
The spleen

Key topics

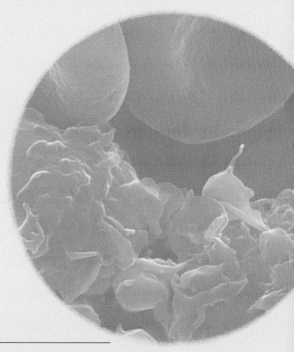

Hoffbrand's Essential Haematology, Eighth Edition. By A. Victor Hoffbrand and David P. Steensma.
© 2020 John Wiley & Sons Ltd. Published 2020 by John Wiley & Sons Ltd.
Companion website: www.wileyessential.com/haematology

The spleen has an important and unique role in the function of the haemopoietic and immune systems. As well as being directly involved in many diseases of these systems, a number of important clinical features are associated with hypersplenic and hyposplenic states.

The anatomy and circulation of the spleen

The spleen lies under the left costal margin, has a normal weight of 150–250 g and a length of between 5 and 13 cm. It is normally not palpable, but becomes palpable when the size is increased to over 14 cm.

Blood enters the spleen through the splenic artery, which then divides into **trabecular arteries**, which permeate the organ and give rise to **central arterioles** (Fig. 10.1). The majority of the arterioles end in **cords**, which lack an endothelial lining and form an open blood system unique to the spleen, with a loose reticular connective tissue network lined by fibroblasts and many macrophages. The blood re-enters the circulation by passing across the endothelium of venous **sinuses**. Blood then passes into the splenic vein and back into the general circulation. The cords and sinuses form the **red pulp**, which is 75% of the spleen and has an essential role in monitoring the integrity of red blood cells (see below). A minority of the splenic vasculature is closed, in which the arterial and venous systems are connected by capillaries with a continuous endothelial layer.

The central arterioles are surrounded by a core of lymphatic tissue known as **white pulp**, which has an organization similar to lymph nodes (Fig. 10.1). The **periarteriolar lymphatic sheath** (PALS) lies directly around the arteriole and is equivalent to the T zone of the lymph node (p. 119). B-cell follicles are found adjacent to the PALS and these are surrounded by the **marginal** and **perifollicular zones**, which are rich in macrophages and dendritic cells. Lymphocytes migrate into white pulp from the sinuses of the red pulp or from vessels that end directly in the marginal and perifollicular zones.

There are both rapid (1–2 min) and slow (30–60 min) blood circulations through the spleen. The slow circulation becomes increasingly important in splenomegaly.

The functions of the spleen

The spleen is the largest filter of the blood in the body and several of its functions are derived from this.

Control of red cell integrity

The spleen has an essential role in the 'quality control' of red cells. Excess DNA, nuclear remnants (**Howell–Jolly bodies**) and **siderotic granules** are removed (Fig. 10.2). In the relatively hypoxic environment of the red pulp, and because of plasma skimming in the cords, the membrane flexibility of aged and abnormal red cells is impaired and they are trapped within the sinus, where they are ingested by macrophages.

Immune function

The lymphoid tissue in the spleen is in a unique position to respond to antigens filtered from the blood and entering the white pulp. Macrophages and dendritic cells in the marginal zone initiate an immune response and then present antigen to B and T cells to start adaptive immune responses. This arrangement is particularly efficient at mounting an immune response to encapsulated bacteria and explains the susceptibility of hyposplenic patients to these organisms.

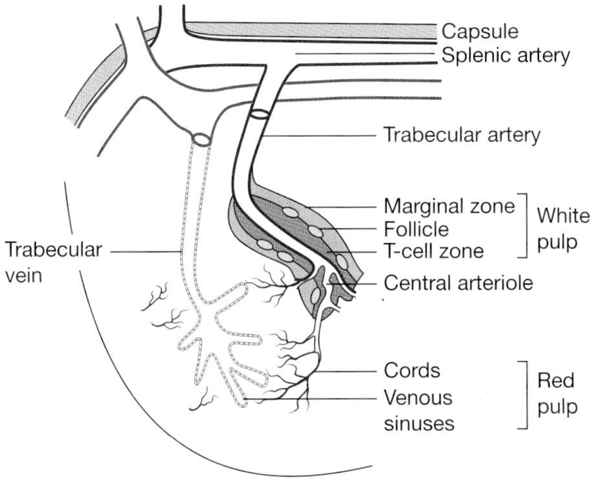

Figure 10.1 Schematic representation of the blood circulation in the spleen. Most blood flows in an 'open' circulation through splenic cords and regains entry into the circulation through the venous sinuses.

Capsule
Splenic artery
Trabecular artery
Marginal zone | White pulp
Follicle
T-cell zone
Central arteriole
Trabecular vein
Cords | Red pulp
Venous sinuses

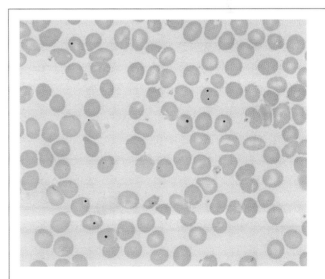

Figure 10.2 Splenic atrophy: peripheral blood film showing Howell–Jolly bodies, Pappenheimer bodies (siderotic granules; see p. 24) and misshapen cells.

Extramedullary haemopoiesis

The spleen, like the liver, undergoes a transient period of haemopoiesis at around 3–7 months of fetal life, but is not a site of erythropoiesis in the normal adult. However, haemopoiesis may be re-established in both organs as **extramedullary haemopoiesis**, in disorders such as primary myelofibrosis or in chronic severe haemolytic and megaloblastic anaemias. Extramedullary haemopoiesis may result either from reactivation of dormant stem cells within the spleen or homing of stem cells from the bone marrow to the spleen.

Imaging the spleen

Ultrasound is the most frequently used technique to image the spleen (Fig. 10.3). This can also detect whether or not blood flow in the splenic, portal and hepatic veins is normal, as well as assessing liver size and consistency. Computed tomography

(CT) is preferable for detecting structural detail and any associated lymphadenopathy (e.g. for lymphoma staging). Magnetic resonance imaging (MRI) also gives improved fine detail structure. Positron emission tomography (PET) is used particularly for initial staging and for detecting residual disease after treatment of lymphoma (Fig. 10.4).

Splenomegaly

Splenic size is increased in a wide range of conditions (Table 10.1). Splenomegaly is usually felt under the left costal margin, but massive splenomegaly may be felt as far as the right iliac fossa (see Fig. 15.11). The spleen moves with respiration and a medial splenic notch may be palpable in some cases. **In developed countries the most common causes of splenomegaly are infectious mononucleosis, haematological malignancy and portal hypertension, whereas malaria and schistosomiasis are more prevalent on a global scale (Table 10.1).** Chronic

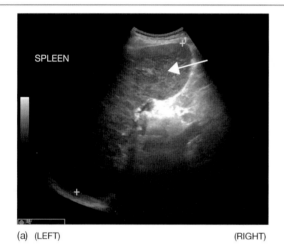

(a) (LEFT)   (RIGHT)

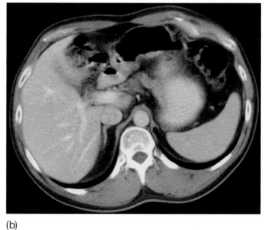

(b)

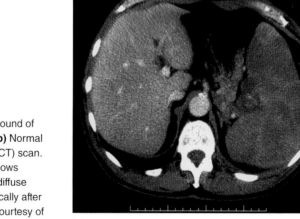

(c)

Figure 10.3 Imaging the spleen. **(a)** Ultrasound of spleen showing splenomegaly (15.3 cm). **(b)** Normal spleen (10 cm) on computed tomography (CT) scan. **(c)** CT scan: the spleen is enlarged and shows multiple low-density areas. A diagnosis of diffuse large B-cell lymphoma was made histologically after splenectomy. Source: Figures (a) and (b) courtesy of Dr T. Ogunremi.

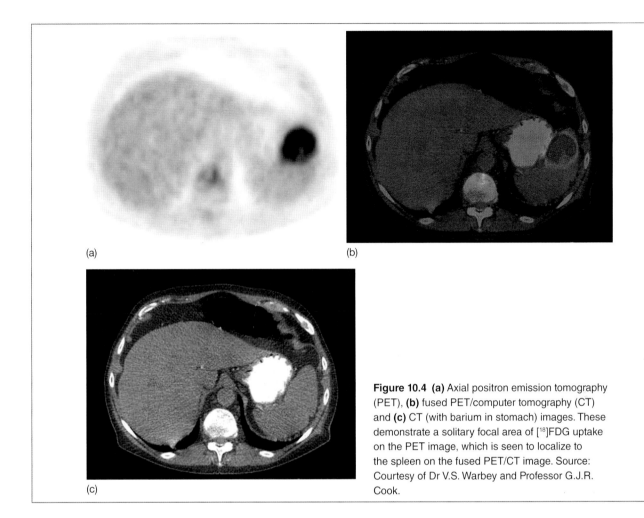

(a)

(b)

(c)

Figure 10.4 **(a)** Axial positron emission tomography (PET), **(b)** fused PET/computer tomography (CT) and **(c)** CT (with barium in stomach) images. These demonstrate a solitary focal area of [^{18}]FDG uptake on the PET image, which is seen to localize to the spleen on the fused PET/CT image. Source: Courtesy of Dr V.S. Warbey and Professor G.J.R. Cook.

myeloid leukaemia, primary myelofibrosis, lymphoma, Gaucher disease, malaria, leishmaniasis and schistosomiasis are potential causes of massive splenomegaly.

Tropical splenomegaly syndrome

A syndrome of massive splenomegaly of uncertain aetiology has been found frequently in many malarious zones of the tropics, including Uganda, Nigeria, New Guinea and the Congo. Smaller numbers of patients with this disorder are seen in southern Arabia, Sudan and Zambia. Previously, such terms as 'big spleen disease', 'cryptogenic splenomegaly' and 'African macroglobulinaemia' have been used to describe this syndrome.

While it seems probable that malaria is the fundamental cause of tropical splenomegaly syndrome, this disease is not the result of active malarial infection, as parasitaemia is usually scanty and malarial pigment is not found in biopsy material from the liver and spleen. An abnormal host response to the continual presence of malarial antigen, which results in a reactive and relatively benign lymphoproliferative

disorder that predominantly affects the liver and spleen, seems more likely.

Splenomegaly is usually gross and the liver is also enlarged. Portal hypertension may be a feature. The anaemia is often severe and leucopenia is usual; some patients develop a marked lymphocytosis. Serum immunoglobulin (Ig) M levels are high and there are high titres of malarial antibody.

Although splenectomy corrects the pancytopenia, there is an increased risk of fulminant malarial infection. Antimalarial therapy has proved successful in the management of many affected patients.

Hypersplenism

Normally, only approximately 5% (30–70 mL) of the total red cell mass is present in the spleen, although up to half of the total marginating neutrophil pool and 30% of the platelet mass may be located there. As the spleen enlarges, the proportion of haemopoietic cells within the organ increases such that up to 40% of the red cell mass, and 90% of platelets (see Fig. 25.9), may be pooled in an enlarged spleen.

Table 10.1 Causes of splenomegaly.

Haematological
Chronic myeloid leukaemia*
Chronic lymphocytic leukaemia
Acute leukaemia
Malignant lymphoma*
Primary myelofibrosis*
Polycythaemia vera
Hairy cell leukaemia
Thalassaemia major or intermedia*
Sickle cell anaemia (before splenic infarction)
Haemolytic anaemias
Megaloblastic anaemia

Portal hypertension
Cirrhosis
Hepatic, portal, splenic vein thrombosis

Storage diseases
Gaucher disease*
Niemann–Pick disease
Histiocytosis X

Systemic diseases
Sarcoidosis
Amyloidosis
Collagen diseases – systemic lupus erythematosus, rheumatoid arthritis
Systemic mastocytosis

Infections
Acute: septicaemia, bacterial endocarditis, typhoid, infectious mononucleosis
Chronic: tuberculosis, brucellosis, syphilis, malaria, leishmaniasis,* schistosomiasis*

*Tropical**
Possibly caused by malaria

*Possible causes of massive (>20 cm) splenomegaly.

Table 10.2 Causes of hyposplenism and blood film features.

Causes	Blood film features
Splenectomy	*Red cells*
Sickle cell disease	Target cells
Essential thrombocythaemia	Acanthocytes
Adult gluten-induced enteropathy	Irregularly contracted or crenated cells
Dermatitis herpetiformis	Howell–Jolly bodies (DNA remnants)
Amyloidosis	
Rarely	Siderotic (iron) granules (Pappenheimer bodies)
Inflammatory bowel disease	*White cells*
Splenic arterial thrombosis	± Mild lymphocytosis, monocytosis
	Platelets
	± Thrombocytosis

Splenectomy

Surgical removal of the spleen may be indicated for treatment of haematological disorders as well as after splenic rupture or for splenic tumours or cysts (Table 10.3). With advances in drug treatment of immune thrombocytopenia, of chemotherapy and immunotherapy for lymphomas and chronic lymphocytic leukaemia, and the introduction of JAK2 inhibitors for treatment of primary myelofibrosis, splenectomy for these conditions is now much less frequently indicated than previously. Splenectomy can be performed by open abdominal laparotomy or by laparoscopic surgery.

The platelet count can often rise dramatically in the early postoperative period, reaching levels of up to 1000×10^9/L and peaking at 1–2 weeks. Thrombotic complications are seen in some patients and prophylactic aspirin or heparin is often required during this period. Long-term alterations in the peripheral blood cell count may also be seen, including a persistent thrombocytosis, lymphocytosis or monocytosis.

Hypersplenism is a clinical syndrome that can be seen in any form of splenomegaly. It is characterized by:

■ Enlargement of the spleen.
■ Reduction of at least one cell line in the blood in the presence of normal bone marrow function.

Depending on the underlying cause, splenectomy may be indicated if the hypersplenism is symptomatic. It is followed by a rapid improvement in the peripheral blood count.

Hyposplenism

Functional hyposplenism is revealed by the blood film findings of Howell–Jolly bodies or Pappenheimer bodies (siderotic granules on iron staining; Fig. 10.2). The most frequent cause is surgical removal of the spleen, e.g. after traumatic rupture, but hyposplenism can also occur in sickle cell anaemia, gluten-induced enteropathy, amyloidosis and other conditions (Table 10.2).

Table 10.3 Indications for splenectomy.

Splenic rupture

Some cases of:

Chronic immune thrombocytopenia

Haemolytic anaemia, e.g. hereditary spherocytosis, autoimmune haemolytic anaemia, thalassaemia major or intermedia

Chronic lymphocytic leukaemia and lymphomas

Primary myelofibrosis

Tropical splenomegaly

Prevention of infection in hyposplenic patients

Patients with hyposplenism are at lifelong increased risk of infection from a variety of organisms. This is seen particularly in children under the age of 5 years and those with sickle cell anaemia. The most characteristic susceptibility is to the encapsulated bacteriae *Streptococcus pneumoniae*, *Haemophilus influenzae* type B and *Neisseria meningitidis*. *Streptococcus pneumoniae* is a particular concern and can cause a rapid and fulminant disease. Malaria and infection caused by animal bites tend to be more severe in splenectomized individuals.

Measures to reduce the risk of serious infection include the following:

1 Patients should be informed about their increased susceptibility to infection and advised to carry a card about their condition. They should be counselled about the increased risk of infection on foreign travel, including that from malaria and tick and animal bites.

2 Prophylactic oral penicillin is recommended, usually for life. High-risk groups include those aged under 16 years or older than 50 years, splenectomy for a haematological malignancy or a history of previous invasive pneumococcal disease. Low-risk adults, if they choose to discontinue penicillin, must be warned to seek immediate medical advice if they develop a high fever. Erythromycin may be prescribed for patients allergic to penicillin. A supply of appropriate antibiotics should also be given for patients to take in the event of onset of fever before medical care is available.

3 Vaccination against pneumococcus, haemophilus, meningococcus and influenza infection is recommended (Table 10.4). All types of vaccine, including live vaccines, can be given safely to hyposplenic individuals, although the immune response to vaccination may be impaired.

Table 10.4 Recommendations for vaccination of patients with hyposplenism.

Vaccine	Time of vaccination	Revaccination schedule	Comments
1 Pneumococcal polyvalent (23) vaccine (PPV) and/or pneumococcal conjugated vaccine (PCV13)	If possible, at least 2 weeks prior to splenectomy. Alternatively 2 weeks post-splenectomy for all three vaccines	5 yearly	Assessment of antibody response may be useful
2 Combined *Haemophilus influenzae* Type b conjugate and meningococcal conjugate		Not required	Not required if previously vaccinated
3 Influenza	As soon as available for seasonal protection	Annual	Standard live vaccine

The more immunogenic pneumococcal conjugate vaccine, PCV13, covers fewer (13 strains) than PPV (23 strains) and is used in those with a poor response to PPV or in some protocols as well as PPV.

SUMMARY

■ The normal adult spleen weighs 150–250 g and is 5–13 cm in diameter. It has a specialized circulation because the majority of arterioles end in 'cords' which lack an endothelial lining. The blood re-enters the circulation via venous sinuses. The cords and sinuses form the red pulp, which monitors the integrity of red blood cells.

■ The central arterioles are surrounded by lymphoid tissue called white pulp, which is similar in structure to a lymph node.

■ The spleen removes aged or abnormal red cells, and excess DNA and siderotic granules, from intact red cells. It also has a specialized immune function against capsulated bacteria, *Pneumococcus*, *Haemophilus influenzae* and *Meningococcus*, against which splenectomized patients are immunized. Splenectomy is needed for splenic rupture and in some haematological diseases.

■ Enlargement of the spleen (splenomegaly) occurs in many malignant and benign haematological diseases, in portal hypertension and with systemic diseases, including acute and chronic infections.

■ Hyposplenism occurs in sickle cell anaemia, gluten-induced enteropathy, amyloidosis and rarely in other diseases.

■ Vaccination against capsulated organisms and prolonged antibiotic prophylaxis is needed for patients with absent splenic function.

Now visit **www.wileyessential.com/haematology** to test yourself on this chapter.

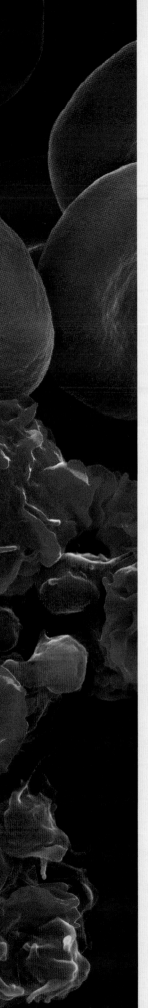

CHAPTER 11

The aetiology and genetics of haematological neoplasia

Key topics

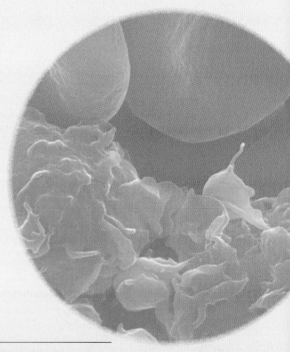

Hoffbrand's Essential Haematology, Eighth Edition. By A. Victor Hoffbrand and David P. Steensma.
© 2020 John Wiley & Sons Ltd. Published 2020 by John Wiley & Sons Ltd.
Companion website: www.wileyessential.com/haematology

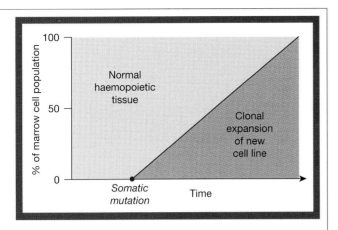

Figure 11.1 Theoretical graph to show the replacement of normal bone marrow cells by a clonal population of malignant cells arising by successive mitotic divisions from a single cell with an acquired genetic alteration.

Haemopoietic malignancies (neoplasms) are **clonal diseases** that derive from a single cell in the marrow or peripheral lymphoid tissue that has undergone genetic alteration (Fig. 11.1). In this chapter, we discuss the aetiology and genetic basis of haematological malignancies. Subsequent chapters discuss the aetiology, diagnosis and management of the individual conditions.

The incidence of haematological neoplasms

Cancer is an important cause of morbidity and mortality, as approximately 50% of, for example, the UK and US population will develop cancer in their lifetime. The majority of cancers are epithelial neoplasms; haematological cancers represent approximately 7% of all malignant disease, if non-melanomatous skin cancer is excluded (Fig. 11.2). There are major geographical variations in the occurrence of some haematological cancers,

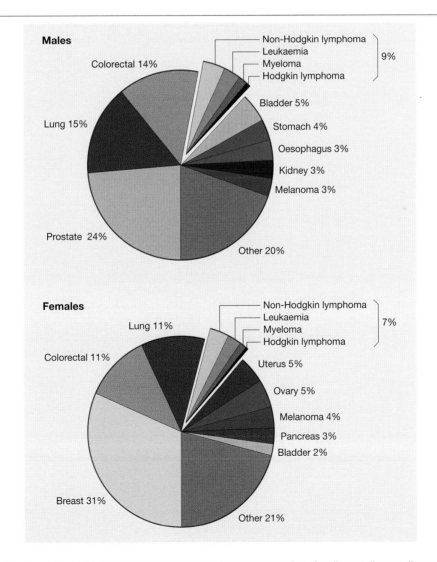

Figure 11.2 The relative frequency of the haematological malignancies as a proportion of malignant disease diagnosed in the UK. Non-melanomatous skin cancers are not included. Source: A. Smith *et al.* (2009) *Br. J. Haematol.* 148: 739–53. Reproduced with permission of John Wiley & Sons.

most notably chronic lymphocytic leukaemia (CLL), which is common in Europe and North America but rare in the Far East.

The aetiology of haemopoietic neoplasia

Cancer results from the accumulation of genetic mutations within a cell. The number of DNA mutations present varies widely from over 100 in some cancers to about 10 in most haematological malignancies (Fig. 11.3). Factors such as genetic inheritance and environmental lifestyle will influence the risk of developing a malignancy, but most cases of leukaemia and lymphoma appear to result simply as a result of the chance acquisition of critical genetic changes.

Inherited factors

The incidence of leukaemia is greatly increased in some genetic diseases such as Down syndrome, where acute leukaemia occurs with a 20- to 30-fold increased frequency. Additional leukaemia-predisposing disorders include Bloom syndrome, Fanconi anaemia, ataxia telangiectasia, neurofibromatosis, Klinefelter syndrome and Wiskott–Aldrich syndrome. Non-syndromic

inherited gene mutations can also predispose to myelodysplastic syndromes (MDS) and acute myeloid leukaemia (AML); these include germline mutations of *GATA2*, *CEBBPA*, *DDX41*, *RUNX1* or *ETV6*.

There is also a weak familial tendency in the diseases CLL, Hodgkin lymphoma and non-Hodgkin lymphoma (NHL), although the genes predisposing to this higher risk are largely unknown. Increasingly it is recognized that germline predispositions to haematological neoplasia may not be detected until adulthood, or may be found in patients with no family history of neoplasia.

Environmental influences

Chemicals

Chronic exposure to industrial solvents or chemicals such as benzene is a known but rare cause of MDS or AML.

Drugs

DNA alkylating agents, such as chlorambucil or melphalan, predispose to later development of MDS or AML, especially

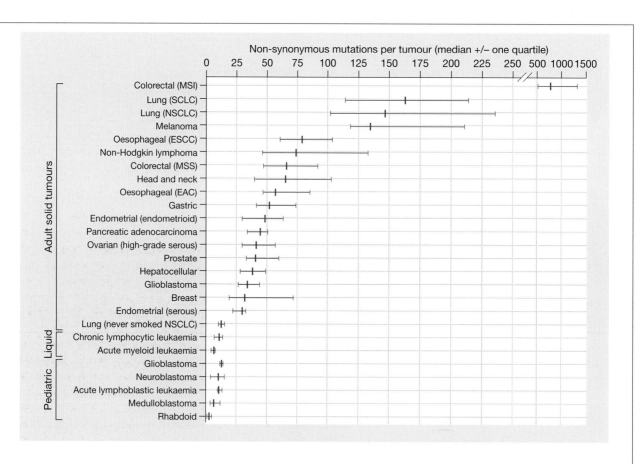

Figure 11.3 Average number of somatic mutations found in different types of cancer. Source: Adapted from Vogelstein B *et al*. (2013) *Science* 339: 1546–58. EAC, oesophageal adenocarcinoma; ESCC, oesophageal squamous cell cancer; MSI, microsatellite instability; MSS, microsatellite stable; NSCLC, non-small cell lung cancer; SCLC, small cell lung cancer.

if combined with radiotherapy. The karyotype in such cases is almost always complex and *TP53* mutations are usually present. Etoposide and other topoisomerase inhibitors including anthracyclines are associated with a risk of the development of secondary leukaemia associated with balanced translocations including that of the *KTM2A (MLL)* gene at 11q23.

Radiation

Radiation, especially to the marrow, is leukaemogenic. This is illustrated by a dose-dependent increased incidence of leukaemia in survivors of the 1945 atom bomb explosions in Japan.

Infection

The World Health Organization estimated in 2002 that infections are responsible for 18% of all cancers. Infectious agents contribute to a range of haematological malignancies.

Viruses

Viral infection is associated with several types of haemopoietic malignancy, especially different subtypes of lymphoma (see Table 20.2). The retrovirus human T-lymphotropic virus type 1 (HTLV-1) is the cause of adult T-cell leukaemia/lymphoma (ATLL, see p. 227), although most people infected with the HTLV-1 virus do not develop a neoplasm. Epstein–Barr virus (EBV) is associated with almost all cases of endemic (African) Burkitt lymphoma, post-transplant lymphoproliferative disease (see p. 303) and a proportion of patients with Hodgkin lymphoma. Human herpes virus 8 infection (HHV-8, Kaposi sarcoma-associated virus) causes Kaposi sarcoma and primary effusion lymphoma (see Table 20.2). Chronic hepatitis C increases the risk of B-cell lymphomas.

HIV infection is associated with an increased incidence of lymphomas at unusual sites such as the central nervous system. These HIV-associated lymphomas are usually of B-cell origin and of high-grade histology. The risk of developing lymphoma increases with lower CD4 lymphocyte counts.

Bacteria

Helicobacter pylori infection has been implicated in the pathogenesis of gastric mucosa B-cell (MALT) lymphoma (see p. 248) and antibiotic treatment may even bring about disease remission without the need for chemotherapy. Chronic *Chlamydia trachomatis* infection predisposes to ocular adnexal lymphoma.

Protozoa

Endemic Burkitt lymphoma occurs in the tropics, particularly in malarial areas. It is thought that malaria may alter host immunity and predispose to tumour formation as a result of EBV infection.

The genetics of haemopoietic neoplasia

Malignant transformation occurs as a result of the accumulation of genetic mutations in cellular genes. The genes that are involved in the development of cancer

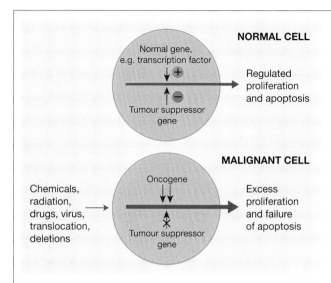

Figure 11.4 Proliferation of normal cells depends on a balance between the action of proto-oncogenes and tumour-suppressor genes. In a malignant cell this balance is disturbed, leading to uncontrolled cell division.

can be divided broadly into two groups: **oncogenes** and **tumour-suppressor genes**.

Oncogenes

Oncogenes arise because of gain-of-function mutations or inappropriate expression pattern in normal cellular genes called **proto-oncogenes** (Fig. 11.4). Oncogenic versions are generated when the activity of proto-oncogenes is increased or they acquire a novel function. This can occur in a number of ways, including translocation, mutation or duplication. In general, these mutations affect the processes of cell signalling, cell differentiation and survival.

One of the striking features of haematological malignancies, in contrast to most solid tumours, is their high frequency of chromosomal translocations. Several oncogenes are involved in the suppression of apoptosis, of which the best example is *BCL2*, which is overexpressed in follicular lymphoma (see p. 248).

The types of mutations that are detected in the neoplastic cells of a patient with cancer fall into two broad groups. **Driver mutations** are those that confer a selective growth advantage to a cancer cell. The sequence in which different driver mutations occur in a tumour may affect the clinical features of the resulting disease. **Passenger mutations** do not confer a growth advantage and may have already been coincidentally present in the cell from which the cancer arose, or may subsequently arise as a neutral genetic change in the proliferating cell. It is important that targeted drug treatments are directed against the activity of driver mutations.

Tyrosine kinases

Tyrosine kinases are enzymes which phosphorylate proteins on tyrosine residues. They are important mediators of intracellular signalling. Mutations or alteration of expression of tyrosine kinases leading to unregulated constitutive activation of the kinase underlie a large number of haematological malignancies. These are the targets of many extremely effective drugs called **tyrosine kinase inhibitors**. Common examples of targetable tyrosine kinases discussed in the relevant disease-specific chapters include **ABL1** in chronic myeloid leukaemia (CML), **JAK2** in myeloproliferative neoplasms, **FLT3** in AML, **KIT** in both systemic mastocytosis and AML, and **Bruton tyrosine kinase (BTK)** in chronic lymphocytic leukaemia and other lymphoproliferative disorders.

Tumour-suppressor genes

Tumour-suppressor genes may acquire loss-of-function mutations, usually by point mutation or deletion, which lead to malignant transformation (Fig. 11.4). Tumour-suppressor genes commonly act as components of control mechanisms that regulate entry of the cell from the G_1 phase of the cell cycle into the S phase or passage through the S phase to G_2 and mitosis (see Fig. 1.7). Examples of oncogenes and tumour-suppressor genes involved in haemopoietic malignancies are shown in Table 11.1. The most significant tumour-suppressor gene in human cancer is *TP53*, which is inactivated by mutation or deletion in over 50% of cases of malignant disease, including many haemopoietic tumours, especially those related to prior exposure to alkylating agents or radiation.

Table 11.1 Some of the more frequent genetic abnormalities within haematological neoplasms (see also individual disease-specific chapters).

Disease	Genetic abnormality	Genes involved
AML (*de novo*)	t(8;21) translocation t(15;17) translocation Nucleotide insertion Mutation	*RUNX1-RUNX1T1 (CBFα)* *PML-RARA* *NPM1, FLT3* *FLT3, DNMT3A, IDH1, IDH2, CEBBPA*
Therapy-related MDS/AML	Chromosome 11q23 translocation Chromosome 17p deletion or mutation	*KMT2A(MLL)* *TP53*
MDS	Loss of chromosome 5 (-5, del (5q)) Mutation	*RPS14, CSKN1A* *SF3B1* or other splicing genes, *TET2, DNMT3A, ASXL1, EZH2*
CML	t(9;22) translocation	*BCR-ABL1*
Myeloproliferative neoplasms	Point mutation Insertion-deletion	*JAK2, MPL* *CALR*
Systemic mastocytosis	Point mutation	*KIT*
B-ALL	t(12;21) translocation t(9;22) translocation 11q23 translocations	*ETV6-RUNX1* *BCR-ABL1* *AF4/KMT2A(MLL)*
T-ALL	Mutation	*NOTCH1*
Non-Hodgkin lymphomas		
Follicular lymphoma	t(14;18) translocation	*BCL2*
Lymphoplasmacytic lymphoma	Mutation	*MYD88, CXCR4*
Burkitt lymphoma	t(8;14) translocation	*MYC*
Hairy cell leukaemia	Mutation	*BRAF*
Large granular lymphocyte leukaemia	Mutation	*STAT3*
CLL	Chromosome 17p deletion Mutations	*TP53* *NOTCH1, SF3B1, ATM*

AML, acute myeloid leukaemia; B-ALL, B-acute lymphoblastic leukaemia; CLL, chronic lymphocytic leukaemia; CML, chronic myeloid leukaemia; MDS, myelodysplastic syndromes; T-ALL, T-acute lymphoblastic leukaemia.

Clonal progression

Malignant cells appear to arise as a multistep process with the acquisition of mutations in different intracellular pathways. This may occur by a **linear evolution**, in which the final clone harbours all the mutations that arose during evolution of the malignancy (Fig. 11.5a), or by **branching evolution**, in which there is more than one clone of cells characterized by different somatic mutations, but which share at least one mutation traceable back to a single ancestral cell (Figure 11.5b). During this progression of the disease, one subclone may gradually acquire a growth advantage. Selection of subclones may also occur during anti-cancer treatment, which may selectively kill some subclones but allow others to survive and new clones to appear (Fig. 11.6). The presence of certain mutations that confer resistance to chemotherapy allows some neoplastic subclones to persist and expand, even as other clonal cells are eliminated. The most frequent of these mutations found in haematological neoplasms are of *TP53* and of *PPM1D*, which encodes a protein phosphatase involved in regulation of DNA damage responses.

Progression of subclinical clonal haematological mutations to clinical disease

The use of sensitive immunological and molecular tests has shown that many healthy individuals harbour clones of cells which have acquired somatic mutations and from which overt haematological clinical disease may arise (Table 11.2). This is particularly frequent in the elderly. Examples include clones of cells identical to those of chronic lymphocytic leukaemia, which can be present in the blood of individuals with a normal lymphocyte count, and the finding of clones of cells harbouring mutations such as *TET2* that are characteristic of myeloid malignancy. Such mutations may be present in a normal-appearing bone marrow at a variant allele frequency of at least 2% in nearly a fifth of elderly healthy subjects. In one study, all healthy subjects exhibiting mutations of *TP53* or of *IDH1/2* in the blood cells eventually developed AML, often many years later, while those who had mutations of *TET2*, *DNMT3A* or *ASXL1* progressed to AML at a rate of less than 1% per year and most never developed AML. The risk of progression is greater with larger clones, as measured by the variant allele frequency (also called allele burden) – a marker of the proportion of genetically abnormal cells in a wild-type background. Progression of monoclonal gammopathy of undetermined significance (MGUS) to myeloma has been well recognised for many decades (see Chapter 21).

Chromosome nomenclature

The normal somatic cell has 46 chromosomes and is called **diploid**; ova or sperm have 23 chromosomes and are called **haploid**. The chromosomes occur in pairs and are numbered 1–22 in approximately decreasing size order (for historical reasons, chromosome 20 is slightly larger than chromosome 19). There are two sex chromosomes, XX in females, XY in males.

Karyotype is the term used to describe the chromosomes derived from a mitotic cell which have been set out in numerical

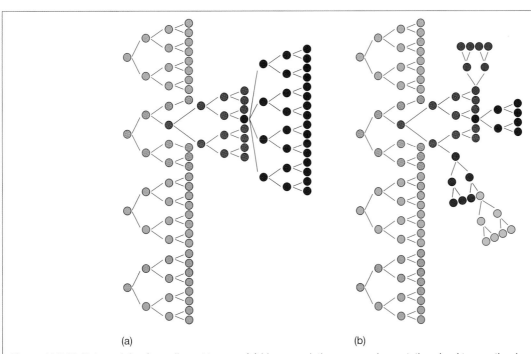

(a)   (b)

Figure 11.5 Multistep origin of a malignant tumour. **(a)** Linear evolution: successive mutations lead to growth advantage of one clone. **(b)** Branching evolution: subclones arise at different stages of the tumour evolution. These subclones share at least one common founder mutation. Green, brown and pink cells are all overtly malignant but may have different phenotypes and behaviour.

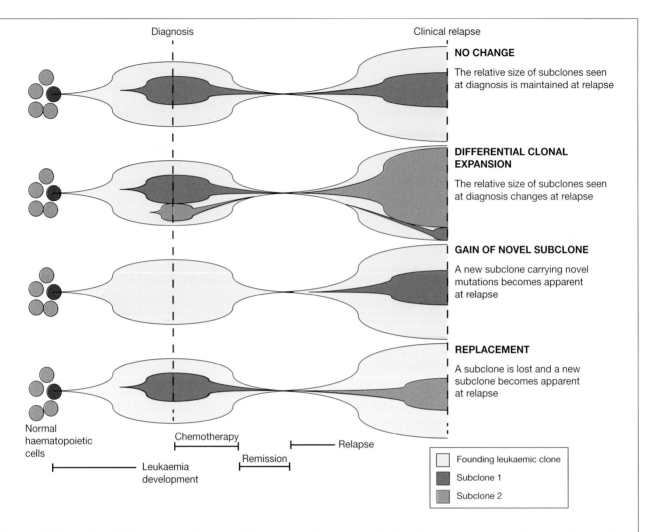

Figure 11.6 Examples of different potential patterns of clonal progression between the development, treatment and relapse of leukaemia. Source: Adapted from N. Bolli, G. Vassiliou. In A.V. Hoffbrand *et al.* (eds) (2016) *Postgraduate Haematology*, 7th edn. Reproduced by permission of John Wiley & Sons.

Table 11.2 Examples of clonal abnormalities which may be detected in otherwise healthy individuals and which may or may not progress to overt clinical disease.

Clonal abnormality	Disease(s)
Monoclonal B lymphocytosis	Chronic lymphocytic leukaemia and non-Hodgkin lymphoma
IgM paraprotein (MGUS)	Waldenstrom macroglobulinaemia
IgG paraprotein (MGUS)	Multiple myeloma
In situ follicular neoplasia	Follicular lymphoma
Mutation in fetal bone marrow, e.g. t(12;21)	Childhood acute lymphoblastic leukaemia
Stem or progenitor cell clone in bone marrow, e.g. mutation of *TET2*, *DNMT3*, *IDH1/2*, *TP53* or *ASXL1*; often called CHIP (clonal haemopoiesis of indeterminate potential; see p. 203)	Myelodysplastic syndromes, acute myeloid leukaemia; less commonly lymphoid neoplasms

MGUS, Monoclonal gammopathy of uncertain significance.

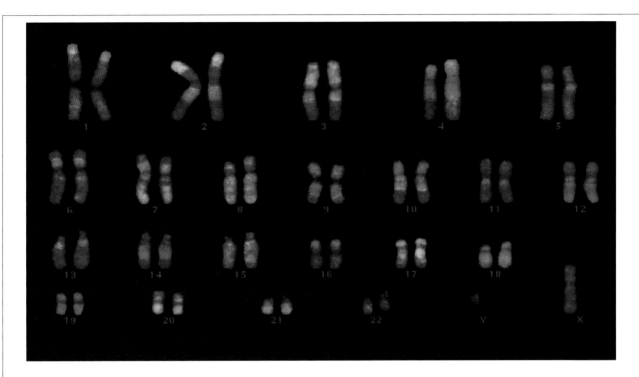

Figure 11.7 A colour-banded karyotype from a normal male. Each chromosome pair shows an individual colour-banding pattern. This involves a cross-species multiple-colour chromosome banding technique. Probe sets developed from the chromosomes of gibbons are combinatorially labelled and hybridized to human chromosomes. The success of cross-species colour banding depends on a close homology between host and human conserved DNA, divergence of repetitive DNA and a high degree of chromosomal rearrangement in the host relative to the human karyotype. Source: Courtesy of Professor C.J. Harrison.

order (Fig. 11.7). A somatic cell with more or fewer than 46 chromosomes is termed **aneuploid**; more than 46 is **hyperdiploid**, fewer than 46 **hypodiploid**; 46 but with chromosome rearrangements, **pseudodiploid**. About 30% of patients with B-ALL have 50–67 chromosomes, which is termed **highhyperdiploid**; less commonly patients with B-ALL have 31–49 chromosomes (**low hypodiploid**).

Each chromosome has two arms: the shorter called 'p', the longer called 'q'. These meet at the **centromere** and the distal ends of the chromosomes are called **telomeres**. On staining with Giemsa (G-banding) or quinacrine (Q-banding), each arm divides into regions numbered outwards from the centromere and each region divides into bands (Fig. 11.8).

When a whole chromosome is lost or gained, a – or + is put in front of the chromosome number. If only part of the chromosome is lost, it is prefixed with **del** (for deletion). If there is extra material replacing part of a chromosome, the prefix **add** (for additional material) is used. Chromosome translocations are denoted by **t**, the chromosomes involved placed in brackets with the lower numbered chromosome first. The prefix **inv** describes an inversion where part of the chromosome has been inverted to run in the opposite direction. An **isochromosome**, denoted by **i**, describes a chromosome with identical chromosome arms at each end; for example, i(17q) would consist of two copies of 17q joined at the centromere.

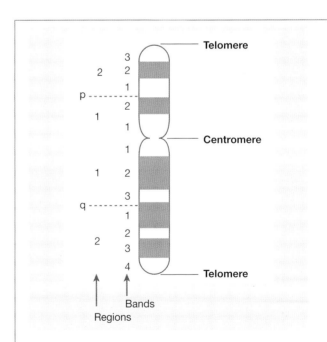

Figure 11.8 A schematic representation of a chromosome. The bands may be divided into sub-bands according to staining pattern. Loci are described orally by noting region and then band (e.g. 'q12' is 'q one-two' rather than 'q twelve'.)

Telomeres

Telomeres are repetitive sequences at the ends of chromosomes. They decrease by approximately 200 base pairs of DNA with every round of cell replication. When they decrease to a critical length, the cell exits from the cell cycle.

Germ cells and stem cells, which need to self-renew and maintain a high proliferative potential, contain the enzyme **telomerase**, which can add extensions to the telomeric repeats and compensate for loss at replication, and so enable the cells to continue proliferation. Telomerase is also often expressed in malignant cells, but this is probably a consequence of the malignant transformation rather than an initiating factor. Germline mutations in components of the telomere complex cause dyskeratosis congenita (p. 275), which predisposes to haematological neoplasms. Patients with dyskeratosis typically have telomere lengths in both lymphocytes and granulocytes that are less than the second percentile for age.

Specific examples of genetic abnormalities in haematological neoplasms

The genetic abnormalities underlying the different types of leukaemia and lymphoma are described with the diseases, which are themselves increasingly classified according to genetic change rather than morphology. The types of gene abnormality include the following (Fig. 11.9).

Point mutation

This is illustrated by the single-nucleotide variant 1849 G>T in the *JAK2* gene resulting in the Val617Phe (V617F) mutation in the JAK2 protein. This leads to constitutive activation of the protein and uncontrolled cell proliferation. JAK2 V617F is present in most cases of myeloproliferative neoplasia (see Chapter 15). Point mutations within the *RAS* oncogenes leading to activation or within the *TP53* tumour-suppressor gene leading to inactivation are common in many haemopoietic malignancies.

A point mutation may involve several base pairs. In 35% of cases of AML with a normal karyotype, the **nucleophosmin** (*NPM1*) gene shows an insertion of four base pairs, resulting in a frameshift change. Internal tandem duplications with varying lengths (ranging from 3 to hundreds of nucleotides, median 39 base pairs) or single-base pair point mutations in the tyrosine kinase domain occur in the *FLT3* gene in 30% of cases of AML. Most cases of MDS with ring sideroblasts have point mutations in the *SF3B1* gene, which alters RNA splicing.

Translocations

These are a characteristic feature of haematological malignancies and there are two main mechanisms whereby they may contribute to malignant change (Fig. 11.10):

1 Fusion of parts of two genes to generate a chimeric fusion gene that is dysfunctional or encodes a novel '**fusion protein**',

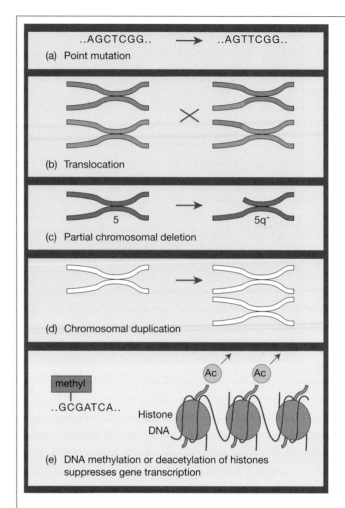

Figure 11.9 Types of genetic abnormality which may lead to haemopoietic malignancy. **(a)** Point mutation; **(b)** chromosomal translocation; **(c)** chromosomal deletion or loss; **(d)** chromosomal duplication; **(e)** epigenetic changes: DNA methylation or deacetylation of histone tails suppresses gene transcription.

e.g. *BCR-ABL1* in t(9;22) in CML (see Fig. 14.1), *RARA-PML* in t(15;17) in acute promyelocytic leukaemia (see Fig. 13.7) or *ETV6-RUNX1* in t(12; 21) in B-ALL.

2 **Overexpression of a normal cellular gene**, e.g. overexpression of *BCL2* in the t(14;18) translocation of follicular lymphoma or of *MYC* in Burkitt lymphoma (Fig. 11.11). Interestingly, this class of translocation nearly always involves an immunoglobulin gene or T-cell receptor (TCR) locus, presumably as a result of aberrant activity of the recombinase enzyme which is involved in immunoglobulin or TCR gene rearrangement in immature B or T cells. Since the immunoglobin gene and TCR gene are actively transcribed in B and T lymphocytes, respectively, the translocated gene that is moved adjacent to these promoters is typically expressed at high levels.

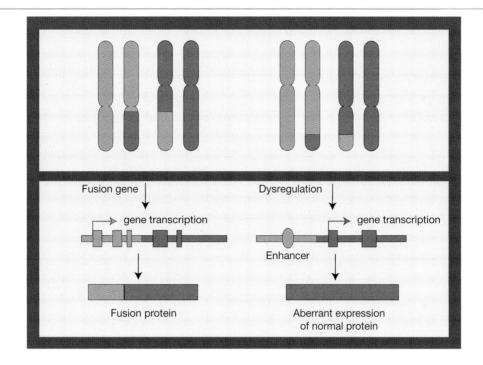

Figure 11.10 The two possible mechanisms by which chromosomal translocations can lead to dysregulated expression of an oncogene.

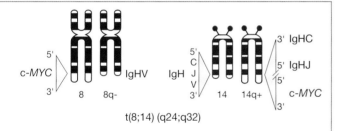

t(8;14) (q24;q32)

Figure 11.11 The genetic events in one of the three translocations found in Burkitt lymphoma and B-cell acute lymphoblastic leukaemia. The oncogene *c-MYC* is normally located on the long arm (q) of chromosome 8. In the (8;14) translocation, *c-MYC* is translocated into close proximity to the immunoglobulin heavy-chain gene on the long arm of chromosome 14. Part of the heavy-chain gene (the V region) is reciprocally translocated to chromosome 8. C, constant region; IgH, immunoglobulin heavy-chain gene; J, joining region; V, variable region.

Deletions

Chromosomal deletions may involve a small part of a chromosome, the entire short or long arm (e.g. 5q–) or the whole chromosome (e.g. monosomy 7). The critical event is probably loss of a tumour-suppressor gene or of a microRNA, as in the 13q14 deletion in CLL (see below). The critical gene or genes in many recurrent deletions associated with haematological malignancies are not understood, in part because these large regions may contain dozens of genes.

Duplication or amplification

In chromosomal duplication (e.g. trisomy 12 in CLL) or gene amplification, gains are common, especially in chromosomes 8, 12, 19, 21 and Y. Gene amplification is increasingly recognized within haemopoietic malignancy and an example is that involving the *KMT2A(MLL)* gene.

Epigenetic alterations

Gene expression in cancer may be dysregulated not only by structural changes to the genes themselves, but also by alterations in the mechanism by which genes are transcribed. These changes are called **epigenetic** and are stably inherited with each cell division, so they are passed on as the malignant cell divides. The most important mechanisms (illustrated in Figure 16.1) are:

1 Methylation of cytosine residues in DNA; and
2 Enzymatic alterations, such as acetylation or methylation, of the histone proteins that package DNA within the cell.

They are particularly important in the myeloid malignancies. Demethylating agents such as azacytidine alter gene transcription and are valuable in treating MDS and AML.

MicroRNAs

Chromosomal abnormalities, both deletions and amplifications, can result in loss or gain of short (micro)RNA sequences. These are normally transcribed but not translated. MicroRNAs (miRNAs) control expression of adjacent or distally located genes. Deletion of the miR15a/miR16-1 locus may be relevant to CLL development with the common 13q14 deletion, and deletions of other microRNAs have been described in AML and other haematological neoplasms.

Diagnostic methods used to study neoplastic haemopoietic cells

Karyotype analysis

Karyotype analysis involves direct morphological analysis of chromosomes from neoplastic cells under the microscope (see Fig. 14.1). This requires neoplastic cells to be in metaphase and so cells are cultured to encourage cell division prior to chromosomal preparation.

Fluorescence *in situ* hybridization analysis

Fluorescence *in situ* hybridization (FISH) analysis involves the use of fluorescent-labelled genetic probes which hybridize to specific parts of the genome. It is possible to label each chromosome with a different combination of fluorescent labels (Fig. 11.12). This is a sensitive technique that can detect extra copies of genetic material in both metaphase and interphase (non-dividing) cells or, by using two different probes, reveal chromosomal translocations (see Fig. 14.1e) or reduced chromosome numbers.

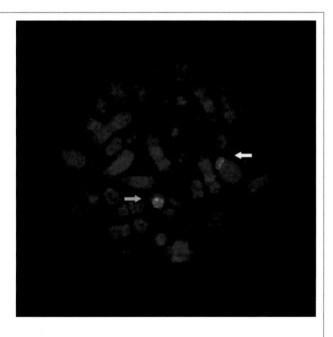

Figure 11.12 An example of fluorescence *in situ* hybridization (FISH) analysis showing the t(12;21) translocation. The green probe hybridizes to the region of the *ETV6* gene on chromosome 12 and the red probe hybridizes to the region of the *RUNX1* gene on chromosome 21. The arrows point to the two derived chromosomes resulting from the reciprocal translocation. Source: Courtesy of Professor C.J. Harrison.

Gene sequencing

Gene sequence analysis is used to detect the genetic mutations that can cause neoplastic disease. **Next generation sequencing (NGS)** can be used to study individual genes of interest; sequencing of the whole exome (3×10^7 base pairs) or genome (3×10^9 base pairs) of the tumour or a specific panel of genes can be performed for moderate cost (Fig. 11.13). The results are then compared to the germline sequence of the patient or a reference sequence to identify the mutations in the tumour. Increasingly, cancer treatment is based on assessment of the patient's germline genome and the genome of their tumour. The bioinformatic analysis of the information that arises from NGS can be challenging and uses sophisticated computer programs. Gene sequencing identifies point mutations such as of *JAK2* in the myeloproliferative neoplasms, *KIT* in systemic mastocytosis (see Chapter 15) and *FLT3* in AML (see Chapter 13).

DNA microarray platforms

DNA microarrays allow a rapid and comprehensive analysis of the pattern of cellular transcription within a cell or tissue by hybridizing labelled cellular mRNA to DNA probes which are immobilized on a slide or microchip (Fig. 11.14). It is valuable in research, but is not widely used for diagnosis. An alternative approach to assessing the profile of RNA within a cell is to use NGS to sequence all RNA transcripts ('RNASeq').

Flow cytometry

In this technique, antibodies labelled with different fluorochromes recognize the pattern and intensity of expression of different antigens on the surface of normal and neoplastic cells (Fig. 11.15). Normal cells each have a characteristic profile, but neoplastic cells often express an aberrant phenotype that can be useful in allowing their detection (see Figs 11.15 and 17.8). In the case of B-cell malignancies such as CLL, expression of only one light chain, κ or λ, by the neoplastic cells distinguishes them from a normal polyclonal population which expresses both κ and λ chains, usually in a κ:λ ratio of 2:1 (see Fig. 20.4). The commonly used markers for the diagnosis of the neoplastic haematological diseases are listed in the relevant chapters.

Immunohistology (immunohistochemistry)

Antibodies can also be used to stain tissue sections. The fixed sections are incubated with an antibody, washed and incubated with a second antibody linked to an enzyme, usually peroxidase. A substrate is added that the enzyme converts to a coloured precipitate, usually brown. The presence and architecture of neoplastic cells can be identified by visualization of stained tissue sections under the microscope (Fig. 11.16). The clonal nature of B-cell malignancies can be shown in tissue sections by staining for κ or λ chains. A malignant clonal population (e.g. in B-cell NHL) will express one or other light chain but not both (see Fig. 20.4).

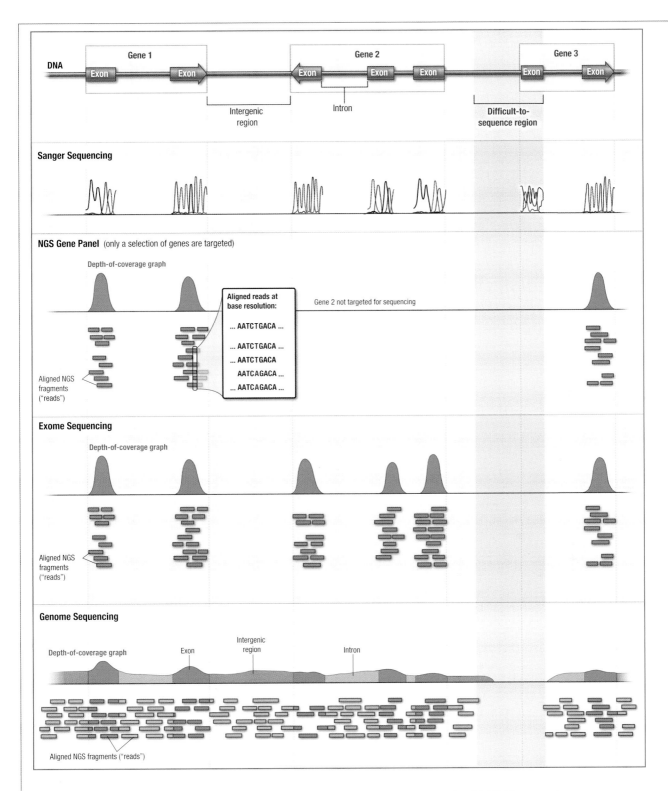

Figure 11.13 Comparison of DNA sequencing techniques, including next generation sequencing (NGS). The genomic coverage characteristics of exome, genome and panel NGS tests are distinct. While NGS panel tests cover a set of genes defined by the clinical diagnostic laboratory, such as those relevant for a specific neoplasm (e.g. acute myeloid leukaemia-associated mutations), exome sequencing covers the majority of known genes regardless of disease association, and genome sequencing includes both coding regions of genes and intergenic regions. Some regions of the genome such as highly repetitive elements are challenging to sequence with any of these methods. Source: D.R. Adams, C.M. Eng (2018) *N. Engl. J. Med.* 379: 1353–62. Reproduced with permission of Massachusetts Medical Society.

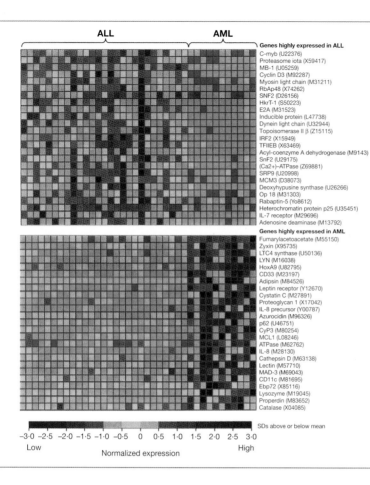

Figure 11.14 Microarray analysis of genes distinguishing acute lymphoblastic leukaemia (ALL) from acute myeloid leukaemia (AML). The 50 genes most highly correlated on gene-expression microarrays with each of these leukaemias are shown. Each row corresponds to a gene; each column corresponds to the expression value in a particular sample. Expression for each gene is normalized across the samples such that the mean is 0 and the standard deviation (SD) is 1. Expression greater than the mean is shaded in red, and that below the mean is shaded in blue. Although the genes as a group appear correlated with the type of leukaemia under study, no single gene is uniformly expressed across the class, illustrating the value of a multigene prediction method. Source: Courtesy of Todd Golub and colleagues.

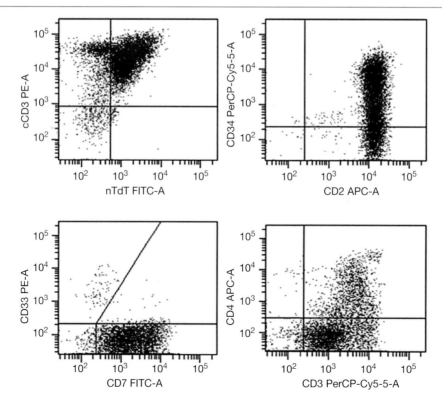

Figure 11.15 Fluorescence-activated cell sorting (FACS) analysis of acute lymphoblastic leukaemia, T lineage. The blast cells express cCD3, TdT, CD34, CD7 and CD2. Source: Courtesy of Immunophenotyping Laboratory, Royal Free Hospital, London.

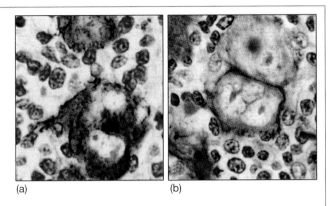

(a)   (b)

Figure 11.16 Immunohistological identification of Reed–Sternberg cells in Hodgkin lymphoma. The binucleate cells stain positively for **(a)** CD15 and **(b)** CD30.

Circulating neoplastic DNA

Cell-free DNA derived from the bone marrow neoplastic cells or from lymphoma cells situated outside the marrow may be found in peripheral blood. This circulating DNA has genomic changes similar to those of the neoplastic disease, can be used to track karyotype and mutations during therapy and is able to detect emerging new clones.

Value of genetic markers in management of haematological neoplasia

The detection of genetic abnormalities is important in several aspects of the management of patients with leukaemia or lymphoma.

Initial diagnosis

Many genetic abnormalities are so specific for a particular disease that their presence determines that diagnosis. An example is the t(11;14) translocation, which defines mantle cell lymphoma. Clonal immunoglobulin or *TCR* gene rearrangements are useful in establishing clonality and determining the lineage of a lymphoid malignancy.

For establishing a treatment protocol

Each major type of haematological malignancy can be further subdivided on the basis of detailed genetic information. For instance, AML is a diverse group of disorders with characteristic genotypes. Individual subtypes respond differently to standard treatment. The t(8;21) and inv(16) subgroups have a favourable prognosis, whereas monosomy 7 carries a poor prognosis. In those with normal cytogenetics, molecular analysis may show *FLT3* internal tandem duplication, an unfavourable marker, or *NPM1* mutation, which is generally favourable. The pattern of genetic changes detected by molecular studies in a new case of AML may distinguish those cases with preceding MDS (and an unfavourable prognosis) from those without

MDS (see p. 161). Treatment strategies are now tailored for the individual and in some instances knowledge of the underlying genetic abnormality can lead to more rational treatment, e.g. the use of all-*trans* retinoic acid in acute promyelocytic leukaemia with t(15;17) (see p. 175).

Genetic information is also valuable for giving a prognosis. For instance, hyperdiploidy in ALL is a favourable finding, whereas for most haematological neoplasias *TP53* mutations or deletion predict for poor prognosis and lack of responsiveness to chemotherapy.

Monitoring the response to therapy

The detection of minimal residual disease (MRD, also called measurable residual disease, i.e. persistent clonal cells that cannot be seen by conventional microscopy of the blood or bone marrow) when the patient is in remission after chemotherapy or stem cell transplantation is possible using the following techniques (in increasing order of sensitivity; Fig. 11.17):

1 Cytogenetic analysis.
2 Fluorescence-activated cell sorting to detect tumour cells using immunological markers that detect 'leukaemia-specific' combinations of antigens (see Figs 11.15 and 17.8).
3 PCR and/or sequence analysis to detect tumour-specific translocations or mutations specific to the original clone (Fig. 11.18). Targeted NGS can also be used to detect and quantify whether mutations found at diagnosis are still present in the bone marrow in clinical remission (Figure 13.11).

Collectively, these approaches have an important role in planning the treatment of many forms of neoplastic haemopoietic disease.

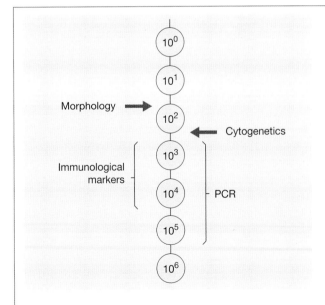

Figure 11.17 Sensitivity of detection of leukaemic cells in bone marrow using four different techniques. 10^1 to 10^6 = 1 cell in 10 to 1 cell in 10^6 detected.

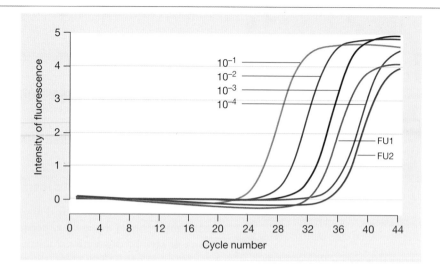

Figure 11.18 Real-time quantitative polymerase chain reaction (PCR) in acute B-lineage lymphoblastic leukaemia for minimal residual disease using the immunoglobulin heavy chain as target. Primers are designed based on DNA from sequence analysis of the presenting leukaemic clone. Bone marrow samples taken in clinical remission are amplified by PCR using these primers and fluorescent labelled using Sybergreen. The intensity of the signal measures the total DNA molecules amplified in successive cycles. In this example, the intensities of amplification of DNA from two follow-up bone marrow samples (FU1 and FU2) are compared with serial deletions of (10^{-1} to 10^{-4}) of the DNA from the presentation bone marrow. FU1 shows a level of residual disease of approximately 1 in 5000 (0.02%) and FU2 of 1 in 12 000 (0.008%). Source: Courtesy of Dr L. Foroni.

SUMMARY

- The haemopoietic neoplasms are clonal diseases that derive from a single cell in the marrow or peripheral lymphoid tissue which has undergone genetic alteration.
- They represent approximately 7% of all malignant disease.
- Inherited and environmental factors both predispose to neoplastic development, but the relative contribution of these is usually unclear.
- Infections (viral and bacterial), drugs, radiation and chemicals can all increase the risk of developing a haemopoietic malignancy.
- Haematological neoplasia occurs because of genetic alterations that lead to increased activation of oncogenes or decreased activity of tumour suppressor genes. They usually show about 10 acquired genetic mutations and progress in a linear or branching manner.
- These genetic alterations may occur through a variety of mechanisms such as point mutation, chromosomal translocation or gene deletion.
- Epigenetic changes are important in the aetiology of many myeloid malignancies
- Important investigations include study of the chromosomes (karyotype analysis), molecular genetics, FISH, mutation analysis, flow cytometry and immunohistochemistry.
- These investigations guide the diagnosis, treatment and monitoring for residual disease of individual cases. They are also an important guide to prognosis.

Now visit **www.wileyessential.com/haematology** to test yourself on this chapter.

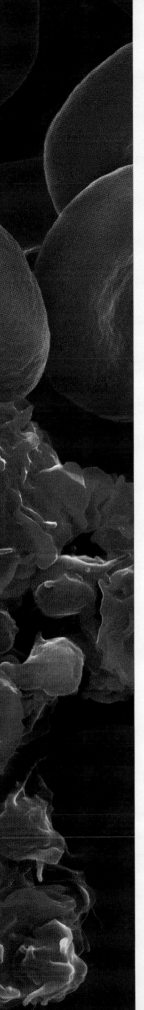

CHAPTER 12
Management of haematological malignancy

Key topics

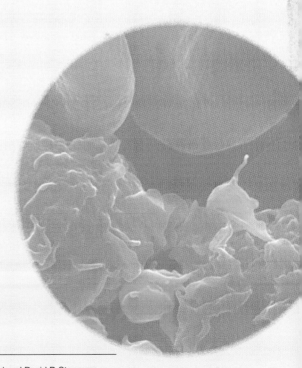

Hoffbrand's Essential Haematology, Eighth Edition. By A. Victor Hoffbrand and David P. Steensma.
© 2020 John Wiley & Sons Ltd. Published 2020 by John Wiley & Sons Ltd.
Companion website: www.wileyessential.com/haematology

The treatment of haematological malignancy has improved greatly since the first effective chemotherapeutic drugs were introduced in the 1940s. This has resulted from developments in both **supportive therapy** and **specific treatment** for each neoplasm. Details of specific treatment of individual diseases are detailed in the appropriate chapter. Supportive care and general aspects of the agents used in the treatment of haematological malignancy are described here.

General supportive therapy

Patients with haematological malignancies often present with medical problems related to suppression of normal haemopoiesis, and this problem is compounded by the treatments given to eradicate the neoplasia. When considering treatment, it is valuable to assess the normal daily living abilities of the patient, using assessments such as the **ECOG (Eastern Cooperative Oncology Group) performance status** (Table 12.1). When formulating a treatment plan, it is also important to consider **co-morbid conditions** such as cardiac, pulmonary and renal disease.

General supportive therapy for patients undergoing intensive treatment often includes the following.

Insertion of a central venous catheter

A central venous catheter is usually inserted for those patients who will need intensive treatment, especially with chemotherapy drugs that can cause damage to the soft tissue if they extravasate from small peripheral blood vessels ('vesicants'). There are several different types of central venous catheter commonly used in clinical practice.

Hickman- or Broviac-style catheters are placed in the operating theatre or interventional radiology suite via a skin

Table 12.1 Eastern Cooperative Oncology Group (ECOG) performance status.

Grade	Description
0	Fully active, able to carry on all pre-disease performance without restriction
1	Restricted in physically strenuous activity, but ambulatory and able to carry out work of a light or sedentary nature, e.g. light housework, office work
2	Ambulatory and capable of all self-care, but unable to carry out any work activities. Up and about more than 50% of waking hours
3	Capable of only limited self-care, confined to bed or chair more than 50% of waking hours
4	Completely disabled. Cannot carry on any self-care. Totally confined to bed or chair
5	Dead

tunnel from the chest into the jugular vein, with the catheter tip terminating in the superior vena cava or at the cavo-atrial junction (Fig. 12.1).

A totally implantable venous access device, sometimes called **Port-a-cath or Mediport**, is similar to a Hickman catheter, but these devices also include a reservoir (port) with a silicone membrane (septum) through which a needle can be inserted. The reservoir and membrane are buried under the skin of the patient's chest wall so that the patient does not have any catheter components protruding from the body. This makes it

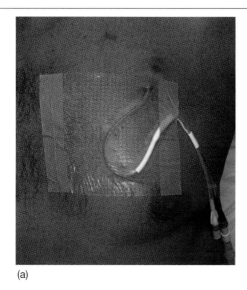
(a)

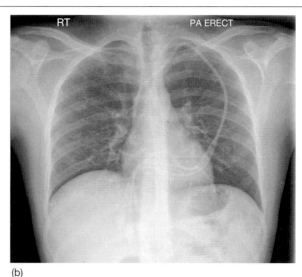
(b)

Figure 12.1 (a) A central venous line in a patient undergoing intensive chemotherapy. **(b)** Chest X-ray showing correct placement of a central venous line, in this case a tunnelled triple lumen left internal jugular line. Source: Courtesy of Dr P. Wylie.

easier for the patient to bathe or swim, but it is more difficult to remove a totally implantable device than a Hickman-style catheter.

Finally, **peripherally inserted central catheters (PICC lines)** are placed in the arm, usually in a cephalic or brachial vein, and then extended up via the axillary and subclavian veins to the superior vena cava. PICC lines have the advantage that they can be placed at the bedside, often by a nurse rather than a surgeon or radiologist, but they typically do not last as long as the other catheter types.

Each of these lines give ease of access for administering chemotherapy, blood products, antibiotics and intravenous feeding. In addition, blood may be taken for laboratory tests through the catheter. However, they require site and line care and are a risk factor for venous thrombosis. In addition, as foreign bodies they may serve as a source of infection.

Blood product support (see also Chapter 30)

Red cell and platelet transfusions are used to treat anaemia and thrombocytopenia. A number of particular issues apply to the support of patients with haematological malignancy:

1 The threshold haemoglobin (Hb) for transfusion will depend on clinical factors such as symptoms and speed of onset of anaemia, but most units give red cell support for an Hb less than 80 g/L, with a higher threshold in older patients or those with ischaemia. In patients needing both red cells and platelets, platelets are given first to reduce the risk of a further fall in the platelet count. Red cell transfusions should be avoided if at all possible in patients with a very high white cell count (above 100×10^9/L) because of hyperviscosity and so the risk of precipitating thrombotic episodes as a result of white cell stasis.

2 Large-volume transfusions, such as 3 units of blood or more, can precipitate pulmonary oedema in older patients and should be given slowly and with clinical monitoring. Diuretics such as furosemide are often given.

3 The trigger for platelet transfusion is typically a platelet count below 10×10^9/L, but the threshold should be increased in the presence of active bleeding or fever.

4 Fresh frozen plasma (FFP) or cryoprecipitate may be needed to reverse coagulation defects.

5 Cytomegalovirus (CMV) negative or leuco-depleted blood should be given to all patients until it has been shown that they are either CMV seropositive or that they will never be candidates for stem cell transplantation (SCT). This is to prevent transmission of CMV to uninfected patients, as the virus is a significant problem in stem cell transplant recipients (see p. 291).

6 Febrile reactions with blood products are not uncommon and should be managed by slowing the infusion and administration of drugs such as antihistamines, pethidine or hydrocortisone. The dosage of steroids should be limited because of concerns with immunosuppression.

7 Granulocyte transfusions may be given for severely neutropenic patients with serious infection not responding to antibiotics as a bridge to endogenous recovery of haemopoiesis, but their efficacy is not proven.

8 Blood products given to highly immunosuppressed patients (such as those who have received fludarabine, with aplastic anaemia, Hodgkin lymphoma or post-allogeneic SCT) should be irradiated prior to administration to prevent transfusion-associated graft-versus-host disease (see p. 382).

9 The use of recombinant erythropoiesis-stimulating agents (ESAs) to reduce the need for blood transfusion (e.g. in myeloma or myelodysplastic syndromes) is discussed on p. 201.

10 Granulocyte-colony stimulating factor (G-CSF) may be given to accelerate neutrophil recovery after certain intensive chemotherapy regimens.

Haemostasis support

A coagulation screen should be performed regularly on patients undergoing intensive chemotherapy; support with vitamin K or FFP may be required. Cryoprecipitate or antithrombin concentrates may be needed for certain coagulation factor deficiency, such as that precipitated by asparaginase in the management of acute lymphoblastic leukaemia. Antiplatelet drugs such as aspirin or clopidogrel are usually discontinued in patients undergoing intensive chemotherapy and patients on long-term warfarin or direct oral anticoagulants can be switched to low molecular weight heparin, which can then itself be stopped if the platelet count falls below 50×10^9/L. Progesterones are given to premenopausal women undergoing intensive chemotherapy to prevent menstruation. Tranexamic acid or aminocaproic acid can be given to reduce haemorrhage in patients with chronic low-grade blood loss despite platelet transfusion or thrombomimetic therapy.

Anti-emetic therapy

Nausea and vomiting are common side-effects of chemotherapy. A key objective is to try to prevent nausea occurring early in the treatment, as it is more difficult to control once the symptom has already arisen. **The 5-HT$_3$ (serotonin) receptor antagonists, such as ondansetron, granisetron and palonosetron**, can control nausea from intensive chemotherapy in over 60% of cases; the addition of dexamethasone can increase this by approximately 20%. Metoclopramide, prochlorperazine or cyclizine, benzodiazepines (e.g. lorazepam), domperidone, neurokinin-1 receptor antagonists (e.g. aprepitant, fosaprepitant) or cannabinoids (e.g. nabilone, dronabinol) can all have a role.

Tumour lysis syndrome

Chemotherapy may trigger an acute rise in plasma uric acid, potassium and phosphate and cause hypocalcaemia because of rapid lysis of tumour cells. This syndrome is seen most commonly with rapidly dividing neoplasias such as lymphoblastic lymphoma or acute leukaemia and can cause acute renal failure. Allopurinol, intravenous fluids and electrolyte replacement are the mainstay of prevention. Rasburicase, an enzyme that oxidizes uric acid to allantoin, is highly effective in controlling hyperuricaemia.

Psychological support

Patients with a diagnosis of malignant disease commonly feel concerns about such issues as the discomfort of treatment, finance, sexuality and fear of mortality. Even when patients achieve a clinical remission, there is understandable concern about the chance of disease relapse. Psychological support should be an integral part of the relationship between physician and patient, and patients should be allowed to express their fears and concerns at the earliest opportunity. Most patients value the opportunity to read more about their disorder and many excellent booklets or websites are now available.

Teamwork is also crucial, and the nursing staff and trained counsellors have a vital role in offering support and information during inpatient and outpatient care. Many units have specialist input from clinical psychologists and psychiatric help may occasionally be required. Inadequate communication is perhaps the most common failing of medical teams. The immediate family should be kept informed of the patient's progress whenever possible and appropriate.

Reproductive issues

Men who are to receive cytotoxic drugs should be offered sperm storage, ideally before treatment commences or, if impossible, within a short period of time thereafter. Ethical issues relating to storage or potential usage of tissue in the event of treatment failure will need to be addressed. Permanent infertility in women is less common after chemotherapy, although premature menopause may occur, and menopause is inevitable with myeloablative allogeneic SCT. Storage of fertilized ova is often impractical and specialist advice should be obtained in relation to storage of eggs.

Nutritional support

Some degree of weight loss is virtually inevitable in patients undergoing inpatient chemotherapy because of the combination of a poor nutritional intake, malabsorption caused by drugs and a catabolic disease state. If a weight loss of more than 10% occurs, nutritional support is often given, either enterally via a nasogastric tube or parenterally through a central venous catheter.

Pain

Pain directly due to the malignancy is rarely a major problem in haematological malignancies except myeloma, although bone pain can be a presenting feature for diseases with extensive marrow involvement such as the leukaemias. Occasionally, lymph nodes in lymphoma will be painful, and lymphoma sometimes also involves bone. The mucositis that follows intensive chemotherapy can cause severe discomfort and continuous infusions of opiate analgesia are often required. Pain is a frequent issue in patients with multiple myeloma and can be managed by a combination of analgesia and chemotherapy/radiotherapy. Advice from palliative care teams or specialist pain management practitioners should be sought when required.

Prophylaxis and treatment of infection

Patients with haematological malignancy are at great risk of infection, which remains the major cause of morbidity and mortality. Immunosuppression may result from neutropenia, hypogammaglobulinaemia and impaired cellular function. These can be secondary to the primary disease or its treatment. Neutropenia is a particular concern and in many patients neutrophils are totally absent from the blood for periods of 2 weeks or more. The use of G-CSF to reduce periods of neutropenia is discussed on p. 100. One potential protocol for the management of infection in an immunosuppressed patient is illustrated in Fig. 12.2.

Bacterial infection

This is the most common problem and usually arises from the patient's own commensal bacterial flora. **Gram-positive skin organisms** (e.g. *Staphylococcus* and *Streptococcus*) commonly colonize central venous lines, whereas **Gram-negative gut bacteria** (e.g. *Pseudomonas aeruginosa*, *Escherichia coli*, *Proteus*, *Klebsiella* and anaerobes) can cause overwhelming septicaemia. Even organisms not normally considered pathogenic, such as *Staphylococcus epidermidis*, may cause life-threatening infection. In the absence of neutrophils, local superficial lesions can rapidly cause severe septicaemia.

Prophylaxis of bacterial infection

Protocols used to limit bacterial infection vary from unit to unit. They usually do not include the use of a prophylactic antibiotic because of resistance developing. During periods of neutropenia, topical antiseptics for bathing and chlorhexidine mouthwashes and a 'clean diet' are recommended. The patient is sometimes nursed in a reverse-barrier room. The severity and length of mucositis may be reduced by treatment with recombinant human keratinocyte growth factor (palifermin). Oral non-absorbed antimicrobial agents, such as neomycin and colistin, reduce gut commensal flora, but many units do not use them in order to avoid bacterial resistance. Regular surveillance cultures can be taken to document the patient's bacterial flora and its sensitivity.

Treatment of bacterial infection

Fever is the main indication that infection is present, because if neutropenia is present pus will not be formed and infections are often not localized. Fever may be caused by blood products or drugs, but infection is the most common cause and fever of over 38°C in neutropenic patients should be investigated and treated very quickly. Cultures should be taken from any likely focus of infection, including blood from central venous lines and peripheral veins, from urine and from mouth swabs. The mouth and throat, intravenous catheter site and perineal

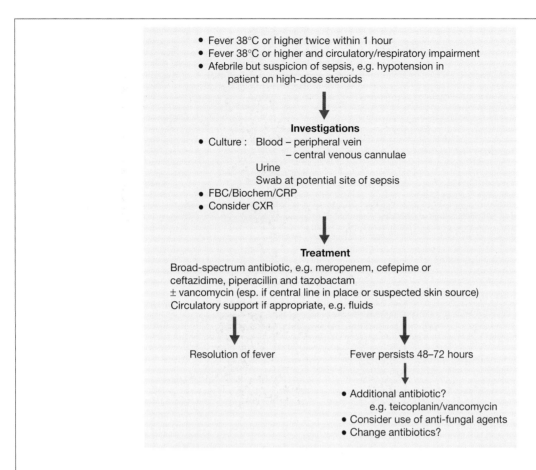

- Fever 38°C or higher twice within 1 hour
- Fever 38°C or higher and circulatory/respiratory impairment
- Afebrile but suspicion of sepsis, e.g. hypotension in patient on high-dose steroids

↓

Investigations

- Culture : Blood – peripheral vein
  – central venous cannulae
  Urine
  Swab at potential site of sepsis
- FBC/Biochem/CRP
- Consider CXR

↓

Treatment

Broad-spectrum antibiotic, e.g. meropenem, cefepime or ceftazidime, piperacillin and tazobactam
± vancomycin (esp. if central line in place or suspected skin source)
Circulatory support if appropriate, e.g. fluids

Resolution of fever   Fever persists 48–72 hours

↓

- Additional antibiotic?
  e.g. teicoplanin/vancomycin
- Consider use of anti-fungal agents
- Change antibiotics?

Figure 12.2 A protocol for the management of fever in the neutropenic patient. CRP, C-reactive protein; CXR, chest X-ray; FBC, full blood count.

and perianal areas are particularly likely foci. A chest X-ray is indicated as chest infections are frequent.

Antibiotic therapy must be started immediately after blood and other cultures have been taken; in many febrile episodes no organisms are isolated. There are many different antibiotic regimes in use and a close link with the microbiology team is essential. A typical regimen might be based on a single agent, such as a broad-spectrum penicillin (e.g. piperacillin/ tazobactam), meropenem or a broad-spectrum cephalosporin with anti-*Pseudomonal* activity. *Staphylococcus epidermidis* is a common source of fever in patients with intravenous lines and an agent such as teicoplanin, vancomycin or linezolid may be needed. If an infective agent and its antibiotic sensitivities become known, appropriate changes in the regimen are made. If no response occurs within 48–72 hours, changing the antibiotics or adding antifungal coverage is considered.

Viral infection

Prophylaxis and treatment of viral infection

Herpes viruses such as herpes simplex, varicella zoster, CMV and Epstein–Barr virus (EBV) undergo latency following primary infection and are never eradicated from the host. Most patients with haematological malignancy have already been infected with these agents and viral reactivation is therefore the most common problem. Aciclovir or valaciclovir is frequently given prophylactically. Herpes simplex is a common cause of oral ulcers, but is usually controlled easily by aciclovir. Varicella zoster frequently reactivates in patients with lymphoproliferative diseases to cause shingles, which requires treatment with high doses of aciclovir or valaciclovir. Primary infection, usually in children, can be very serious and immunoglobulin can be used to prevent infection following recent exposure. While the live attenuated varicella vaccine (Zostavax®) is contraindicated for many patients with haematological malignancy, the new non-live recombinant adjuvant-enhanced vaccine (Shingrix®) represents a safer and more effective alternative. Reactivation of CMV infection is particularly common following SCT (see Chapter 23), but may occur following intensive chemotherapy. Failure of immune control of EBV following allogeneic transplantation can lead to outgrowth of a B-cell tumour known as post-transplant lymphoproliferative disease (see p. 293).

Fungal infection

Prophylaxis and treatment of fungal infection

Because of the intensity of current chemotherapy, fungal infections are a major cause of morbidity and mortality. The two major subtypes are yeasts, such as *Candida* species, and moulds, of which *Aspergillus fumigatus* is the most common.

Invasive aspergillosis is a common cause of infectious death in intensively immunocompromised patients (Fig. 12.3). Infection occurs through inhalation of *Aspergillus* spores (conidia) and air filtration systems are used in many haematology wards. The major risk factor is neutropenia – nearly 70% of patients become infected if they are neutropenic for over 34 days. Steroid use is also important, as is age, chemotherapy and antimicrobial history.

The diagnosis of invasive aspergillosis can be difficult. Definitive diagnosis requires demonstration of invasive growth on a biopsy specimen, but such evidence is rarely available. Polymerase chain reaction for fungal DNA or enzyme-linked immunosorbent assay (ELISA) for *Aspergillus* galactomannan or β1–3 d-glucan is useful. High-resolution computed tomography (HRCT) chest scan is valuable and early features are nodular lesions with a 'ground glass' halo appearance. Later on,

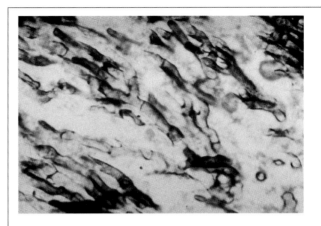

Figure 12.3 Cytology of sputum illustrates the branching septate hyphae of *Aspergillus* (methenamine silver stain).

wedge lesions and the air crescent sign are seen (Fig. 12.4). A high index of suspicion for fungal infection should be maintained, and treatment is often started empirically for a fever that has failed to resolve after 2–4 days of antibiotic treatment.

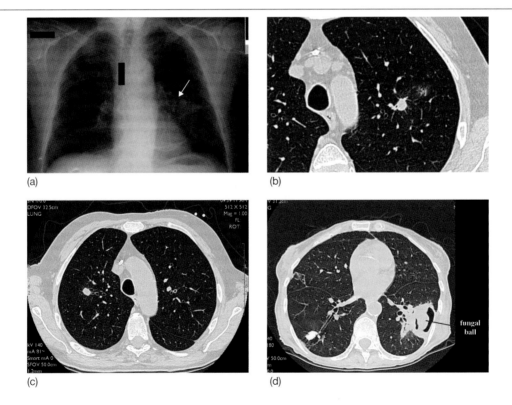

(a)

(b)

(c)

(d)

Figure 12.4 (a) Chest X-ray of patient with pulmonary aspergillosis which shows an area of cavitation containing a central fungal ball (arrow), leading to the typical 'air-crescent' sign. **(b)** and **(c)** Computed tomography (CT) scans in *aspergillosis* show hazy ground-glass shadowing with bronchiolar dilatation. **(d)** Nodules are seen in early aspergillosis, whereas a fungal ball with surrounding air is typical of more advanced disease.

Prophylaxis or treatment for patients at risk of *Aspergillus* infection is usually performed with itraconazole, caspofungin, micafungin, voriconazole, posaconazole, isavuconazium or lipid formulation amphotericin. Surgery to remove lung lesions may be needed.

Candida species are a common hospital pathogen and frequently cause oral infection. *Candida* is significant when isolated from normally sterile body fluids such as blood or urine. Prophylaxis or treatment is usually with fluconazole, itraconazole or caspofungin. Anidulafungin and micafungin are also licensed. *Pneumocystis jirovecii (carinii)* is an important cause of pneumonitis. Prophylaxis is with co-trimoxazole or atovaquone (highly effective) or with nebulized pentamidine (less effective) and is given to those who have received intensive (combination) chemotherapy or fludarabine. Treatment is with high-dose co-trimoxazole.

Drugs used in the treatment of haemopoietic malignancies

Specific therapy is aimed at reducing the neoplastic cell burden by the use of drugs or radiotherapy. The hope in some diseases is to eradicate the neoplasia completely, and cure rates for haematological malignancy are gradually improving. However, cure is often not achievable, so palliation can also be an important aim.

A wide variety of drugs is used in the management of haemopoietic malignancies. Several drugs acting at different sites (Fig. 12.5) are often combined together in regimens that minimize the potential for resistance to occur against a single agent. Many act specifically on dividing cells and their selectivity is dependent on the high proliferation rate within the tumour. Not all neoplastic cells will be killed by a single course of treatment and it is usual to give several courses of treatment, which gradually eradicate the neoplastic cell burden. This 'log kill' hypothesis also gives the residual normal haemopoietic cells the opportunity to recover between treatment courses.

Cytotoxic drugs (Table 12.2)

Alkylating agents, such as chlorambucil, cyclophosphamide and melphalan, are activated to expose reactive alkyl groups which make covalent bonds to molecules within the cell. These have a particular affinity for purines and are thus able to

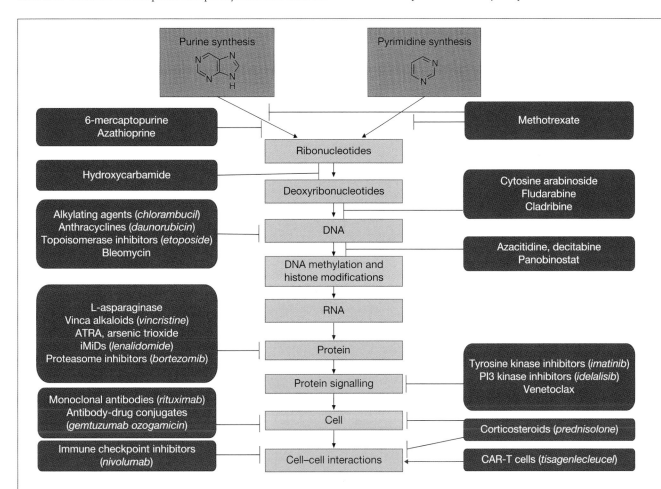

Figure 12.5 The site of action of some drugs used in the treatment of haemopoietic malignancies. One example of the drugs in each of the different major classes is given. ATRA, all-*trans* retinoic acid; CAR, chimeric antigen receptor.

Table 12.2 Drugs used in the treatment of leukaemia and lymphoma.

Drug/drug class	Mechanism of action	Particular side-effects*
Alkylating agents		
Cyclophosphamide	Cross-link DNA, impede RNA formation	Marrow aplasia, haemorrhagic cystitis, cardiomyopathy, loss of hair
Chlorambucil		Marrow aplasia, hepatic toxicity, dermatitis, alopecia
Busulphan		Marrow aplasia, pulmonary fibrosis, hyperpigmentation, seizures, hepatic toxicity, alopecia
Melphalan		Marrow aplasia, alopecia
Bendamustine	Cross-link DNA as for other alkylating agents, and also purine nucleoside analogue	Myelosuppression
Antimetabolites		
Hydroxycarbamide (hydroxyurea)	Inhibit ribonucleotide reductase	Pigmentation, nail dystrophy, skin keratosis, epitheliomas
Methotrexate	Inhibit pyrimidine or purine synthesis or incorporation into DNA	Mouth ulcers, gut toxicity
Cytosine arabinoside (Ara-C)	Inhibits DNA synthesis	CNS, especially cerebellar toxicity and conjunctivitis at high doses
6-mercaptopurine,† 6-thioguanine†	Purine analogue	Jaundice, gut toxicity
Clofarabine	Purine analogue	Myelosuppression
Fludarabine, 2-chlorodeoxyadenosine (2-CDA, cladribine), deoxycoformycin (pentostatin)	Purine analogues; inhibit adenosine deaminase or other purine pathways	Immunosuppression (low CD4 counts); renal and neurotoxicity (at high doses)
Cytotoxic antibiotics		
Anthracyclines (e.g. daunorubicin, idarubicin; mitoxantrone)	Bind to DNA and interfere with mitosis	Cardiac toxicity, hair loss
Bleomycin	Induce DNA breaks	Pulmonary fibrosis, skin pigmentation
Amasacrine (m-AMSA)	Topoisomerase inhibitor	Hair loss, mucositis
Plant derivatives		
Vincristine (Oncovin®), vinblastine	Spindle damage	Neuropathy (peripheral or bladder or gut)
Etoposide	Mitotic inhibitor	Hair loss, oral ulceration
Epigenetic modifiers		
Demethylating (hypomethylating) agents: azacytidine, decitabine	Inhibit DNA methlytransferase	Myelosuppression, injection site reactions (for subcutaneous azacytidine)
Histone deacetylase inhibitors (panobinostat, romidepsin)	Inhibit histone deacetylase	Fatigue, thrombocytopenia
Signal transduction inhibitors		
Imatinib, dasatinib, nilotinib, bosutinib, ponatinib, asciminib	Inhibit ABL tyrosine kinase	Myelosuppression, fluid retention, pancreatitis, GI upset, thrombosis (ponatinib)
Midostaurin, gilteritinib, crenolanib, quizartinib, sorafenib	Inhibit FLT3 kinase	Myelosuppression, GI upset
Ibrutinib, acalbrutinib	Inhibit BTK protein	Bleeding, disease flare
Idelalisib, duvelisib, copanlisib	Inhibit PI3K delta	Colitis, atrial dysrhythmia
Ruxolitinib, pacritinib, fedratinib	Inhibit JAK2	Marrow suppression
Crizotinib	Inhibit ALK	Visual disturbance, hepatic enzyme elevation, GI effects
Gladesgib	Inhibit Hedgehog pathway	Marrow suppression, myalgias, nausea, embryo-fetal toxicity

Miscellaneous

Corticosteroids	Lymphoblast lysis	Diabetes, osteoporosis, psychosis,
Trans-retinoic acid	Induces differentiation	Skin hyperkeratosis, leucocytosis and pleural effusion
Arsenic trioxide	Induces differentiation or apoptosis	Hyperleucocytosis, prolonged QTc interval, neuropathy
α-Interferon	Activation of RNAase and natural killer activity	Flu-like symptoms, thrombocytopenia, leucopenia, weight loss
Enasidenib, ivosidenib	Inhibit mutated isocitric dehydrogenase (IDHI)	Differentiation syndrome, cytopenias
Venetoclax	Inhibit BCL2 signalling	Tumour lysis
Panobinostat	Histone deacetylase inhibitor	Fatigue, thrombocytopenia
Omacetaxine	Inhibits protein translation	Injection site reactions, GI effects, myelosuppression
Bortezomib, ixazomib, carfilzomib	Proteasome inhibition	Neuropathy
L-asparaginase, PEG-asparaginase	Deprive cells of asparagine	Hypersensitivity, low albumin and coagulation factors, pancreatitis
Thalidomide, lenalidomide, pomalidomide	Immunomodulation, alteration of protein degradation	Neuropathy, constipation, thrombosis

Monoclonal antibodies

Rituximab, ofatumumab, obinutuzumab (all anti-CD20)	Induction of apoptosis	Infusion reactions, immunosuppression
Alemtuzumab (anti-CD52)	Lysis of target cell by complement fixation	Infusion reactions, immunosuppression
Ibritumomab (Zevalin®) (anti-CD20 with ^{90}Y radioisotope)	Toxicity to bound cell	Myelosuppression, nausea
Gemtuzumab (Mylotarg®) (anti-CD33 with calicheamicin cytotoxin)	Kill myeloid cells	Myelosuppression, hepatic sinusoidal occlusive syndrome
Inotuzumab (Besponsa®) (anti-CD22 with calicheamicin cytotoxin)	Kill neoplastic B cells	Cytokine release syndrome, hepatic sinusoidal occlusive syndrome
Tagraxofusp (Elzonristm®) (anti-CD123 with diphtheria toxin)	Kill myeloid cells or blastic plasmacytoid dendritic cells	Oedema and capillary leak syndrome, nausea, fever, hepatotoxicity, hypoalbuminemia, myelosuppression
Blinatumomab (Blincyto®) (bispecific CD20/CD3)	Recruit cytotoxic T cells to neoplastic B cells	Neurotoxicity, cytokine release syndrome
Brentuximab (Adcetris®) (anti-CD30)	Kill CD30+ lymphocytes	Myelosuppression, neuropathy
Daratumumab (Darzalex®) (anti-CD38)	Kill malignant plasma cells	Infusion reactions, myelosuppression, difficulty matching for transfusion
Elotuzumab (Empliciti®) (anti-SLAMF7)	Kill malignant plasma cells	Fatigue, GI effects, neuropathy, myelosuppression

Immune checkpoint inhibitors

Nivolumab, pembrolizumab, ipilimumab	Inhibit PD-1, PDL-1 or CTLA4 signalling and activate cytotoxic T cells	Autoimmune manifestations (myocarditis, colitis, thyroid disease, iridocyclitis, hepatic injury, kidney dysfunction), infection

Chimeric antigen receptor T cells

Tisagenlecleucel, axicabtagene ciloleucel	Kill CD19+ cells directly	Cytokine release syndrome, neurotoxicity

*Many of the drugs cause nausea, vomiting, mucositis and bone marrow toxicity, and in large doses infertility. Tissue necrosis is a problem if the drugs are extravasated during infusion.
† Allopurinol potentiates the action and side-effects of 6-mercaptopurine.
CNS, central nervous system; GI, gastrointestinal.

crosslink DNA strands and impair DNA replication, resulting in a block at G_2 and death of the cell by apoptosis (see Fig. 1.9). Bendamustine is a unique drug in this class, as it also appears to have activity associated with purine analogue function.

Antimetabolites block metabolic pathways used in DNA synthesis. There are four major groups:

1 **Inhibitors of *de novo* DNA synthesis**. Hydroxycarbamide (hydroxyurea) is used widely in the treatment of myeloproliferative disorders. It inhibits the enzyme ribonucleotide reductase, which converts ribonucleotides to deoxyribonucleotides. It is not thought to permanently damage DNA and is also used in non-malignant disorders such as sickle cell anaemia (p. 93).

2 **Folate antagonists**, such as methotrexate (see p. 54). Methotrexate is widely used alone or in combination with cytosine arabinoside as intrathecal prophylaxis of central nervous system (CNS) disease in patients with acute lymphoid leukaemia (ALL), acute myeloid leukaemia (AML) or high-grade non-Hodgkin lymphoma. High systemic doses may also penetrate the CNS. Folinic acid (formyl THF) is able to overcome the activity of methotrexate and is sometimes administered to 'rescue' normal cells after high-dose methotrexate therapy.

3 **Pyrimidine analogues** include cytosine arabinoside (cytarabine; ara-C), which is an analogue of 2′-deoxycytidine and is incorporated into DNA, where it inhibits DNA polymerase and blocks replication.

4 **Purine analogues** include fludarabine (which inhibits DNA synthesis in a manner similar to ara-C), mercaptopurine, azathioprine, bendamustine, clofarabine and pentostatin.

Cytotoxic antibiotic drugs include the anthracyclines, such as doxorubicin, daunorubicin, idarubicin and the chemically similar anthracenedione mitoxantrone. These are able to intercalate into DNA and then bind strongly to topoisomerases, which are critical for relieving torsional stress in replicating DNA by nicking and resealing DNA strands. If topoisomerase activity is blocked, DNA replication cannot take place.

Bleomycin is a metal chelating antibiotic that generates superoxide radicals within cells that degrade preformed DNA. It is active on non-cycling cells.

Plant derivatives include the vinca alkaloids such as vincristine, which is derived from the periwinkle plant. It binds to tubulin and prevents its polymerization to microtubules. This blocks cell division in metaphase. Etoposide inhibits topisomerase action.

Targeted drugs

A wide range of targeted drugs which block specific proteins are now in use and are likely to eventually replace the cytotoxic agents described above.

ABL1 inhibitors such as imatinib and nilotinib bind to the BCR-ABL1 fusion protein. They block binding of adenosine triphosphate (ATP) and thus prevent the overactive tyrosine kinase from phosphorylating substrate proteins, leading to apoptosis of the cell (see Fig. 14.4). They are used in chronic myeloid leukaemia (CML) and BCR-ABL1+ ALL.

Inhibitors of B cell signalling pathways such as ibrutinib and acalbrutinib, which block Bruton kinase (BTK), or idelalisib or duvelisib, which inhibit the delta isoenzyme of PI3 kinase, are valuable in the management of a range of B-cell disorders (Fig. 9.4).

A wide range of **additional kinase inhibitors** is being introduced into therapy, such as JAK2 inhibitors, effective in primary myelofibrosis and polycythaemia vera; crizotinib, which blocks ALK activity; and inhibitors of the FLT3 kinase such as midostaurin, gilteritinib and crenolanib for treatment of AML. Glasdegib inhibits Hedgehog signalling, an important survival pathway for neoplastic cells.

Ivosidenib and **enasidenib** inhibit mutant isocitrate dehydrogenase 1 and 2, respectively, and are useful in the ~25% of AML cases that have one of these mutations.

Bortezomib, **ixazomib** and **carfilzomib** are proteasome inhibitors used widely in the treatment of myeloma and some lymphomas.

Monoclonal antibodies are highly effective and are particularly well established against B-cell malignancies. Rituximab binds to CD20 on B cells and mediates cell death, primarily through direct induction of apoptosis and opsonization (see p. 247). Other anti-CD20 antibodies, e.g. obinutuzumab and ofatumumab, are available. Alemtuzumab binds to CD52 and is highly efficient at fixing complement, which lyses the target B and T cells. Anti-CD30 (brentuximab) is effective in Hodgkin lymphoma. Antibodies may also carry attached toxins (e.g. gemtuzumab, anti-CD33, inotuzumab, anti-CD22, or tagraxofusp, anti-CD123) or radioactive isotopes (e.g. Zevalin®, anti-CD20). Bispecific antibodies (e.g. blinatumomab) recruit CD3+ T cells to tumour cells.

Other agents

Corticosteroids have a potent lymphocytotoxic activity and have an important role in many chemotherapeutic regimens used in the treatment of lymphoid malignancy and myeloma.

All-*trans* retinoic acid (ATRA) is a vitamin A derivative that acts as a differentiation agent in acute promyelocytic leukaemia (APML). Tumour cells in APML are arrested at the promyelocyte stage as a result of transcriptional repression resulting from the PML-RARA fusion protein (see p. 165). ATRA relieves this block and may lead to a brisk neutrophilia within a few days of treatment, with other side-effects known as the 'ATRA' or 'differentiation' syndrome (see p. 166).

Demethylation agents (e.g. azacytidine, decitabine) act to increase transcription by reducing methylation on cytosine residues within DNA. However, the precise mechanism of their clinical activity is unclear.

Interferon-α is an antiviral and antimitotic substance produced in response to viral infection and inflammation. It has proven useful in CML, myeloma and myeloproliferative neoplasms.

Immunomodulatory drugs include thalidomide, lenalidomide and pomalidomide. They are effective in myeloma and in some types of myelodysplasia.

Asparaginase is an enzyme derived from bacteria that breaks down the amino acid asparagine within the circulation. ALL cells lack asparagine synthase and thus need a supply of exogenous asparagine for protein synthesis. Intramuscular asparaginase is an important agent in the treatment of ALL, although hypersensitivity reactions are not uncommon and blood clotting may be disturbed. PEGylation of asparaginase increases half-life and decreases frequency of required injection.

Platinum derivatives (e.g. cisplatin) are used in combinations for treating lymphoma.

Arsenic is useful in treatment of acute promyelocytic leukaemia. It induces differentiation and apoptosis.

Immune checkpoint inhibitors are antibodies designed to overcome T cell self-tolerance to neoplastic cells. Approved checkpoint inhibitors block PD-1, PD-L1 or CTLA4 molecules that mediate self-tolerance. They can be useful in some cases of relapsed Hodgkin lymphoma or in leukaemias relapsed after allogeneic SCT.

Chimeric antigen receptor (CAR)-T cells

Chimeric antigen receptors are T-cell receptors that are bioengineered using retroviral vectors to give T cells the antigen specificity of a monoclonal antibody (Chapter 9). The receptors are called 'chimeric' because the components of the engineered T-cell receptor construct include both tumour antigen-reactive and T-cell-activating functions. CAR-T cells can be derived either from the patient's own immune cells (autologous) or a donor (allogeneic); the latter offers the possibility of an off-the-shelf product. Autologous CAR-T cells targeting CD19 are approved for B-cell ALL (Chapter 17), for relapsed/refractory B-cell large cell lymphoma (Chapter 20), and are proving effective also in refractory multiple myeloma (Chapter 21) and refractory acute myeloid leukaemia (Chapter 13).

Toxicities include **cytokine release syndrome**, with fever, hypotension, hypoxia, vomiting, diarrhoea, skin rashes, renal failure, tremor, confusion and delirium due to encephalitis. The cytokines released from the neoplastic and normal cells include tumour necrosis factor, interferon-gamma and many interleukins (ILs). The plasma levels of some of these ILs may be measured to assess the severity and progress. Treatment is with corticosteroids and with anti-interleukin-6 antibodies such as toclizumab. As the cells also destroy normal B cells, treated patients require lifelong immunoglobulin infusions.

SUMMARY

- Progress in the treatment of haemopoietic malignancies has been the result of improvements in both supportive therapy and specific tumour treatments.
- Initial assessment includes a performance score and tests for co-morbidities.
- Supportive treatments often include insertion of a central venous catheter; appropriate use of red cell, platelet transfusions; early administration of drugs to treat infection; optimization of the blood coagulation system; drugs to reduce side-effects such as nausea or pain; psychological support.
- Gram-positive skin organisms such as *Staphylococcus* are common infections and often colonize central venous catheters.
- Gram-negative bacteria are usually derived from the gut and can cause severe septicaemia.
- The use of air filters, handwashing and prophylactic antibiotics can reduce infection rates.
- Neutropenic patients who develop a fever should be treated urgently with broad-spectrum antibiotics.
- Herpes viruses are a common cause of infection in patients who are significantly immunosuppressed.
- Fungal infections are a major clinical problem for patients undergoing chemotherapy. Oral and intravenous antifungal drugs may be used for either prevention or treatment of disease.
- A wide range of drugs is now available for the treatment of haemopoietic malignancy: alkylating agents; antimetabolites; anthracyclines; signal transduction inhibitors, including tyrosine kinase inhibitors; monoclonal antibodies; immune modulators; proteasome inhibitors; others, e.g. corticosteroids, ATRA, demethylating agents, interferon, asparaginase, arsenic, platinum derivatives.
- CAR-T cells have entered clinical practice for therapy of resistant B-lymphoid and plasma cell malignancies. They may cause a cytokine release syndrome including neurotoxicity.

Now visit **www.wileyessential.com/haematology** to test yourself on this chapter.

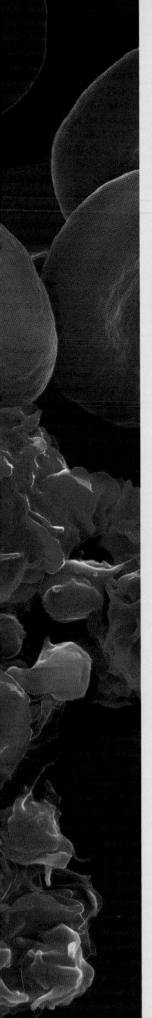

CHAPTER 13
Acute myeloid leukaemia

Key topics

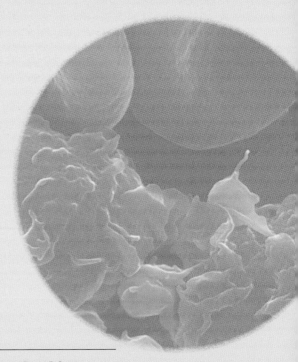

Hoffbrand's Essential Haematology, Eighth Edition. By A. Victor Hoffbrand and David P. Steensma.
© 2020 John Wiley & Sons Ltd. Published 2020 by John Wiley & Sons Ltd.
Companion website: www.wileyessential.com/haematology

The leukaemias are a group of disorders characterized by the accumulation of malignant white cells in the bone marrow and blood. These abnormal cells cause symptoms because of (i) bone marrow failure (e.g. anaemia, neutropenia, thrombocytopenia); and, less commonly, (ii) infiltration of organs (e.g. liver, spleen, lymph nodes, meninges, brain, skin or testes).

Classification of leukaemia

The main classification is into four types: **acute or chronic leukaemias,** which are further subdivided into **lymphoid or myeloid leukaemias**. Acute leukaemias are usually aggressive diseases in which malignant transformation occurs in a haemopoietic stem cell or early progenitor. Acquired genetic damage results in an increased rate of proliferation, reduced apoptosis and a block in cellular differentiation. Together these events cause accumulation in the bone marrow of early haemopoietic cells known as **blast cells**. The dominant clinical feature of acute leukaemia is usually bone marrow failure caused by accumulation of blast cells, although organ infiltration also can occur. If untreated, acute leukaemias are usually rapidly fatal, although with modern treatments most younger patients are ultimately cured of their disease.

Diagnosis of acute leukaemia

Acute leukaemia is normally defined as the presence of at least 20% of blast cells in the bone marrow or blood at clinical presentation. However, it can be diagnosed with less than 20% blasts if certain leukaemia-specific cytogenetic or molecular genetic abnormalities are present (Table 13.1; see also Table 17.1).

The **lineage of the blast cells** is defined by microscopic examination (morphology; see Fig. 13.5 and Fig. 17.3), immunophenotypic (flow cytometry; Fig. 13.1), cytogenetic and molecular analysis (see Table 13.4 and Table 11.1). These assessments define whether the blasts are of myeloid or lymphoid lineage and also localize the stage of cellular differentiation (Table 13.2). A typical 'myeloid' immunophenotype is CD13⁺, CD33⁺ and TdT⁻ (Table 13.2; Fig. 13.1). Special antibodies are helpful in the diagnosis of the rare undifferentiated, erythroid or megakaryoblastic subtypes (Table 13.2). Acute lymphoblastic leukaemia is discussed in Chapter 17. Occasionally, a case of leukaemia will express both myeloid and lymphoid markers.

Cytogenetic and **molecular** analysis is essential and is usually performed on marrow cells, although blood may be used if the circulating blast cell count is high. Cytochemistry can also be useful in determining the blast cell lineage (see Fig. 13.2), but is no longer performed in centres where the newer and more definitive tests are available.

Table 13.1 Classification of acute myeloid leukaemia (AML) according to the World Health Organization classification 2016 (this does not include AML with germline predisposition; see Appendix).

Acute myeloid leukaemia with recurrent genetic abnormalities

AML with t(8;21)(q22;q22); *RUNX1-RUNX1T1*

AML with inv(16)(p131q22) or t(16;16)(p13.1;q22); *CBFB-MYH11*

Acute promyelocytic leukaemia (APL) with t(15;17)(q22;q12); *PML-RARA*

AML with t(9;11)(p21.3;q23.3); *MLLT3-KMT2A (MLL)*

AML with t(6;9)(p23;q34.1); *DEK-NUP214*

AML with inv(3)(q21.3q26.2) or t(3;3)(q21.3;q26.2); *GATA2, MECOM*

AML (megakaryoblastic) with t(1;22)(p13.3;q13.3); *RBM15-MKL1*

AML with mutated *NPM1*

AML with biallelic mutations of *CEBPA*

Provisional entities: AML with mutated *RUNX1*, AML with *BCR-ABL1*

Acute myeloid leukaemia with myelodysplasia-related changes

Therapy-related myeloid neoplasms (t-AML/MDS)

Acute myeloid leukaemia, not otherwise specified

AML with minimal differentiation

AML without maturation

AML with maturation

Acute myelomonocytic leukaemia

Acute monoblastic/monocytic leukaemia

Acute erythroid leukaemia

Acute megakaryoblastic leukaemia

Acute basophilic leukaemia

Acute panmyelosis with myelofibrosis

Myeloid sarcoma

Myeloid proliferations related to Down syndrome

Transient abnormal myelopoiesis

Myeloid leukaemia

Acute myeloid leukaemia (AML)

Pathogenesis

The AML genome contains an average of about 10 mutations within protein-coding genes in each case, among the smallest number of any adult cancer (see Fig. 11.3). Many AML 'driver mutations' promoting clonal expansion have been identified, with the most common being within *FLT3*, *NPM1* and

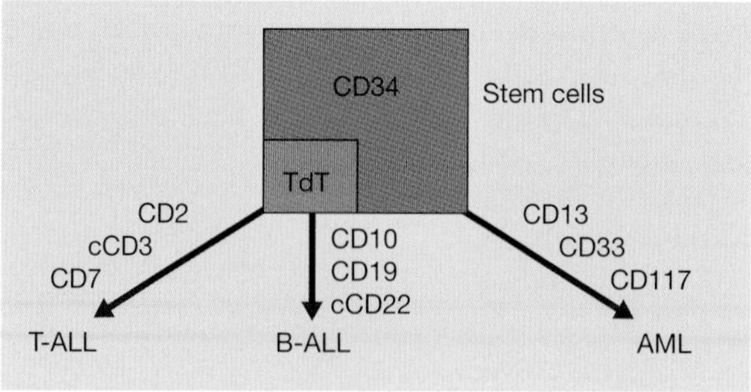

Figure 13.1 Development of three cell lineages from pluripotential stem cells giving rise to the three main immunological subclasses of acute leukaemia. CD34 is expressed on most stem cells, whereas TdT expression defines a lymphoid lineage. Three examples of surface markers which are seen characteristically in T-ALL, B-ALL and AML are shown; others are described in the relevant sections of this chapter and Chapter 17. AML, acute myeloid leukaemia; B-ALL, B-cell acute lymphoblastic leukaemia; c, cytoplasmic; CD, cluster of differentiation; HLA, human leucocyte antigen; T-ALL, T-cell acute lymphoblastic leukaemia; TdT, terminal deoxynucleotidyl transferase.

Table 13.2 Specialized tests for acute myeloid leukaemia (AML).	
Immunological markers (flow cytometry)	*Indicates*
CD13, CD33, CD34, CD117	Usually positive in AML
CD11c, 14, 64	Monoblastic differentiation
Glycophorin (CD235a), CD36	Erythroid differentiation
CD41, CD61	Megakaryoblastic differentiation
Myeloperoxidase, CD65	Granulocytic differentiation
Chromosome and genetic analysis (see Tables 13.1 and 13.4)	
Cytochemistry	
Myeloperoxidase	Myeloid differentiation (usually bright in Auer rods)
Sudan black	Myeloid differentiation (usually bright in Auer rods)
Non-specific esterase	Monocytic differentiation

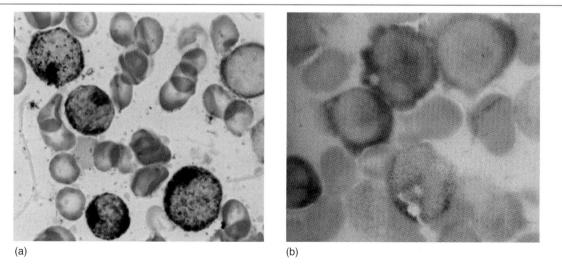

(a)   (b)

Figure 13.2 Cytochemical staining in acute myeloid leukaemia. **(a)** Sudan black B shows black staining in the cytoplasm. **(b)** Myelomonocytic: non-specific esterase/chloracetate staining shows orange-staining monoblast cytoplasm and blue-staining (myeloblast) cytoplasm.

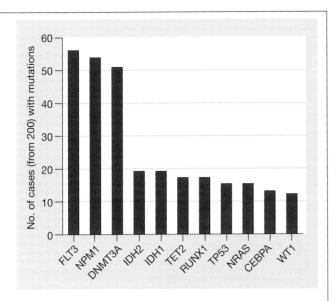

Figure 13.3 The most commonly mutated genes within an analysis of 200 cases of acute myeloid leukaemia. Source: Adapted from The Cancer Genome Atlas Research Network (2013) *N. Engl. J. Med.* 368(22): 2059–74.

DNMT3A (Fig. 13.3). Some other mutations, e.g. of *ASXL1* or mutations in splicing-associated genes, are frequent in myelodysplastic syndromes (MDS) and when found in AML suggest that it is secondary to MDS, which may not have been recognized clinically.

The mutations usually occur on only one of the two alleles for the gene and, depending on the gene, may be 'loss of function', 'gain of function' or 'neomorphic' (i.e. conferring a novel function). Some AML cases are characterized by a gene-fusion event, which usually arises from translocations, with the most common being *PML-RARA*, *CBFB-MYH11* and *RUNX1-RUNX1T1* (Table 11.1), which are found in around 15%, 12% and 8% of cases, respectively. The wide variety of cytogenetic abnormalities and molecular mutations is such that there are hundreds of patterns of mutations. Mutations of genes *DNMT3A*, *TET2*, *ASXL1* and less commonly *IDH1*, *IDH2*, *TP53* or spliceosome genes may be found in the blood cells of healthy subjects, especially after age 60 years (age-related clonal haemopoiesis or clonal haemopoiesis of indeterminate potential). Patients with these mutations can develop AML, which may present many years later. The likelihood of AML development is higher in those with *IDH1*, *IDH2*, *TP53* or spliceosome gene mutations, more than one mutation, high mutation allele burden, or an elevated red cell distribution width.

Incidence

AML is the most common form of acute leukaemia in adults and becomes increasingly common with age, with a median onset of 65 years. It forms only a minor fraction (10–15%) of the leukaemias in childhood. Cytogenetic and molecular abnormalities and response to initial treatment have a major influence on prognosis (see Table 13.4).

Classification

AML is classified according to the World Health Organization (WHO; 2016) scheme (Table 13.1). There is an increasing focus on the genetic abnormalities within the malignant cells, and it is likely that ultimately all AML cases will be classified by specific genetic subtype. Currently this is not yet possible, but many genetic subtypes have been determined. Approximately 60% of AML cases exhibit karyotypic abnormalities on cytogenetic analysis and most cases with a normal karyotype carry mutations in genes such as *FLT3*, *NPM1*, *CEBPA* or *DNMT3A*, detected only by molecular methods (see below).

Six main groups of AML are recognized (Table 13.1):

1 **AML with recurrent genetic abnormalities** encompasses subtypes with specific chromosomal translocations or gene mutations. The detection of a subset of these abnormalities – t(8;21), inv(16), or t(15;17) – defines the neoplasm as AML, and so the diagnostic criteria for this subgroup are relaxed in that the bone marrow blast cell count does not need to exceed 20% in order to make a diagnosis.

2 **AML with myelodysplasia-related changes.** In this group the AML is associated with microscopic features of dysplasia in at least 50% of cells in at least two lineages. The clinical outcome of these patients is impaired in relation to the first subgroup.

3 **Therapy-related myeloid neoplasms (t-AML)** arise in patients who have been previously treated with drugs such as etoposide or alkylating agents or with radiation. They commonly exhibit mutations in the *TP53* or *KMT2A(MLL)* gene and the clinical response is usually poor.

4 **AML, not otherwise specified.** This group is defined by the absence of any of the subset of recurrent cytogenetic or molecular genetic abnormalities that are distinctly classified by the WHO, and comprises around 20% of all cases.

5 **Myeloid sarcoma** is rare, but refers to a disease that resembles a solid tumour but is composed of clustered myeloid blast cells. This is often called 'extramedullary leukaemia', 'granulocytic sarcoma' or 'chloroma'.

6 **Myeloid proliferations related to Down syndrome.** Children with Down syndrome have a greatly increased risk of acute leukaemia, especially megakaryoblastic leukaemia. Two myeloid variants are recognized: (i) transient abnormal myelopoiesis, in which there is a self-limiting leucocytosis; and (ii) AML.

In addition, **acute leukaemias of ambiguous lineage (mixed phenotype acute leukaemias)** are rare cases that express two markers for both myeloid and lymphoid differentiation, either on the same blast cells or on two different cell populations in the same patient. They usually have a poor prognosis.

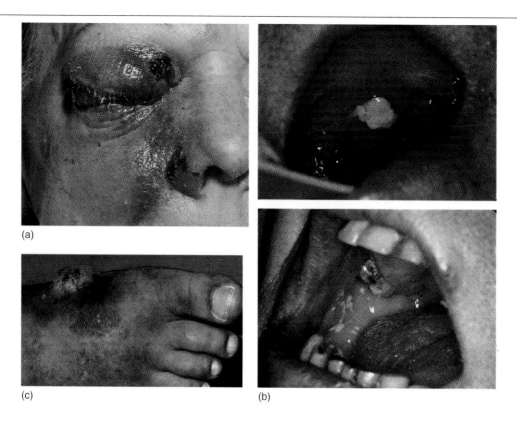

(a)

(b)

(c)

Figure 13.4 (a) An orbital infection in a female patient (aged 68 years) with acute myeloid leukaemia and severe neutropenia (haemoglobin 83 g/L, white cells 15.3 × 10⁹/L, blasts 96%, neutrophils 1%, platelets 30 × 10⁹/L). **(b)** Acute myeloid leukaemia: top: plaque *Candida albicans* on soft palate; lower: plaque *Candida albicans* in the mouth, with lesion of herpes simplex on the upper lip. **(c)** Skin infection (*Pseudomonas aeruginosa*) in a female patient (aged 33 years) with acute lymphoblastic leukaemia receiving chemotherapy and with severe neutropenia (haemoglobin 101 g/L, white cells 0.7 × 10⁹/L, neutrophils <0.1 × 10⁹/L, lymphocytes 0.6 × 10⁹/L, platelets 20 × 10⁹/L).

Clinical features

The clinical features of AML are dominated by the pattern of bone marrow failure caused by the accumulation of malignant cells within marrow (Fig. 13.4). Infections are frequent, and anaemia and thrombocytopenia are often profound. A bleeding tendency caused by thrombocytopenia and disseminated intravascular coagulation (DIC) is characteristic of the promyelocytic variant of AML. Tumour cells can infiltrate a variety of tissues. Gum hypertrophy and infiltration (Fig. 13.5), skin involvement (leukaemia cutis) and central nervous system (CNS) disease are characteristic of the myelo-monocytic and monocytic subtypes.

Investigations

Table 13.3 lists the initial clinical and laboratory tests to be performed in newly diagnosed cases of AML; similar work-up is needed for all new haematological malignancies.

Haematological investigations reveal a normochromic normocytic anaemia with thrombocytopenia in most cases. The total white cell count is usually increased, and blood film examination typically shows a variable numbers of blast cells. The bone marrow is hypercellular and typically contains many

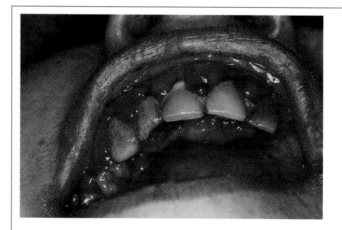

Figure 13.5 Monocytic acute myeloid leukaemia: the gums are swollen and haemorrhagic because of infiltration by leukaemic cells.

leukaemic blasts (Fig. 13.6). Blast cells are characterized by morphology, immunological (flow cytometric) cytogenetic and molecular genetic analysis for confirming the diagnosis, determining prognosis and developing a treatment plan (Table 13.4).

Table 13.3 The initial evaluation of a new patient with suspected acute myeloid leukaemia.

Assessment of medical history, examination and performance status; analysis for co-morbidities (see Chapter 12)

Full blood count and differential

Bone marrow aspirate and trephine biopsy

Immunophenotyping of bone marrow (and/or blood if blast cells present)

Cytogenetic analysis by karyotype

Mutation analysis

Cytochemical analysis (performed in some countries instead of immunophenotyping)

Biochemistry (liver, renal, uric acid, calcium, LDH)

Coagulation

Pregnancy test

Information on oocyte or sperm storage

Assessment of eligibility for stem cell transplantation

Hepatitis B, C and HIV test

CXR with ECG and ECHO

CXR, chest X-ray; ECG, electrocardiography; ECHO, echocardiography; HIV, human immunodeficiency virus; LDH, lactate dehydrogenase.

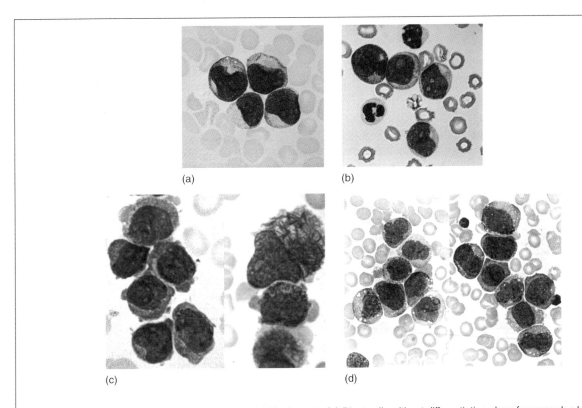

(a) (b)

(c) (d)

Figure 13.6 Morphological examples of acute myeloid leukaemia. **(a)** Blast cells without differentiation show few granules but may show Auer rods, as in this case; **(b)** cells in differentiation show multiple cytoplasmic granules; **(c)** Acute promyelocytic leukaemia blast cells contain prominent granules or multiple Auer rods; **(d)** myelomonocytic blasts have some monocytoid differentiation;

(Continued)

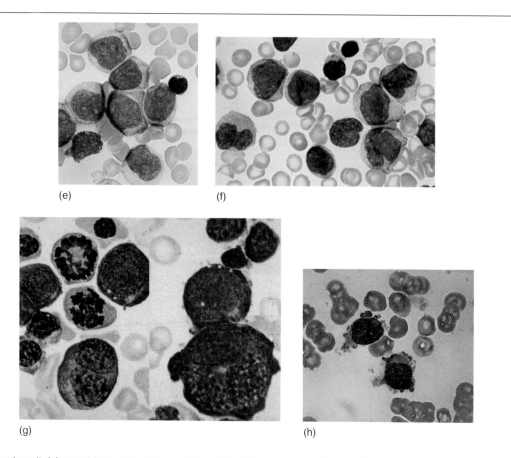

(e)

(f)

(g)

(h)

Figure 13.6 *(Continued)* **(e)** monoblastic leukaemia in which >80% of blasts are monoblasts; **(f)** monocytic with <80% of blasts monoblasts; **(g)** erythroid showing preponderance of erythroblasts; **(h)** megakaryoblastic showing cytoplasmic blebs on blasts.

Table 13.4 Drugs used for treatment of acute myeloid leukaemia (AML) or acute promyelocytic leukaemia (APML)

Class	Examples
Anti-metabolites/nucleoside analogues	Cytosine arabinoside (Ara-C), 6-mercaptopurine, methotrexate, hydroxycarbamide
Cytotoxics	Daunorubicin, idarubicin, mitoxantrone, CPX-351 (Vyxeos®)
Topoisomerase inhibitors	Etoposide, daunorubicin, idarubicin
DNA hypomethylating agents	Azacytidine, decitabine
Isocitrate dehydrogenase (IDH) inhibitors	Ivosidenib (IDH1), enasidenib (IDH2)
Signalling inhibitors	Midostaurin (multiple tyrosine kinases including FLT3), sorafenib (multiple tyrosine kinases including FLT3), gilterinib (FLT3), crenolanib (FLT3), quizartinib (FLT3), ventoclax (BCL2), glasdegib (Hedgehog pathway)
Differentiating agents	All-*trans* retinoic acid (ATRA), arsenic trioxide
Monoclonal antibodies	Gemtuzumab ozogamicin (anti-CD33 conjugated to calicheamicin cytotoxin), tagraxofusp (anti-CD123 conjugated to toxin)

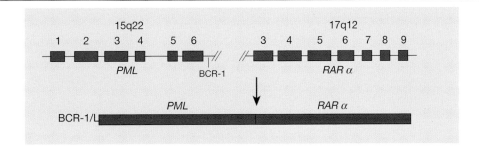

Figure 13.7 Generation of the t(15;17) translocation. The *PML* gene at 15q22 may break at one of three different breakpoint cluster regions (BCR-1, -2 and -3) and joins with exons 3–9 of the *RAR*α gene at 17q12. Three different fusion mRNAs are generated – termed long (L), variable (V) or short (S) – and these give rise to fusion proteins of different size. In this diagram only the long version resulting from a break at BCR-1 is shown.

Tests for DIC are often positive in patients with the promyelocytic variant of AML, and in some cases with monocytic differentiation (see below). Biochemical tests are performed as a baseline before treatment begins and may reveal raised uric acid or lactate dehydrogenase.

Cytogenetics and molecular genetics

Genetic abnormalities are used to classify the majority of cases of AML (Table 13.1). Two of the most common – t(8;21) and inv(16) – are associated with a good prognosis. **Acute promyelocytic leukaemia** (APML) is a variant of AML that contains the t(15;17) translocation in which the gene *PML* on chromosome 15 is fused to the retinoic acid receptor α gene, *RARA*, on chromosome 17 (Fig. 13.7). The resultant PML-RARα fusion protein functions as a transcriptional repressor, whereas normal (wild-type) *RARα* is an activator. Normally, the PML protein forms homodimers with itself, whereas the RARα protein forms heterodimers with the retinoid X receptor protein, RXR. The PML-RARα fusion protein binds to PML and RXR, preventing them from linking with their natural partners. This results in the cellular phenotype of arrested differentiation.

Point mutations affecting the genes *FLT3*, *NPM1*, *DNMT3A*, *IDH1*, *IDH2 TET2*, *RUNX1*, *TP53* and others are frequent in AML, especially in those cases without a cytogenetic abnormality (Fig. 13.3). They may be used to subclassify the disease (see Table 11.1) and have prognostic significance (Table 13.5). Some of these genes are involved in DNA methylation or histone methylation or acetylation (see Fig 16.1), and are also mutated in cases of myelodysplasia and myeloproliferative neoplasms (see Chapters 15 and 16). The presence in *de novo* AML of an MDS-associated mutation, e.g. *ASXL1* or *SF3B1*, is unfavourable.

Treatment

Management is both supportive and specific:
1 **General supportive therapy** for bone marrow failure is described in Chapter 12 and includes the insertion of a central venous cannula, blood product support and prevention of tumour lysis syndrome. The platelet count is generally maintained above 10×10^9/L and the haemoglobin above 80 g/L. Any episode of fever must be treated promptly. APML needs special support, as described below.
2 The **aim of treatment** in acute leukaemia in younger, fit patients is to induce complete remission (less than 5% blasts in the bone marrow, with recovery of normal blood counts and improved clinical status) and then to consolidate this with intensive therapy, hopefully eliminating the disease (Fig. 13.8). Allogeneic stem cell transplantation is considered in poor prognosis cases (Table 13.5) or for patients who have relapsed.
3 **Specific therapy of AML** is determined by the age and performance status of the patient, as well as the genetic lesions within the tumour. Drugs used for AML are summarized in Table 13.4. In younger patients, intensive chemotherapy is usual. This is given in several blocks, each of approximately 1 week. The most frequently used drugs are cytosine arabinoside and daunorubicin (Fig. 13.9). A standard induction regimen is 3 days of daunorubicin and 7 days of cytosine arabinoside (3+7). Other chemotherapy drugs including idarubicin, mitoxantrone and etoposide are also used in various regimens, but none is consistently superior to 3+7. The aim of induction is to achieve a complete remission, which occurs after one or two courses in up to 80% of younger patients and 60% of those over 60 and fit for intensive therapy. Depending on whether or not stem cell transplantation (SCT) is planned and on the age of the patient, one to four courses of consolidation with e.g. high-dose cytosine arabinoside are given. Initial therapy with a liposomal nanoparticle preparation of a fixed 5 : 1 ratio of cytosine arabinoside and daunorubicin, CPX-351, improved survival in 60–75-year-old patients with secondary AML or AML with myelodysplasia-related changes compared to intensive therapy with cytosine arabinoside and daunorubicin, and is now approved for initial therapy of AML. For older, frailer patients, treatment is usually palliative (see below).

Table 13.5 Prognostic factors in acute myeloid leukaemia.

	Favourable	Intermediate	Unfavourable
Cytogenetics	t(15;17)	Normal	Deletions of chromosome 5 or 7 or 17p, inv (3), t(6;9), *KMT2A* rearranged
	t(8;21) inv(16)	Other non-complex changes	Complex rearrangements (>3 unrelated abnormalities)
Molecular genetics	*NPM1* mutation *CEBPA* mutation (biallelic only)	Wild type	*FLT3* internal tandem repeat, mutations of *TP53*, *RUNX1*, *ASXL1* and splicing mutations; high *NPM1* – mutant allele burden
Bone marrow response to remission induction	<5% blasts after first course		>20% blasts after first course
Age	Child	<60 years	>60 years
Performance status	Good		Bad
Co-morbidities	Absent		Present
White cell count	<10 × 10⁹/L		>100 × 10⁹/L
Secondary leukaemia	Absent		Present, e.g. to previous chemotherapy or marrow disease
Minimal residual disease in remission	Absent	Present but only mutation detected is *DNMT3A*, *TET2* or *ASXL1* at low variant allele frequency	Present (>0.1% of cells) by flow cytometry or molecular genetics with genes other than *DNMT3A*, *TET2* or *ASXL1* (Fig. 13.12)

A typical good response in AML is shown in Fig. 13.10. The drugs are myelotoxic with limited selectivity between leukaemic and normal marrow cells, so marrow failure resulting from the chemotherapy is severe and prolonged, and intensive supportive care is required. Maintenance therapy is of no proven value except in promyelocytic AML with all-*trans* retinoic acid (ATRA). CNS prophylaxis is not usually given.

Midostaurin, a multikinase inhibitor that inhibits FLT3, improves survival when combined with chemotherapy in AML with *FLT3* mutations. Another FLT3 inhibitor, gilteritinib, is useful in relapsed cases, and several other FLT3 inhibitors are in development. Monoclonal immunoconjugates targeted against CD33 (e.g. gemtuzumab ozogamicin, Mylotarg®) provide an additional therapeutic option in combination with e.g. 3+7 chemotherapy for initial or consolidation AML therapy, particularly in patients with favourable risk features including t(8;21) and inv(16), where it has become standard of care. The BCL2 inhibitor ventoclax in combination with chemotherapy shows promise for relapsed cases and in older patients as initial therapy with hypomethylating drugs.

APML has its own treatment protocol. A haemorrhagic syndrome can lead to catastrophic haemorrhage and may be present either at diagnosis or develop in the first few days of treatment. It is treated as for disseminated intravascular coagulation (DIC) with multiple platelet transfusions and replacement of clotting factors with cryoprecipitate or fresh frozen plasma (see p. 335). In addition, ATRA therapy is given for this disease subtype and is combined initially with either arsenic trioxide or anthracycline. The arsenic combination gives a better clinical response with fewer side-effects. The **differentiation syndrome** (also known as ATRA syndrome though it can occur with arsenic and other agents) is a specific complication that may arise after ATRA treatment. Clinical problems, which result from the neutrophilia that follows differentiation of promyelocytes, include fever, hypoxia with pulmonary infiltrates and fluid overload. Treatment is with steroids and ATRA is only discontinued in very severe cases.

Prognosis and treatment stratification

The outcome for an individual patient with AML will depend on a number of factors, including age and white cell count at presentation (Table 13.4). However, the genetic abnormalities in the tumour are the most important determinant.

The initial goal is to achieve a complete remission. Complete remission is defined as less than 5% marrow blasts without Auer rods, neutrophil count greater than 1.0 × 10⁹/L, platelets

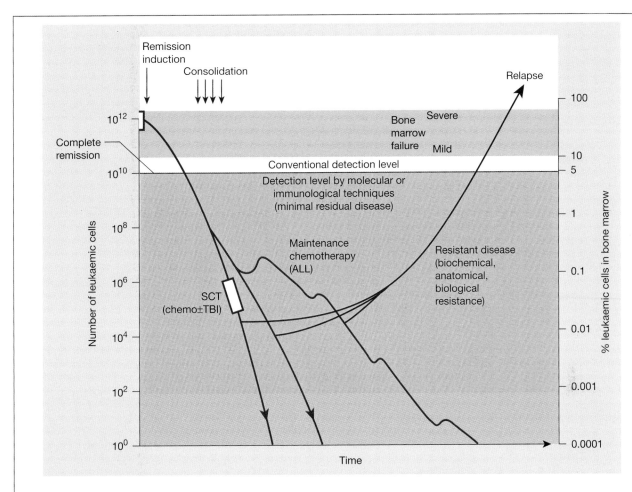

Figure 13.8 Acute leukaemia: principles of therapy for acute myeloid leukaemia or acute lymphoid leukaemia (ALL). The decision for stem cell transplantation (SCT) in remission is based on prognostic factors as well as tests for minimal residual disease. TBI, total body irradiation.

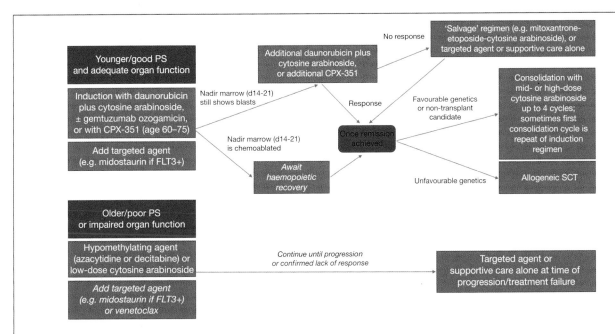

Figure 13.9 Acute myeloid leukaemia: flow chart illustrating typical treatment regimens. A key consideration is whether the patient is likely to tolerate an intensive induction or not. For patients receiving intensive therapy who still have disease on a nadir marrow during induction, a repeat induction is typically administered. PS, performance status; SCT, stem cell transplantation.

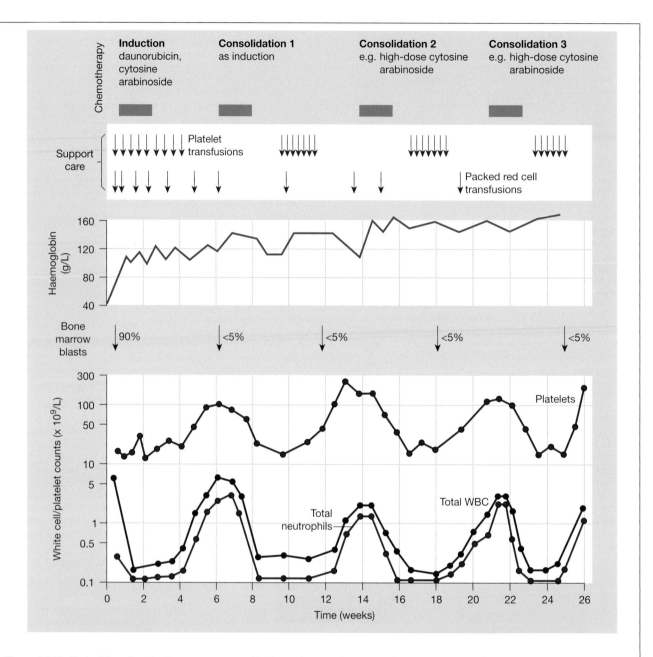

Figure 13.10 Typical flow chart for the management with chemotherapy of acute myeloid leukaemia. WBC, white blood cells.

greater than 100×10^9/L, independence of red cell transfusions and no extramedullary disease.

An important development in AML therapy is that of basing treatment according to the individual patient's **risk group**. Favourable cytogenetics and remission after one course of chemotherapy both predict for a better prognosis. In contrast, chromosome 5 or 7 abnormalities, blast cells with the *FLT3* internal tandem duplication mutation or other mutations including *TP53*, or poorly responsive disease places patients in poor-risk groups which need more intensive treatments (Table 13.4).

Monitoring of **minimal (measurable) residual disease** (MRD) during and after chemotherapy, for example detection of a positive FLT3 mutation test in otherwise complete remission, is being investigated as a means to guide appropriate treatment. It may be performed by molecular tests (Fig 13.11) or flow cytometry of the abnormal 'leukaemia-associated immunophenotype' seen in over 90% of cases. If the only mutation detected after induction on a molecular genetic MRD assay is *DNMT3A*, *TET2* or *ASXL1* at low variant allele frequency, akin to clonal haemopoiesis of indeterminate potential (CHIP), the relapse risk is lower than for detection of other mutations.

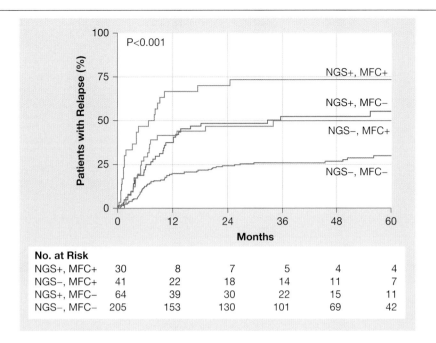

Figure 13.11 Minimal residual disease is a risk factor for relapse in AML. Depicted here is the cumulative incidence of relapse for patients in clinical complete remission, stratified by positive (+) or negative (–) results for persistent non-*DTA* (*DNMT3A*, *TET2*, *ASXL1*) mutations on next generation sequencing (NGS) and multiparameter flow cytometry (MFC). Source: M. Jongen-Lavrencic *et al.* (2018) *N. Engl. J. Med.* 378: 1189–99. Reproduced with permission of Massachusetts Medical Society.

Stem cell transplantation

Allogeneic SCT reduces the rate of AML relapse and is offered in selected intermediate- and high-risk cases in first remission. It carries risk of morbidity and mortality, so is not used for patients in the favourable risk group unless they have disease relapse. Reduced-intensity conditioning regimens have raised the age at which patients may be considered for SCT. Potential donors are discussed in Chapter 23. Autologous transplantation confers no benefit above that of post-remission chemotherapy.

Treatment of relapse

Most patients suffer relapse and the outlook will then depend on age, the duration of the first remission and the cytogenetic risk group. In addition to further chemotherapy to try to obtain a second remission, allogeneic SCT with either standard or reduced-intensity conditioning is usually performed in those patients who can tolerate the procedure and who have a suitable donor. Arsenic trioxide, if it has not been used initial treatment or it has been several years since its prior use, is useful in management of relapse in the promyelocytic variant. For patients with mutations of *IDH2*, enasidenib is approved and leads to complete remission in up to 20% of cases, while for those with mutations of *IDH1*, ivosidenib is approved and has a similar remission rate. Gladesgib, an inhibitor of the Hedgehog pathway, is approved, as are gemtuzumab, ozogamicin and ventoclax.

Patients over 70 years old

The median age for presentation of AML is approximately 65 years and treatment outcomes in the elderly are poor because of primary disease resistance and poor tolerability of intensive treatment protocols. Death from haemorrhage, infection or failure of the heart, kidneys or other organs is more frequent than in younger patients. In elderly patients with serious disease of other organs, the decision may be made to use supportive care with or without gentle single-drug chemotherapy, e.g. with low-dose cytarabine, azacytidine or hydroxycarbamide. Ventoclax alone or in combination with one of these drugs appears beneficial in early trials. In those who are otherwise well, combination chemotherapy similar to that used in younger patients may produce long-term remissions, and reduced-intensity SCT is increasingly being offered.

Outcome

The prognosis for patients with AML has been improving steadily, particularly for those under 60 years of age, and approximately one-third of this group can expect to achieve long-term cure (Fig. 13.12a). For the elderly the situation is poor, and less than 10% of those over 70 years of age achieve long-term remission (Fig. 13.12b).

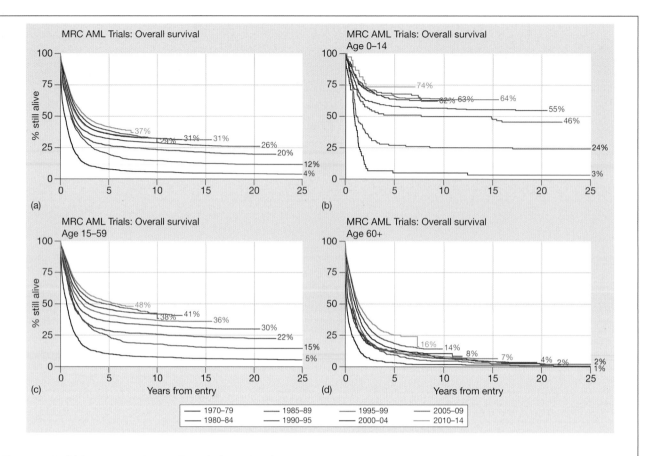

Figure 13.12 (**a**) Improvement in overall survival over time for patients with acute myeloid leukaemia (AML) in UK MRC/NCRI AML Trials; (**b**) age 0–14 years; (**c**) age 15–59 years; (**d**) age 60+ years. Courtesy of Professor Robert Hills, University of Oxford.

SUMMARY

- The leukaemias are a group of disorders characterized by the accumulation of malignant white cells in the bone marrow and blood. They can be classified into four subtypes on the basis of being either *acute* or *chronic*, and *myeloid* or *lymphoid*.
- Acute leukaemias are aggressive diseases in which transformation of a haemopoietic stem cell leads to accumulation of >20% blast cells in the bone marrow.
- The clinical features of acute leukaemia mainly result from bone marrow failure and include anaemia, infection and bleeding. Tissue infiltration can also occur.
- AML is rare in childhood, but becomes increasingly common with age, with a median onset of 65 years.
- The disease may arise *de novo* or result from transformation of a previous bone marrow neoplastic disease.

- The diagnosis is made by analysis of blood and bone marrow using microscopic examination (morphology) as well as immunophenotypic, cytogenetic and molecular studies.
- Cytogenetic and molecular abnormalities are used to classify and indicate prognosis in the majority of cases of AML.
- In younger patients treatment is primarily with the use of intensive chemotherapy. This is usually given in three or four blocks, each of approximately 1 week, using drugs such as cytosine arabinoside and daunorubicin. The blood count must be given time to recover before the next block of therapy can be given and this can typically take 4–6 weeks.
- Acute promyelocytic leukaemia is a variant of AML that carries a t(15;17) chromosomal translocation. It commonly presents with bleeding and is treated with retinoic acid (ATRA) and arsenic or chemotherapy.

- The prognosis for patients with AML has been improving steadily, particularly for those under 60 years of age, and approximately one-third of this group can expect to achieve long-term cure. The outcome for elderly people remains disappointing.

- New drugs targeting specific signal transduction pathways are being introduced for treating relapsed disease and into up-front therapy
- Allogeneic stem cell transplantation is useful in treating some subsets of patients and may also be curative for patients with relapsed disease.

Now visit **www.wileyessential.com/haematology** to test yourself on this chapter.

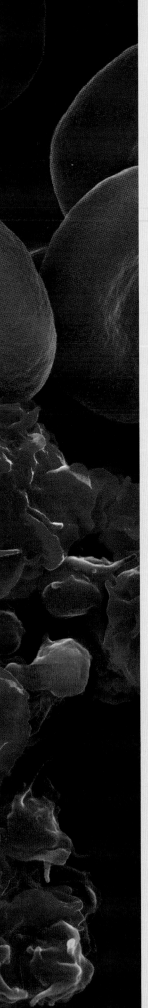

CHAPTER 14
Chronic myeloid leukaemia

Key topics

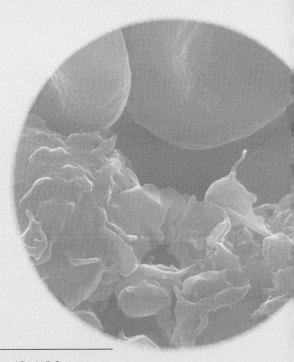

Hoffbrand's Essential Haematology, Eighth Edition. By A. Victor Hoffbrand and David P. Steensma.
© 2020 John Wiley & Sons Ltd. Published 2020 by John Wiley & Sons Ltd.
Companion website: www.wileyessential.com/haematology

The chronic leukaemias are distinguished from acute leukaemias by their slower progression; with currently available treatments, most patients with chronic leukaemias will live many years. Chronic leukaemias can be broadly subdivided into myeloid (Table 14.1) and lymphoid groups (see Chapter 18). The World Health Organization (WHO) 2016 classification of the myeloproliferative neoplasms (Table 14.1) includes chronic myeloid leukaemia *BCR-ABL1* positive (CML), discussed here, the non-leukaemic myeloproliferative neoplasms and rare chronic neutrophilic and eosinophilic leukaemias, described in Chapter 15, and the myelodysplastic/myeloproliferative neoplasms, covered in Chapter 16.

Chronic myeloid leukaemia

Chronic myeloid leukaemia, BCR-ABL1 rearrangement positive (CML) is a clonal disorder of a pluripotent stem cell. The disease accounts for around 15% of leukaemias and may occur at any age. The diagnosis of CML is rarely difficult and is assisted by the characteristic presence of the **Philadelphia (Ph) chromosome**. This results from the t(9;22) (q34;q11) translocation between chromosomes 9 and 22, as a result of which part of the oncogene *ABL1* is moved to the *BCR* gene on chromosome 22 (Fig. 14.1a) and part of chromosome 22 moves to chromosome 9. The abnormal chromosome 22 is the Ph chromosome; the variant chromosome 9 does not have a specific name. In the Ph translocation 5' exons of *BCR* are fused to the 3' exons of *ABL1* (Fig. 14.1b, c).

The resulting chimeric *BCR-ABL1* gene usually codes for a fusion protein of size 210 kDa (p210). This has constitutively active tyrosine kinase activity in excess of the normal 145 kDa ABL1 product, resulting in uncontrolled cell proliferation.

The Ph translocation is also seen in a minority of cases of acute lymphoblastic leukaemia (ALL), and in some of these

Table 14.1 World Health Organization 2016 classification of myeloproliferative neoplasms (MPN), including chronic myeloid leukaemia (CML), and myelodysplastic/myeloproliferative (MDS/MPN) neoplasms, including those with eosinophilia and recurrent genetic rearrangements (see also Chapters 15 and 16; see also Appendix). For classification of MDS without MPN features, see Chapter 16.

Type
Myeloproliferative neoplasms
Chronic myeloid leukaemia, *BCR-ABL1* rearrangement positive
Chronic neutrophilic leukaemia (CNL)
Polycythaemia vera (PV)
Primary myelofibrosis (PMF) – including prefibrotic/early stage and overt fibrotic stage
Essential thrombocythaemia (ET)
Chronic eosinophilic leukaemia, not otherwise specified (NOS)
MPN, unclassifiable
Myelodysplastic/myeloproliferative (MDS/MPN) neoplasms
Atypical CML, *BCR-ABL1* rearrangement negative
Chronic myelomonocytic leukaemia (CMML)
Juvenile myelomonocytic leukaemia (JMML)
MDS/MPN with ring sideroblasts and thrombocytosis (MDS/MPN-RS-T)
MDS/MPN, unclassifiable
Myeloid/lymphoid neoplasms with eosinophilia and rearrangement of PDGFRA, PDGFRB or FGFR1, or with PCM1-JAK2
Myeloid/lymphoid neoplasms with *PDGFRA* rearrangement
Myeloid/lymphoid neoplasms with *PDGFRB* rearrangement
Myeloid/lymphoid neoplasms with *FGFR1* rearrangement
Provisional entity: Myeloid/lymphoid neoplasms with *PCM1-JAK2*

N.B. All the diseases in this table except BCR-ABL1-positive CML, ET, PV and PMF are quite rare, with <100 cases per year in the UK and <700 per year in the USA.

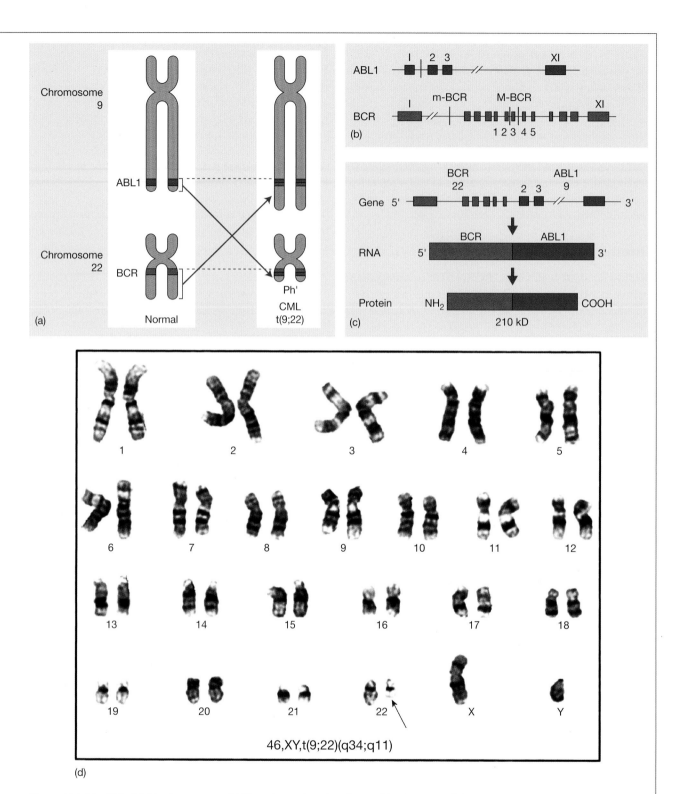

Figure 14.1 The Philadelphia chromosome. **(a)** There is translocation of part of the long arm of chromosome 22 to the long arm of chromosome 9 and reciprocal translocation of part of the long arm of chromosome 9 to chromosome 22 (the Philadelphia chromosome). This reciprocal translocation brings most of the *ABL1*-gene into the *BCR* region on chromosome 22 (and part of the *BCR* gene into juxtaposition with the remaining portion of *ABL* on chromosome 9). **(b)** The breakpoint in *ABL1* is between exons 1 and 2. The breakpoint in *BCR* is at one of the two points in the major breakpoint cluster region (M-BCR) in chronic myeloid leukaemia (CML) or in some cases of Ph+ acute lymphoblastic leukaemia (ALL). **(c)** This results in a 210-kDa fusion protein product derived from the *BCR-ABL1* fusion gene. In other cases of Ph+ ALL, the breakpoint in *BCR* is at a minor breakpoint cluster region (m-BCR), resulting in a smaller *BCR-ABL1* fusion gene and a 190 kDa protein. **(d)** Karyotype showing the t(9;22) (q34;q11) translocation. The Ph chromosome is arrowed.

(Continued)

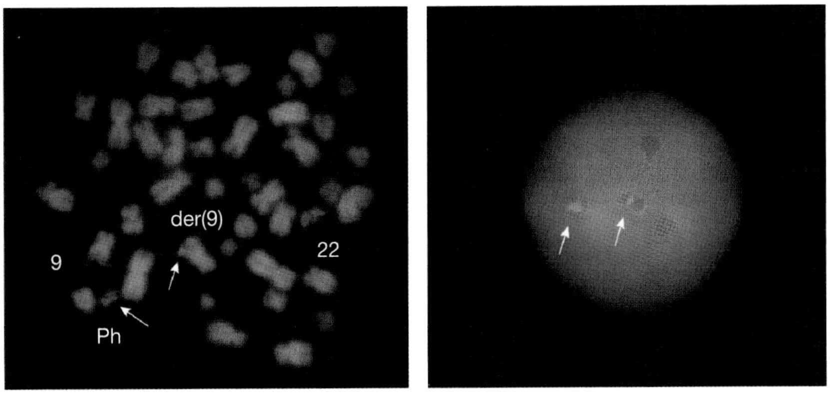

Figure 14.1 *(Continued)* **(e)** Visualization of the Ph chromosome on (i) dividing (metaphase); and (ii) quiescent (interphase) cells by fluorescence *in situ* hybridization (FISH) analysis (ABL probe in red and BCR probe in green) with fusion signals (red/green which shows as yellow) on the Ph (BCR-ABL1) and der(9) (ABL1-BCR) chromosomes. Source: Courtesy of Dr Ellie Nacheva.

the breakpoint in *BCR* occurs in the same region as in CML. However, in other cases of ALL, the breakpoint in *BCR* is further upstream, in the intron between the first and second exons, leaving only the first *BCR* exon intact. This chimeric *BCR-ABL1* gene is expressed as a p190 protein which, like p210, has enhanced tyrosine kinase activity. The p190 protein is not seen in CML. Rarely, other fusions occur from different fusions, such as a p230 variant, but many clinical laboratories are unable to test for these.

In most patients the Ph chromosome is seen by karyotypic examination of neoplastic cells (Fig. 14.1d), but in a few the Ph abnormality cannot be seen under the microscope, although the same molecular rearrangement is detectable by more sensitive techniques: fluorescence *in situ* hybridization (FISH; Fig. 14.1e) or reverse transcriptase PCR (RT-PCR) for *BCR-ABL1* transcripts. This Ph-negative *BCR-ABL1*-positive CML behaves clinically like Ph-positive CML, since the molecular driver is identical. *BCR-ABL1*-negative atypical chronic myeloid leukaemia is a distinct disease, classified with the myelodysplastic/myeloproliferative syndromes (see Chapter 16).

The Ph chromosome is an acquired abnormality of haemopoietic stem cells, so it is typically found in cells of both the myeloid (granulocytic, erythroid and megakaryocytic) and lymphoid (B and T cell) lineages. The main cause of death in CML is transformation to a blast phase, which may have myeloid or lymphoid markers, and may be preceded by an accelerated phase. These are discussed later in this chapter.

Clinical features

CML occurs in either sex (male:female ratio of 1.4:1), most frequently between the ages of 40 and 60 years. However, it may occur in children and neonates, as well as in the very old. In up to 50% of cases the diagnosis is made incidentally from a routine blood count. In those cases where the disease presents clinically, the following features may be seen:

1 Symptoms related to hypermetabolism (e.g. weight loss, lassitude, anorexia or night sweats).
2 Splenomegaly is nearly always present and may be massive. In some patients, splenic enlargement is associated with considerable abdominal discomfort, pain or indigestion.
3 Features of anaemia may include pallor, dyspnoea and tachycardia.
4 Bruising, epistaxis, menorrhagia or haemorrhage from other sites because of abnormal platelet function.
5 Gout or renal impairment caused by hyperuricaemia from excessive purine breakdown may be a problem.
6 Rare symptoms include visual disturbances and priapism.

Laboratory findings

1 Leucocytosis is the main feature and may reach levels greater than 200×10^9/L (Fig. 14.2). A complete spectrum of myeloid cells is seen in the peripheral blood film. The levels of neutrophils and myelocytes exceed those of blast cells and promyelocytes (Fig. 14.3).
2 Increased circulating basophils is a characteristic feature.
3 Normochromic normocytic anaemia is usual.
4 Platelet count may be increased (most frequently), normal or decreased.
5 Bone marrow is hypercellular with granulocytic predominance.
6 Presence of the *BCR-ABL1* gene fusion by RT-PCR analysis and in 98% of cases Ph chromosome on cytogenetic analysis (Fig. 14.1d).
7 In addition to *BCR-ABL1*, some patients have mutations in neoplasia-associated genes, e.g. *ASXL1*, *IKZF1* and *RUNX1*, or other fusions or rearrangements at diagnosis. These patients are more likely to transform to acute leukaemia than those with only *BCR-ABL1*.
8 Serum uric acid is usually raised.

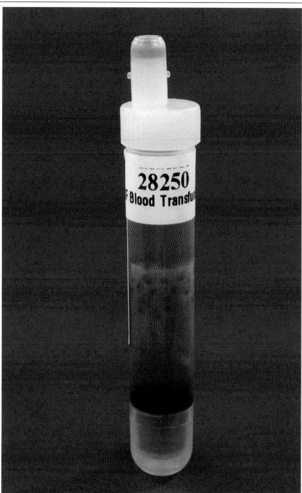

Figure 14.2 Chronic myeloid leukaemia: peripheral blood film showing a vast increase in buffy coat. The white cell count was 532×10^9/L.

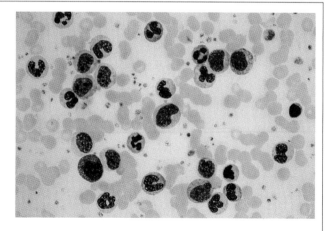

Figure 14.3 Chronic myeloid leukaemia: peripheral blood film showing various stages of granulopoiesis including promyelocytes, myelocytes, metamyelocytes and band and segmented neutrophils.

Prognostic scores (stages)

Attempts have been made to stage CML at presentation in order to predict prognosis. In the past, the most frequently used were the Sokal, Hasford and EUTOS scores, which took into account factors such as age, blast cell percentage, spleen size and platelet count. However, the rate of response to a tyrosine kinase inhibitor (TKI) is now a more useful measure of prognosis.

Treatment

Treatment of chronic phase

Tyrosine kinase inhibitors

TKIs are the mainstay of the treatment of CML and several different drugs are now available (Table 14.2).

First-line therapy for patients with chronic phase CML is usually imatinib, nilotinib or dasatinib. Most experience exists with imatinib (Fig. 14.4), which is also the cheapest. Overall around 60% of patients given imatinib achieve an excellent response and remain on the drug long-term, whereas 40% proceed to a second-line agent due to intolerance or inadequate response.

Nilotinib and dasatinib achieve more rapid responses as first-line therapy and are therefore used first in some centres, although side-effects are somewhat more common. They are also used as second-line therapy after imatinib (Fig. 14.5). Bosutinib is also an effective therapy, while ponatinib has the unique advantage that it is effective against CML that carries the T315I mutation within ABL1, but ponatinib is associated with the highest risk of thrombotic events. Asciminib has a distinct pattern of binding to ABL kinase and may be useful either in combination with another TKI or in the event of resistance mediated by a mutation of the ABL kinase.

Monitoring of response to tyrosine kinase inhibitors

TKIs are highly effective at reducing the number of neoplastic cells in the bone marrow and should be monitored by RT-PCR analysis for *BCR-ABL1* transcripts in marrow or blood and/or karyotypic analysis of the bone marrow, typically at 3, 6 and 12 months. Molecular response is assessed as the ratio of *BCR-ABL1* transcripts to *ABL1* transcripts and it is expressed as *BCR-ABL1%* on a log scale, where 10%, 1%, 0.1%, 0.01% and 0.001% correspond to a decrease of 1, 2, 3, 4 and 5 logs, respectively, below the standard baseline. A major goal of therapy is achievement of a 'major molecular remission', defined as 3-log reduction (<0.1%) or better. A complete cytogenetic response (CCyR) is defined as the absence of Ph-positive metaphases within bone marrow.

Treatment responses can be defined as **optimal** or **failure**, with an intermediate area termed **warning** (Table 14.3). Patients with optimal responses continue their original treatment, whereas those with treatment failure are treated with second-generation TKI therapy or stem cell transplantation (SCT). Patients in the warning zone should be monitored

Table 14.2 The tyrosine kinase inhibitors (TKIs) used for treatment of chronic myeloid leukaemia (CML).

	Action	Side-effects	Role in clinical therapy
Imatinib	The first TKI, designed as a specific inhibitor of the BCR-ABL1 fusion protein. It blocks tyrosine kinase activity by competing with adenosine triphosphate (ATP) binding (Fig. 14.4).	Rash, nausea, myelosuppression, fluid retention, muscle cramps	First-line therapy. Occasional use in resistance/intolerance to other TKIs
Nilotinib	Second-generation inhibitor that has increased affinity for BCR-ABL1. Achieves molecular remission more rapidly than imatinib	Myelosuppression, peripheral vascular disease, headache, nausea, prolonged QT interval	First-line or resistance/intolerance to first-line TKI
Dasatinib	Inhibits BCR-ABL and SRC family kinases, which play a role in driving CML progression	Headache, pleural effusion, pulmonary hypertension, cough, prolonged QT interval	First-line or resistance/intolerance to first-line TKI
Bosutinib	BCR-ABL1 inhibitor with additional inhibitory effect on SRC family kinases	Diarrhoea, liver test abnormalities, nausea, low platelet count	First-line or resistance/intolerance to first-line TKI
Ponatinib	Multitargeted TKI inhibitor	Low platelets, rash, dry skin, arterial and venous thrombosis	Resistance/intolerance to first-line TKI. The only TKI able to treat CML with the T315I mutation
Asciminib (ABL-001)	TKI inhibitor that, unlike others which bind to the ATPase site of ABL kinase, binds to the myristoyl site and thus may be active in treatment of patients with resistance to other TKIs	Rash, gastrointestinal upset, low counts	Resistance to other TKIs; may be used in combination with other TKIs

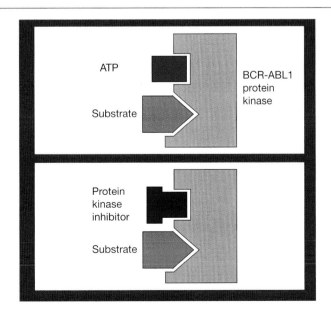

Figure 14.4 Mode of action of the tyrosine kinase inhibitor imatinib. It blocks the enzyme's adenosine triphosphate (ATP) binding site.

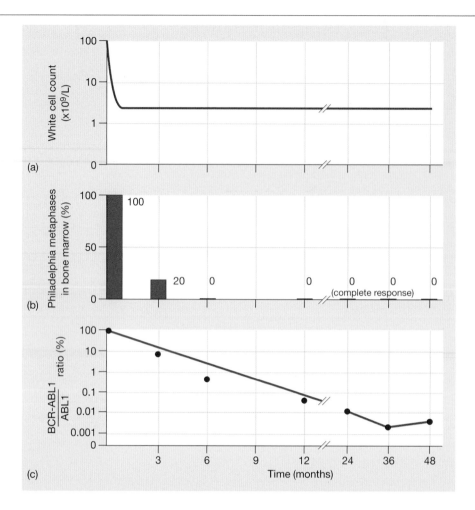

Figure 14.5 Example of an optimal haematological and cytogenetic response in a patient with chronic myeloid leukaemia who achieves complete remission with imatinib therapy. **(a)** The white cell count returns to normal within days. **(b)** Karyotypic examination of the bone marrow reveals a gradual reduction in the number of Ph+ chromosomes over the 6 months. **(c)** Polymerase chain reaction analysis of the bone marrow or blood shows a reduction in the number of *BCR-ABL1* transcripts in comparison with the normal ABL1 transcript. *BCR-ABL1* transcripts continue to be detected at a very low level, but can become negative in some patients. In this case analysis was performed on bone marrow for the first 6 months and on peripheral blood thereafter.

more regularly and might be considered for an early change in therapy or increase in the dose of first-line therapy. Patients who fail to achieve a *BCR-ABL1* transcript level of <10% (normalized to the International Standard) at the 3-month time point, so-called early molecular response (EMR), have a less favourable outlook.

BCR-ABL1 mutation screening

One mechanism of disease resistance to TKI therapy is selection for clones carrying mutations within the *BCR-ABL1* fusion gene, e.g. T315I. These mutations may be detected by sequencing the *ABL1* gene. The pattern of mutation can be useful for determining which treatment to choose as second-line therapy, since certain mutations confer specific resistance to one TKI while sensitivity to other TKIs persists.

Response to TKI therapy and stopping therapy

TKI therapy is highly effective and after 5 years of treatment the progression-free survival is 85–90%, with overall survival over 90% (Fig. 14.6). For patients becoming *BCR-ABL1* transcript negative, about 60% will remain negative on stopping TKI therapy or remain in remission with a stable low level of the transcripts, and these patients are likely to be cured. For those who do become *BCR-ABL1* positive again after stopping with a rising level of transcripts, treatment with the TKI will usually result in restoration of disease control.

Additional forms of treatment for CML

Chemotherapy

Hydroxycarbamide (hydroxyurea) treatment can control and maintain the white cell count in the chronic phase, but does

Table 14.3 Definition of the response to tyrosine kinase inhibitors as first-line treatment in chronic myeloid leukaemia. As examples, BCR-ABL1 ≤10% refers to the fact that the *BCR-ABL1* transcript level has been reduced to less than 10% of the *ABL1* level. Ph+ ≤35% indicates that the number of Philadelphia-positive chromosomes in cells in the bone marrow is less than 35% of the total number that are examined. Source: M. Baccarani *et al.* (2013) *Blood*, 122: 872–84. Reproduced with permission of the American Society of Hematology.

	Optimal	Warning	Failure
3 months	BCR-ABL1 ≤10% ('EMR') and/or Ph+ ≤35%	BCR-ABL1 >10% and/ or Ph+ 36–95%	Non-CHR and/or Ph+ >95%
6 months	BCR-ABL1 <1% and/or Ph+ 0	BCR-ABL1 1–10% and/or Ph+ 1-35%	BCR-ABL1 >10% and/or Ph+ >35%
12 months	BCR-ABL1 ≤0.1%	BCR-ABL1 >0.1–1%	BCR-ABL1 >1% and/or Ph+ >0
Then, and at any time	BCR-ABL1 ≤0.1%	CCA/Ph– (–7, or 7q–)	Loss of complete haematological response Loss of complete cytogenetic response Loss of major molecular response (BCR-ABL1 expression of ≤0.1%) ABL1 mutations Clonal chromosome abnormalities in Ph+ cells

CCA, complex cytogenetic abnormalities; CHR, complete haematological response, EMR, early molecular response.

not reduce the percentage of *BCR-ABL1*-positive cells. TKIs have now largely replaced its use and that of DNA alkylating drugs such as busulphan. Omacetaxine is a subcutaneously administered inhibitor of protein translation that has achieved regulatory approval for relapsed/refractory CML in several countries.

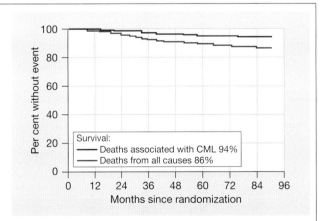

Figure 14.6 Clinical outcome of patients given imatinib therapy for treatment of chronic myeloid leukaemia (CML) in chronic phase. After 7 years only 6% of patients died due to CML and overall survival is 86%. Source: S.G. O'Brien *et al.* (2008) *Blood* 112: 76a. Reproduced with permission.

α-Interferon

Formerly, this was used after the white cell count had been controlled by hydroxycarbamide, often in combination with the nucleoside analogue cytarabine, but has now been replaced by imatinib and other TKIs. It is still used in pregnant patients, however, since TKIs are not known to be safe in pregnancy and hydroxycarbamide is teratogenic. Almost all patients treated with interferon have symptoms of a 'flu-like' illness in the first few days of treatment, which responds to paracetamol and gradually wears off. More serious complications include anorexia, depression and cytopenias (see Table 12.2). A minority (approximately 15%) of patients may achieve long-term remission with loss of the Ph chromosome on cytogenetic analysis, although the *BCR-ABL1* fusion gene can usually still be detected by PCR.

Stem cell transplantation

Allogeneic SCT is a potentially curative treatment for CML, but because of the risks associated with the procedure, it is usually reserved for TKI failures (Fig. 14.7) or patients presenting in accelerated or acute phases. The results are, however, better when it is performed in chronic rather than these later phases. The 5-year survival is approximately 50–70%. Relapse of CML after the transplant is a significant problem, but donor leucocyte infusions are highly effective in CML (see p. 293), particularly if relapse is diagnosed early by molecular detection of the *BCR-ABL1* transcript.

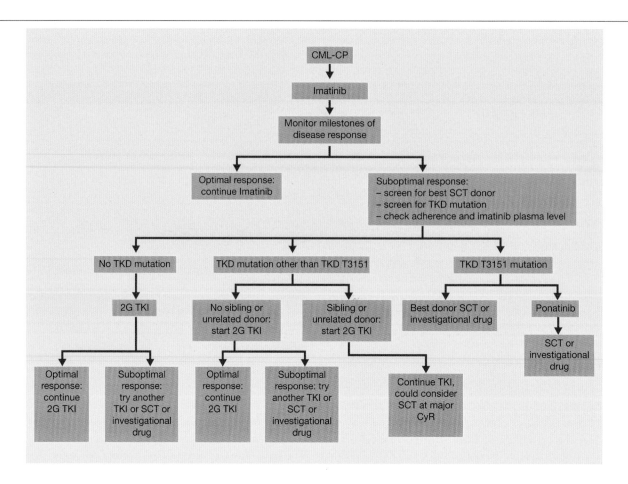

Figure 14.7 A potential algorithm for the management of young patients with chronic myeloid leukaemia in chronic phase (CML-CP). Imatinib is suggested as first-line therapy for many patients, since it is inexpensive and the only agent now available in a generic form. The role of stem cell transplantation (SCT) is diminishing as more TKIs become available. Source: Adapted from J. de la Fuente *et al.* (2014) *Br. J. Haematol.* 167(1): 33–47. 2G TKI, second generation tyrosine kinase inhibitor.

Accelerated phase disease and blast transformation

Acute transformation (greater than 20% blasts in blood or marrow, either lymphoblasts or myeloblasts) may occur rapidly over days or weeks (Fig. 14.8). More commonly there is an **accelerated phase** with anaemia, thrombocytopenia (platelets less than 100×10^9/L), increase in blood basophils to greater than 20% or marrow blast cells 10–19% with blast cells in the blood. The spleen may be enlarged despite control of the blood count and the marrow may be fibrotic. New clonal chromosomal or molecular abnormalities may appear. The patient may be in this phase for several months, during which the disease is less easy to control than in the chronic phase.

In approximately one-fifth of cases of acute transformation this is lymphoblastic and patients may be treated in a similar way to ALL, with a number of patients returning to the chronic phase for months or even a year or two. In the majority, transformation is into acute myeloid leukaemia or mixed types. These are more

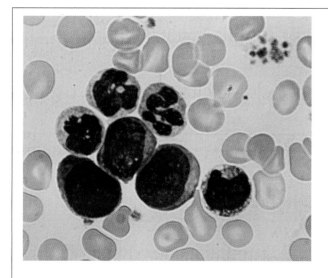

Figure 14.8 Chronic myeloid leukaemia: acute myeloblastic transformation. Peripheral blood film showing frequent myeloblasts.

difficult to treat and survival is rare beyond 1 year without SCT. TKIs are valuable in the management of blastic transformation, but resistance to treatment usually occurs within a few weeks. Allogeneic SCT is a valuable option where possible.

SUMMARY

- Chronic myeloid leukaemia is a clonal disorder of a pluripotent stem cell. The disease accounts for around 15% of leukaemias and may occur at any age.
- All cases of CML have a translocation between chromosomes 9 and 22. This leads to the oncogene *ABL1* being moved to the *BCR* gene on chromosome 22 and generates the Philadelphia (Ph) chromosome.
- The resulting chimeric *BCR-ABL1* gene codes for a fusion protein with increased tyrosine kinase activity.
- In most patients the Ph chromosome is seen by karyotypic examination of blood or bone marrow cells, but the molecular rearrangement may rarely only be detected by FISH or PCR.
- The disease can occur at any age, but is most common between the ages of 40 and 60 years.

- The clinical features include loss of weight, sweating, anaemia, bleeding and splenomegaly. There is usually a marked neutrophilia, with myelocytes and basophils seen in the blood film.
- Transformation to an accelerated phase or acute leukaemia may occur.
- Treatment is with tyrosine kinase inhibitors such as imatinib, dasatinib or nilotinib. Neoplastic cells can acquire resistance to treatment and drug therapy is tailored in response to this.
- Stem cell transplantation can be curative and may also be useful for advanced disease.
- The clinical outlook is now very good for patients diagnosed in chronic phase and more than 90% of patients can expect long-term control of disease.

Now visit **www.wileyessential.com/haematology** to test yourself on this chapter.

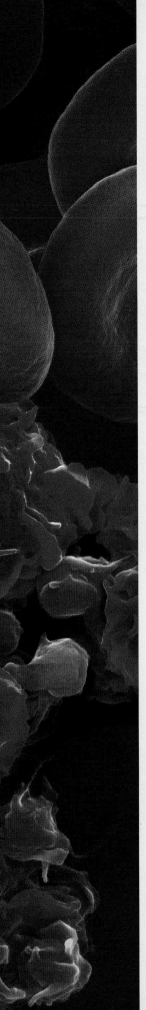

CHAPTER 15
Myeloproliferative neoplasms

Key topics

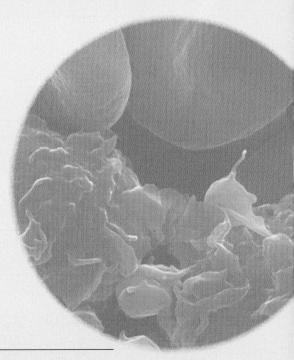

Hoffbrand's Essential Haematology, Eighth Edition. By A. Victor Hoffbrand and David P. Steensma.
© 2020 John Wiley & Sons Ltd. Published 2020 by John Wiley & Sons Ltd.
Companion website: www.wileyessential.com/haematology

The term myeloproliferative neoplasms (MPN) describes a group of conditions arising from transformed marrow stem cells or haemopoietic progenitors and characterized by clonal proliferation of one or more haemopoietic components in the bone marrow and, in many cases, the liver and spleen.

The three major disorders included in this classification are:

1 Polycythaemia vera (PV).
2 Essential thrombocythaemia (ET).
3 Primary myelofibrosis (PMF).

Mastocytosis is also discussed in this chapter, as are **chronic eosinophilic leukaemia** and **chronic neutrophilic leukaemia**, rare disorders classified as MPN. *BCR-ABL1-* positive chronic myeloid leukaemia (CML) is described in Chapter 14, and the myelodysplastic syndromes (MDS) and mixed MDS/MPN (overlap syndromes) in Chapter 16. Classification of MPN is shown in Table 14.1.

Genetic drivers of myeloproliferation

MPN are closely related to each other, and transitional forms can occur with evolution from one entity into another during the course of the disease (Fig. 15.1). These diseases are associated with acquired mutations of genes that encode tyrosine kinases or kinase-associated proteins, primarily Janus-associated kinase 2 (*JAK2*), calreticulin (*CALR*) or *MPL* (the receptor for thrombopoietin; Table 15.1).

Table 15.1 Driver genetic mutations in myeloproliferative neoplasms.

Disease	Gene mutations or fusions
Chronic myeloid leukaemia	*ABL1* (fusion with *BCR*)
Polycythaemia vera	*JAK2*
Primary myelofibrosis	*JAK2, CALR, MPL*
Essential thrombocythaemia	*JAK2, CALR, MPL*
Mastocytosis	*KIT*
Myeloid neoplasm with eosinophilia	*PDGFRA, PDGFRB, FGFR1, PCM1-JAK2*

Mutation of *JAK2* (*JAK2 V617F*) occurs in a heterozygous, hemizygous (i.e. loss of the normal allele) or homozygous state, in the marrow and blood of almost all patients with PV and in approximately 60% of those with ET or PMF, showing the common aetiology of these three diseases (Fig. 15.2). The mutation occurs in a highly conserved region of the pseudokinase domain, which normally negatively regulates JAK2 signalling. JAK2 has a major role in normal myeloid development

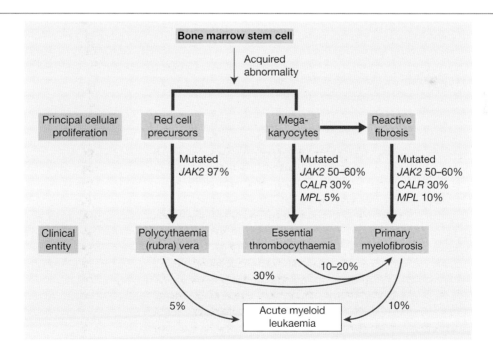

Figure 15.1 Relationship between the three myeloproliferative neoplasms. They may all arise by somatic mutation in the pluripotential stem and progenitor cells. Many transitional cases occur showing features of two conditions and, in other cases, the disease transforms during its course from one of these diseases to another or to acute myeloid leukaemia. The three diseases, polycythaemia rubra vera, essential thrombocythaemia and primary myelofibrosis, are characterized by *JAK2*, *MPL* or *CALR* mutation in a varying proportion of cases.

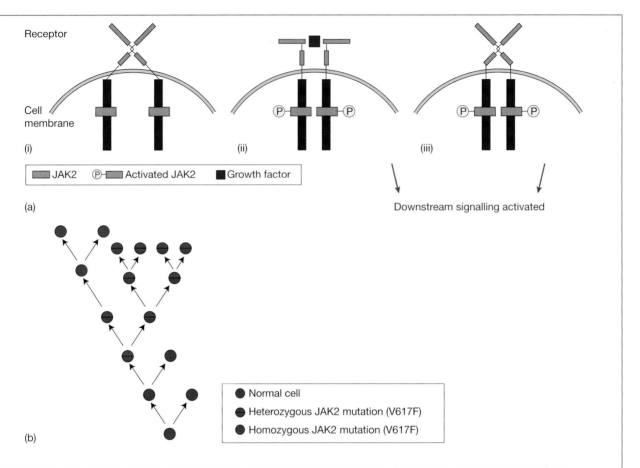

Figure 15.2 The role of *JAK2* mutation in the generation of myeloproliferative neoplasms. **(a)** (i) Most haemopoietic growth factor receptors do not have intrinsic kinase activity, but associate with a protein kinase such as JAK2 in the cytoplasm. (ii) When the receptor binds a growth factor (e.g. erythropoietin or thrombopoietin), the cytoplasmic domains move closer together and the JAK2 molecules can activate each other by phosphorylation and subsequently phosphorylate downstream proteins, e.g. STAT (signal transducer and activator of transcription) proteins (Fig. 1.7). (iii) The V617F *JAK2* and the *MPL* mutations allow the JAK protein to become activated even when no growth factor is bound. **(b)** A model for the development of myeloproliferative neoplasm following *JAK2* mutation. The primary event appears to predispose to an acquired heterozygous mutation of *JAK2* (V617F). This leads to a survival advantage. In some patients, a mitotic recombination event leads to a homozygous *JAK2* mutation state.

by transducing signals from cytokines and growth factors including erythropoietin, granulocyte-colony stimulating factor receptor and thrombopoietin (see Fig. 1.7). Why the same mutation is associated with different myeloproliferative neoplasms is unclear, but depends partly on the dosage of the mutant allele, this being usually higher in PV than ET. Cooperating mutations and the cell differentiation stage at which the mutations developed may also influence the phenotype. A minority of PV patients show a variant *JAK2* mutation in exon 12 rather than a V617F mutation.

In those patients with ET or PMF who do not demonstrate a *JAK2* mutation, a mutation in *CALR* is observed in most cases. CALR is a multifunction protein involved in signal transduction and gene transcription. Mutated CALR is abnormally secreted from the cell, where it interacts with the

thrombopoietin receptor. Constitutively activating mutations in the *MPL* gene encoding thrombopoietin receptor are found in about 5% of ET and 10% PMF cases.

A mutation in one of these three genes is seen in 99% of cases of PV and around 85–90% of cases of ET or PMF (Fig. 15.3). Some patients also show mutations of epigenetic regulator genes, e.g. *TET2* and *DNMT3A* involved in disease initiation, or *ASXL1* and *EZH2* in disease progression. These mutations as well as those of other driver genes are also found recurrently in myelodysplastic syndromes (MDS) and acute myeloid leukaemia (AML; see Fig. 16.1).

There is a five-fold increased incidence of myeloproliferative neoplasm in close relatives of patients, implying a genetic predisposition to the diseases. A germline polymorphism in *JAK2*, *JAK2 46/1*, increases the risk of MPN.

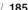

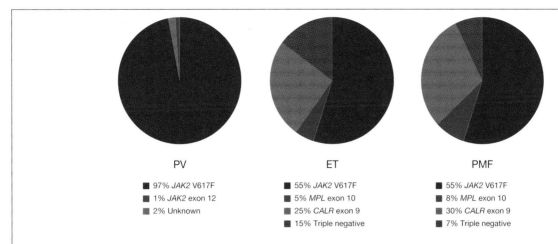

Figure 15.3 Phenotype driver mutations in classic BCRABL1−negative myeloproliferative neoplasms. ET, essential thrombocythemia; PMF, primary myelofibrosis; PV, polycythaemia vera. Source: K. Zoi, N.C.P. Cross (2017) *J. Clin. Oncol*. 35: 947–54. Reproduced with permission of the American Society of Clinical Oncology.

Polycythaemia

Polycythaemia is defined as an increase in the haemoglobin concentration above the upper limit of normal for the patient's age and sex.

Classification of polycythaemia

Polycythaemia is classified according to its pathophysiology, but the major subdivision is into **absolute polycythaemia** or erythrocytosis, in which the red cell mass (volume) is raised to greater than 125% of that expected for body mass and gender, and **relative** or **pseudopolycythaemia**, in which the red cell volume is normal but the plasma volume is reduced. If the haematocrit is higher than 0.60 there will always be a raised red cell mass and absolute polycythaemia. A haemoglobin (Hb) >185 g/L or haematocrit >0.52 in men, and Hb >165 g/L or haematocrit >0.48 in women, indicates that erythrocytosis is likely.

Formerly, radioisotope studies (Table 15.2) were often performed to document a raised red cell mass, but with the advent of molecular genetic testing to confirm the presence of a clonal neoplasm, these are much less commonly done today and such testing is no longer available in many regions.

Once established, absolute polycythaemia can be subdivided into **primary polycythaemia,** or **secondary polycythaemia** in which the bone marrow is driven by an increase in erythropoietin as a result of factors such as smoking, sleep apnoea or altitude (Table 15.3). Primary polycythaemia includes both rare congenital causes of polycythaemia related to genetic changes in oxygen sensing or erythropoietin signalling, and the more common acquired myeloproliferative neoplasm **polycythaemia vera** (in which there is an intrinsic overactivity in the bone marrow).

Table 15.2 Radiodilution methods for measuring red cell and plasma volume.

	Normal	Primary or secondary polycythaemia	Relative polycythaemia
Total red cell volume (^{51}Cr)	Men 25–35 mL/kg Women 22–32 mL/kg	Increased	Normal
Total plasma volume (^{125}I-albumin)	40–50 mL/kg	Normal	Decreased

Table 15.3 Causes of polycythaemia (erythrocytosis).

Primary erythrocytosis
Congenital
Erythropoietin receptor mutations
Acquired
Polycythaemia vera

Secondary erythrocytosis
Congenital
Defects of the oxygen-sensing pathway
   VHL gene mutation (Chuvash erythrocytosis)
   PHD2 mutations
   HIF2A mutations
Other congenital defects
   High oxygen-affinity haemoglobin
Acquired
Erythropoietin-mediated
   Central hypoxia
   Chronic lung disease
   Right-to-left cardiopulmonary vascular shunts
   Carbon monoxide poisoning
   Smoking
   Obstructive sleep apnoea
   High altitude
Local hypoxia
   Renal artery stenosis
   End-stage renal disease
   Hydronephrosis
   Renal cysts (polycystic kidney disease)
   Post-renal transplant erythrocytosis
Pathological erythropoietin production
   Tumours – cerebellar haemangioblastoma, meningioma,
   parathyroid tumours, hepatocellular carcinoma, renal
   cell cancer, Wilms tumour, phaeochromocytoma, uterine
   leiomyoma
Drug-associated
   Erythropoietin analogue administration
   Androgen administration

Primary polycythaemia (erythrocytosis): polycythaemia vera (PV)

In PV, the increase in red cell volume is caused by a clonal malignancy of a marrow stem cell. The disease results from somatic mutation of a single haemopoietic stem cell which gives its progeny a proliferative advantage. The JAK2 V617F mutation is present in haemopoietic cells in about 95% of patients and a mutation in exon 12 is seen in most of the remainder. Although the increase in red cells is the diagnostic finding, in many patients there is also an overproduction of granulocytes and platelets. Some families have an inherited predisposition to MPN, but *JAK2* or *CALR* mutations are not present in the germline.

Diagnosis

Making the diagnosis of PV in a patient who presents with polycythaemia can be difficult. Current WHO criteria are

Table 15.4 World Health Organization 2016 diagnostic criteria for polycythaemia vera (PV).

Major criteria

1	High haematocrit (>49% in men, >48% in women) or high haemoglobin (>165 g/L in men, >160 g/L in women) or raised red cell mass (>25% above predicted)
2	Bone marrow (BM) biopsy showing hypercellularity for age with trilineage growth (panmyelosis) including prominent erythroid, granulocytic, and megakaryocytic proliferation with pleomorphic mature megakaryocytes
3	Presence of *JAK2 V617F* or *JAK2* exon 12 mutation

Minor criterion

Subnormal serum erythropoietin test

Diagnosis of PV requires meeting either all three major criteria, or the first two major criteria and the minor criterion. Criterion number 2 (BM biopsy) may not be required in cases with sustained absolute erythrocytosis: haemoglobin levels 185 g/L in men (haematocrit 55.5%) or 165 g/L in women (haematocrit 49.5%) if major criterion 3 and the minor criterion are present. However, initial myelofibrosis (present in up to 20% of patients) can only be detected by performing a BM biopsy; this finding may predict a more rapid progression to overt myelofibrosis (post-PV MF).

listed in Table 15.4. The identification of the *JAK2* mutation has rationalized the approach to diagnosis of polycythaemia. A three-stage approach to diagnosis has been suggested:

1 **Stage 1**
- History and examination.
- Arterial oxygen saturation (pulse oximetry).
- Full blood count/film.
- *JAK2(V617F)* mutation.
- Serum erythropoietin level.
- Serum ferritin.
- Renal and liver function tests.

If JAK2(V617F) is negative and there is no clear secondary cause, consider investigations in stage 2.

2 **Stage 2**
- Abdominal ultrasound.
- Bone marrow aspirate and trephine.
- Cytogenetic analysis.

Specialized tests may then be required.

3 **Stage 3**
- Arterial oxygen dissociation (high oxygen-affinity haemoglobin).
- Sleep study.
- Lung function studies.
- Gene mutations found in congenital polycythaemia (e.g. *EPOR, VHL, PHD2, HIF2A*).

Clinical features

PV is usually a disease of older people and has an equal sex incidence. Clinical features result from hyperviscosity, hypervolaemia, hypermetabolism or thrombosis.

1 Headaches, dyspnoea, blurred vision and night sweats. Generalised pruritus, characteristically after a hot bath or shower, can be a severe problem.
2 Plethoric appearance: ruddy cyanosis (Fig. 15.4), conjunctival suffusion and retinal venous engorgement.
3 Splenomegaly in 75% of patients, usually not massive (Fig. 15.5).

4 Haemorrhage or thrombosis, either arterial or venous, may be seen.
5 Gout (as a result of raised uric acid production; Fig. 15.6).

Laboratory findings

1 The haemoglobin, haematocrit and red cell count are increased. The total red cell volume (Table 15.2) is increased.
2 A neutrophil leucocytosis is seen in >50% of patients and some have increased basophils.
3 A raised platelet count is present in about 50% of patients.
4 A *JAK2* mutation is present in the bone marrow and peripheral blood granulocytes in over 95% of patients.
5 The bone marrow is hypercellular with trilineage growth, as assessed by trephine biopsy (Fig. 15.7).
6 Serum erythropoietin is low.
7 Plasma urate is often increased; the serum lactate dehydrogenase (LDH) is normal or slightly raised.
8 Circulating erythroid progenitors (erythroid colony-forming unit, CFU_E, and erythroid burst-forming unit, BFU_E; see p. 12) are increased compared to normal and grow *in vitro* independently of added erythropoietin (endogenous erythroid colonies).

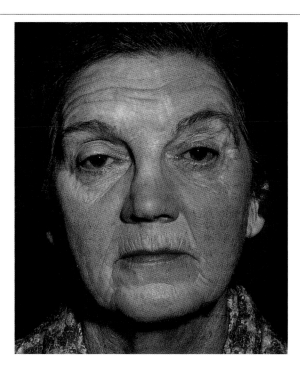

Figure 15.4 Polycythaemia vera: facial plethora and conjunctival suffusion in a 63-year-old woman. Haemoglobin 180 g/L; total red cell volume 45 mL/kg.

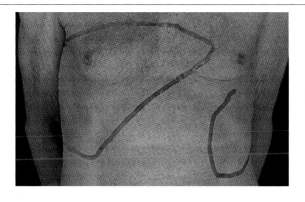

Figure 15.5 Splenomegaly: enlarged liver and spleen in a patient with polycythaemia vera.

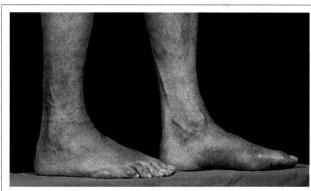
(a)

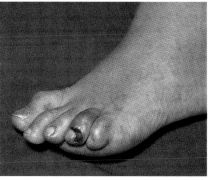
(b)

Figure 15.6 (a) The feet of a 72-year-old man with polycythaemia rubra vera. There is inflammation of the right metatarsophalangeal and other joints caused by uric acid deposits. **(b)** Gangrene of the left fourth toe in essential thrombocythaemia.

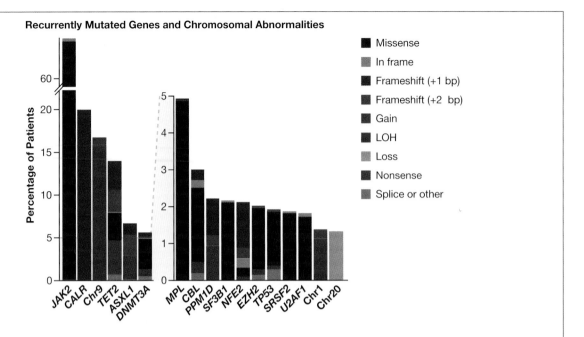

Figure 15.7 Distribution of recurrent gene mutations and chromosome (Chr) changes in myeloproliferative neoplasms. Point mutations include insertions and deletions, some of which (e.g. of calreticulin) result in a frame-shift. Chromosomal changes include whole or partial gains or losses, and copy-neutral loss of heterozygosity (LOH). Source: J. Grinfield *et al.* (2018) *N. Engl. J. Med.* 379: 1416. Reproduced with permission of Massachusetts Medical Society.

9 Chromosome abnormalities (e.g. deletions of 9p or 20q) are found in a minority of subjects. Mutations in genes *TET2, ASXL1, DNMT3A, MPL, CBL, PPMID, SF3B1, NFE2, EZH2, SRSF2* (many involved in epigenetic reactions, see Fig. 16.1) and others occur in 10–20% of patients with PV and also in patients with ET and PMF (Figure 15.7). They are more frequent in older patients and are associated with more rapid progression and transformation to myelofibrosis. *TP53* and *RUNX1* mutations predict for transformation to AML.

Treatment

Treatment is aimed at maintaining a normal blood count. The haematocrit should be strictly maintained below 0.45 and the platelet count below 600 and ideally below 400×10^9/L. Cardiovascular risk factors such as hypertension, diabetes mellitus and hyperlipidaemia should be controlled.

Venesection

Venesection to reduce the haematocrit to less than 0.45 is particularly useful when a rapid reduction of red cell volume is required (e.g. at the start of therapy). It is indicated especially in younger patients and those with mild disease. The resulting iron deficiency may limit erythropoiesis. Unfortunately, venesection does not control the platelet count and with iron deficiency the platelet count may even increase.

Hydroxycarbamide (hydroxyurea)

This is used in patients who are high risk (i.e. over age 60, prior history of thrombosis), as well as if there is poor control or intolerance of venesection, or symptomatic or progressive splenomegaly, thrombocytosis, weight loss or night sweats. Daily treatment can control the blood count and may need to be continued for many years (Fig. 15.8). The *JAK2* mutation affects platelet function, leading to thrombosis or haemorrhage, and it is therefore necessary to control both the platelet count and haematocrit to reduce the risk. Side-effects of hydroxycarbamide include myelosuppression, nausea and toxicity to the skin, especially in areas exposed to ultraviolet light.

JAK inhibitors

Drugs such as ruxolitinib inhibit JAK2 activity and are effective in many patients. At present ruxolitinib is used in patients who are not controlled adequately or have side-effects with hydroxycarbamide therapy, or those with severe constitutional symptoms that hydroxycarbamide does not adequately treat. Other JAK2 inhibitors including fedratinib and pacritinib are in development.

Interferon

Injectable α-interferon suppresses excess proliferation in the marrow and has produced good haematological responses in some patients. It is less convenient than the oral agents and

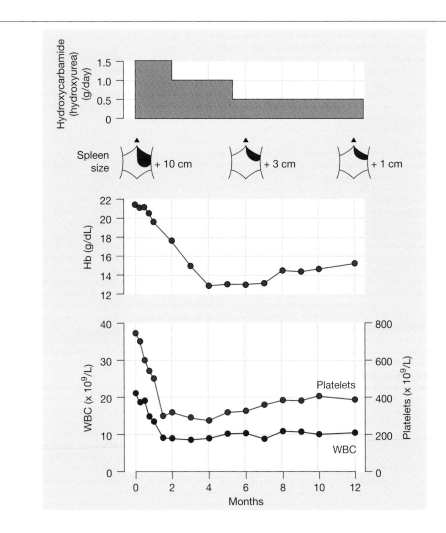

Figure 15.8 Haematological response to therapy with hydroxycarbamide (hydroxyurea) in polycythaemia vera. Hb, haemoglobin; WBC, white blood cells.

side-effects are frequent. It may be particularly valuable in controlling itching and is often used in its long-acting form for younger patients to avoid early exposure to other drugs, and for those who might become pregnant, since ruxolitinib is not known to be safe in pregnancy and hydroxycarbamide is teratogenic.

Aspirin

Low-dose aspirin reduces thrombotic complications without significant increased risk of major haemorrhage and is used in almost all patients.

Angiotensin-converting-enzyme (ACE) inhibitors

These drugs can be useful if there is hypertension, since they also mildly inhibit red cell production.

Course and prognosis

Typically, the prognosis is good, with a median survival over 10 years. Thrombosis and haemorrhage are the major clinical problems. Increased viscosity, vascular stasis and high platelet levels and altered platelet function may all contribute to thrombosis, whereas defective platelet function may promote haemorrhage. Transition from PV to myelofibrosis occurs in approximately 30% of patients, especially those with a *JAK2* mutation allele burden >50%, and approximately 5% of patients progress to acute myeloid leukaemia (AML). Cooperating mutations of myeloid genes also predict for these outcomes.

Congenital causes of primary polycythaemia

Congenital causes are relatively rare and include cases caused by mutations in the genes that regulate oxygen sensing (*VHL*,

PHD2 or *HIF2A*; see Chapter 2) as well as mutation of the erythropoietin receptor gene (*EPOR*) and haemoglobin mutations that lead to high oxygen-affinity variants with subsequent tissue hypoxia. These patients often have a family history of polycythaemia and present at a young age.

Secondary polycythaemia

The causes of secondary polycythaemia are listed in Table 15.3. Acquired causes are due to an increase in the erythropoietin level. Hypoxia caused by smoking, sleep apnoea or chronic obstructive airway disease is a common cause, and measurement of arterial oxygen saturation is a valuable test. Renal and tumour causes of inappropriate erythropoietin secretion are less common.

There is little evidence on which to guide a treatment plan, but one approach is to advise venesection if the haematocrit is above 0.54, with the aim of reducing to a target of around 0.50. A lower target for venesection may be used if there is hypertension, diabetes, dyspnoea, angina or a previous thrombotic episode.

Apparent polycythaemia

Apparent polycythaemia, also known as pseudopolycythaemia, is the result of plasma volume contraction. By definition, the red cell mass is normal. Diuretic therapy, extreme volume loss (e.g. severe diarrhoea), anasarca, smoking, hypertension, obesity and alcohol consumption are frequent associations. Management includes volume replacement and correction of the underlying cause. Phlebotomy is not of benefit.

Essential thrombocythaemia

In this condition there is a sustained increase in the platelet count due to megakaryocyte proliferation and overproduction of platelets. The haematocrit is normal and the Philadelphia chromosome or *BCR-ABL1* rearrangement is absent. The bone marrow shows no collagen fibrosis. A persisting platelet count of greater than 450×10^9/L is the central diagnostic feature, but other causes of a raised platelet count (particularly iron deficiency, inflammatory or malignant disorder and myelodysplasia) need to be fully excluded before the diagnosis can be made.

From 50% to 60% of patients show the *JAK2 V617F* mutation and these cases tend to resemble more closely PV with higher haemoglobin and white cell counts than *JAK2*-negative cases (Table 15.5). The *JAK2* mutation also affects platelet and neutrophil function (including increasing production of neutrophil extracellular traps, NETs, structures formed from DNA expelled by activated neutrophils), leading to a pro-thrombotic state. *JAK2 exon 12* mutation is associated with erythrocytosis and is not seen in ET.

Mutations in the *CALR* gene are seen in around 75% of *JAK2*-negative ET patients, in total representing about a third of all patients. These patients tend to be younger and have higher platelet counts, but a lower incidence of thrombosis

Table 15.5 Typical clinical and laboratory features of essential thrombocythaemia associated with *JAK2* or *CALR* mutation.

Feature	*JAK2* mutated	*CALR* mutated
Age	Older	Younger
Haemoglobin	Higher	Lower
White cell count	Higher	Lower
Platelet count	Lower	Higher
Serum erythropoietin	Lower	Higher
Thrombosis risk	Higher	Lower
Transformation to polycythaemia vera	Yes	No
Risk of transformation to myelofibrosis	Equal	Equal
Approximate survival	17 years	>25 years

(Table 15.5). Mutations within the *MPL* gene are seen in ~5% of cases. Mutations in other driver genes described in MPN occur in a minority of cases of ET with similar prognostic implications (see below and Figure 15.7). Rare primary familial cases in children have been associated with germline mutations in the genes for thrombopoietin or its receptor MPL.

Diagnosis

This used to be based on the exclusion of other causes of chronic thrombocytosis, but now that specific genetic lesions have been identified, a positive diagnosis can be made in most cases (see Table 15.6).

Clinical and laboratory findings

The dominant clinical features are thrombosis and haemorrhage. Most cases are asymptomatic and are diagnosed on a routine blood count. Thrombosis may occur in the venous or arterial systems (Fig. 15.6), whereas haemorrhage, as a result of abnormal platelet function, may cause either chronic or acute bleeding. Some patients, particularly those with the *JAK2* mutation, present with Budd–Chiari syndrome, when the platelet count may be normal because of splenomegaly. A characteristic symptom is erythromelalgia, a burning sensation felt in the hands or feet and promptly relieved by aspirin. Up to 40% of patients will have palpable splenomegaly, whereas in others there may be splenic atrophy because of infarction.

Abnormal large platelets and megakaryocyte fragments may be seen on the blood film (Fig. 15.9). The bone marrow is similar to that in PV, but an excess of abnormal megakaryocytes is typical. Cytogenetics and molecular analysis are performed

Table 15.6 World Health Organization 2016 diagnostic criteria for essential thrombocythaemia.

Major criteria

1	Sustained platelet count above 450×10^9/L
2	Bone marrow biopsy showing proliferation mainly of the megakaryocyte lineage with increased numbers of enlarged, mature megakaryocytes with hyperlobulated nuclei. No significant increase or left shift in neutrophil granulopoiesis or erythropoiesis and very rarely minor (grade 1) increase in reticulin fibre
3	No other myeloid malignancy, polycythaemia vera, primary myelofibrosis, chronic myeloid leukaemia (*BCR-ABL1* positive) or myelodysplastic syndrome
4	Presence of an acquired pathogenetic mutation (in *JAK2*, *CALR* or *MPL*)

Minor criteria

1	Presence of a clonal marker
2	Absence of evidence for reactive thrombocytosis

Diagnosis of essential thrombocythaemia requires meeting all four major criteria or the first three major criteria and both the minor criteria.

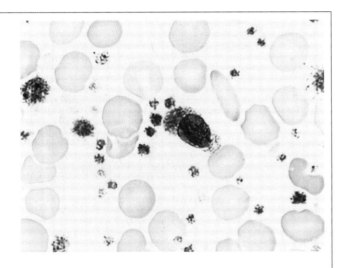

Figure 15.9 Peripheral blood film in essential thrombocythaemia showing increased numbers of platelets and a nucleated megakaryocytic fragment.

Table 15.7 Causes of a raised platelet count.

Reactive

Haemorrhage, trauma, postoperative

Chronic iron deficiency

Malignancy

Chronic infections

Connective tissue diseases (e.g. rheumatoid arthritis)

Post-splenectomy

Endogenous

Essential thrombocythaemia (*JAK2* mutation + or –)

Some cases of polycythaemia vera, primary myelofibrosis, BCR-ABL1+ chronic myeloid leukaemia, myelodysplastic syndromes (5q– syndrome or myelodysplastic syndromes/ myeloproliferative neoplasms with ring sideroblasts and thrombocytosis)

to exclude *BCR-ABL1*+ CML and to detect the underlying mutation of *JAK2*, *CALR* or *MPL* or any additional mutations (Fig. 15.7) which, as for PV, have prognostic significance. The condition must be distinguished from other causes of a raised platelet count (Table 15.7). Platelet function tests are rarely needed, but are consistently abnormal, with failure of aggregation with adrenaline being particularly characteristic.

Prognosis and treatment

The principle is to reduce the risk of the major clinical problems of thrombosis or haemorrhage. Standard cardiovascular risk factors, such as cholesterol, smoking, diabetes, obesity and hypertension, should be identified and treated. Low-dose aspirin at 75 mg/day is generally recommended in all cases.

Patients at **high risk** include those over 60 years of age, and/or with previous thrombosis and/or with platelet count $>1500 \times 10^9$/L, and this group should be treated with hydroxycarbamide or another cytoreductive agent to reduce the platelet count. **Low-risk** patients are those aged below 60 years without a history of thrombosis or extreme thrombocytosis, and here aspirin alone is sufficient.

Hydroxycarbamide is the most widely used treatment and is well tolerated, although after prolonged therapy some patients develop skin keratosis, epitheliomas, ulceration or pigmentation. Anagrelide is a good second-line treatment but has cardiovascular side-effects, and a possible increased risk of myelofibrosis is also of concern. These two drugs can be combined at low doses to reduce side-effects. α-Interferon is also effective and is often used in younger patients or during pregnancy. A long-acting PEGylated preparation of interferon is preferred, since it allows once-weekly dosing. JAK2 inhibitors are also being assessed.

Course

Often the disease is stationary for 10–20 years or more. The disease may transform after a number of years to myelofibrosis, but the risk of transformation to AML is relatively low (less than 5%).

Primary myelofibrosis

The predominant feature of PMF is a progressive generalized reactive fibrosis of the bone marrow in association with megakaryocyte atypia and proliferation (Fig. 15.10), and with the development of haemopoiesis in the spleen and liver (known as myeloid metaplasia or extra-medullary haemopoieisis). Clinically this leads to anaemia and massive splenomegaly (Fig. 15.11). In some patients there is osteosclerosis. The fibrosis of the bone marrow is secondary to the hyperplasia of abnormal megakaryocytes. Fibroblasts are stimulated by platelet-derived growth factor and other cytokines secreted by megakaryocytes and platelets. Up to 50% of PMF present in a **prefibrotic/early stage** with no significant increase in reticulin or collagen, but markedly abnormal megakaryocytes in a hypercellular marrow. In prefibrotic PMF, the subjects tend to be younger, include more females, to have smaller spleens, fewer cytopenias and fewer additional mutations (other than of *JAK2*, *CALR* or *MPL*) and more thrombocytosis than those with overt PMF.

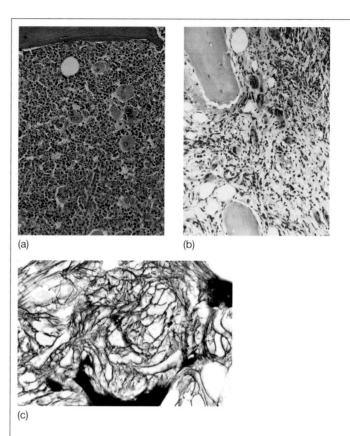

(a)

(b)

(c)

Figure 15.10 Iliac crest trephine biopsies. **(a)** Polycythaemia vera: fat spaces are almost completely replaced by hyperplastic haemopoietic tissue. All haemopoietic cell lines are increased, with megakaryocytes particularly prominent. **(b)** Primary myelofibrosis: normal marrow architecture is lost and haemopoietic cells are surrounded by increased fibrous tissue and intercellular substance. Atypical megakaryocytes are prominent. **(c)** Primary myelofibrosis: Silver staining shows a dense reticulin network. Source: (c) A.V. Hoffbrand *et al.* (2019) *Color Atlas of Clinical Hematology*, 5th edn. Reproduced with permission of John Wiley & Sons.

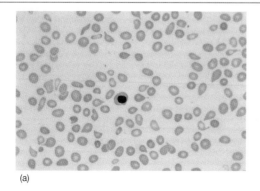

(a)

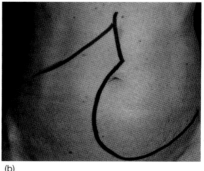

(b)

Figure 15.11 **(a)** Peripheral blood film in primary myelofibrosis. Leucoerythroblastic change with 'tear-drop' cells and an erythroblast. **(b)** Massive splenomegaly in a patient with myelofibrosis.

When myelofibrosis evolves after polycythaemia vera or essential thrombocythaemia, it is termed 'post-polycythaemic' or 'post-thrombocythaemic' myelofibrosis, respectively, and behaves similarly to primary myelofibrosis.

The *JAK2*, *CALR* and *MPL* mutations occur in approximately 55%, 25% and 10% of patients respectively (Fig. 15.2). One-third of patients with similar features have a previous history of PV or ET and some patients present with clinical and laboratory features of both disorders.

Clinical features

1 An insidious onset in older people is usual with symptoms of anaemia.
2 Symptoms resulting from massive splenomegaly are frequent and include abdominal discomfort, pain or indigestion. Splenomegaly is the main physical finding (Fig. 15.5b).
3 Hypermetabolic symptoms such as loss of weight, anorexia, fever and night sweats are common.
4 Bleeding problems, bone pain or gout occur in a minority of patients.

Laboratory findings

1 Anaemia is usual, but a normal or increased haemoglobin level may be found in some patients.
2 The white cell and platelet counts are frequently high at the time of presentation. Later in the disease leucopenia and thrombocytopenia are common. In the prefibrotic disease, leukocytosis and thrombocytosis tend to be more marked and anaemia less than in overt disease.
3 A leucoerythroblastic blood film is found. The red cells show characteristic 'tear-drop' poikilocytes (Fig. 15.11).
4 Bone marrow is usually unobtainable by aspiration. Trephine biopsy (Fig. 15.8b) shows a fibrotic, hypercellular marrow. Silver staining shows a dense reticulin network (Fig 15.8c), except in prefibrotic PMF. The degree of fibrosis can be semi-quantitatively divided into four grades. Increased megakaryocytes are frequently seen. In 10% of cases there is increased bone formation (osteosclerosis) with increased bone density on X-ray.
5 *JAK2* is mutated in approximately 60% of cases, *CALR* in ~25% and *MPL* in ~10%. The *CALR*-mutated patients have lower white cell and higher platelet counts and longest survival, while triple-negative patients have the shortest survival.
6 High serum urate and LDH levels reflect increased, although ineffective, haemopoiesis.
7 Transformation to AML occurs in 10–20% of patients. Certain chromosome abnormalities, e.g. loss of the long arms of chromosomes 5 or 7, an extra copy of chromosome 8 (trisomy 8) or rearrangements of 11q23 predict for this transformation. As for PV, additional genetic mutations (Fig. 15.7) predict for progression of the myelofibrosis, while mutations of *TP53* and *RUNX1* predict for transformation to AML. Overall, survival is reduced in those with mutations of two or more of these additional 'high-risk' driver genes.

Table 15.8 A dynamic international prognostic scoring system (DIPSS) for patients with primary myelofibrosis. Median survival times are 185, 78, 35 and 16 months for the low (0 points), intermediate-1 (1 point), intermediate-2 (2–3 points) and high-risk (4–6 points) categories, respectively. Source: N. Gangat *et al.* (2011) *J. Clin. Oncol.* 29(4): 392–7. Reproduced with permission of the American Society of Clinical Oncology.

Variable	IPSS*	DIPSS	DIPSS Plus
Age >65 years	✓	✓	✓
Constitutional symptoms	✓	✓	✓
Haemoglobin (Hb) <100 g/L	✓	✓	✓
Leucocyte count >25 × 10⁹/L	✓	✓	✓
Circulating blasts ≥1%	✓	✓	✓
Platelet count <100 × 10⁹/L			✓
Red blood cell transfusion need			✓
Unfavourable karyotype	1 point each	1 point each but Hb = 2	✓ 1 point each

*Unfavourable karyotype includes +8, +–7/7 q, –5/5q, complex and others.

Treatment

Therapy for PMF is aimed at reducing the effects of anaemia and splenomegaly. Useful prognostic information may be obtained by analysis of prognostic scoring systems (Table 15.8). Blood transfusions and regular folic acid therapy are useful in severely anaemic patients.

Ruxolitinib is an oral JAK2 inhibitor that can reduce spleen size, improve constitutional symptoms and quality of life and increase survival. As mentioned under PV, other JAK2 inhibitors are in development. Hydroxycarbamide may reduce splenomegaly and hypermetabolic symptoms. Thalidomide and corticosteroids or androgens improve anaemia in some cases. Erythropoiesis-stimulating agents can be tried, but may cause splenic enlargement.

Splenectomy is considered for patients with severe symptomatic splenomegaly: mechanical discomfort, thrombocytopenia, portal hypertension or excessive transfusion requirements. Splenectomy is associated with a high morbidity and mortality, even with experienced surgeons. Allopurinol may be indicated to prevent gout and urate nephropathy from hyperuricaemia. Allogeneic stem cell transplantation may be curative for young patients.

The median survival is 3–5 years and causes of death include heart failure, infection and leukaemic transformation.

For prefibrotic disease, if there are no symptoms a watch-and-wait approach may be taken, but if symptoms are present, vascular complications, marked thrombocytosis or splenomegaly, therapy may be needed.

Mastocytosis

Mastocytosis is a clonal neoplastic proliferation of mast cells that accumulate in one or more organ systems. Mast cells are similar to basophils and survive for months or years in vascular tissues and most organs. **Cutaneous mastocytosis** with the skin lesions of urticarial pigmentosa (Fig. 15.12) is much more common than systemic forms of mastocytosis and tends to run an indolent course.

Systemic mastocytosis is a clonal myeloproliferative neoplasm with diverse presentations involving bone marrow, heart, spleen, lymph nodes and skin. The bone marrow or other organs than skin show multifocal dense (>15 per aggregate) mast cell infiltrates. The cells are CD2 and/or CD25 positive. Systemic mastocytosis is often seen in association with other haemopoietic conditions including MDS, MPN or AML. The most aggressive form of mastocytosis is **mast cell leukaemia**, in which large numbers of clonal, atypical mast cells circulate in the blood; median survival in mast cell leukaemia is only a few months.

The somatic KIT mutation Asp816Val (D816V) is detected in the majority of patients and is responsible for autonomous growth and enhanced survival of the neoplastic mast cells. Kit is a tyrosine kinase cell membrane receptor for the growth factor stem cell factor (SCF).

Symptoms are either related to organ infiltration or histamine and prostaglandin release, and include flushing, pruritus, abdominal pain and bronchospasm. The skin usually shows urticaria pigmentosa (Fig. 15.12). Serum tryptase is increased and can be used to monitor treatment. Midostaurin is approved for treatment of systemic mastocytosis and avipritinib is also highly active; both inhibit the KIT tyrosine kinase. Antihistamine drugs and cromolyn are valuable in reducing mast cell mediator symptoms, and interferon or chemotherapies such as chlorodeoxyadenosine can be helpful in resistant cases. Additional mutations similar to those found in advanced PV, ET and PMF are also found in advanced cases of systemic mastocytosis.

Chronic neutrophilic leukaemia

These patients have a raised white cell count of $>25 \times 10^9$/L with at least 80% mature neutrophils. They have no inflammatory or other causes of neutrophilia, no evidence for any other myeloproliferative neoplasm and no increase in blast cells. They may have mild splenomegaly. Activating mutations in the gene encoding the receptor for colony-stimulating factor 3 (*CSF3R*) are found in most patients and kinase inhibitors may be useful. The prognosis is variable.

Chronic eosinophilic leukaemia

Chronic eosinophilic leukaemia is a clonal persistent eosinophilia (greater than 1.5×10^9/L). An interstitial lesion in chromosome 4 resulting in *FIP1L1-PDGFRA* fusion gene if present predicts for a response to tyrosine kinase inhibitors. In other cases there are less frequent cytogenetic or molecular defects (Table 15.1). There may be greater than 5% but less than 20% blasts in the marrow. The cells may infiltrate various organs, causing damage, e.g. endomyocardial fibrosis, lung fibrosis, central nervous system, skin (with pruritus) and gastrointestinal tract. If clonality cannot be shown and blasts are less than 5%, the condition is diagnosed as hypereosinophilic syndrome (see p. 106). For those not responding to tyrosine kinase inhibitors, treatment is with steroids, hydroxycarbamide, interferon and chlorodeoxyadenosine may be tried.

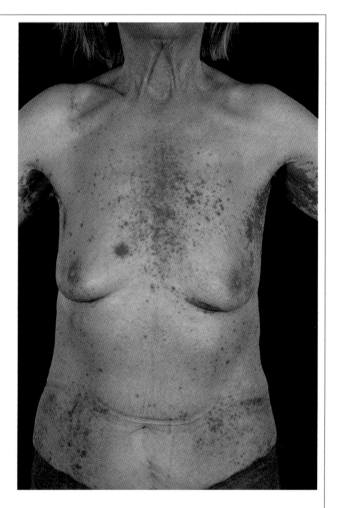

Figure 15.12 Systemic mastocytosis: female 72 years; widespread erythematous, confluent plaques of urticaria pigmentosa over chest, abdomen and upper arms. Source: Courtesy of Professor M. Rustin.

- Myeloproliferative neoplasms are a group of conditions arising from marrow stem cells and characterized by clonal proliferation of one or more haemopoietic components in the bone marrow. The three major subtypes are polycythaemia vera (PV), essential thrombocythaemia (ET) and primary myelofibrosis (PMF).
- These subtypes are closely related to each other. Mutation of the *JAK2* gene is detected in almost all patients with PV and approximately 60% of those with ET and primary myelofibrosis. Mutations in *CALR* or *MPL* are present in most cases of ET or PMF without a *JAK2* mutation.
- Polycythaemia is defined as an increase in the haemoglobin concentration above normal for the age and sex. The major subdivision is into **absolute polycythaemia**, in which the red cell mass is raised, and **relative polycythaemia**, in which the red cell volume is normal but the plasma volume is reduced.
- Absolute polycythaemia is divided into primary polycythaemia, known as polycythaemia vera (PV) or the much rarer congenital types, or secondary polycythaemia.
- The diagnosis of PV is made by finding polycythaemia together with a *JAK2* mutation. It occurs in older patients and the increase in blood viscosity leads to headaches, plethoric appearance, thrombosis and splenomegaly.
- Treatment of PV aims to maintain the haematocrit around 45%. Useful approaches include venesection, hydroxycarbamide and *JAK2* inhibitors. Aspirin is also given. Survival is usually over 10 years, but there may be progression to AML or myelofibrosis.
- Secondary polycythaemia can arise from rare congenital causes or acquired disorders such as lung disease or tumours that secrete erythropoietin. Venesection may be needed.
- Essential thrombocythaemia is diagnosed by persistent raised platelet count >450 × 10⁹/L in the absence of other causes. *JAK2*, *CALR* or *MPL* genes are mutated in most cases.
- The predominant feature of primary myelofibrosis is a progressive generalized reactive fibrosis of the bone marrow in association with the development of haemopoiesis in the spleen and liver. Symptoms usually result from anaemia and a grossly enlarged spleen.
- Diagnosis of myelofibrosis is made on blood film, which shows a leuco-erythroblastic appearance, together with bone marrow biopsy and *JAK2*, *CALR* and *MPL* mutation screen. Treatment is mainly with red cell transfusion and JAK2 inhibition. Stem cell transplantation offers a chance of cure in younger patients.
- Systemic mastocytosis is a clonal proliferation of mast cells with involvement of bone marrow, skin (as urticaria pigmentosa) and other organs. There is usually an underlying *KIT* mutation, most commonly D816V, and the disease may respond to tyrosine kinase inhibitors.
- Chronic neutrophilic leukaemia and chronic eosinophilic leukaemia are rare MPN that sometimes respond to tyrosine kinase inhibitors.

Now visit **www.wileyessential.com/haematology** to test yourself on this chapter.

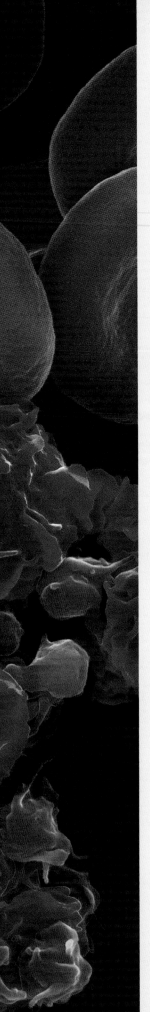

CHAPTER 16
Myelodysplastic syndromes

Key topics

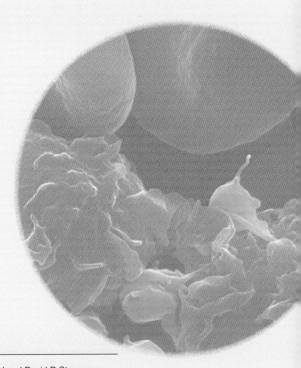

Hoffbrand's Essential Haematology, Eighth Edition. By A. Victor Hoffbrand and David P. Steensma.
© 2020 John Wiley & Sons Ltd. Published 2020 by John Wiley & Sons Ltd.
Companion website: www.wileyessential.com/haematology

Myelodysplastic syndromes (MDS)

MDS includes a group of clonal disorders of haemopoietic stem cells characterized by bone marrow failure in association with dysplastic cell morphology in one or more cell lineages (Table 16.1).

A hallmark of these diseases is simultaneous proliferation and apoptosis of haemopoietic cells (**ineffective haemopoiesis**), leading to the paradox of a hypercellular bone marrow but pancytopenia in peripheral blood. There is a tendency for MDS to progress to acute myeloid leukaemia (AML), although death from complications of cytopenias or from unrelated causes often occurs before this develops.

In most cases, the disease is *de novo* (**primary**), but in a proportion of patients it is a result of chemotherapy or radiotherapy given for treatment of another disorder. This latter type is termed **therapy-related MDS (t-MDS)** and is now classified together with therapy-related AML, since the marrow blast proportion has little influence on outcome in this poor-prognosis form of myeloid neoplasm. **Secondary MDS** describes MDS arising from germline mutations or inherited marrow failure syndromes.

Pathogenesis

The pathogenesis of the MDS begins with genetic changes in a multipotent haemopoietic progenitor cell. The immune system may have a role in suppressing bone marrow function once an abnormal clone is present and immunosuppression is sometimes used in treatment (see below). The marrow microenviroment (stromal cells) probably also contributes to abnormal haemopoiesis, though the microenvironmental defects are not yet well defined.

Acquired chromosome abnormalities in marrow cells are frequent, detectable in more than half of cases (Table 16.2). Most of these are numerical abnormalities or segmental chromosomal deletions, rather than the balanced translocations that are common in AML.

In addition, molecular analysis shows that clonally derived cells in MDS typically carry several point mutations. More than 40 different driver mutations have been identified in MDS and usually involve genes involved in epigenetic processes such as DNA methylation (*TET2* and *DNMT3A*) and chromatin modification (*ASXL1* and *EZH2*), as well as in RNA splicing

Table 16.1 The World Health Organization (2016) classification of myelodysplastic syndromes (MDS). Therapy-related myeloid neoplasms and MDS arising as a consequence of a germline mutation are classified separately.

Subtype	Peripheral blood	Bone marrow	% blasts in marrow	Relative proportion (%)
MDS with single-lineage dysplasia (MDS-SLD)	Anaemia, neutropenia or thrombocytopenia	Unilineage dysplasia (in >10% cells), <5% blasts	<5	10–20
MDS with single-lineage dysplasia and ring sideroblasts (MDS-RS-SLD)	Anaemia	Unilineage erythroid dysplasia, ≥15% erythroid precursors are ring sideroblasts or if ≥5% are ring sideroblasts *SF3B1* mutation is present, <5% blasts	<5	3–10
MDS with multilineage dysplasia (MDS-MLD)	Cytopenia(s)	Multilineage dysplasia +/– ring sideroblasts (if ≥15% ring sideroblasts present or ≥5% with *SF3B1* mutation, may designate as MDS-RS-MLD), <5% blasts, no Auer rods	<5	30
MDS with excess blasts type 1 (MDS-EB1)	Cytopenia(s)	Unilineage or multilineage dysplasia	5–9	20
MDS with excess blasts type 2 (MDS-EB2)	Cytopenia(s)	Unilineage or multilineage dysplasia	10–19	20
Myelodysplastic syndrome associated with isolated del(5q)	Anaemia, normal or high platelet count	5q31 chromosome deletion Anaemia, hypolobulated megakaryocytes	<5	<5
MDS-unclassifiable	Cytopenia(s)	Variable; not meeting criteria for other subtypes	<5	2–3
Provisional entity: refractory cytopenia of childhood	Pancytopenia	Multilineage dysplasia; no known germline syndrome or mutation	<5	<1

Table 16.2 Examples of recurrent cytogenetic abnormalities in MDS and their prognostic implications.

Prognosis	Cytogenetic abnormality
Very good	–Y or del(11q)
Good	Normal or del(5q)
Intermediate	del(7q) or double independent clones
Poor	inv(3) or double including –7 or del(7q)
Very poor	Complex: ≥3 abnormalities

Source: Based on P.L. Greenberg et al. (2012) Blood 120: 2454–65.

(*SF3B1*, *SRSF2*, *U2AF1*) (Figs 16.1 and 16.2). Most of these gene mutations, e.g. of *TET2*, may be found in other myeloid malignancies, including AML and the myeloproliferative neoplasms (MPN). However, in MDS, common AML-associated mutations including *FLT3* or *NPM1* are rare, probably because these are strong leukaemia drivers that result when they are acquired in rapid progression to AML. The molecular mutations have prognostic significance. At the time MDS progresses to AML, additional mutations are often acquired.

A striking example of genotype–phenotype correlation is mutation in the *SF3B1* gene, which encodes a component of the RNA spliceosome. *SF3B1* mutations are seen in almost all cases of MDS with ring sideroblasts (ring sideroblasts are abnormal erythroid precursors, discussed in Chapter 3 and further below). *TP53* mutations are detected most commonly in patients with t-MDS and are often associated with complex chromosome rearrangements, chemotherapy resistance and a poor prognosis.

Classification

MDS are classified on the basis of the blood count, marrow morphological appearance, the proportion of blast cells in blood or bone marrow, and cytogenetic and molecular genetic analysis (Table 16.1). Although the classification appears complex, the principles are as follow:

■ Cell morphological abnormalities (dysplasia) may be present solely in a single myeloid cell lineage ('single-lineage dysplasia') – red cells, neutrophils or platelets – or present in two or more myeloid lineages (**multilineage dysplasia**).

■ Erythroid dysplasia can also be associated with **ring sideroblasts** to define a unique subtype. The definition of a pathological ring sideroblast is an erythroid precursor with five or more iron granules encircling at least one-third of the nucleus. Most of these patients have mutations in *SF3B1*.

■ If the blast cell count is increased in the bone marrow, the diagnosis is made of **MDS with excess blasts** (**MDS-EB**) and these subtypes tend to have a poorer prognosis.

■ **5q– syndrome,** also called **MDS with isolated del(5q)**, is considered a distinct entity. A key gene that is deleted is

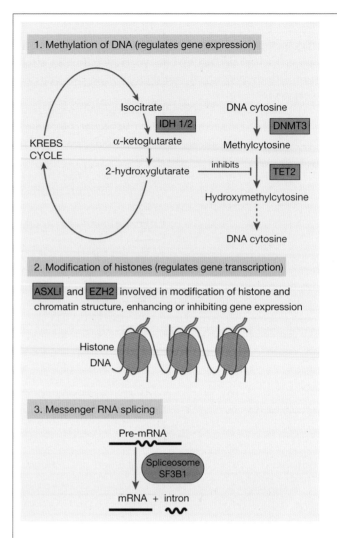

Figure 16.1 Genes involved in DNA methylation, histone modification and in mRNA splicing are frequently mutated (loss of function or gain in function) in myelodysplastic syndromes, acute myeloid leukaemia or myeloproliferative neoplasms.

RPS14, encoding a ribosomal protein (see Fig. 22.3). This subtype is more common in women and typically there is a macrocytic anaemia with thrombocytosis in 50% of cases. This subtype has a favourable prognosis and responds well to lenalidomide therapy (Tables 16.3 and 16.4).

Clinical features

The disease has an incidence of at least 1 in 10000 persons per year and a slight male predominance. The median age is 70 years and fewer than 5% of patients are under 50 years of age. The evolution is often slow and the disease may be found by chance when a patient has a blood count for some unrelated reason. The symptoms, if present, are those of anaemia, infections from neutropenia or functional neutrophil defects, or of

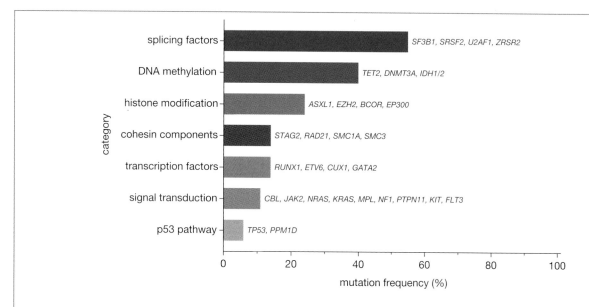

Figure 16.2 Recurrently mutated genes in MDS can be organized into biological categories. Estimated mutation frequencies and examples of the most commonly implicated genes in each category are depicted. Source: J.A. Kennedy, B.L. Ebert (2017) *J. Clin. Oncol.* 35(9): 968–74. Reproduced with permission of Journal of Clinical Oncology: American Society of Clinical Oncology. Data also from E. Papaemmanuil *et al.* (2013) *Blood* 122: 3616–27 and T. Haferlach *et al.* (2014) *Leukemia* 28: 241–47.

Table 16.3 Revised International Prognostic Scoring System (IPSS-R) prognostic risk categories/scores and clinical outcomes.

Prognostic variable	0	0.5	1	1.5	2	3	4
Cytogenetics (see Table 16.2)	Very good		Good		Intermediate	Poor	Very poor
Bone marrow blast %	≤2		>2–<5		5–10	>10	
Haemoglobin (Hb) concentration (g/L)	≥100		80–<100	<80			
Platelet count	≥100	50–<100	<50				
Neutrophil count (×10⁹/L)	≥0.8	<0.8					

Time taken for 25% of cases to evolve to acute myeloid leukaemia (AML)

Risk category	Risk score	Survival (median in years)	Median time to evolution of AML in 25% + of cases (years)
Very low	≤1.5	8.8	Not reached
Low	>1.5–3	5.3	10.8
Intermediate	>3–4.5	3.0	3.2
High	>4.5–6	1.6	1.4
Very high	>6	0.8	0.73

Source: Based on P.L. Greenberg *et al.* (2012) *Blood* 120: 2454–65.

Table 16.4 Acronyms describing clonal haemopoiesis and related states.

Acronym	State	Description
CHIP	Clonal haemopoiesis of indeterminate potential	Somatic mutation of myeloid malignancy-associated genes in blood or bone marrow at ≥2% variant allele frequency in people without a haematological neoplasm. Conveys a risk of subsequent haematological neoplasm diagnosis or acute vascular events.
ARCH	Ageing-related clonal haemopoiesis	Clonal haemopoiesis defined by presence of somatic mutations in blood and marrow and an expanded haemopoietic clone, with or without a leukaemia-associated driver mutation. Incidence increases with age. No specific variant allele frequency.
ICUS	Idiopathic cytopenia(s) of undetermined significance	Patient with one or more cytopenias but no evidence of myelodysplastic syndromes or another haematological neoplasm or specific disorder. Either no somatic mutation is detected or a mutation has not been sought.
IDUS	Idiopathic dysplasia of undetermined significance	Unexplained morphological dysplasia of blood or marrow cells with normal blood count.

easy bruising or bleeding from thrombocytopenia or functional platelet defects (Fig. 16.3).

In some patients transfusion-dependent anaemia dominates the course, while in others recurring infections or spontaneous bruising and bleeding are the major clinical problems. The function of the neutrophils, monocytes and platelets is often impaired, so that infections and bleeding may occur out of proportion to the severity of the cytopenia. The spleen is not usually enlarged.

Dysplastic cell morphology features in bone marrow may be seen in a wide range of conditions, such as excess alcohol intake, megaloblastic anaemia, parvovirus or HIV infection,

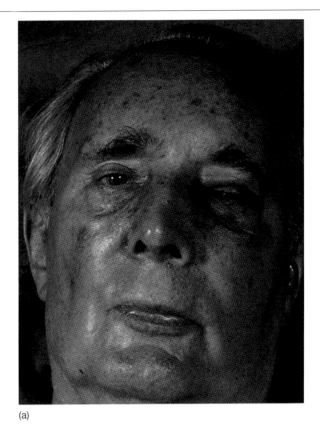

(a)

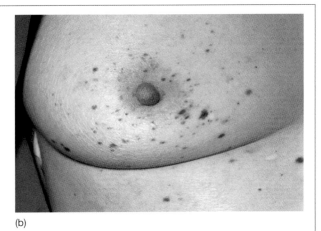

(b)

Figure 16.3 Physical signs seen in myelodysplastic syndromes (MDS). **(a)** A 78-year-old male patient with MDS with multilineage dysplasia (MDS-MLD) had recurring infections of the face and maxillary sinuses associated with neutropenia (haemoglobin 98 g/L; white cells 1.3×10^9/L; neutrophils 0.3×10^9/L; platelets 38×10^9/L). **(b)** Purpura of the skin of the breast in a 58-year-old female with MDS-MLD (haemoglobin 105 g/L; white cells 2.3×10^9/L; platelets 8×10^9/L).

recovery from cytotoxic chemotherapy, other myeloid neoplasms, and granulocyte colony-stimulating factor (G-CSF) therapy. These alternative conditions must be ruled out before making a diagnosis of MDS, and diagnostic tests may need to be repeated over time in some patients.

Laboratory findings

Peripheral blood

Pancytopenia is a frequent finding. The red cells are usually macrocytic but occasionally hypochromic; normoblasts may be present. The reticulocyte count is low. Granulocytes are often reduced in number and frequently show lack of granulation (Fig. 16.4). Their chemotactic, phagocytic and adhesive functions are impaired. The pseudo-Pelger abnormality (i.e. single or bilobed nucleus of neutrophils) is often present. The platelets may be unduly large or small and are usually decreased in number, but in ~10% of cases are elevated. In poor-prognosis cases, variable numbers of myeloblasts (<20%) are present in the blood.

Bone marrow

The cellularity is usually increased. A small number of dysplastic cells may be seen in marrow from healthy elderly individuals, so at least 10% of the cells in a lineage should be dysplastic in order to consider the diagnosis of MDS. Typical dysplastic features are:

- **Erythroid** Multinucleate normoblasts, internuclear bridges and nuclear budding (Fig. 16.4). Ring sideroblasts are seen in a specific subset of MDS and are caused by iron deposition in the mitochondria of erythroblasts.
- **Myeloid** The granulocyte precursors often show defective granulation and may be difficult to distinguish from monocytes.
- **Megakaryocytes** Dysplastic megakaryocytes may show micronuclear, small binuclear or polynuclear forms (Fig. 16.4).

In a minority of cases (about 10%) the marrow is hypocellular and may resemble aplastic anaemia; in others there is fibrosis that may cause confusion with primary myelofibrosis.

Genetic abnormalities

Cytogenetic analysis is essential in cases of unexplained cytopenias or suspected MDS. Common abnormalities include 5q–, partial or total loss of chromosomes 5 or 7, or trisomy 8 (Table 16.2). Several cytogenetic abnormalities such as 5q– are considered so diagnostic of MDS that they allow diagnosis of MDS even in the absence of morphological abnormalities within cells.

The mutations that may be found by molecular testing have been described on page 199 and summarized in Fig. 16.2, while Fig. 16.1 illustrates those involved in epigenetic processes.

Treatment

A key subdivision for considering treatment of MDS is stratifying into patients with lower-risk or higher-risk disease. 'Risk' here describes risk of progression to leukaemia or death from complications of cytopenias.

The Revised International Prognostic Scoring System (IPSS-R) classifies patients according to the proportion of marrow blasts, the type of karyotype abnormality, and the number and severity of cytopenias (Table 16.3). For ease, 'clinical calculators' are now available online at http://www.mds-foundation.org/ipss-r-calculator. At this stage it is not clear if patients with IPSS-R 'intermediate-risk' prognosis should be treated according to lower-risk or higher-risk approaches, and molecular genetic findings may help risk stratify this group.

Lower-risk myelodysplastic syndromes

Patients with less than 5% blasts in the marrow, only one cytopenia and favourable cytogenetics are defined as having lower-risk MDS. Those with mild cytopenias and minimal symptoms can often be observed with serial blood counts or, if necessary, attempts may be made to improve marrow function with haemopoietic growth factors, either singly or in combination. **Erythropoiesis-stimulating agents (ESAs)** may improve anaemia in 40–50% of cases with an endogenous erythropoietin level <500 U/L, although the haemoglobin should not be raised above 120 g/L. G-CSF shows synergy with ESAs and may increase the erythroid response rate. Thrombomimetics, such as **eltrombopag or romiplostim**, can be given for severe thrombocytopenia or bleeding, but may stimulate blast growth. Ciclosporin or anti-thymocyte globulin occasionally helps, particularly for those with a hypocellular bone marrow and normal karyotype.

For patients with ring sideroblasts who have not responded to an ESA or are not good candidates for an ESA, an antibody fusion protein/ligand trap called **luspatercept** may improve effective erythropoiesis. Luspatercept binds to members of the transforming growth factor superfamily, including growth differentiation factor 11 (GDF11), which inhibits erythropoiesis. Binding to these factors by the antibody fusion protein may decrease inhibitory signalling and allow erythropoiesis to improve. A randomized trial in patients with ring sideroblasts indicated benefit, and trials are in place for other types of MDS as well as in thalassaemia and primary myelofibrosis.

Transfusion support with red cells or platelets is often needed. Antibiotics may be required either prophylactically or to treat infections. In the long term, iron overload may be a problem after multiple transfusions; iron chelation therapy should be considered after 20–50 units have been transfused or if the ferritin rises above 1000 μg/L. Measurement of liver and cardiac iron by magnetic resonance imaging (MRI) is helpful in deciding whether or not chelation therapy is indicated.

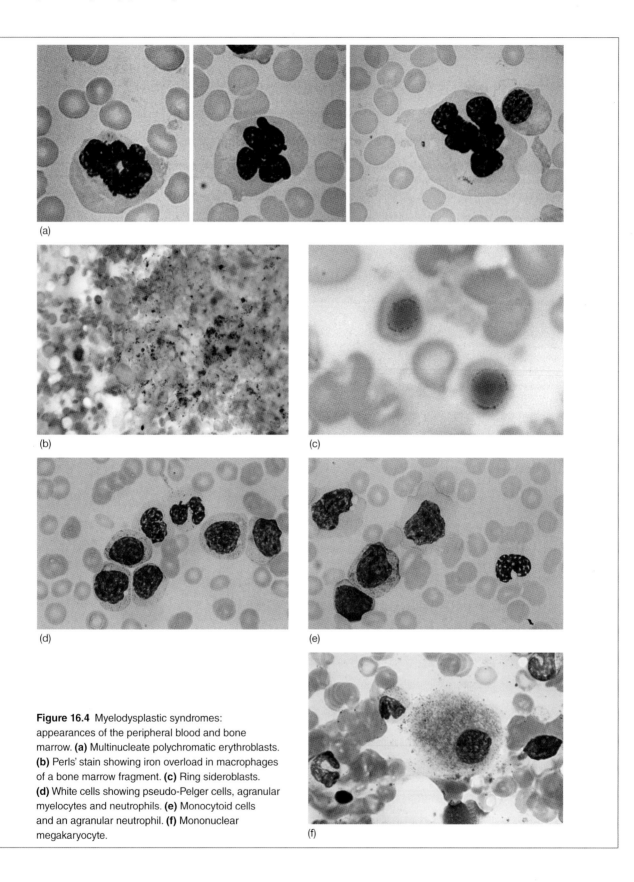

Figure 16.4 Myelodysplastic syndromes: appearances of the peripheral blood and bone marrow. **(a)** Multinucleate polychromatic erythroblasts. **(b)** Perls' stain showing iron overload in macrophages of a bone marrow fragment. **(c)** Ring sideroblasts. **(d)** White cells showing pseudo-Pelger cells, agranular myelocytes and neutrophils. **(e)** Monocytoid cells and an agranular neutrophil. **(f)** Mononuclear megakaryocyte.

Lenalidomide is particularly effective in MDS associated with del(5q), where it can often reduce the size of the del(5q) clone and reduce transfusion requirements in the majority of patients. Lenalidomide's mechanism of action includes binding to the E3 ubiquitin ligase-associated protein cereblon and augmentation of ubiquitin-mediated degradation of casein kinase 1. Casein kinase 1, a serine/threonine kinase involved in regulation of signal transduction pathways, is encoded on chromosome 5q. It is haploinsufficient in del5q cells, so del5q cells exposed to lenalidomide experience a greater reduction in casein kinase 1 compared to healthy cells, and del5q cells are selectively killed.

In selected patients standard or more frequently reduced-intensity allogeneic haemopoietic stem cell transplantation (SCT) offers the chance of a permanent cure.

Higher-risk myelodysplastic syndromes

In these patients a variety of treatments have been attempted to improve the overall prognosis, with varying degrees of success.

Stem cell transplantation

SCT offers the prospect of a complete cure for MDS and the advent of reduced-intensity conditioning is increasing the age range of patients who may be treated. Patients who lack *TP53* mutations have a >50% chance of long-term disease-free survival, while those with *TP53* mutations have a <20% chance of a favourable outcome. Chemotherapy should be given prior to the transplant in patients with >10% blasts in the marrow.

Intensive chemotherapy

Chemotherapy as given in AML (see p. 165) is occasionally tried in higher-risk patients, usually as a bridge to SCT. Although the majority may obtain a remission, relapse is likely and frequently occurs within a few months. The risks of intensive chemotherapy are great because prolonged pancytopenia may occur in some cases without normal haemopoietic cell regeneration, presumably because normal stem cells are much reduced.

Hypomethylating agents

Azacytidine (azacitidine) and decitabine are DNA methyltransferase inhibitors which inhibit methylation of newly formed DNA. They are nucleoside analogues that irreversibly bind to DNA methyltransferase and also are incorporated into DNA and RNA, causing DNA double-strand breaks. They improve blood counts in 40–50% of higher-risk MDS patients. Azacitidine is given for 7 days every month and is continued for as long as the patient is responding. It can improve survival by approximately 9 months compared to supportive care alone. Decitabine is typically given for 5 days per month and can delay progression to AML. The exact mechanism of the clinical activity of these drugs in MDS is unknown.

General supportive care only

This is most suitable in elderly patients with other major medical problems. Transfusions of red cells and platelets, and therapy with antibiotics and antifungals, are given as needed (see Chapter 12).

Clonal haemopoiesis of indeterminate potential (CHIP)

By age 65, at least 10% of the population have acquired a clone of haemopoietic cells with a single acquired mutation in a leukaemia driver gene at a variant allele frequency (mutation allele burden) of ≥2%, but without evidence of a haematological malignancy. These age-associated mutations are primarily mutations in *DNMT3A*, *TET2* and *ASXL1* (DTA; see Table 11.2). This phenomenon has been termed clonal haemopoiesis of indeterminate potential (CHIP; Table 16.4). CHIP becomes more frequent with ageing and affects >30% of the population over age 85 years. Because of the association with ageing, some investigators use the term 'ageing-related clonal haemopoiesis' (ARCH).

CHIP carries a ~1% risk per year of development of an overt haematological neoplasm meeting World Health Organization (WHO) diagnostic criteria. The risk is higher in those with larger clone size, multiple mutations or mutations of *TP53*, of genes for splicing factors, e.g. *SRSF2*, *SF3B1*, or of genes coding for proteins involved in DNA methylation, e.g. *TET2*, *DNMT3A* or *IDH1/2*. More importantly from a public health standpoint, CHIP is associated with an increased risk of acute vascular events including myocardial infarction and stroke, and it increases overall mortality. This cardiovascular risk is a result of clonally derived monocytes in the peripheral blood interacting with endothelial cells and differentiating into macrophages that induce progression in atherosclerotic plaques by releasing pro-inflammatory cytokines such as interleukin-1β.

Some patients have blood cytopenias, but no specific diagnosis is apparent even after extensive evaluation. There is insufficient dysplasia in blood or marrow cells to warrant a diagnosis of MDS. These patients' haematological abnormalities are termed 'idiopathic cytopenias of undetermined significance' (ICUS). In time the diagnosis often becomes clear in people with ICUS: some patients will evolve to overt MDS. If a clonal mutation is present, the term CCUS (clonal cytopenias of undetermined significance) can be used. These patients have a risk of developing MDS or AML exceeding 75% by 4 years. Finally, dysplastic cells are rarely seen in a peripheral blood film even though the blood counts are normal and there is no evidence of MDS. This state has been termed idiopathic dysplasia of undetermined significance (IDUS).

Myelodysplastic syndromes/ myeloproliferative 'overlap' neoplasms

These disorders are classified distinctly by WHO 2016 as they show the presence of dysplastic features and usually at least one cytopenia similar to MDS, but also an increased number of circulating cells in one or more lineages similar to myeloproliferative neoplasms (MPN; Table 16.5). They share common clinical and genetic features, such as mutations of the *TET2* tumour suppressor gene in about 20% of cases and of *JAK2* in a smaller proportion of patients.

Chronic myelomonocytic leukaemia (CMML)

This is defined by a persistent monocytosis of more than 1.0×10^9/L with blasts <20% in the marrow, dysplasia in other lineages and negative for the *BCR-ABL1* translocation. The total white cell count (WBC) is usually raised and may exceed 100×10^9/L. CMML may be separated into 'dysplastic' and 'proliferative' subtypes depending on WBC < or $\geq 13 \times 10^9$/L, respectively. Patients may develop skin rashes and around half have splenomegaly. Bruising is frequent and gum hypertrophy and lymphadenopathy may also be present. *TET2*, *ASXL1*, *SRSF2*, *JAK2*, Ras pathway and other mutations (Fig. 16.1) are frequent and the pattern of mutations differs from MDS without proliferative features. Treatment is difficult, although azacitidine or decitabine, hydroxycarbamide, ruxolitinib or etoposide may be useful. SCT may be tried in younger patients. Median survival is approximately 2 years, with transfusion dependency, white cells >13.0×10^9/L, increased marrow blasts, complex cytogenetics and mutation status predictors of poor outcome.

Atypical chronic myeloid leukaemia (aCML)

These patients have an increased white cell count with mainly granulocytes and granulocyte precursors in the blood and hypercellular bone marrow, but the Philadelphia chromosome and *BCR-ABL1* fusion gene are not present. Despite the name, this condition has no relation to CML. There are usually some morphological features in the blood or bone marrow of MDS. Treatment is difficult and the outlook is poor.

Juvenile myelomonocytic leukaemia (JMML)

This presents in the first 4 years of life and has features of both myelodysplasia and a myeloproliferative neoplasm. There is often an eczematous skin rash, hepatosplenomegaly and lymphadenopathy. There is monocytosis to more than 1.0×10^9/L and clonal cytogenetic change. The only curative treatment is allogeneic SCT. If untreated, death usually occurs within 4 years, often from acute transformation with leukaemic infiltration (e.g. of the lungs). Co-mutations in the *TET2* and *SRSF2* genes are commonly found.

Children with two genetic disorders, Noonan syndrome and neurofibromatosis, are at increased risk of JMML, and mutations in the genes *PTPN11* and *NF1*, which respectively underlie these genetic disorders, are frequent in the haemopoietic cells of cases of JMML not associated with these genetic disorders.

MDS/MPN with ring sideroblasts and thrombocytosis

This rare syndrome resembles MDS with single-lineage dysplasia with ring sideroblasts, but the anaemia is accompanied by a platelet count >450×10^9/L and usually mutations of *SF3B1* and of *JAK2* or *MPL*.

Table 16.5 World Health Organization 2016 classification of myelodysplastic/ myeloproliferative neoplasms (MDS/MPN)

Subtype	Diagnostic features
Chronic myelomonocytic leukaemia (CMML)	Monocytosis >1×10^9/L and monocytes represent $\geq$10% of circulating white cells *SRSF2*, *TET2*, *ASXL1* mutations common
Atypical chronic myeloid leukaemia (aCML), *BCR-ABL1* negative	WBC >13×10^9/L *BCR-ABL1* absent; *SETBP1* mutations in 30%
Juvenile myelomonocytic leukaemia (JMML)	Monocytosis to more than 1.0×10^9/L and clonal cytogenetic change, elevated fetal haemoglobin, often mutations of Ras pathway
MDS/MPN, unclassifiable (MDS/MPN-U)	MDS and MPN features without specific findings of other disorders in this group
MDS/MPN with ring sideroblasts associated with marked thrombocytosis (MDS/MPN-RS-T)	Platelet count >450×10^9/L Large atypical megakaryocytesUsually *SF3B1* mutation plus *JAK2* or *MPL* mutation

SUMMARY

- MDS includes a group of clonal disorders of haemopoietic stem cells that lead to bone marrow failure and low blood cell counts. A hallmark of the disease is increased proliferation and apoptosis of haemopoietic cells, leading to the paradox of a hypercellular bone marrow with pancytopenia. There is a tendency to progress to AML.
- In most cases the disease is *primary (de novo)*, but it may be *therapy-related* due to chemotherapy or radiotherapy given for treatment of another malignancy.
- The main clinical features of anaemia, infection and bleeding are caused by a reduction in the blood count. Most patients are over 70 years of age.
- Diagnosis is made by examination of the blood and bone marrow together with cytogenetic and molecular genetic studies of the neoplastic cells. They are classified into eight major subtypes.

- Scoring systems can divide patients into those with low-grade or high-grade disease.
- Lower-risk MDS may not need treatment. Haemopoietic growth factors, lenalidomide or blood product support are useful when required. Luspatercept is a promising new agent to treat the anaemia in some patients.
- Higher-risk MDS may be treated by intensive chemotherapy, demethylating drugs or stem cell transplantation. Allogeneic transplantation is the only curative procedure.
- MDS/MPN are a group of disorders classified between myelodysplasia and myeloproliferative neoplasms and show the presence of dysplastic features, but also an increased number of circulating white cells or platelets.

Now visit **www.wileyessential.com/haematology** to test yourself on this chapter.

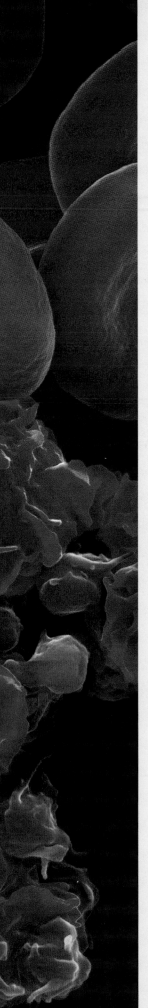

CHAPTER 17
Acute lymphoblastic leukaemia

Key topics

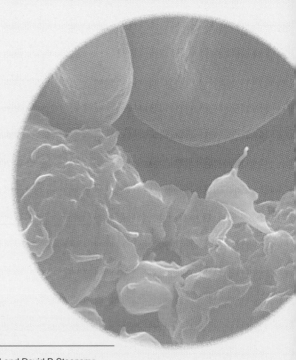

Hoffbrand's Essential Haematology, Eighth Edition. By A. Victor Hoffbrand and David P. Steensma.
© 2020 John Wiley & Sons Ltd. Published 2020 by John Wiley & Sons Ltd.
Companion website: www.wileyessential.com/haematology

Acute lymphoblastic leukaemia (ALL) is caused by an accumulation of lymphoblasts in the bone marrow and is the most common malignancy of childhood, although it can occur at any age. The definition of acute leukaemia and differentiation of ALL from acute myeloid leukaemia are described in Chapter 13.

Incidence and pathogenesis

The incidence of ALL is highest at 3–7 years, with 75% of cases occurring before the age of 6. There is a secondary incidence rise after the age of 40 years. B-cell lineage represents 85% of cases and these have an equal sex incidence; there is a male predominance for the 15% of T-cell ALL (T-ALL).

The pathogenesis is varied. **A proportion of cases of childhood ALL are initiated by genetic mutations that occur during development in utero** (Fig. 17.1). Studies in identical twins have shown that both may be born with the same chromosomal abnormality, e.g. the t(12;21), *ETV6-RUNX1* translocation. This has presumably arisen spontaneously in a haemopoietic progenitor cell that has passed from one twin to the other as a result of shared placental circulation. Environmental exposure during pregnancy may be important for this first event. One twin may develop ALL early (e.g. at age 4) because of a second transforming event affecting the copy numbers of several genes, including those

in B-cell development (see below). The other may remain well or develop ALL later, perhaps as a result of a different transforming event. The *ETV6-RUNX1* translocation is present in the blood of approximately 10% of newborn infants, but only 1 in 100 of these go on to develop ALL at a later date. The mechanism of the 'second genetic hit' within the neoplastic cell is unclear, but an abnormal response of the immune system to infection is suggested by epidemiological studies. In other cases, the disease seems to arise as a postnatal mutation in an early lymphoid progenitor cell.

Children with a high level of social activity, notably those attending early nursery daycare, have a reduced incidence of ALL, whereas those living in more isolated communities and who have a reduced exposure to common infections in the first years of life have a higher risk.

Certain germline polymorphisms in a group of genes mainly involved in B-cell development (e.g. *IKZF1*) appear to predispose to ALL, since they are more frequent in children with B-cell ALL (B-ALL) than controls. *IKZF1* is also deleted in the leukaemic cells in 30% of high-risk B-ALL and 95% of ALL *BCR-ABL1* positive cases.

In general, the genomic landscape in ALL is characterized by primary chromosomal abnormalities and a wide range of secondary deletions and mutations involving key pathways implicated in leukaemogenesis. These are described in more detail below. For childhood ALL, an average of 11 somatically acquired structural variations are present (Fig 11.1).

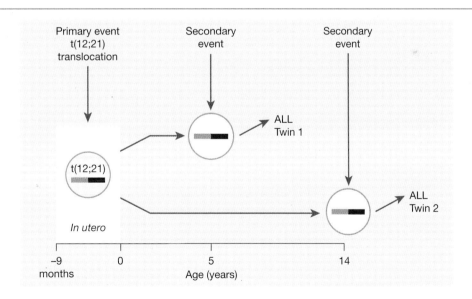

Figure 17.1 Prenatal origin of acute lymphoblastic leukaemia (ALL) in a pair of identical twins. Both tumours had an identical t(12;21) translocation. ALL was diagnosed in the first twin at age 5 years and in the second at age 14 years, indicating probable origin of the leukaemic clone *in utero* and dissemination to both twins via a shared placental blood supply. Because of the prolonged latency of the ALL, it is presumed that a secondary event is required to initiate the development of overt leukaemia. At the time of the diagnosis of ALL in twin 1 the t (12;21) translocation could be detected in the bone marrow of twin 2. It is likely that such a 'fetal origin' of childhood ALL occurs in a significant number of sporadic ALL cases. Source: Adapted from J.L. Wiemels *et al*. (1999) *Blood*, 94(3): 1057–62.

Classification

Acute lymphoblastic leukaemia, B cell or T cell, is sub-classified by the World Health Organization (WHO 2016) according to the underlying genetic defect (Table 17.1). Within B-ALL there are several specific genetic subtypes, such as those with the t(9;22) [*BCR-ABL1*] or t(12;21) [*ETV6-RUNX1*] translocations, rearrangements of the *KMT2A(MLL)* gene or alteration in chromosome number (aneuploidy; Table 17.1). The subtype in both B-ALL and T-ALL is an important guide to the optimal treatment protocol and to prognosis.

Among *BCR-ABL1* (Philadelphia chromosome) negative cases, some patients have a gene expression signature similar to *BCR-ABL1* positive cases. These 'Ph-like' cases comprise about 15% of children with ALL (more common in those with Down syndrome), 20–25% of adolescents and young adults, and at least 10–15% of older adults. About half of patients with Ph-like ALL have overexpression of *CRLF2* and half of those have JAK-STAT pathway mutations, most commonly JAK2 R683G (a different JAK2 mutation from the one recurrently observed in myeoproliferative neoplasms and one that is not effectively inhibited by ruxolitinib).

IKZF1 deletions are also common in this subtype. In Ph-like ALL without *CRLF2* overexpression, fusions involving *JAK2*, *ABL1* (with partners other than *BCR*), *PDGFRB* or *ABL2* are common, and these patients (especially those with *PDGFRB* translocations) may benefit from TKI therapy, but this is under study in trials.

In T-ALL an abnormal karyotype is found in 50–70% of cases and the NOTCH signalling pathway is activated in most cases. Early T-precursor (ETP) ALL leukaemia has a unique immunophenotype. Blasts in ETP ALL express T-cell marker CD7, but lack CD1a and CD8 that characterize more mature T cells, and they express at least one myeloid/stem cell-associated marker. The genetic profile of ETP ALL is also distinct. Common T-cell-associated gene alterations such as of *NOTCH1* or *CDKN1/2* are rare in this subtype, but myeloid-associated gene mutations are common. The prognostic significance is controversial, with early reports suggesting poorer outcomes, but more recent series showing no difference from other patients with T-ALL.

Clinical features

Clinical features are a result of the following.

Table 17.1 Classification of acute lymphoblastic leukaemia (ALL)/lymphoblastic lymphoma according to the World Health Organization (modified from WHO 2016); see also Appendix.

B cell
B acute lymphoblastic leukaemia NOS
B-lymphoblastic leukaemia/lymphoma with recurrent genetic abnormalities
B-lymphoblastic leukaemia/lymphoma with t(9;22)(q34.1;q11.2); *BCR-ABL1*
B-lymphoblastic leukaemia/lymphoma with t(v;11q23.3); *KMT2A(MLL)* rearranged
B-lymphoblastic leukaemia/lymphoma with t(12;21)(p13.2;q22.1); *ETV6-RUNX1*
B-lymphoblastic leukaemia/lymphoma with hyperdiploidy (>50 chromosomes)
B-lymphoblastic leukaemia/lymphoma with hypodiploidy (<45 chromosomes)
B-lymphoblastic leukaemia/lymphoma with t(5;14)(q31.1;q32.3); *IL3-IGH*
B-lymphoblastic leukaemia/lymphoma with t(1;19)(q23;p13.3); *TCF3-PBX1*
Provisional entity: B-lymphoblastic leukaemia/lymphoma, *BCR-ABL1*-like
Provisional entity: B-lymphoblastic leukaemia/lymphoma with *IAMP21*
T cell
T-lymphoblastic leukaemia/lymphoma
Provisional entity: Early T-cell precursor lymphoblastic leukaemia

N.B. A minority of patients present with nodal or extranodal masses and <20% blasts in the marrow, and are called lymphoblastic lymphoma if the tumour cells resemble those of ALL. They are approached similarly to ALL.
NOS, not otherwise specified.

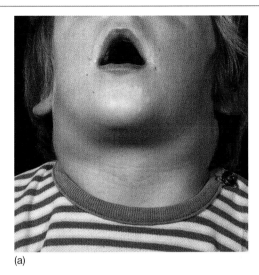
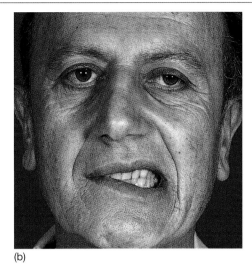

(a)   (b)

Figure 17.2 Acute lymphoblastic leukaemia. **(a)** Marked cervical lymphadenopathy in a boy. **(b)** Facial asymmetry in a 59-year-old man due to a right lower motor neurone seventh nerve palsy resulting from meningeal leukaemic infiltration. Source: V.A. Hoffbrand *et al.* (2019) *Color Atlas of Clinical Hematology*, 5th edn. Reproduced with permission of John Wiley & Sons.

Bone marrow failure

- Anaemia (pallor, lethargy and dyspnoea).
- Neutropenia (fever, malaise, features of mouth, throat, skin, respiratory, perianal or other infections).
- Thrombocytopenia (spontaneous bruises, purpura, bleeding gums and menorrhagia).

Organ infiltration

This can cause tender bones, lymphadenopathy (Fig. 17.2), moderate splenomegaly, hepatomegaly and meningeal syndrome (headache, nausea and vomiting, blurring of vision and diplopia). Fundal examination may reveal papilloedema and sometimes haemorrhage. Many patients have a fever at presentation, which usually resolves after starting chemotherapy. Less common manifestations include testicular swelling or signs of mediastinal compression, which is more common in T-ALL (Fig. 17.3).

If lymph node or solid extranodal masses predominate with <20% blasts in the marrow, the disease can be called lymphoblastic lymphoma, but is treated as ALL. The WHO 2016 classifies these cases identically.

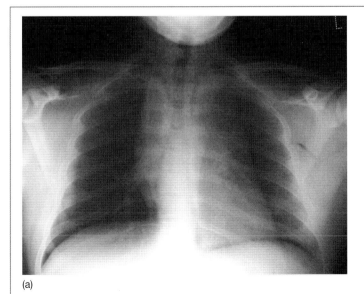
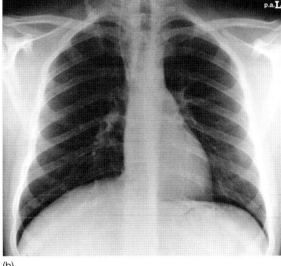

(a)   (b)

Figure 17.3 Chest X-ray of a boy aged 16 years with acute lymphoblastic leukaemia (T-ALL). **(a)** There is a large mediastinal mass caused by thymic enlargement at presentation. **(b)** After 1 week of therapy with prednisolone, vincristine and daunorubicin, the mass has resolved.

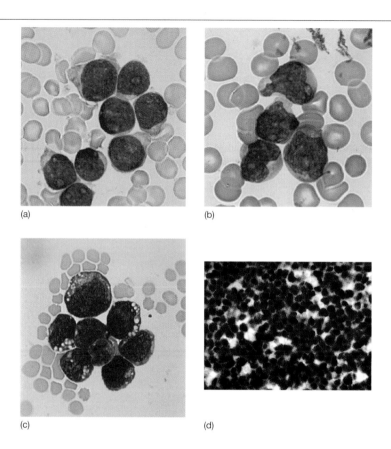

Figure 17.4 Morphology and immunophenotyping of acute lymphoblastic leukaemia. **(a)** Lymphoblasts show scanty cytoplasm without granules. **(b)** Lymphoblasts are large and heterogeneous with abundant cytoplasm. **(c)** Lymphoblasts are deeply basophilic with cytoplasmic vacuolation. **(d)** Acute lymphoblastic leukaemia: bone marrow cells staining positive for TdT by immunoperoxidase. Source: A.V. Hoffbrand *et al.* (2019) *Color Atlas of Clinical Hematology*, 5th edn. Reproduced with permission of John Wiley & Sons.

Investigations

Haematological investigations reveal a normochromic, normocytic anaemia with thrombocytopenia in most cases. The total white cell count may be decreased, normal or increased, sometimes to 200×10^9/L or more. The blood film typically shows a variable number of blast cells. The bone marrow is hypercellular with >20% leukaemic blasts. The blast cells are characterized by morphology (Fig. 17.4), immunological tests (Table 17.2) and cytogenetic analysis (Table 17.1). Identification of the immunoglobulin or T-cell receptor (TCR) clonal gene rearrangement (Fig 9.7), (aberrant) immunophenotype, and molecular genetics of the neoplastic cells is important to determine treatment and to detect minimal residual disease (MRD) during follow-up (Table 17.3).

Lumbar puncture for cerebrospinal fluid (CSF) examination is important in disease staging, but should be performed only by experienced physicians, as a traumatic procedure may promote the spread of neoplastic cells from blood to the central nervous system (CNS). Initial assessment of the CSF should always be combined with the concurrent administration of intrathecal chemotherapy.

Biochemical tests may reveal a raised serum uric acid, serum lactate dehydrogenase or, less commonly, hypercalcaemia. Liver and renal function tests are performed as a baseline before treatment begins. Radiography may reveal lytic bone lesions and a mediastinal mass caused by enlargement of the thymus and/or mediastinal lymph nodes characteristic of T-ALL (Fig. 17.3).

The diagnosis is usually obvious, but differential diagnosis includes acute myeloid leukaemia (AML), aplastic anaemia (with which ALL sometimes presents), marrow infiltration by other malignancies (e.g. rhabdomyosarcoma, neuroblastoma and Ewing sarcoma), infections such as infectious mononucleosis and pertussis, juvenile rheumatoid arthritis and immune thrombocytopenic purpura.

Table 17.2 Immunological markers for classification of acute lymphoblastic leukaemia (ALL; see also Fig. 11.14). Markers that distinguish the early T-cell precursor subtype are described in the text.

Marker	ALL	
	B	T
B lineage-associated		
CD19	+	−
cCD22	+	−
cCD79a	+	−
CD10	+ or −	−
cIg	+ (pre-B)	−
sIg	−	−
TdT	+	+
T lineage-associated		
CD7	−	+
cCD3	−	+
CD2	−	+
TdT	+	+
CD1a	−	+
CD4, CD8	−	+
Myeloid or stem cell lineage-associated		
CD34, CD117, HLADR, CD13, CD33, CD11b, or CD65	Negative except in multilineage	Negative except in early T-cell precursor subtype or multilineage

c, cytoplasmic; s, surface.

Table 17.3 Specialized tests for acute lymphoblastic leukaemia (ALL).

Immunological markers (flow cytometry)*	See Table 17.3; Fig. 11.14
Immunoglobulin and TCR genes *	B-ALL: clonal rearrangement of immunoglobulin genes
	T-ALL: clonal rearrangement of TCR genes
Chromosomes and genetic analysis	See Table 17.1

*Tests needed at diagnosis for subsequent monitoring for minimal residual disease.
B-ALL, B-cell acute lymphoblastic leukaemia; T-ALL, T-cell acute lymphoblastic leukaemia; TCR, T-cell receptor.

Cytogenetics and molecular genetics

Cytogenetic analysis shows differing frequencies of abnormalities in infants, children and adults, which partly explains the different prognoses of these groups (Fig. 17.5). Cases are stratified according to the number of chromosomes in the neoplastic cell (**ploidy**) or by specific molecular abnormalities. The two parameters define good- and poor-prognosis disease.

Hyperdiploid cells have more than 50 chromosomes and generally have a good prognosis, whereas **hypodiploid** cases (44 or fewer chromosomes) carry a poor prognosis. The most common specific chromosome abnormality in childhood

B-ALL is the t(12;21)(p13;q22) *ETV6-RUNX1* translocation. The RUNX1 protein plays an important part in transcriptional control of haemopoiesis and is repressed by the *ETV6-RUNX1* fusion protein. The frequency of the Ph translocation t(9;22) increases with age and carries an unfavourable prognosis (although improving with the addition of *BCR-ABL1* kinase inhibitors to therapy); Ph-like also has an unfavourable prognosis and the role of TKIs is in trials. Translocations of chromosome 11q23 involve the *KMT2A(MLL)* gene and are seen particularly in cases of infant leukaemia.

Using more sensitive molecular genetic tests, as well as fluorescence *in situ* hybridization (FISH) analysis, some cases,

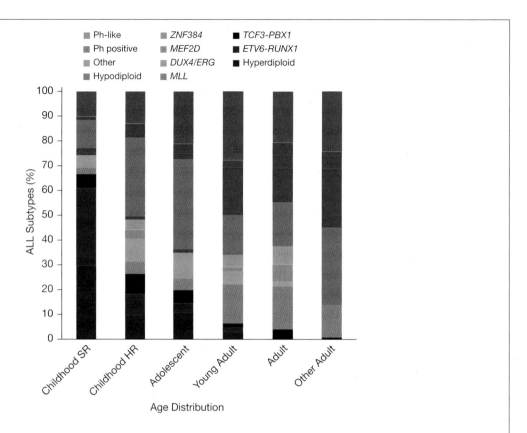

Figure 17.5 Age distribution of cytogenetically or molecularly defined acute lymphoblastic leukaemia (ALL) subtypes. The incidence of Ph-positive and Ph-like increases with ageing; ETV6-RUNX1 and hyperdiploid genotypes dominate in childhood standard-risk disease. *MLL(KMT2A)*, *ZN384*, *MEF2D* and *DUX4/ERG* indicate rearrangements of these genes. Source: I. Iacobucci, C.G. Mullighan (2017) *J. Clin. Oncol.* 35: 975–83. Reproduced with permission of the American Society of Clinical Oncology.

normal by conventional cytogenetic testing, are found to have fusion genes, e.g. *BCR-ABL1*. These molecular genetic changes carry prognostic significance whether or not a corresponding chromosomal change is present.

T-ALL accounts for 15% of childhood and 25% of adult ALL and the clinical picture is often dominated by a very high white cell count, mediastinal mass or pleural effusion. TCR genes (and in 20% the *IGH* gene) show clonal rearrangement. Cytogenetic changes often involve the TCR loci with different partner genes. The majority of cases have acquired genetic abnormalities that lead to constitutive activation of the *NOTCH* signalling pathway and drugs that target these abnormalities are being developed (Fig. 17.6).

Treatment

This may be conveniently divided into **supportive** and **specific** treatment.

General supportive therapy

General supportive therapy for bone marrow failure is described in Chapter 12 and includes the insertion of a central venous cannula, blood product support and prevention of tumour lysis syndrome. The risk of tumour lysis syndrome is highest in children with a high white cell count, T-cell disease or concurrent renal impairment at presentation. Any episode of fever must be treated promptly.

Specific therapy of ALL in children

Specific therapy of ALL is with chemotherapy and sometimes radiotherapy (Fig. 17.7) and treatment protocols are complex. There are several phases in a treatment course, which usually has four components (Fig. 17.7). The protocols are **risk adjusted** to reduce the treatment given to patients with good prognosis. The factors that guide treatment include age, gender and white cell count at presentation. The initial response to therapy is also important, as slow clearance of blood or marrow blasts after a week or two of induction therapy or persistence of minimal residual disease (MRD, see below) is associated with a relatively high risk of relapse. ALL in infants (<1 year) has a poor clinical outcome, with cure rates of only 20–50%. The disease is associated with chromosomal translocation involving the *KMT2A(MLL)* gene in 80% of cases and is treated by unique protocols.

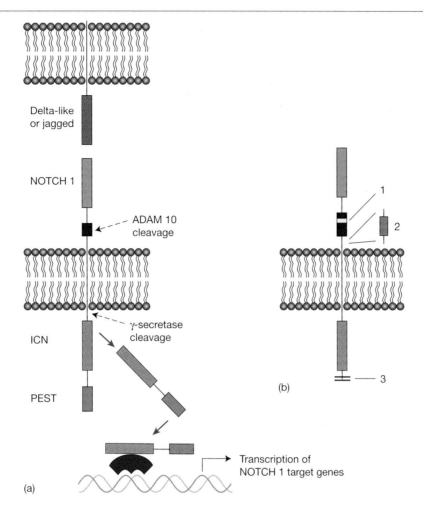

Figure 17.6 The molecular basis of activation of NOTCH signalling in T-cell acute lymphoblastic leukaemia (T-ALL). **(a)** The molecular basis of NOTCH signalling. NOTCH is expressed at the cell membrane and after binding to a ligand (Delta-like or Jagged) on a neighbouring cell, the protein is cleaved in two places – first by extracellular ADAM 10 and then by an intracellular γ-secretase complex. The portion of intracellular NOTCH that is released is then translocated to the nucleus, where it leads to activation of NOTCH1 target genes. **(b)** Several types of genetic abnormalities are seen in the NOTCH signalling pathway in patients with T-ALL. These include (1) mutations in the extracellular cleavage site, (2) insertion of an internal tandem duplications in the juxtamembrane region or (3) deletion of the intracellular PEST domain. The net result of all these mutations is to increase the rate of cleavage and nuclear translocation of the NOTCH domain.

Minimal (measurable) residual disease

Even when the blood and bone marrow appear to be clear of leukaemia by light microscopy, small numbers of neoplastic cells may sometimes be detected by fluorescence-activated cell sorter (FACS) analysis or molecular methods (Chapter 11; Fig. 17.8). A positive result indicates **minimal (also called 'measurable') residual disease** and the analysis of children for the presence of MRD at day 29 or adults after 3 months of treatment has prognostic significance and is now used in planning therapy (see below; Fig. 17.9). The value of tests for MRD at the end of induction or during consolidation with respect to subsequent therapy continues to be explored in trials, in which the intensity of consolidation or maintenance therapy is reduced in those who rapidly become MRD negative, whereas more intensified therapy, or even allogeneic stem cell transplantation (SCT), is given to those with persistent MRD. Good-prognosis children become MRD negative as early as day 29 of therapy, whereas in adults the findings on MRD testing at 3 months have greater prognostic importance (Table 17.4). One example is the reduction in the number of intensification blocks in children with no evidence of MRD at day 29 within the UK ALL 2003 trial. This reduction did not impair the excellent prognosis in these low-risk children and is now standard therapy.

Remission induction

At presentation, the patient with acute leukaemia has a very high tumour burden and is at great risk from the complications

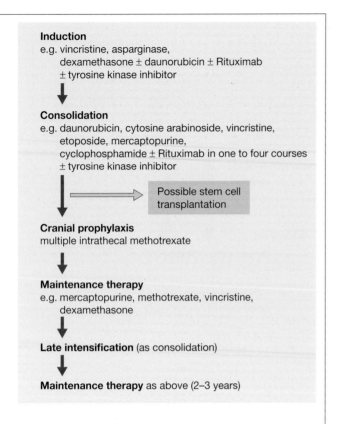

Induction
e.g. vincristine, asparginase,
    dexamethasone ± daunorubicin ± Rituximab
    ± tyrosine kinase inhibitor

↓

Consolidation
e.g. daunorubicin, cytosine arabinoside, vincristine,
    etoposide, mercaptopurine,
    cyclophosphamide ± Rituximab in one to four courses
    ± tyrosine kinase inhibitor

↓ → Possible stem cell transplantation

↓

Cranial prophylaxis
multiple intrathecal methotrexate

↓

Maintenance therapy
e.g. mercaptopurine, methotrexate, vincristine,
    dexamethasone

↓

Late intensification (as consolidation)

↓

Maintenance therapy as above (2–3 years)

Figure 17.7 Flow chart illustrating typical treatment regimen of acute lymphoblastic leukaemia (ALL).

of bone marrow failure and leukaemic infiltration (Fig. 17.1). The aim of **remission induction** is to rapidly kill most (>99%) of the tumour cells and get the patient into remission. This is defined as less than 5% blasts in the bone marrow, normal or near-normal peripheral blood count and no other symptoms or signs of the disease. Steroids (dexamethasone or prednisolone), vincristine and asparaginase are the drugs usually used and they are very effective – achieving remission in over 95% of children and in 80–90% of adults (in whom daunorubicin is also usually added). Rituximab is added in CD20 positive cases (defined as >20% blast cells expressing CD20) and trials are in progress to determine whether it is of benefit in all B-ALL cases. In remission, however, a patient may still be harbouring large numbers of neoplastic cells and, without further chemotherapy, virtually all patients will relapse (see Fig. 13.8). Nevertheless, achievement of remission is a valuable first step in the treatment course. Patients who fail to achieve remission need to change to a more intensive protocol with the goal of reaching SCT.

Intensification (consolidation)

These courses use high doses of multidrug chemotherapy in order to eliminate the disease or reduce the tumour burden to very low levels. The doses of chemotherapy are near the limit of patient tolerability and during intensification blocks patients may need substantial support. Typical protocols involve the use of vincristine, cyclophosphamide, cytosine arabinoside, daunorubicin, etoposide or mercaptopurine, given as blocks in different combinations. Rituximab and a TKI are included for

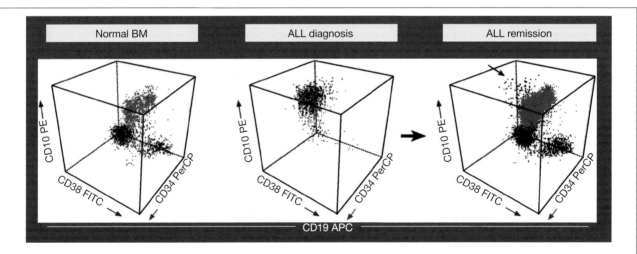

Figure 17.8 Detection of minimal residual disease (MRD) by four-colour flow cytometry in normal bone marrow mononuclear cells (BM), BM from a patient with B-lineage ALL at diagnosis and in remission 6 weeks after diagnosis. The cells were detected with four different antibodies (anti-CD10, anti-CD19, anti-CD34, anti-CD38) attached to fluorescent labels abbreviated as PE, APC, PerCP and FITC, respectively. The tridimensional plot shows the immunophenotype of CD19$^+$ lymphoid cells in the three samples. MRD of 0.03% of cells expressing the leukaemia-associated phenotype (CD10$^+$, CD34$^+$, CD38$^-$) were detected at 6 weeks, confirmed by polymerase chain reaction (PCR) analysis. Source: D. Campana, E. Coustan-Smith (1999) *Commun. Clin. Cytometry* 38: 139–52. Reproduced with permission of John Wiley & Sons.

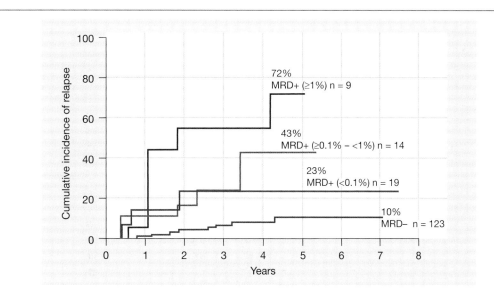

Figure 17.9 Cumulative incidence of relapse according to minimal residual disease (MRD) levels at the end of remission induction in children with acute lymphoblastic leukaemia (ALL) treated at St Jude Children's Research Hospital. Source: Courtesy of Dr D. Campana.

those for whom these drugs were indicated in induction. The numbers of blocks given in children depends on the child's risk category and varies between one and three.

Central nervous system-directed therapy

Few of the drugs given systemically reach the CSF and specific treatment is required to prevent or treat CNS disease. Intrathecal methotrexate, cytosine arabinoside and corticosteroids are usually used. CNS relapses still occur and present with

headache, vomiting, papilloedema and blast cells in the CSF. Treatment of such relapses is also with intrathecal methotrexate, cytosine arabinoside and hydrocortisone, with or without cranial irradiation and systemic chemotherapy, because bone marrow disease is often also present.

Maintenance

Maintenance therapy with daily oral mercaptopurine and once-weekly oral methotrexate prevents late relapses. Intravenous

Table 17.4 Prognosis in acute lymphoblastic leukaemia (ALL).

	Good	Poor
WBC	Low (<50 × 10/9/L)	High (e.g. >50 × 10^9/L B-ALL, >100 × 10^9/L T-ALL)
Sex	Female	Male
Age	Child (1–10 years)	Adult (or infant <1 year)
Immunophenotype (in children)	B-cell	T-cell
Cytogenetics	Normal or hyperdiploidy; *ETV6* rearrangement	t(9;22), most translocations involving 11q23 (MLL), hypodiploidy (<44 chromosomes)
Molecular genetics	Absence of high-risk mutations	Mutations of *TP53, NRAS, NR3C1, BTG*; Ph-like expression pattern
Time to clear blasts from blood	<1 week	>1 week
Time to remission	<4 weeks	>4 weeks
CNS disease at presentation	Absent	Present
Minimal (measurable) residual disease (MRD)	Negative or <0.01% at 1 month (children); 3 months (adults)	Still positive (>0.01%) at 3–6 months

CNS, central nervous system; WBC, white blood cell count.

vincristine with a short course (5 days) of oral corticosteroid is added at monthly or 3-monthly (in adults) intervals. There is a high risk of varicella or measles during maintenance therapy in children who lack immunity to these viruses. If exposure to these infections occurs, prophylactic immunoglobulin should be given. In addition, oral co-trimoxazole or atovaquone is given to reduce the risk of *Pneumocystis jirovecii* infection. Adults also receive antiviral and pneumocystis prophylaxis. Maintenance may in some protocols begin soon after remission induction and is interrupted by the periods of intensification chemotherapy. In typical regimens, intensive chemotherapy finishes around 38 weeks and then maintenance begins again and lasts until week 112 in girls or 164 in boys.

Treatment of *BCR-ABL1* positive ALL

The introduction of TKIs has transformed the management of patients with BCR-ABL1 positive (Ph-positive) ALL. Imatinib or another TKI is given continuously in combination with chemotherapy and is able to obtain remission of the disease in most patients. However, relapse is common because of the appearance of resistant subclones containing mutations in the *BCR-ABL1* gene, as well as additional gene mutations. Allogeneic SCT is therefore usually recommended wherever possible once remission has been obtained. For older patients in whom SCT is not feasible, prolonged maintenance with the TKI may result in disease-free remission of several years. Current trials will show which Ph-like cases benefit from TKI therapy to the same degree as Ph-positive cases.

Treatment of relapse

If relapse, detected by MRD tests or by reappearance of ALL cells in the blood or marrow, occurs during or soon after maintenance chemotherapy, the outlook is poor. Reinduction with combination chemotherapy may result in a second remission, but without allogeneic transplant these remissions are typically brief.

Chimeric antigen receptor (CAR)-T cells are another approach to targeting refractory neoplastic B cells. B-ALL is one of the first diseases for which this treatment has been successful. The patient's own T cells are programmed to kill B cells expressing CD19 (Chapter 9). CAR-T cell therapy is approved for patients with refractory B-ALL or large B cell non-Hodgkin lymphoma expressing CD19. The side-effects of CAR-T cell therapy are described in Chapter 12. Relapses of ALL with CD19 negative blast cell subsets may occur after CAR-T cell therapy. CAR-T cells for treating B-cell malignancies with different antigen specificity such as CD22 are in development.

The anti-CD22 monoclonal antibody–cytotoxic drug conjugate **inotuzumab ozogamicin** may also help in cases of ALL that express CD22, though it increases the risk of hepatic veno-occlusive disease after subsequent SCT. Epratuzumab, another humanized anti-CD22, is being studied in relapsed cases. Chemotherapy or immunotherapy including CAR-T cell therapy for relapsed disease is usually followed, where possible, by allogeneic SCT. If relapse occurs after years off all therapy, the outlook is better, but allogeneic SCT is usually also recommended in this setting.

Although patients with persistently positive MRD have a poorer prognosis and high relapse risk, optimal management of these patients is unclear, as they do not necessarily have improved overall survival with allogeneic SCT. One new drug useful in this setting is **blinatumomab**, a CD19 antibody conjugated to an antibody against CD3. This recruits cytotoxic T cells into the proximity of neoplastic B cells and can convert MRD positive disease to MRD negative. Adverse effects of blinatumomab include neurotoxicity and, like CAR-T cells, cytokine release syndrome.

Late toxicity

The long-term toxicity of therapy is a major concern of those treating children with ALL. Specific concerns are the large risk of avascular bone necrosis, seen in teenagers and young adults in association with high doses of dexamethasone, the potential long-term cardiac risk of even modest anthracycline doses, the impact of alkylating agents on fertility and the small risk of second tumours. New generation clinical trials in children are aimed at reducing the risk of toxicity while preserving anti-leukaemic activity.

Specific therapy of ALL in adults

Treatment for ALL in adults has proved less successful compared to children. The initial control of the leukaemia (remission induction) is comparable in both groups, but the rate of disease relapse is much higher in adults than in children. Although cure rates in children now approach 90%, no more than 40% of adult patients remain free of leukaemia after 5 years and this rate is much lower in patients over age 50. A significant factor is that the genetic subtypes of the ALL differ according to age. Hyperdiploidy and t(12;21), which carry a good prognosis and together make up 50% of childhood cases, are both rare in adult patients. In contrast, the presence of the Ph-positive and Ph-like disease becomes more common with age (Fig. 17.5).

An additional factor that has contributed to the relatively poor outcome for ALL in adults is the lower doses of chemotherapy that have traditionally been used in adult patients. This is now being addressed in younger adult patients, especially those under age 40 years, where many are now being treated within 'childhood' protocols with higher-intensity chemotherapy regimens. Cranial prophylaxis in adults usually involves intrathecal methotrexate, with or without intrathecal cytosine arabinoside and steroids, and with high-dose methotrexate and cytosine arabinoside given systemically.

The presence of MRD after 3 months or more of therapy in adults is an unfavourable prognostic sign. Many patients are treated by allogeneic SCT if a suitable sibling or matched unrelated donor is available. It is not clear if SCT improves outcomes for persistently MRD positive patients, who tend to do poorly regardless of the approach.

Prognosis

There is a great variation in the chance of individual patients achieving a long-term cure based on a number of biological variables (Table 17.4). Approximately 25% of children relapse after first-line therapy and need further treatment, but overall 90% of children can expect to be cured (Fig. 17.10). The cure rate in adults drops significantly to less than 5% over the age of 70 years. The challenge in both adults and children over the next few years is to better define risk groups and individualize therapy. This may be accomplished using both existing MRD technology and also newer assessment of molecular patterns; these patterns may, for example, define subgroups with specific drug sensitivities or children at particular risk of a specific drug toxicity.

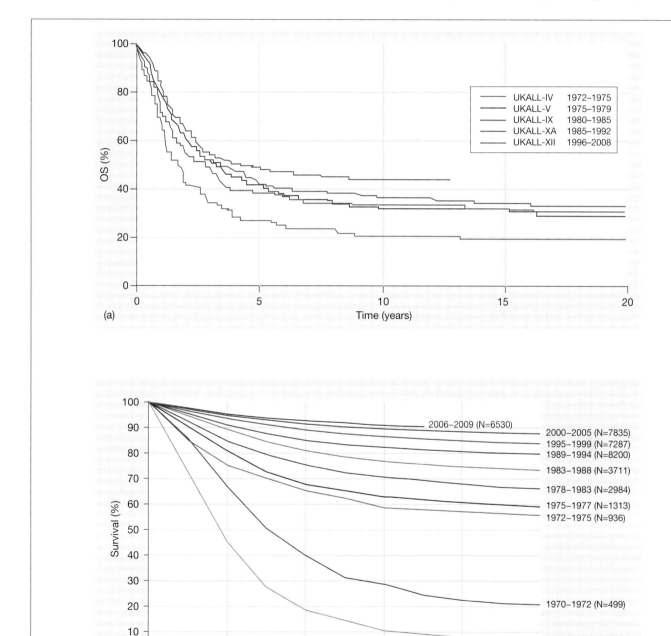

Figure 17.10 Overall survival rates for (a) adult and (b) paediatric acute lymphoblastic leukaemia (ALL). (a) UK ALL trials; (b) Children's Cancer Group and Children's Oncology Group trials. Source: (a) Courtesy of Dr Adele Fielding. (b) S.P. Hunger, C.G. Mullighan (2016) *N. Engl. J. Med.* 376: 1541. Reproduced with permission of the Massachusetts Medical Society.

SUMMARY

- Acute lymphoblastic leukaemia is caused by an accumulation of lymphoblasts in the bone marrow. It is the most common malignant disease of childhood – 75% of cases occur before the age of 6 years; 85% of cases are of B-cell lineage with the rest of T-cell lineage.
- The first genetic mutation occurs in many cases *in utero*, with a secondary genetic event occurring later in childhood, possibly as a reaction to an infection.
- The clinical presentation is with the features of bone marrow failure (anaemia, infection and bleeding) together with symptoms of tissue infiltration by tumour cells, leading to bone pain, enlarged lymph nodes, meningeal and testicular infiltration in some cases.
- Diagnosis is by examination of blood and bone marrow. Important tests include microscopic examination of the neoplastic cells, immunophenotyping, chromosome and genetic analysis.
- ALL is subclassified according to the underlying genetic defect and a wide variety of genetic lesions are seen. The number of chromosomes in the neoplastic cell has prognostic importance: *hyperdiploid* cells have >50 chromosomes and generally have a good prognosis, whereas *hypodiploid* cases (<44 chromosomes) carry a poor prognosis. Other cytogenetic abnormalities are also of prognostic

- significance, e.g. t(9;22), increasingly frequent with age, which is unfavourable, though it can be targeted with specific tyrosine kinase inhibitors.
- Treatment protocols for ALL are complex and usually have four components – remission induction, intensification or consolidation, CNS-directed therapy and maintenance.
- Treatment is *risk adjusted* to reduce the treatment given to patients with good prognosis. This is based on age, gender, white cell count and cytogenetics at presentation.
- Small numbers of neoplastic cells may sometimes be detected by flow cytometry or molecular analysis even when the blood and bone marrow appear to be clear of leukaemia. This *minimal residual disease* at specific time points has prognostic significance and is used in planning therapy.
- If relapse occurs during chemotherapy the outlook is poor, but if it happens after years off all treatment the outlook is better. Further chemotherapy and allogeneic SCT should be considered. CAR-T cells and bispecific antibodies that recruit T cells are active therapies in the setting of relapsed/refractory disease.
- Overall, >90% of children can now expect to be cured. The cure rate in adults is about 40%, but drops significantly with advancing age to less than 5% over the age of 70 years.

 Now visit **www.wileyessential.com/haematology** to test yourself on this chapter.

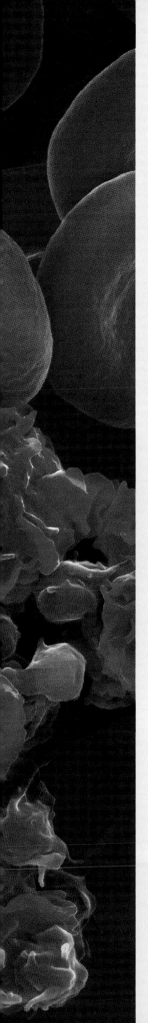

CHAPTER 18
The chronic lymphocytic leukaemias

Key topics

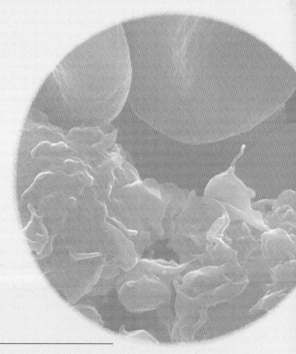

Hoffbrand's Essential Haematology, Eighth Edition. By A. Victor Hoffbrand and David P. Steensma.
© 2020 John Wiley & Sons Ltd. Published 2020 by John Wiley & Sons Ltd.
Companion website: www.wileyessential.com/haematology

Several disorders are included in the chronic lymphocytic leukaemias group. All are characterized by accumulation in the blood of mature lymphocytes of either B- or T-cell type (Table 18.1). In general, these diseases are not cured, but available treatments are highly effective, and they tend to run a chronic and fluctuating course.

Diagnosis

Patients with chronic lymphocytic leukaemias are often asymptomatic and discovered by a full blood count done for another clinical indication. Alternatively, they may have constitutional symptoms, or may have local signs and symptoms related to lymph node or spleen enlargement. The usual laboratory finding is chronic persistent blood lymphocytosis, in some cases accompanied by anaemia or thrombocytopenia. Reactive lymphocytosis should be ruled out (see Chapter 9). The clonal nature of the lymphocytosis in chronic lymphocytic leukaemias can be proven with flow cytometry or DNA analysis. Subtypes of chronic lymphocytic leukaemias are distinguished by morphology, immunophenotype and genetic analysis.

There is some overlap between chronic lymphocytic leukaemias and the non-Hodgkin lymphomas, as lymphoma cells may be found circulating in the blood, while chronic leukaemias may involve lymph nodes and other lymphatic tissue. In particular, distinction between chronic lymphocytic leukaemia (CLL) and small lymphocytic lymphoma (SLL) can be somewhat arbitrary, depending on the relative proportion of the disease in soft tissue masses compared to blood and bone marrow; CLL and SLL cells have an identical immunophenotype and genetic abnormalities.

Monoclonal B-cell lymphocytosis

Clonal B cells with the same phenotype as CLL are found at low levels in the blood of many older people. Indeed, this monoclonal B-cell lymphocytosis (MBL) has been demonstrated in >10% of persons over the age of 50 years and becomes more frequent with advancing age. It is believed that all cases of clinical CLL progress from this precursor clonal state, which is usually undetected. Similar genetic changes to these found in CLL may be present in MBL. If CLL is to be diagnosed, there must be a monoclonal B-cell count of $>5 \times 10^9$/L or tissue involvement outside the bone marrow.

B-cell diseases

Chronic lymphocytic leukaemia

Pathogenesis

CLL is the most common of the chronic lymphocytic leukaemias and has a peak incidence between 60 and 80 years of age. There are geographical variations in incidence. It is the most common form of leukaemia within Europe and the USA, but less frequent elsewhere, especially in Asia. There is a seven-fold increased risk of CLL in the close relatives of patients, which indicates a genetic predisposition to the disease

The CLL neoplastic cell is a mature B cell with weak surface expression of immunoglobulin (IgM or IgD). CLL cells exhibit impaired apoptosis and a prolonged lifespan, and this is reflected in their accumulation in the blood, bone marrow, liver, spleen and lymph nodes. The proliferative rate is usually not markedly increased, but clonal cells accumulate because they survive longer than normal lymphocytes. SLL (see Chapter 20) is the tissue equivalent of CLL and SLL cells have the same immunophenotype and cytogenetics as CLL. The difference is that in SLL the neoplastic cells accumulate almost exclusively in the lymph nodes, and by definition there are fewer than 5×10^9/L circulating monoclonal B cells.

Cytogenetic and molecular genetic abnormalities that may be present at diagnosis are listed below. Multiple clones from linear or branching evolution may be present at diagnosis. At later stages, after chemotherapy one or other resistant subclone may become dominant (see Chapter 11).

Clinical features

1 The mean age at diagnosis is 72 years, with only 15% of cases before 50 years of age. The male : female ratio is approximately 2 : 1.
2 Over 80% of cases are diagnosed from the results of a routine blood test taken for another reason.
3 Enlargement of cervical, axillary or inguinal lymph nodes is the most frequent clinical sign (Fig. 18.1). The nodes are usually discrete and non-tender. Chest X-ray is performed routinely. Abdominal ultrasound may help in evaluation of deep lymphadenopathy, but CT scans are generally not required for initial evaluation or follow-up.
4 Clinical features of anaemia such as pallor and dyspnea may be present and patients with thrombocytopenia may show bruising or purpura.

Table 18.1 Classification of the chronic lymphocytic leukaemias (World Health Organization, 2016).

B-cell	T-cell
■ Chronic lymphocytic leukaemia (CLL)/small lymphocytic lymphoma (SLL)	■ T-cell large granular lymphocytic leukaemia (T-LGL)
■ B-cell prolymphocytic leukaemia (B-PLL)	■ T-cell prolymphocytic leukaemia (T-PLL)
■ Hairy cell leukaemia (HCL)	■ Adult T-cell leukaemia/lymphoma (ATLL)
	■ Sézary syndrome (see Chapter 20)

Note that this classification includes these disorders within the category of lymphoid malignancies and does not distinguish mature B-cell leukaemias separately (see Appendix).

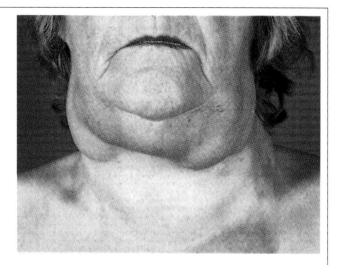

Figure 18.1 Chronic lymphocytic leukaemia: bilateral cervical lymphadenopathy in a 67-year-old woman. Haemoglobin 125 g/L; white blood count 150×10⁹/L (lymphocytes 146×10⁹/L); platelets 120×10⁹/L.

5 Splenomegaly and, less commonly, hepatomegaly are often seen in later stages.

6 Immunosuppression is often a significant problem resulting from hypogammaglobulinaemia and cellular immune dysfunction. Early in the disease course, bacterial infections such as sinus and chest infections predominate, but with advanced disease, viral infections such as herpes zoster (Fig. 18.2) and fungal infections are also seen.

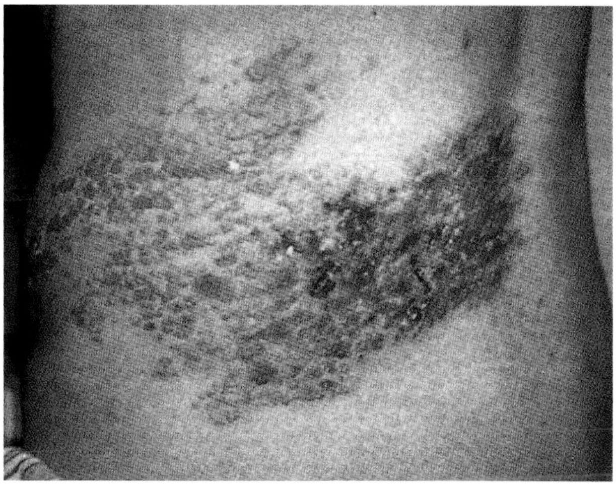

Laboratory findings

1 Lymphocytosis. The absolute clonal B-cell lymphocyte count is $\geq 5 \times 10^9$/L by definition and may be 300×10^9/L or more. Typically, between 70% and 99% of white cells in the blood film appear as small lymphocytes. 'Smudge' or 'smear' cells are also present (Fig. 18.3). These result from altered expression of cytoskeletal proteins such as vimentin in clonal cells, leading to fragility of the cells.

2 Immunophenotyping of the lymphocytes shows them to be B cells (surface CD19⁺) with expression of only one light chain (known as 'light chain restriction'; see Fig. 20.4). Characteristically, the cells are also brightly positive for CD5 and CD23, but show low levels of surface immunoglobulin, CD20, CD22 and CD79b (Table 18.2). CD10 and FMC7 are usually negative.

3 Two surface proteins that can be detected by flow cytometry and have prognostic significance are CD38, a marker of differentiation, and ZAP70, a protein kinase involved in signalling (Table 18.3).

4 Normochromic normocytic anaemia is present in later stages as a result of marrow infiltration or hypersplenism. Usually the marrow must be at least 60–70% involved by CLL cells before cytopenias due to marrow replacement develop. Autoimmune haemolysis may also occur (see below). Thrombocytopenia occurs in many patients and may also have an autoimmune basis.

5 Bone marrow aspiration shows lymphocytic replacement of normal marrow elements. Trephine biopsy reveals nodular, diffuse or interstitial involvement by lymphocytes (Fig. 18.4).

Figure 18.2 Chronic lymphocytic leukaemia: dermatomal herpes zoster infection in a 68-year-old female.

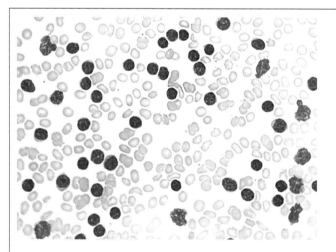

Figure 18.3 Chronic lymphocytic leukaemia: peripheral blood film showing lymphocytes with thin rims of cytoplasm, coarse condensed nuclear chromatin and rare nucleoli. Typical smudge cells are present.

Table 18.2 Immunophenotype of the chronic B-cell leukaemias/lymphomas (all cases CD19⁺).

	CLL	Hairy cell leukaemia	Follicular lymphoma	Mantle cell lymphoma
SIg	Weak	++	++	+
CD5	+	–	–	+
CD22/FMC7	–	+	+	++
CD23	+	–	–	–
CD79b	–	–/+	++	++
CD103*	–	+	–	–

*CD103 is positive only in classic hairy cell leukaemia (HCL); a variant form of HCL is negative for CD103 (as well as for CD25, also typically expressed in classical HCL).
CLL, chronic lymphocytic leukaemia; SIg, surface immunoglobulin.

Table 18.3 Prognostic factors in chronic lymphocytic leukaemia.

Variable	Good	Bad
Stage	Binet A (Rai 0–I)	Binet B, C (Rai II–IV)
Lymphocyte doubling time	Slow (>12 months)	Rapid
Bone marrow biopsy appearance	Nodular	Diffuse
Chromosomes	Deletion 13q14	Deletion 17p;11q23*
Genetic mutations	High-risk mutations absent	*NOTCH1*, *SF3B1*, *TP53*
VH immunoglobulin genes	Hypermutated	Unmutated; use of VH3.21
ZAP expression	Low	High
CD38 expression	Negative	Positive
LDH	Normal	Raised

*Mutation in the *ATM* gene is also unfavourable if associated with 11q23 deletion.
LDH, lactate dehydrogenase; VH, heavy chain variable. See Table 18.4 for Binet/Rai staging.

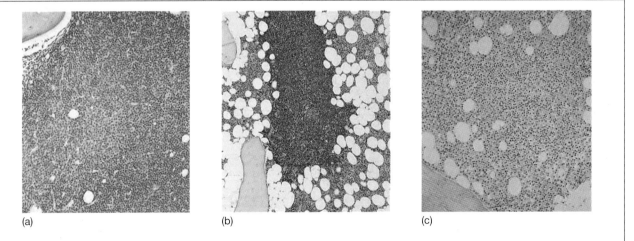

(a)　　　　　(b)　　　　　(c)

Figure 18.4 Chronic lymphocytic leukaemia: trephine biopsies showing **(a)** a marked diffuse increase in marrow lymphocytes (closely packed cells with small dense nuclei); **(b)** a nodular pattern of lymphocyte accumulation (in a different patient); and **(c)** interstitial infiltration.

6 Reduced concentrations of serum immunoglobulins are found, and this becomes more marked with advanced disease. Rarely, a paraprotein (M-spike) is present.

7 Autoimmunity directed against cells of the haemopoietic system is common. Autoimmune haemolytic anaemia is most frequent but immune thrombocytopenia, neutropenia and red cell aplasia are also seen.

Molecular tests

Genetics and molecular genetics

The four most common chromosomal abnormalities in CLL, listed from best prognosis to poorest, are deletion of 13q14, trisomy 12, deletion at 11q23 (involving the *ATM* gene) and 17p deletion (involving the *TP53* gene). More than 80% of patients with CLL have one of these findings. Normal karyotype has an outlook similar to trisomy 12. The 13q14 deletion leads to loss of microRNAs (see p. 141) that normally control expression of proteins that regulate B-cell survival.

The most common genetic point mutations at presentation are found in *ATM*, *NOTCH1* and *SF3B1* (all at around 10% prevalence). In addition, point mutations in *TP53* can be seen in up to 5% of patients, and these have negative prognostic value and confer resistance to cytotoxic chemotherapy (Table 18.3).

Somatic hypermutation of the immunoglobulin genes

When B cells recognize antigen in the germinal centre of secondary lymphoid tissues, they undergo a process called **somatic hypermutation** in which random mutations occur in the immunoglobulin heavy-chain gene (Chapter 9). In CLL the *IGVH* gene shows evidence of this hypermutation in approximately 50% of cases, whereas in the other cases the *VH* genes are unmutated. CLL with unmutated immunoglobulin genes has an unfavourable prognosis and may respond less well to initial and subsequent therapy (Table 18.3).

Staging

It is useful to stage patients at presentation both for prognosis and for deciding on therapy. The **Rai and Binet staging systems** are shown in Table 18.4. Typical survival ranged historically from 12 years for Rai stage 0 to less than 4 years for stage IV, but there is considerable variation between patients, and with current therapies survival rates have improved substantially. Many patients in Rai stage 0 or Binet stage A have a normal life expectancy.

Treatment

It is difficult to cure CLL except with allogeneic stem cell transplant (rarely employed due to the advanced age of most patients and the availability of excellent safer therapies). **Therefore, the approach to therapy is generally conservative, aiming for symptom control rather than a normal blood count.** Indeed, cytotoxic chemotherapy given too early in the disease can shorten rather than prolong life expectancy.

Many patients will never need treatment. Treatment is given for troublesome enlarged lymph nodes or spleen, constitutional symptoms such as weight loss, or cytopenias as a result of bone marrow suppression. The lymphocyte count alone is not a good guide to the need for treatment, but if it doubles in <6 months, treatment will usually be required soon. As a general guide, patients in Binet stage C will need treatment, as will some in stage B, and patients in Rai stages III or IV will need treatment, as will a smaller proportion of patients in stages I or II (Table 18.5).

Table 18.4 Staging of chronic lymphocytic leukaemia.

(a) Rai classification

Stage	
0	Absolute lymphocytosis ≥5 × 10^9/L without adenopathy, organomegaly or cytopenias due to replacement of marrow by clonal cells
I	Enlarged lymph nodes (adenopathy)
II	Enlarged liver or spleen ± adenopathy
III	Anaemia (Hb <100 g/L) [†] ± adenopathy ± organomegaly
IV	Thrombocytopenia (platelets <100 × 10^9/L) [†] ±adenopathy ± organomegaly

(b) International Working Party classification (Binet)

Stage	Organ enlargement*	Haemoglobin[†] (g/L)	Platelets[†] (× 10^9/L)
A (50–60% of patients)	0, 1 or 2 areas	≥100	≥100
B (30%)	3, 4 or 5 areas	≥100	≥100
C (<20%)	Not considered	<100	or <100

* One area = lymph nodes >1 cm in neck (including Waldeyer's ring), axillae, groins or spleen, or liver enlargement.
[†] Secondary causes of anaemia (e.g. iron deficiency) or autoimmune haemolytic anaemia or autoimmune thrombocytopenia must be treated before staging. For example, a patient may have Stage 0 disease but be anaemic due to autoimmune haemolysis.
Hb, haemoglobin.
Source: (b) Adapted from J.L. Binet *et al.* (1981) *Cancer* 48: 198.

Table 18.5 Treatment of chronic lymphocytic leukaemia.
Source: Modified from Professor Michael Hallek, 2019 Presidential Address for the 24th annual meeting of the European Hematology Association, Amsterdam, Netherlands, 14 June 2019.

Disease stage	Are del(17p) or *TP53* mutation present?	Is the patient fit for and willing to undergo intensive therapy?	IgVH mutation status	Suggested therapy
Binet A or B, Rai 0–II stages; Inactive disease	Irrelevant	Irrelevant	Irrelevant	None (observation)
Active disease or Binet C or Rai III–IV stages	Yes	Irrelevant	Irrelevant	Ibrutinib or venetoclax+obinutuzumab or idelalisib+rituximab (if contraindications for ibrutinib)
	No	Yes	Mutated	FCR (BR if above 60–65 years) or ibrutinib
			Unmutated	Ibrutinib or FCR (BR if above 60–65 years)
		No	Mutated	Venetoclax+obinutuzumab or chlorambucil+obinutuzumab or ibrutinib
			Unmutated	Venetoclax+obinutuzumab or chlorambucil+obinutuzumab or ibrutinib

Consider and discuss with the patient long-term versus fixed length (e.g. 6–12 month duration) therapy, specific adverse effects of each option (e.g. myelo-suppression, infections, and secondary malignancy risk for chemoimmunotherapy; cardiac toxicity, bleeding risk and autoimmune disease for ibrutinib; tumour lysis syndrome and infections for venetoclax+obinutuzumab; autoimmune disease (diarrhoea) and opportunistic infections for idelalisib).
FCR, fludarabine, cyclophosphamide, rituximab; BR, bendamustine and rituximab.

Chemotherapy

For many years the treatment for CLL was based on the combination of cytotoxic drugs (such as fludarabine, chlorambucil, cyclophosphamide or bendamustine) together with a monoclonal antibody against CD20, usually rituximab. However, there are now several effective new targeted drugs (Table 18.5) which are being combined with these regimens and may in some cases replace them, e.g. initial therapy with ibrutinib or ventoclax. These are discussed below.

Beginning in the 1990s, the most commonly used first-line **treatment for younger patients** was R-FC (also known as FCR), which combines rituximab with fludarabine and cyclophosphamide. This regimen, given every 4 weeks, is able to control the white cell count and reduce organ swelling in most cases. Four to six courses are usually given and treatment can be stopped after a satisfactory response has been achieved. The average 'time to disease progression' after treatment with R-FC is around 4.5 years. The regimen has several potential serious side-effects, including myelosuppression and immunosuppression with risk of severe infection. A large randomized study showed that ibrutinib was more effective than R-FC for most patients 70 years or younger (the exception were those with mutated immunoglobulin heavy chain), and practice is shifting to incorporation of ibrutinib alone in front-line therapy.

Bendamustine with rituximab (BR) is an alternative approach that is less myelosuppressive, but progression-free survival is inferior to R-FC. It has therefore been more commonly used for patients over 60 years rather than for younger patients. However, randomized comparison of ibrutinib to BR in older patients with CLL also shows superiority for ibrutinib.

New agents in the treatment of B-CLL

In recent years several new and highly effective therapies have emerged in the treatment of lymphoid disorders (Table 18.5). They are used for treating relapsed, resistant patients but, as mentioned earlier, trials of their use as initial therapy show they may be superior for first-line therapy.

1 **Drugs which suppress signalling through the B-cell receptor** (BCR; Chapter 9). The surface immunoglobulin on a B cell acts as the BCR for antigen and B cells need to receive stimulatory signals through the BCR in order to remain alive. Drugs have been introduced that block two of the signalling proteins, Bruton kinase (BTK) and phospho-inositide 3-kinase (PI3K), both of which act 'downstream' of the BCR (Fig. 9.4).

■ **Ibrutinib** and **acalabrutinib** are oral drugs which inactivate BTK and lead to B-cell apoptosis. Inherited inactivating mutations of the *BTK* gene are a cause of immunodeficiency with B-cell lymphopenia (Chapter 9). The drugs are highly effective in the treatment of CLL as single agents, either as single agents or in combination with monoclonal antibodies or chemotherapy.

Remarkably, they are also effective for cases in which the leukaemic cells have a chromosome 17p deletion or *TP53* mutation, genetic changes which confer resistance to chemotherapy. BTK inhibitors are also active in Richter transformation (see below). Patients treated with ibrutinib in combination with chemo-immuno-therapy can achieve minimal residual disease negativity, and some may prove to be cured. Increased susceptibility to atrial fibrillation, bleeding due to an anti-platelet effect, or Aspergillus infection are potential side-effects. The drugs need to be discontinued several days before elective surgical procedures.

- **Idelalisib** is an oral drug which blocks PI3Kδ activity, an isoenzyme particularly important for B-cell survival. It is effective in CLL. Adverse events including colitis can occur and have limited its use. **Duvelisib**, which inhibits both the delta and gamma isoenzymes of PI3K, is as effective as idelalisib, but has a better safety profile. Other PI3K inhibitors are in development.

- A feature of both BTK inhibitors and PI3K inhibitors is that, like steroids, they initially cause an increase in the lymphocyte count in peripheral blood. This reflects a redistribution from lymph nodes and marrow and does not represent disease progression. An anti-CD20 monoclonal antibody which lowers the lymphocyte count is sometimes given initially with these drugs.

2 **Drugs which suppress the activity of BCL-2**. BCL-2 is expressed at a high level in most CLL cells and has potent anti-apoptotic effects, leading to abnormally prolonged cell survival. Venetoclax, a direct inhibitor of BCL-2, is highly active. Due to the risk of tumour lysis, hospitalization with careful monitoring is often required initially and during dose escalation of venetoclax.

3 **Effective monoclonal antibodies** include ofatumumab and obinutuzumab, which are CD20 specific (see Chapter 17). The combination of obinutuzumab with chlorambucil is excellent first-line treatment for older and less fit patients, while cytoreduction with obinutuzumab and ibrutinib, with subsequent addition of venetoclax, is extremely effective against relapsed or refractory disease.

Other forms of treatment

- *Corticosteroids* Prednisolone or other corticosteroids are given for autoimmune haemolytic anaemia, thrombocytopenia and red cell aplasia.
- *Radiotherapy* This is valuable in reducing the size of bulky lymph node groups that are unresponsive to chemotherapy.
- *Lenalidomide* This immune-modulating agent (see Chapter 16) has therapeutic activity in CLL. Initial treatment is sometimes associated with a disease 'flare' at affected tissue sites, which has limited its use.
- *Ciclosporin* Red cell aplasia may respond to ciclosporin or other calcineurin inhibitors.

- *Immunoglobulin replacement* Immunoglobulin (e.g. 400 mg/kg/21–28 days by intravenous infusion) is useful for patients with severe hypogammaglobulinaemia and recurrent infections, especially during winter months.
- *Vaccination* Patients should be vaccinated with a conjugated pneumococcal vaccine and with the Shingrix™ recombinant adjuvanted zoster vaccine, and should receive annual influenza vaccination.
- *Allogeneic stem cell transplantation (SCT)* SCT may be curative but has a significant mortality rate. It is typically employed only in younger patients with multiply relapsed disease.
- *Chimeric antigen receptor (CAR)-T cell therapy* CLL cells often express CD19 to which CAR-T cells may be infused. CAR-T cells and their adverse effects, including neurotoxicity and cytokine release syndrome, are further described in Chapters 9, 12 and 17.

Course of disease

Many patients in Binet stage A or Rai stage 0 or I never need therapy, and this is particularly likely for females and those with favourable prognostic markers (Table 18.3). For those who do need treatment, a typical pattern is that of response to several courses of therapy with a prolonged disease-free interval, before the gradual onset of extensive bone marrow infiltration or bulky disease. Molecular and cytogenetic tests often show that initially small subclones with genetic characteristics that confer treatment resistance, e.g. chromosome 17p deletion or *TP53* mutations, now form the bulk of the resistant disease. The new oral therapies (BTK and PI3K inhibitors, BCL-2 inhibitors) are proving effective even at these late stages and in patients with *TP53*-mutant disease.

CLL, like low-grade lymphomas, may transform into a high-grade lymphoma (Richter transformation). This usually resembles a diffuse large B-cell lymphoma with mutations of *TP53*, *MYC*, *NOTCH1* and *CDKN2A* genes. Less frequently, transformation resembles Hodgkin lymphoma. Richter transformation is often signalled by a dominant node that is brighter on positron emission tomography (PET) scans than other nodes. Richter transformation requires therapy as for other high-grade B-cell lymphomas. Prognosis is usually poor.

B-cell prolymphocytic leukaemia

Although B-cell prolymphocytic leukaemia (B-PLL) may initially appear similar to CLL, the diagnosis is made by the appearance of a majority of prolymphocytes in the blood. The prolymphocyte is around twice the size of a CLL lymphocyte and has a large central nucleolus (Fig. 18.5). **B-PLL typically presents with splenomegaly without lymphadenopathy and with a high and rapidly rising lymphocyte count.** Anaemia is a poor prognostic feature. Treatment is difficult and prognosis is worse than for CLL (median survival 3–5 years), but in general similar strategies are used for B-PLL as for CLL,

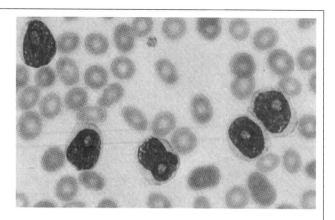

Figure 18.5 Prolymphocytic leukaemia: blood film showing prolymphocytes that have prominent central nucleoli and an abundance of pale cytoplasm.

The blood film reveals a variable number of unusual large lymphocytes with villous cytoplasmic projections (Fig. 18.6). Immunophenotyping shows CD11c, CD19, CD25, CD103 and CD123 positivity in most cases (see Table 20.3). **A mutation in exon 15 of the gene for the protein kinase *BRAF* (V600E) underlies the most frequent 'classical' variant of the disease.** The bone marrow trephine shows a characteristic appearance of mild fibrosis and a diffuse cellular infiltrate (Fig. 18.6).

There are several highly effective treatments for HCL and the median relapse-free survival after initial chemotherapy is more than 10 years. The treatment of choice is **2-chlorodeoxyadenosine (CDA, cladribine) or deoxycoformycin (DCF, pentostatin)**; both agents achieve complete responses in over 80% of cases. In two-thirds of cases a long-term remission is achieved. Alpha-interferon is also effective and is sometimes used first for those with severe cytopenias to improve these before the more effective drugs, which initially tend to lower the neutrophil and platelet counts, are given. Rituximab can be combined with CDA or DCF for relapsed cases. BRAF inhibitors such as vemurafenib are potentially useful in refractory disease, as is moxetumomab pasudotox, an anti-CD22 antibody conjugated to a bacterial toxin.

For the HCL variant, where BRAF mutation is absent, monocytopenia is less common and the immunophenotype is distinct (e.g. these cases typically lack CD123, CD25 or CD103 expression). The outlook is poorer than for classic HCL. Responsiveness to chemotherapy is decreased and the disease-free interval is shorter. Splenectomy may be required in some cases.

Lymphocytosis in non-Hodgkin lymphomas

Some cases of splenic marginal zone lymphoma show circulating monoclonal B lymphocytes with a villous cell outline and were previously termed 'splenic lymphoma with villous lymphocytes'. Lymphocytosis may also be

including ibrutinib and chemotherapy combined with a monoclonal antibody.

Alemtuzumab is an anti-CD52 monoclonal antibody that is effective at killing B and T lymphocytes by complement fixation, but can lead to serious infectious complications. It has been used in resistant and relapsed disease, but has mostly been replaced by the newer agents.

Hairy cell leukaemia

Hairy cell leukaemia (HCL) is an uncommon B-cell lymphoproliferative disease with a male:female ratio of 4:1 and a peak incidence at 40–60 years. **Patients typically present with infections, anaemia or splenomegaly. Lymphadenopathy is uncommon. Pancytopenia is usual at presentation and the lymphocyte count is rarely over 20×10^9/L. Monocytopenia is a distinctive feature.**

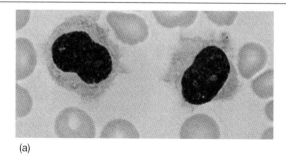

(a)

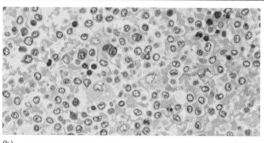

(b)

Figure 18.6 Hairy cell leukaemia: **(a)** peripheral blood film showing typical 'hairy' cells with oval nuclei and finely mottled pale grey-blue cytoplasm with an irregular edge; **(b)** bone marrow trephine.

seen in other types of non-Hodgkin lymphoma (e.g. follicular, mantle cell, diffuse large B cell), discussed further in Chapter 20.

T-cell diseases

T-cell prolymphocytic leukaemia

T-cell prolymphocytic leukaemia (T-PLL) presents similar to B-PLL with a high white cell count, but lymphadenopathy is more marked and skin lesions and serous effusions are common. Most cases express CD4$^+$. Treatment is with alemtuzumab (anti-CD52) followed by SCT in appropriate patients. There is an association with ataxia-telangiectasia syndrome due to germline mutations in *ATM* and faulty DNA repair.

Large granular lymphocytic leukaemia

Large granular lymphocytic (LGL) leukaemia is characterized by the presence of **circulating lymphocytes with abundant cytoplasm and large azurophilic granules (Fig. 18.7a)**. Such cells may be either T or natural killer (NK) cells and show variable expression of CD16, CD56 and CD57. *STAT3* mutations are present in 50% of cases and patients may respond to JAK-STAT inhibitors, including ruxolitinib or tofacitinib. Cytopenia, especially neutropenia, is the main clinical problem. Anaemia, splenomegaly and arthropathy with

positive serology for rheumatoid arthritis are also common. The median age is 50 years.

Treatment may not be needed, but if required, steroids, cyclophosphamide, ciclosporin/tacrolimus or methotrexate may relieve the cytopenia. A randomized trial of cyclophosphamide versus methotrexate is ongoing. Granulocyte colony-stimulating factor (G-CSF) has been used in cases associated with neutropenia.

Adult T-cell leukaemia/lymphoma

Adult T-cell leukaemia/lymphoma (ATLL) was the first malignancy to be associated with a human retrovirus, human T-cell leukaemia/lymphoma virus type 1 (HTLV-1). The virus is endemic in parts of Japan and the Caribbean and the disease is very rare in people who have not lived in these areas. ATLL lymphocytes have a bizarre morphology with a convoluted 'clover-leaf' nucleus and a consistent CD4$^+$ phenotype (Fig. 18.7b).

Most subjects infected with the HTLV-1 virus do not develop the disease. The clinical presentation is often acute and dominated by hypercalcaemia, skin lesions, hepatosplenomegaly and lymphadenopathy. Diagnosis is by morphology and serology. Zidovudine, an anti-retroviral drug, and alpha interferon are first-line therapy if leukaemia is dominant, but combination chemotherapy is used if the presentation is more like a lymphoma. Allogeneic SCT may be used, but the cure rate is only about 35%. The prognosis is poor.

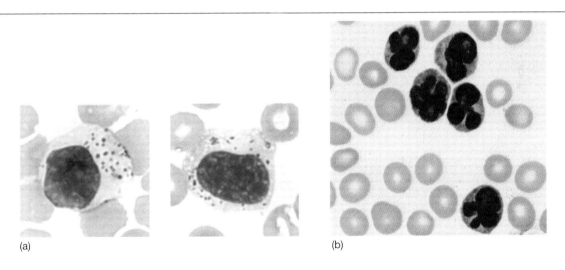

(a) (b)

Figure 18.7 (a) Large granular lymphocytes in the peripheral blood. **(b)** Adult T-cell leukaemia/lymphoma. Typical convoluted lymphoid cells in peripheral blood.

SUMMARY

- Chronic lymphocytic leukaemias are characterized by the accumulation of mature B or T lymphocytes in the blood.
- Individual subtypes are distinguished on the basis of morphology, immunophenotype and cytogenetics.
- Chronic lymphocytic leukaemia (CLL, B cell) represents 90% of cases and has a peak incidence between 60 and 80 years of age. There is genetic predisposition to development of the disease. It is preceded by monoclonal B-cell lymphocytosis.
- Most cases of CLL are identified when a routine blood test is performed. As the disease progresses the patient may develop enlarged lymph nodes, splenomegaly, hepatomegaly or bone marrow failure.
- Immunosuppression is a significant problem in CLL because of hypogammaglobulinaemia and cellular immune dysfunction.
- In CLL, anaemia may develop because of autoimmune haemolysis or bone marrow infiltration.
- Diagnosis of CLL is usually performed by immunophenotypic analysis of peripheral blood, which reveals a clonal population of CD5$^+$ CD23$^+$ light-chain restricted B cells.

- The best guide to prognosis is the stage of the disease. CLL that has acquired somatic mutations in the immunoglobulin genes has a relatively good prognosis compared to unmutated cases. Lymphocyte doubling time, immunological markers, cytogenetics and molecular genetics also provide useful prognostic information.
- Treatment for CLL is usually given only when clinical symptoms start to develop. Many patients require no therapy.
- Use of a combination of chemotherapy and immunotherapy, e.g. with fludarabine, cyclophosphamide and an anti-CD20 monoclonal antibody, establishes disease remission but is not curative. Drugs which block the activity of BTK (ibrutinib, acalabrutinib), PI3K (idelalisib, duvelisib) or BCL-2 (venetoclax) are new highly effective treatments even in otherwise resistant patients, and ibrutinib is now an established first-line therapy.
- Less common subtypes of chronic lymphocytic leukaemias include prolymphocytic leukaemia, hairy cell leukaemia and T-cell disorders.

Now visit **www.wileyessential.com/haematology** to test yourself on this chapter.

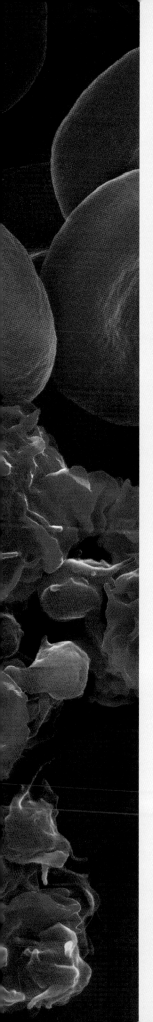

CHAPTER 19
Hodgkin lymphoma

Key topics

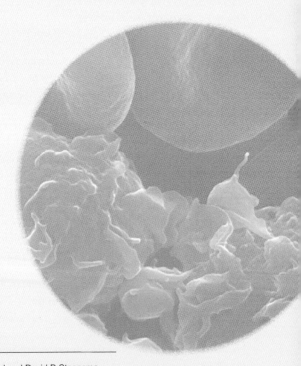

Hoffbrand's Essential Haematology, Eighth Edition. By A. Victor Hoffbrand and David P. Steensma.
© 2020 John Wiley & Sons Ltd. Published 2020 by John Wiley & Sons Ltd.
Companion website: www.wileyessential.com/haematology

Lymphomas are a group of neoplastic diseases caused by malignant lymphocytes that accumulate in lymph nodes and other lymphoid tissue and cause the characteristic clinical feature of lymphadenopathy. Occasionally, clonal lymphocytes may spill over into blood ('leukaemic phase') or infiltrate organs outside the lymphoid tissue.

The major subdivision of lymphomas is into Hodgkin lymphoma (HL) and non-Hodgkin lymphoma (NHL), and this is based on the histological presence of Reed–Sternberg (RS) cells in Hodgkin lymphoma.

History and pathogenesis

Thomas Hodgkin was curator of the Anatomy Museum at Guy's Hospital in London and described the disease in 1832. Carl von Sternberg in Vienna identified the abnormal cell that defines this subtype of lymphoma in 1898, and in 1902 Dorothy Reed, who was then a pathology trainee at Johns Hopkins, was the first to distinguish the cell from granulomas found in nodal tuberculosis. The characteristic RS cells, and the associated abnormal mononuclear cells, are neoplastic, whereas the infiltrating inflammatory cells are reactive.

Immunoglobulin gene rearrangement studies show that the **RS cell is of B-lymphoid lineage and that it is often derived from a B cell with a 'crippled' immunoglobulin gene** caused by the acquisition of mutations that prevent synthesis of full-length immunoglobulin. Human leukocyte antigen (HLA) class I expression is usually lost on the neoplastic cells and mutation of the β2-microglobulin gene is frequent. The Epstein–Barr virus (EBV) genome has been detected in over 50% of cases in Hodgkin tissue, but its exact role in the pathogenesis is unclear.

Clinical features

The disease can present at any age, but is rare in children and has a peak incidence in young adults. There is an almost 2 : 1 male predominance. The following symptoms are common:

1 **Most patients present with painless, asymmetrical, firm and discrete enlargement of superficial lymph nodes** (Fig. 19.1). The cervical nodes are involved in 60–70% of patients, axillary nodes in approximately 10–15% and inguinal nodes in 6–12%. In some cases, the size of the nodes decreases and increases spontaneously; they may also become matted. Typically, the disease is localized initially to a single peripheral lymph node region and its subsequent progression is by contiguity within the lymphatic system. Retroperitoneal nodes are also often involved, but usually only diagnosed by computed tomography (CT) scan.

2 Modest splenomegaly occurs during the course of the disease in 50% of patients. The liver may also be enlarged because of liver involvement.

3 Mediastinal involvement is found in up to 10% of patients at presentation. This is a feature of the nodular sclerosing type, particularly in young women. There may be

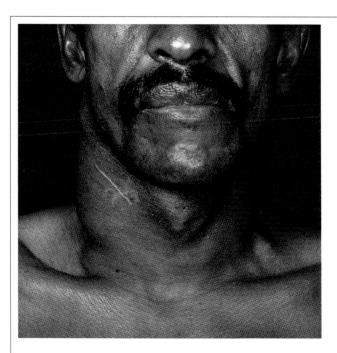

Figure 19.1 Cervical lymphadenopathy in a patient with Hodgkin lymphoma.

associated pleural effusions or superior vena cava obstruction (Fig. 19.2).

4 Cutaneous Hodgkin lymphoma occurs as a late complication in approximately 10% of patients. Other organs may also be involved, even at presentation, but this is unusual.

5 Constitutional symptoms are prominent in patients with widespread disease. The following may be seen:
  (a) fever occurs in approximately 30% of patients and is continuous or cyclic;
  (b) pruritus, which is often severe, occurs in approximately 25% of cases;
  (c) alcohol-induced pain in the areas where disease is present occurs in some patients;
  (d) other constitutional symptoms include weight loss, profuse sweating (especially at night), weakness, fatigue, anorexia and cachexia. Haematological and infectious complications are discussed below.

Haematological and biochemical findings

1 Normochromic normocytic anaemia is most common. Bone marrow involvement is unusual in early disease, but if it occurs bone marrow failure may develop with a leuco-erythroblastic anaemia.

2 One-third of patients have a neutrophilia; eosinophilia is frequent.

3 Advanced disease is associated with lymphopenia and loss of cell-mediated immunity.

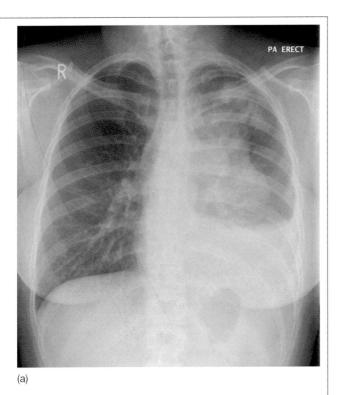

(a)

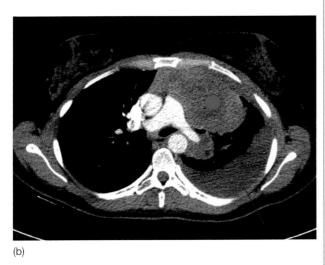

(b)

Figure 19.2 (a) Chest X-ray in Hodgkin lymphoma showing enlargement of left hilar lymph nodes, abnormal soft tissue projected over the upper left lung and a large left pleural effusion. **(b)** Axial computer tomography (CT) scan with intravenous contrast in the same patient. There is a large anterior mediastinal mass (yellow circle) with left hilar nodes enlarged (red circle) and left pleural effusion. Source: Courtesy of Dr Peter Wylie and Dr N. Nir.

4 The platelet count is normal or increased during early disease and reduced in later stages.

5 The erythrocyte sedimentation rate (ESR) and C-reactive protein are usually raised. The ESR is useful in monitoring disease progress.

6 Serum lactate dehydrogenase (LDH) is raised initially in 30–40% of cases.

7 The HIV status should be determined.

Diagnosis and histological classification

The diagnosis is made by histological examination of an excised lymph node. **The distinctive multinucleate polyploid RS cell is central to the diagnosis of the four classic types (Figs 19.3 and 19.4)** and mononuclear Hodgkin cells are also part of the malignant clone. These cells stain with CD30 and CD15, but are usually negative for B-cell antigen expression such as CD10, CD19 or CD20. Inflammatory components consist of lymphocytes, neutrophils, eosinophils, plasma cells and variable fibrosis. CD68 detects infiltrating macrophages and if this is strongly positive it is an unfavourable feature.

Histological classification is into four classical types and nodular lymphocyte predominant disease (Table 19.1). There is no difference in the prognosis or management of the different subtypes of classical HL. **Nodular sclerosis** is the most frequent in Europe and the USA, whereas **lymphocyte depleted** is more common in developing countries and has a particularly strong association with EBV infection and malnutrition.

Nodular lymphocyte predominant (LP) Hodgkin lymphoma does not show RS cells and has many features of non-Hodgkin lymphoma, the tumour cells being polylobated ('popcorn') B cells (Fig. 19.4d). It is usually treated like other small cell non-Hodgkin lymphomas. The prognosis is good.

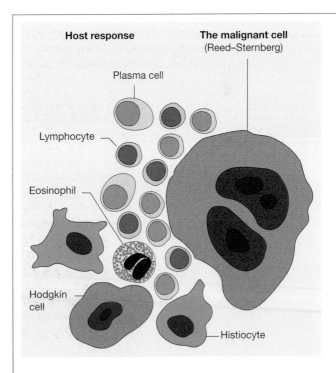

Figure 19.3 Diagrammatic representation of the different cells seen histologically in Hodgkin lymphoma.

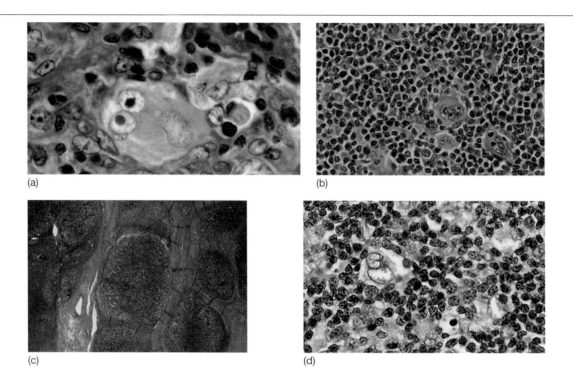

Figure 19.4 Hodgkin lymphoma: **(a)** high-power view of a lymph node biopsy showing two typical multinucleate Reed–Sternberg cells, one with a characteristic owl eye appearance, surrounded by lymphocytes, histiocytes and an eosinophil; **(b)** mixed cellularity; and **(c)** nodular sclerosing Hodgkin lymphoma; **(d)** microscopic appearance of nodular lymphocyte-predominant (LP) Hodgkin lymphoma: 'popcorn-like' LP cells surrounded by small lymphocytes. Source: (d) A.V. Hoffbrand *et al.* (2019) *Color Atlas of Clinical Hematology*, 5th edn. Reproduced with permission of John Wiley & Sons.

Table 19.1 World Health Organization (2016) classification of Hodgkin lymphoma.

Classical Hodgkin lymphoma (95% of cases)

Nodular sclerosis	Collagen bands extend from the node capsule to encircle nodules of abnormal tissue. A characteristic lacunar cell variant of the Reed–Sternberg cell is often found. The cellular infiltrate may be of the lymphocyte-predominant, mixed cellularity or lymphocyte-depleted type; eosinophilia is frequent
Lymphocyte rich	Scanty Reed–Sternberg cells; multiple small lymphocytes with few eosinophils and plasma cells; nodular and diffuse types
Mixed cellularity	The Reed–Sternberg cells are numerous and lymphocyte numbers are intermediate
Lymphocyte depleted	There is either a reticular pattern with dominance of Reed–Sternberg cells and sparse numbers of lymphocytes, or a diffuse fibrosis pattern where the lymph node is replaced by disordered connective tissue containing few lymphocytes. Reed–Sternberg cells may also be infrequent in this latter subtype

Nodular lymphocyte-predominant (5% of cases)

Reed–Sternberg cells are absent. Scattered lymphocyte-predominant (LP) tumour cells with polylobated (popcorn-like) nuclei are present in a background of small lymphocytes with an absence of inflammatory cells (Fig. 19.4d). The disease arises in lymphoid follicles and there is a vaguely nodular appearance. In contrast to classical Hodgkin lymphoma, the LP cells are positive for B cell markers and strongly positive with the B cell transcription factor antibody OCT2.

Table 19.2 Techniques for staging of lymphoma.	
Laboratory	Full blood count, ESR, bone marrow aspirate and trephine biopsy (not routine), liver tests, LDH, C-reactive protein, albumin
Radiology	Chest X-ray; PET/CT of thorax, abdomen, chest and pelvis; MRI

CT, computed tomography; ESR, erythrocyte sedimentation rate; LDH, lactate dehydrogenase; MRI, magnetic resonance imaging; PET, positron emission tomography.

Clinical staging

Selection of appropriate treatment depends on accurate staging of the extent of disease (Table 19.2). Figure 19.5 shows the scheme that is used. Staging is performed by clinical examination together with **combined positron emission tomography (PET) and CT scans**. CT scan alone can be used if PET is not available (Figs 19.5 and 19.6). The criteria by which a lymph node is considered normal or abnormal are described in Chapter 9, page 124. Magnetic resonance imaging (MRI) scanning may be needed for particular sites (Table 19.2). Bone marrow trephine is sometimes carried out and liver biopsy may also be needed in difficult cases. **PET/CT scanning is useful in monitoring response to treatment and for detection of small foci of residual disease** (Fig. 19.7).

Patients are also classified as A or B according to whether or not constitutional features (fever, drenching night sweats or weight loss) are present (Fig. 19.5).

Positron emission tomography

[18]F-fluorodeoxyglucose positron emission tomography (FDG-PET) is now used widely in the management of lymphoma and other haematological malignancies. It utilizes the fact that

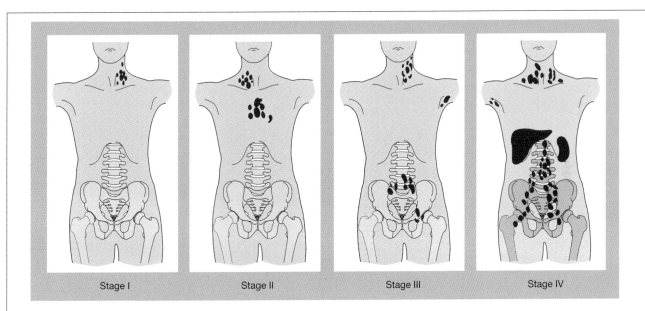

Figure 19.5 Staging of Hodgkin lymphoma. Stage I indicates node involvement in one lymph node area. Stage II indicates disease involving two or more lymph nodal areas confined to one side of the diaphragm. Stage III indicates disease involving lymph nodes above and below the diaphragm. Splenic disease is included in stage III, but this has special significance (see below). Stage IV indicates involvement outside the lymph node areas and refers to diffuse or disseminated disease in the bone marrow, liver and other extranodal sites. N.B. The stage number in all cases is followed by the letter A or B, indicating the absence (A) or presence (B) of one or more of the following: unexplained fever above 38°C; night sweats; or loss of more than 10% of body weight within 6 months. Localized extranodal extension from a mass of nodes does not advance the stage, but is indicated by the subscript E. Thus, mediastinal disease with contiguous spread to the lung or spinal theca would be classified as I_E. As involvement of the spleen is often a prelude to widespread haematogenous spread of the disease, patients with lymph node and splenic involvement are staged as III_S. Bulky disease (widening of the mediastinum by more than one-third, or the presence of a nodal mass >10 cm in diameter) is relevant to therapy at any stage.

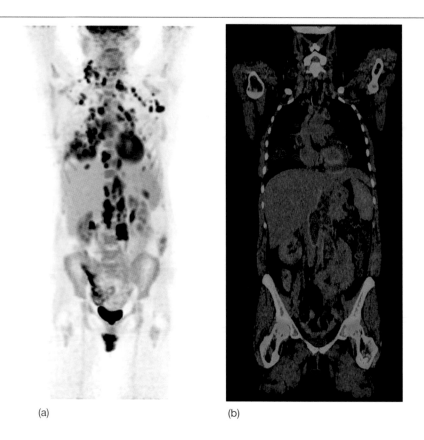

(a)   (b)

Figure 19.6 Hodgkin lymphoma. Staging positron emission tomography (PET)/computed tomography (CT): 35-year-old female who had disease above and below the diaphragm at presentation. **(a)** Coronal PET image shows multiple foci of uptake above and below the diaphragm. **(b)** Coronal fused PET/CT scan image shows multiple foci of uptake above and below the diaphragm corresponding to nodes, spleen and lung nodules. PET stage IV. Source: Courtesy of Dr Thomas Wagner and the Department of Nuclear Medicine, Royal Free Hospital, London.

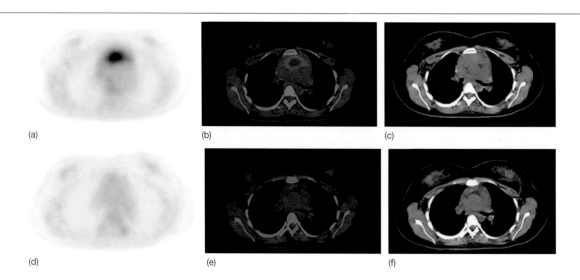

(a)   (b)   (c)

(d)   (e)   (f)

Figure 19.7 Example of the value of imaging in the management of Hodgkin lymphoma. **(a)** Axial positron emission tomography (PET), **(b)** fused PET/computer tomography (CT) and **(c)** CT images at diagnosis demonstrate intense [^{18}]FDG uptake in an anterior mediastinal mass. Following two cycles of ABVD chemotherapy, **(d)** the axial PET, **(e)** fused PET/CT and **(f)** CT images demonstrate no significant [^{18}]FDG uptake in the residual mediastinal mass, in keeping with a complete metabolic response. Source: Courtesy of Dr V.S. Warbey and Professor G.J.R. Cook.

rapidly dividing malignant cells readily take up glucose from their environment. Radiolabelled glucose is infused into the patient and the tissues that have taken up the label can then be visualized by the PET scanner. As well as detecting the presence of active disease at the time of diagnosis, PET/CT scans can also be used to assess the response to treatment and to potentially guide the treatment course.

Deauville score

Interim PET/CT scans are reported according to the Deauville 5-point criteria, which uses the uptake in the mediastinum and liver as an internal control, from which to assess the activity of the tumour. Scores 1 and 2 are generally considered 'negative', whereas 4 and 5 are 'positive' and a score of 3 must be interpreted according to the clinical context.

- ■ Score 1 no abnormal uptake.
- ■ Score 2 nodal uptake present but ≤ mediastinum uptake.
- ■ Score 3 nodal uptake > mediastinum but ≤ liver.
- ■ Score 4 moderately increased nodal uptake > liver.
- ■ Score 5 markedly increased nodal uptake > liver.

Treatment

Treatment is either with chemotherapy alone or a combination of chemotherapy with radiotherapy. The choice depends primarily on the stage, clinical state A or B (Fig. 19.5) and prognostic factors (Table 19.3). Semen storage for males, if appropriate, should be carried out before therapy is begun. For females it is advisable that fertility advice is sought from a specialist. If blood transfusion is needed, this must be irradiated to avoid graft-versus-host disease due to the infusion of live donor lymphocytes, which can engraft due to the impaired cellular immunity of the HL patient.

Table 19.3 Prognosis of stage 1–2 disease (EORTC criteria).

Favourable	Unfavourable
	Any one of:
No large mediastinal lymphadenopathy*	Large mediastinal lymphadenopathy
ESR <50 without B symptoms	ESR ≥50 without B symptoms
ESR <30 with B symptoms	ESR ≤30 with B symptoms
Age ≤50 years	Age >50 years
1–3 lymph node sites involved	4 or more lymph node sites involved

*Large is defined as mediastinal thoracic ratio >0.35 at the level of T5/6. EORTC, European Organization for the Research and Treatment of Cancer; ESR, erythrocyte sedimentation rate.

Early-stage disease

The outcome for early-stage disease is excellent and an important aim is to avoid over-treatment and the risk of late complications. Two broad options are chemotherapy alone or 'combined modality treatment' (CMT) using chemotherapy and radiotherapy. CMT achieves better short-term disease control, but in the longer term there is no clear increase in overall survival. Individual treatment decisions will depend on local regimens and patient choice. The most widely used regimen is with two courses of A (Adriamycin = Doxorubicin), B (Bleomycin), V (Vinblastine), D (Dacarbazine) (ABVD) chemotherapy followed by 20Gy radiotherapy to the involved field. If lymph nodes are not bulky radiotherapy can be omitted, but then at least three courses of ABVD are given.

In contrast, unfavourable disease (1B or 2B) could be treated with four to six courses of ABVD followed by 30Gy radiotherapy for bulky disease. Alternatively, the first two cycles of ABVD can be replaced by more intensive chemotherapy, such as escalated BEACOPP (Bleomycin, Etoposide, Adriamycin, Cyclophosphamide, Vincristine = Oncovin, Procarbazine and Prednisolone).

Advanced-stage disease

Cyclical chemotherapy is used for stage III and IV disease. Six courses of ABVD are most widely used, but this in most centres depends on PET scan findings after the first two courses (discussed below). Escalated BEACOPP gives a higher complete remission rate at the expense of greater short- and long-term toxicity, so is usually used as initial therapy only for young patients with the highest risk. Subsequent radiotherapy is given if residual nodes are more than 1.5 cm diameter, or smaller but remain PET positive, or to sites of originally bulky disease.

Because bleomycin causes pulmonary toxicity, there is interest in alternative agents that might offer comparable cure rates to ABVD or BEACOPP but with fewer adverse effects. A randomized trial compared ABVD to the combination of the anti-CD30 monoclonal antibody–drug conjugate brentuximab (Adcetris®) with doxorubicin, vinblastine and dacarbazine (AAVD regimen). The complete response rate was slightly better and progression-free survival was improved with AAVD compared to ABVD, but there was more febrile neutropenia with AAVD and brentuximab is more costly than bleomycin.

Assessment of response to treatment

Clinical examination and imaging (PET/CT scans) are used to assess response to treatment and plan further therapy. Regular pulmonary function assessment is needed in older patients and those receiving bleomycin. Patients with HL often show residual masses following treatment, which may be because of the large degree of fibrosis present within lymph nodes.

PET/CT scanning reveals the areas of residual active disease (Fig. 19.7). PET/CT can be used to define the management of individual patients. It is widely used after the first two cycles of ABVD and if there is residual active disease, treatment might be switched to more intensive chemotherapy such as BEACOPP. Alternatively, if the PET scan is negative, bleomycin might be omitted from subsequent chemotherapy and there is generally no need to repeat the PET/CT scan at the end of therapy if the interim PET scan was negative. For patients PET/CT positive at the end of therapy, repeat biopsy and close clinical and imaging assessment are needed. Inflammatory tissue may cause a false positive PET scan.

Relapsed cases

Approximately 25% of patients suffer from disease relapse or are refractory to initial therapy. Treatment is generally given as an alternative combination chemotherapy to the initial regimen and, if necessary, with radiotherapy to sites of bulky disease. As described above, brentuximab vedotin is an anti-CD30 antibody linked to a microtubule-disrupting agent and may produce favourable responses if it has not been used for first-line therapy. If the disease remains chemosensitive, high-dose chemotherapy and autologous stem cell transplantation improve the probability of cure and are given for most fit patients below the age of 70 years. Allogeneic transplantation may be curative in a minority of patients who fail other therapies. The deacetylase inhibitor panobinostat is also an active agent.

A new therapy is the use of antibodies which block the inhibitory molecules PD-1 or PD-L1 on T cells (checkpoint inhibitors; Fig. 19.8). Hodgkin lymphoma often expresses high levels of PD-1 or its ligand PD-L1, and this acts as a mechanism for evading the T cell immune response. PD-1 blockade with immune checkpoint inhibitor antibodies such as nivolumab or pembrolizumab has proven to be highly effective in management of relapsed HL and is now being investigated earlier in treatment.

Prognosis

The prognosis depends on age, stage and histology. Overall approximately 85% of patients are cured.

The late effects of Hodgkin lymphoma and its treatment

Long-term follow-up of patients has revealed a considerable burden of late disease following treatment, especially those treated with radiation. Secondary cancers, such as lung and breast cancer, appear to be related to radiotherapy, whereas

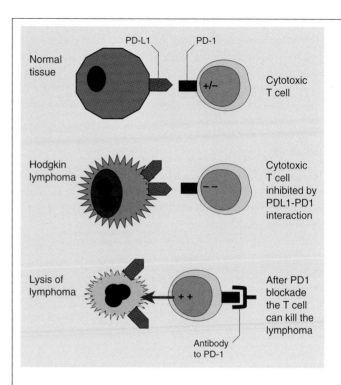

Figure 19.8 Potential mechanism whereby Hodgkin lymphoma is controlled after treatment with antibodies to block PD-1. PD-1 and PD-L1 are natural molecules that limit the attack of normal tissues by cytotoxic T cells. Hodgkin lymphoma overexpresses PD-L1 due to gene amplification or effects of Epstein–Barr virus infection. This delivers a strong negative signal to the T cells around the tumour. If antibody-mediated blockade of PD-1 is used, the T cells can then recognize and kill the tumour.

myelodysplastic syndromes or acute myeloid leukaemia, more common after escalated BEACOPP than after ABVD, are more associated with the use of alkylating agents and radiotherapy. Non-Hodgkin lymphoma and other cancers also occur with greater frequency than in controls. Non-malignant complications include sterility, intestinal complications, coronary artery disease and pulmonary complications of the mediastinal radiation or bleomycin chemotherapy. Vinblastine may cause a permanent neuropathy. These features are the main reason why less intensive treatment regimens guided by interim PET/CT results are now being explored for this disease.

SUMMARY

- Lymphomas are a group of diseases caused by malignant lymphocytes that accumulate in lymph nodes (and in other tissues) and cause lymphadenopathy.
- The major subdivision of lymphomas is into Hodgkin lymphoma and non-Hodgkin lymphoma and this is based on the presence of Reed–Sternberg cells in Hodgkin lymphoma.
- Reed–Sternberg cells are neoplastic B cells, but most cells in the lymph node are reactive inflammatory cells.
- The usual clinical presentation is with painless asymmetrical lymphadenopathy – most commonly in the neck.
- Constitutional symptoms of fever, weight loss and sweating are prominent in patients with widespread disease.
- Blood tests may show anaemia, neutrophilia and raised erythrocyte sedimentation rate (ESR) and lactate dehydrogenase (LDH).

- Diagnosis is made by histological examination of an excised lymph node and there are four classical subtypes and a fifth type nodular predominant disease.
- Staging of the disease is important for determining treatment and prognosis. History, examination, blood tests, CT and PET scan are typically used.
- Treatment is with radiotherapy, chemotherapy or a combination of both. The choice depends on the stage and grade of the disease.
- The response to treatment can be monitored by CT and PET scans. The treatment may be modified according to interim PET/CT findings.
- Disease relapse can be treated with chemotherapy, sometimes with stem cell transplantation.
- The prognosis is excellent and over 85% of patients can expect to be cured. Late side-effects of treatment are a concern.

Now visit **www.wileyessential.com/haematology** to test yourself on this chapter.

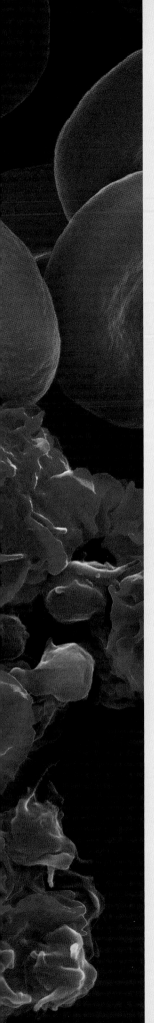

CHAPTER 20
Non-Hodgkin lymphomas

Key topics

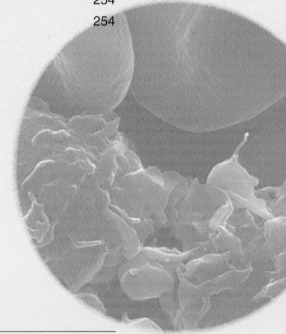

Hoffbrand's Essential Haematology, Eighth Edition. By A. Victor Hoffbrand and David P. Steensma.
© 2020 John Wiley & Sons Ltd. Published 2020 by John Wiley & Sons Ltd.
Companion website: www.wileyessential.com/haematology

Introduction to non-Hodgkin lymphomas

The non-Hodgkin lymphomas (NHL) are a large group of clonal lymphoid tumours, about 85% of B cell and 15% of T or NK (natural killer) cell origin (Table 20.1). Their clinical presentation and natural history are much more variable than those of Hodgkin lymphoma. NHL are characterized by an irregular pattern of spread and a significant proportion of patients develop disease outside the lymph nodes. Their frequency has increased markedly over the last 50 years and, with an incidence of approximately 17 in 100 000 in the UK, they now represent the fifth most common malignancy in some developed countries (see Fig 11.2).

Classification

The lymphomas are classified within a group of **mature B-cell and T-cell neoplasms**, which also includes chronic lymphoid leukaemias and myeloma (Table 20.1). The World Health Organization (WHO) classification incorporates age (paediatric or elderly) and site of involvement (e.g. skin, central nervous system, intestine, spleen, mediastinal) as well as the disease histology, immunophenotype and genotype. In this chapter, we consider the more common B-cell and T-cell lymphoma subtypes (Fig. 20.1 and Fig. 20.18).

Cell of origin

The normal B-cell development stages are illustrated in Fig. 9.11. B-cell lymphomas tend to mimic normal B cells at different stages of development (Fig. 20.2). This is shown by their phenotypic patterns on immune histology or flow cytometry (see Table 20.3). They can be divided into those resembling precursor B cells found in the bone marrow, and those which resemble germinal centre (GC) cells or post-GC cells from lymph nodes. T-cell lymphomas resemble precursor T cells in the bone marrow and thymus, or peripheral mature T cells.

Low- versus high-grade NHL

NHL includes a diverse group of diseases that vary from highly proliferative and potentially rapidly fatal conditions to some very indolent and well-tolerated malignancies.

For many years, clinicians have subdivided lymphomas into 'low-grade' and 'high-grade' disease. This approach is valuable as, in general terms, the low-grade disorders are relatively indolent, respond well to chemotherapy or immunotherapy, and have a lengthy median survival but are very difficult to cure, whereas high-grade lymphomas are aggressive and need urgent treatment, but are more often curable.

Table 20.1 The 2016 World Health Organization (WHO) classification of mature B-cell and T-cell neoplasms (modified), which includes the non-Hodgkin lymphomas. B-cell disorders comprise 85% of cases. T cell and NK cell together comprise 15% of cases. A few rare or provisional subtypes have been omitted (see Appendix).

Mature B-cell neoplasms	Mature T-cell and NK-cell neoplasms
■ Chronic lymphocytic leukaemia/small lymphocytic lymphoma ■ Monoclonal B-cell lymphocytosis ■ B-cell prolymphocytic leukaemia ■ Splenic marginal zone lymphoma ■ Hairy cell leukaemia ■ Lymphoplasmacytic lymphoma (Waldenström macroglobulinaemia) ■ Monoclonal gammopathy of undetermined significance (IgM and IgG/IgA subtypes) ■ Heavy-chain diseases ■ Plasma cell myeloma ■ Plasmacytoma (solitary plasmacytoma of bone, extraosseous) ■ Extranodal marginal zone lymphoma of mucosa-associated lymphoid tissue (MALT lymphoma) ■ Follicular lymphoma ■ Mantle cell lymphoma ■ Diffuse large B-cell lymphoma (germinal centre B-cell type, activated B-cell type) ■ Primary diffuse large cell lymphoma of the central nervous system ■ EBV+ diffuse large cell lymphoma ■ High-grade B-cell lymphoma, with MYC and BCL2 and/or BCL6 rearrangements ■ Burkitt lymphoma	■ T-cell prolymphocytic leukaemia ■ T-cell large granular lymphocytic leukaemia ■ Chronic lymphoproliferative disorder of NK cells ■ Aggressive NK-cell leukaemia ■ Adult T-cell leukaemia/lymphoma ■ Extranodal NK/T-cell lymphoma, nasal type ■ Enteropathy-associated T-cell lymphoma ■ Hepatosplenic T-cell lymphoma ■ Subcutaneous panniculitis-like T-cell lymphoma ■ Mycosis fungoides ■ Sézary syndrome ■ Peripheral T-cell lymphoma NOS ■ Angioimmunoblastic T-cell lymphoma ■ Anaplastic large cell lymphoma, *ALK* positive ■ Anaplastic large cell lymphoma, *ALK* negative ■ Breast implant-associated anaplastic large cell lymphoma

ALK, anaplastic lymphoma kinase, the gene on chromosome 2 which is overexpressed; EBV, Epstein–Barr virus; Ig, immunoglobulin; NK, natural killer; NOS, not otherwise specified.

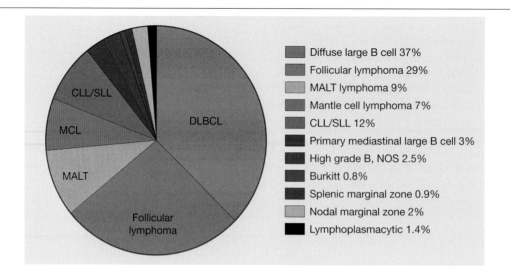

Figure 20.1 The relative frequencies of B-cell non-Hodgkin lymphomas. CLL, chronic lymphocytic lymphoma; DLBCL, diffuse large B-cell lymphoma; MALT, mucosa-associated lymphoid tissue; MCL, mantle cell lymphoma; NOS, not otherwise specified; PMLBCL, primary mediastinal large B-cell lymphoma; SLL, small lymphocytic lymphoma.

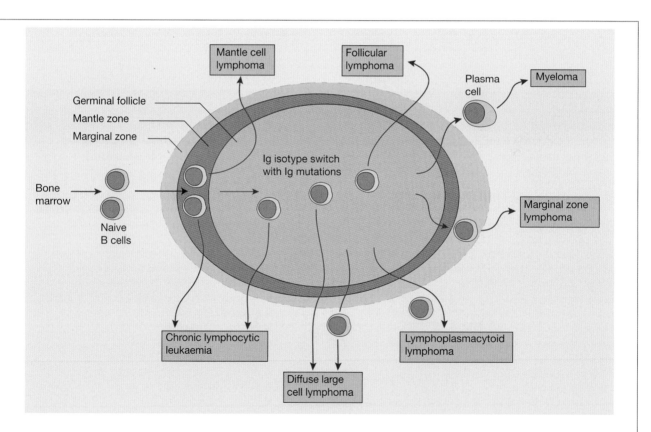

Figure 20.2 Proposed cellular origin of B-lymphoid malignancies. Normal B cells migrate from the bone marrow and enter secondary lymphoid tissue. When they encounter antigen, a germinal centre is formed and B cells undergo somatic hypermutation of the immunoglobulin (Ig) genes. Finally, B cells exit the lymph node as memory B cells or plasma cells. The cellular origin of the different lymphoid malignancies can be inferred from immunoglobulin gene rearrangement status and membrane phenotype. Mantle cell lymphoma and a proportion of B-cell chronic lymphocytic leukaemia (B-CLL) cases have unmutated immunoglobulin genes, whereas marginal zone lymphoma, diffuse large cell lymphoma, follicle cell lymphoma, lymphoplasmacytoid lymphoma and some B-CLL cases have mutated immunoglobulin genes.

Leukaemias versus lymphomas

The difference between **lymphomas**, in which lymph nodes, spleen or other solid organs are involved, and **leukaemias**, with predominant bone marrow and circulating neoplastic cells, may be blurred. Chronic lymphocytic leukaemia and small lymphocytic lymphoma (Chapter 18) are identical lymphoproliferative diseases that show predominantly leukaemic and lymph node distribution, respectively. Acute lymphoblastic leukaemia (Chapter 17) and lymphoblastic lymphoma are also similar and have comparable treatment regimens. Small numbers of malignant cells circulate in the blood in many forms of NHL.

Pathogenesis

The aetiology of the majority of cases of NHL is unknown, although infectious agents are an important cause in particular subtypes (Table 20.2). There are also considerable geographical variations in incidence and distribution of subtypes (Table 20.2). **Cytogenetic abnormalities are frequent, often translocations involving the immunoglobulin genes in the B-cell neoplasms.** Translocations of oncogenes to the immunoglobulin loci on chromosomes 2, 14 or 22 may result in overexpression of the oncogene under the influence of the highly active promoter elements of an immunoglobulin locus,

leading to alteration of the cell cycle, failure of apoptosis or aberrant expression of survival genes (see Chapter 11 and Table 20.4). Specific signalling pathways may be affected and next generation sequencing has revealed point mutations in genes involved in, for example, chromatin remodelling, the NFκB pathway of B-cell activation, and pre-mRNA splicing. As many as 80 somatic mutations may be present in NHL at presentation (see Fig. 11.3) and further mutations may appear as the disease progresses.

Clinical features of NHL

1 **Superficial lymphadenopathy** The majority of patients present with asymmetrical painless enlargement of lymph nodes in one or more peripheral lymph node regions.
2 **Constitutional symptoms** Fever, night sweats and weight loss can occur, but are less frequent than in Hodgkin lymphoma. Their presence is usually associated with more advanced, disseminated disease.
3 **Oropharyngeal involvement** In 5–10% of patients there is disease of the oropharyngeal lymphoid structures (Waldeyer's ring), which may cause complaints of a 'sore throat' or noisy or obstructed breathing.
4 **Symptoms due to anaemia, infections due to neutropenia or purpura with thrombocytopenia** These may be presenting features in patients with diffuse bone marrow involvement. Cytopenias may also be autoimmune in origin or due to sequestration in an enlarged spleen.
5 **Abdominal disease** The liver and spleen are often enlarged and involvement of retroperitoneal or mesenteric nodes is frequent. The gastrointestinal tract is the most commonly involved extranodal site after the bone marrow, and patients may present with acute or subacute abdominal symptoms.
6 **Other organs** Involvement of the skin, brain, testis or thyroid is not infrequent. The skin is also primarily involved in two closely related T-cell lymphomas: mycosis fungoides and Sézary syndrome.

Investigations

Histology

Whole lymph node excisional biopsy, or more usually core needle (e.g. Trucut) biopsy of lymph node or of other involved tissue (e.g. bone marrow or extranodal tissue), is the definitive investigation (Fig. 20.3). Fine needle aspiration of lymph node or involved tissue is rarely sufficient to establish a definitive diagnosis of lymphoma due to loss of diagnostic node architectural features, and for this reason is unreliable and a biopsy should instead be obtained.

Morphological examination of the biopsy is assisted by immunophenotypic and, in some cases, genetic analysis

Table 20.2 Infections associated with lymphoid neoplasms.

Infection	Neoplasm
Virus:	
HTLV-1	Adult T-cell leukaemia/lymphoma
Epstein–Barr virus	Burkitt and Hodgkin lymphomas; PTLD; extranodal NK/T-cell lymphoma, nasal type
HHV-8	Primary effusion lymphoma; multicentric Castleman disease
HIV	High-grade B-cell lymphoma, primary CNS lymphoma, Hodgkin lymphoma
Hepatitis C	Splenic marginal zone lymphoma
Bacteria:	
Helicobacter pylori or *Chlamydia trachomatis*	Gastric lymphoma or ocular adnexal lymphoma (MALT)
Protozoan: Malaria	Burkitt lymphoma (endemic variant)

CNS, central nervous system; HHV-8, human herpesvirus 8; HIV, human immunodeficiency virus; HTLV-1, human T-lymphotropic virus type 1; MALT, mucosa-associated lymphoid tissue; PTLD, post-transplant lymphoproliferative disease.

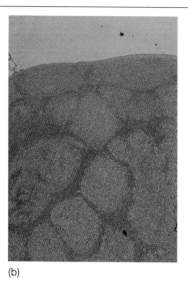

(a) (b)

Figure 20.3 Histological sections of lymph nodes in non-Hodgkin lymphoma showing **(a)** a diffuse pattern of involvement in lymphocytic lymphoma with the normal architecture totally replaced by neoplastic lymphocytic cells; **(b)** a follicular or nodular pattern in follicular lymphoma – the 'follicles' or 'nodules' of neoplastic cells compress surrounding tissue and lack a mantle of small lymphocytes seen in healthy nodal biopsy specimens.

(Tables 20.3 and 20.4). For B-cell lymphomas, expression of either only κ or only λ light chains by lymphoid cells confirms clonality and distinguishes neoplastic disease from a reactive node in which both κ and λ light chains are expressed (Fig. 20.4).

Laboratory investigations

1 In advanced disease with marrow involvement there may be anaemia, neutropenia or thrombocytopenia.

2 Lymphoma cells (e.g. mantle zone cells, 'cleaved follicular lymphoma' or 'blast' cells) may be found in the peripheral blood in some patients (Fig. 20.5).

3 Trephine biopsy of marrow may be valuable in staging if risk of involvement is high, e.g. high-grade lymphomas, if positron-emission tomography (PET) scan shows marrow uptake or if cytopenias are present (Fig. 20.6).

4 The serum lactate dehydrogenase (LDH) level is raised in rapidly proliferating and extensive disease and is used as a

Table 20.3 Characteristic immunophenotype of common B-cell lymphomas. Compare also Table 18.2.

	SIg	CD20	CD5	CD10	CD23	BCL6	MUM1
Small lymphocytic lymphoma/CLL	weak	+	+	–	+	–	–
Hairy cell leukaemia (classical subtype)	+	+	–	–	–	–	–
Lymphoplasmacytic lymphoma	+	+	–	–	–	–	+
MALT lymphoma	+	+	–	–	+/–	–	+/–
Follicular lymphoma	+	+	–	+	+/–	+	–
Mantle cell lymphoma	+	+	+	–	–	–	–
Diffuse large B-cell lymphoma, GCB	+/–	+	–	+		+	–
Diffuse large B-cell lymphoma, ABC	+/–	+	–	–		–	+
Burkitt lymphoma	+	+	–	+	–	+	–

ABC, activated B-cell type; CLL, chronic lymphocytic leukaemia; GCB, germinal centre B-cell type; MALT, mucosa-associated lymphoid tissue; MUM1, a lymphocytic-specific transcription factor; SIg, surface immunoglobulin.

Table 20.4 Examples of cytogenetic abnormalities and gene mutations found in cases of lymphoid malignancies.

	Cytogenetics	Gene mutations
Chronic lymphocytic leukaemia	Chromosome 13p, 11q or 17p deletions; trisomy 12	*TP53, ATM, NOTCH1, SF3B1*
Hairy cell leukaemia	Non-specific	*BRAF* (>99% in classic subtype)
Lymphoplasmacytic lymphoma	Non-specific	*MYD88* (>90%), *CXCR4* (30%)
MALT lymphoma	t(11;18) *[BIRC3-MALT1]*, t(1;14) *[BCL9-IGH]*	Activation of NFκB pathway
Follicular lymphoma	t(14;18) *[IGH-BCL2]*	Mutations in genes such as *CREBBP*, *EZH2* and *KMT2D* (*MLL2*), which influence chromatin remodelling
Mantle cell lymphoma	t(11;14) *[IGH-CCND1]*	*ATM, CCND1, TP53* and genes influencing chromatin modification
Diffuse large B-cell lymphoma	t(14;18) *[IGH-BCL2]* and others	*MYD88, CD79B, NOTCH1/2, EZH2, BCL2, BCL6, MYC*
Burkitt lymphoma	t(8;14) *[MYC-IGH]*, t(2;8) *[IGK-MYC]*, t(8;22) *[MYC-IGL]*	Various
Anaplastic large cell lymphoma	t(2;5) *[NPM1-ALK]*	*ALK*

MALT, mucosa-associated lymphoid tissue.

prognostic marker (Table 20.5). Elevation of serum uric acid may also occur.

5 Immunoglobulin electrophoresis may reveal a paraprotein.

6 HIV status should be tested as indicated. HIV positivity influences prognosis in certain lymphoma subtypes, such as Burkitt lymphoma.

Cytogenetic and genetic analysis

The subtypes of NHL are associated with characteristic chromosomal translocations and genetic mutations which are of

diagnostic and prognostic value (Table 20.3). Particularly characteristic translocations are t(14;18) in follicular lymphoma, t(11;14) in mantle cell lymphoma, t(8;14) in Burkitt lymphoma and t(2;5) in anaplastic large cell lymphoma. Genetic analysis reveals mutation of *MYD88* in virtually all cases of lymphoplasmacytic lymphoma.

In B-cell lymphomas the immunoglobulin genes are clonally rearranged, whereas in T-cell lymphomas there is clonal rearrangement of the T-cell receptor genes (see Chapter 11).

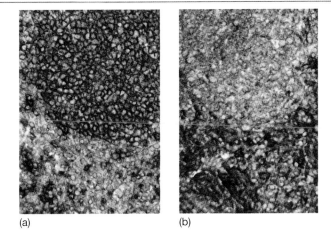

(a)   (b)

Figure 20.4 Non-Hodgkin lymphoma: lymph node stained by immunoperoxidase shows **(a)** brown ring staining for κ in the malignant lymphoid nodule; and **(b)** no labelling for λ, confirming the monoclonal origin of the lymphoma.

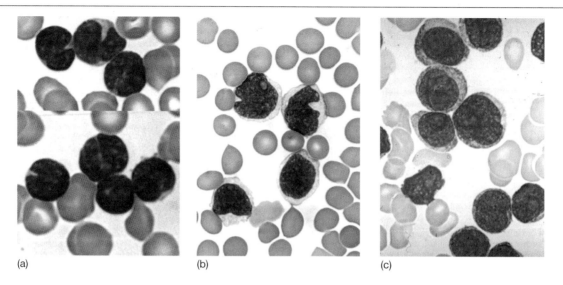

Figure 20.5 Blood involvement by malignant lymphoma: **(a)** small cleaved lymphoid cells in follicle centre cell lymphoma; **(b)** mantle cell lymphoma; **(c)** large B-cell lymphoma.

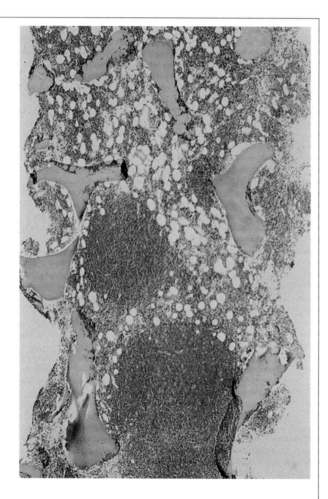

Figure 20.6 Iliac crest trephine biopsy in lymphocytic lymphoma. Prominent nodules of lymphoid tissue are seen in the intertrabecular space and paratrabecular areas.

Table 20.5 The National Comprehensive Cancer Network-International Prognostic Index (NCCN-IPI) for patients with high-grade non-Hodgkin lymphoma.

	Score
Age, years	
>40 to ≤60	1
>60 to ≤75	2
>75	3
LDH, normalized	
>1 to ≤3	1
>3	2
Ann Arbor stage III–IV	1
Extranodal disease*	1
Performance status ≥2	1

*Disease in bone marrow, CNS, liver/gastrointestinal tract, or lung.
LDH, lactate dehydrogenase.

Staging

The staging system is the same as that described for Hodgkin lymphoma (Chapter 19), but is less clearly related to prognosis than the histological subtype. Staging procedures usually include chest X-ray and PET/CT scanning (Fig. 20.7). **The criteria by which a lymph node is considered normal or abnormal by CT are described in Chapter 9 (p. 124).** PET/CT can also be used to follow treatment response (Fig. 20.8). Bone marrow aspiration and trephine are often performed. PET/CT may detect marrow disease when the biopsy is negative. The **Deauville criteria** by which a lymph node is considered normal or abnormal on PET/CT scanning have been described in Chapter 19.

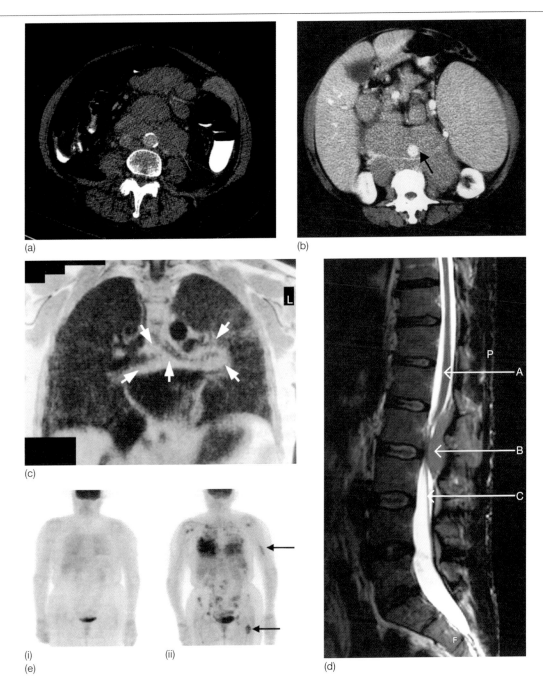

Figure 20.7 Non-Hodgkin lymphoma. **(a)** Computed tomography (CT) examination performed for weight loss and abdominal pain in an 86-year-old female showing enlarged para-aortic (yellow arrow) and mesenteric lymph nodes (blue circle). Histology revealed diffuse large B-cell non-Hodgkin lymphoma. Source: Courtesy of Dr P. Wylie. **(b)** CT scan of the abdomen: enlarged retroperitoneal and mesenteric nodes from a man causing the 'floating aorta' (arrowed) appearance. Source: Courtesy of Professor A. Dixon and Dr R.E. Marcus. **(c)** Magnetic resonance imaging (MRI) scan of the chest showing large mediastinal lymph nodes (white and arrowed) adjacent to the great vessels (black). **(d)** MRI T_2-weighted midline sagittal image of a lumbosacral spine showing compression of the dural sac by an extradural mass. A, spinal cord; B, extradural mass; C, roots of corda equina. Source: Courtesy of Dr A. Valentine. **(e)** Positron emission tomography (PET) body scan of a 59-year-old woman with high-grade non-Hodgkin lymphoma. (i) The first scan showed no evidence of disease prior to allogeneic transplant. Normal physiological uptake is seen in the brain and bladder. Two months post-transplant the patient relapsed clinically with a mass on the anterior chest wall. (ii) The PET scan showed evidence of widespread relapse in nodal (para-aortic and iliac nodes) and extranodal sites including the lung and bone. The uptake in bone is clearly demonstrated in the left humerus and femur (arrowed). This scan illustrates how well PET can detect both nodal and extranodal disease and allows whole body assessment at a single scanning session. Source: Courtesy of Dr S.F. Barrington.

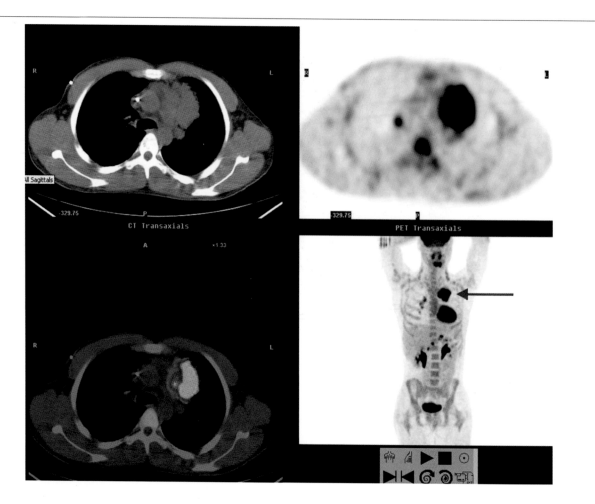

Figure 20.8 Non-Hodgkin lymphoma. Positron emission/computed tomography (PET/CT) scan of a male aged 26 years. Red arrow shows the level at which trans-axial section is performed. Upper right-hand panel showing fluorodeoxyglucose (FDG) uptake in anterior mediastinal mass and right hilar node. Upper left-hand panel shows corresponding CT section, bottom left-hand panel shows the CT and PET fused image of the corresponding section. Bottom right-hand panel, coronal section showing FDG uptake in mediastinal mass and right hilar node. There is also FDG uptake in the thyroid, heart, bowel, kidneys and bladder. Source: Courtesy of the Department of Nuclear Medicine, University College London.

General principles of treatment of NHL

When treatment is started, it is usually in the form of a combination of chemotherapy drugs together with a monoclonal antibody directed against the tumour cell. However, various new targeted drugs have been developed which have changed the management of disease. These include:

- Oral agents that block activity of the BTK or PI3Kδ proteins, as used for B-cell chronic lymphocytic lymphoma (BLL; Chapter 18), or other kinases, such as anaplastic lymphoma kinase (ALK), activity of which is increased in patients with anaplastic large cell lymphoma.
- Drugs that inhibit BCL-2 activity e.g. venetoclax.

Bioengineered chimeric antigen receptor (CAR)-T cells have been developed against specific B-cell-associated targets such as CD19 and are now approved for use for relapsed or refractory patients with some subtypes of lymphoma. Other types of CAR-T cells are in development.

Monoclonal antibody therapy

In the 85% of cases of NHL that are of B-cell origin, antibodies against CD20 have proven of great benefit. Rituximab was the first such agent and can be given intravenously or subcutaneously. Ofatumumab and obinutuzumab are also anti-CD20 antibodies that have a distinct binding pattern to the receptor and may be somewhat more effective than rituximab, but they cost more. Antibodies against CD30 such as brentuximab are often used for anaplastic large cell lymphoma and other NHL, as well as for Hodgkin lymphoma (see Chapter 19).

Specific subtypes of non-Hodgkin lymphoma

Low-grade non-Hodgkin lymphoma

Small lymphocytic lymphoma

This term is used for cases with the same morphology and immunophenotype as B-CLL, but with less than 5×10^9/L peripheral blood B cells and no cytopenias due to bone marrow involvement. Lymphadenopathy is typical. Treatment is as for patients with B-CLL (Chapter 18).

Lymphoplasmacytoid lymphoma (Waldenström macroglobulinaemia)

This is an uncommon condition, seen most frequently in men over 50 years of age. **There is usually a monoclonal immunoglobulin (Ig) M paraprotein and the lymphoplasmacytoid lymphoma (LPL) may then be termed Waldenström macroglobulinaemia.** The cell of origin is a post-germinal centre B cell with the characteristics of an IgM-bearing memory B cell.

LPL or its precursor, IgM monoclonal gammopathy of undetermined significance (MGUS; see Chapter 21), may be diagnosed by chance in symptomless patients (see Fig. 21.3). The disease usually presents clinically with an insidious onset, often with fatigue and weight loss. Hyperviscosity syndrome (see Fig. 21.15) is a common complication as the IgM paraprotein increases blood viscosity more than equivalent concentrations of IgG or IgA. Visual upset is frequent and the retina may show a variety of changes, such as engorged veins, haemorrhages, exudates and a blurred disc (Fig. 21.15). If the macroglobulin is a cryoglobulin, features of cryoprecipitation, such as Raynaud phenomenon, may be present.

Anaemia is usually a significant problem and a bleeding tendency may result from macroglobulin interference with coagulation factors and platelet function. Neurological symptoms, dyspnoea and heart failure may be presenting symptoms. Moderate lymphadenopathy and enlargement of the liver and spleen are frequently seen.

Diagnosis is made by the finding of a monoclonal serum IgM together with bone marrow or lymph node infiltration with lymphoplasmacytoid cells (Fig. 20.9). **Mutation of MYD88 is present in nearly all cases.** About 30% of patients have *CXCR4* mutations, almost all also with the *MYD88* mutation. These patients tend to have more cytopenias and more extensive disease. CXCR4 signalling is usually upregulated whether or not *CXCR4* is mutated. The erythrocyte sedimentation rate (ESR) is raised and there may be peripheral blood lymphocytosis.

Treatment

No treatment is required for patients without symptoms, but treatment should be started if there are features such as organomegaly, symptomatic anaemia or hyperviscosity. Combination treatment with an anti-CD20 antibody such as rituximab (Fig. 20.10) and chemotherapy is generally given. If rituximab

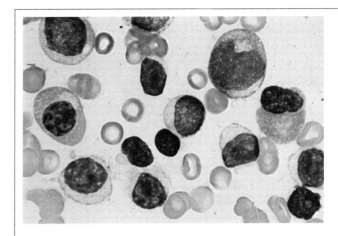

Figure 20.9 Lymphoplasmacytoid lymphoma associated with Waldenström macroglobulinaemia. Bone marrow shows cells with features of lymphocytes and plasma cells.

is given alone, the IgM level may transiently rise ('flare'), which can cause hyperviscosity. Chemotherapy options include cyclophosphamide, fludarabine, bendamustine or bortezomib. Ibrutinib and acalabrutinib are effective in cases refractory to other drugs and are also becoming first-choice initial therapy, either alone or in combination with rituximab or another CD20 antibody. Autologous or allogeneic stem cell transplantation (SCT) is considered for advanced disease. Erythropoiesis-stimulating agents or regular transfusions may be required for chronic anaemia.

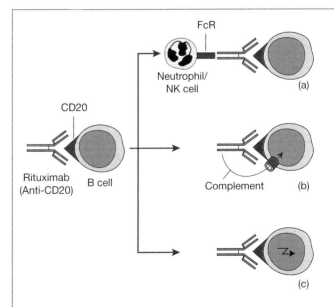

Figure 20.10 The potential mechanisms of action of rituximab. Rituximab binds to CD20 on the surface of B cells. It can elicit a number of effector mechanisms, including **(a)** antibody-dependent cell-mediated cytotoxicity; **(b)** complement-mediated lysis of tumour cells; and **(c)** direct apoptosis of the target cell.

Acute hyperviscosity syndrome (see p. 269) is treated with repeated plasmapheresis until the underlying disease can be brought under control. As IgM is mainly present in the intravascular space, plasmapheresis is more effective than for IgG or IgA paraproteins, where much of the protein is extravascular and so rapidly replenishes the plasma compartment after plasmapheresis.

Marginal zone lymphomas

Marginal zone lymphomas are low-grade lymphomas that arise from the marginal zone of B cell germinal follicles. It is thought that lymphoid hyperplasia initially occurs in response to antigen or inflammation and then cells acquire secondary genetic damage that leads to lymphoma. Cytogenetic analysis may reveal translocations involving the immunoglobulin loci and molecular tests show point mutations particularly involving the NF-κB pathway. Marginal zone lymphomas are classified according the anatomical site at which they arise, such as the **spleen, mucosa (MALT)** or **lymph node (nodal)**.

Mucosa-associated lymphoid tissue (MALT) lymphomas usually arise in the stomach (Fig. 20.11), respiratory tract, skin and salivary glands. Gastric MALT lymphoma is the most common form and is preceded by *Helicobacter pylori* infection. In the early stages it may respond to antibiotic therapy aimed at eliminating *H. pylori*. Ocular adnexal lymphoma may result from *Chlamydia* infection.

Splenic marginal zone lymphoma usually presents as splenomegaly and may be associated with circulating 'villous' lymphocytes that may be mistaken for hairy cells. Localized stage Ia disease may be cured by local radiotherapy. If chemotherapy is needed, it is usually based on regimens used in other low-grade lymphomas such as follicular lymphoma. Splenectomy maybe useful for symptomatic patients, but is becoming less frequently needed with improved drug therapy.

Follicular lymphoma

This represents around 25% of NHL, with a median age of onset of 60 years. It is associated with the t(14;18) translocation in the great majority of cases. The translocation leads to constitutive expression of the *BCL2* gene with increased survival of cells because of reduced apoptosis. Additional molecular abnormalities are usually present (Table 20.3). The cells are typically CD10, CD19, CD20, BCL2 and BCL6 positive (Table 20.3, Fig 20.12).

Patients are likely to be middle-aged or elderly and their disease is often characterized by a benign course for many years. The median survival from diagnosis is approximately 10 years. Rarely the disease presents in a benign form in children or as an *in situ* form, e.g. as an incidental finding on duodenal biopsy. The histological appearances are graded as I–III according to the relative proportion of centrocytes and centroblasts. Grade IIIb patients have the worst prognosis and are generally treated according to diffuse large B-cell lymphoma (DLBCL) guidelines. Bone marrow involvement is frequent.

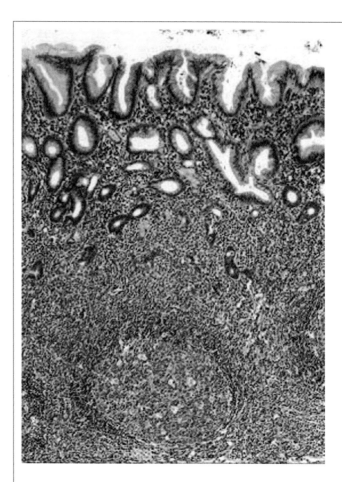

Figure 20.11 Gastric mucosa-associated lymphoid tissue (MALT) lymphoma: the tumour cells surround reactive follicles and infiltrate the mucosa. The follicle has a 'starry sky' appearance. Source: Courtesy of Professor P. Isaacson.

Presentation is usually with painless lymphadenopathy, often widespread, and the majority of patients will have stage III or IV disease. However, sudden transformation may occur at a rate of about 3% a year to aggressive diffuse tumours.

Around 10% of patients have initially localized (stage I) disease and may achieve cure with radiotherapy alone. Those with disseminated (stage II–IV) disease are generally not treated in the absence of symptoms ('watch and wait'), but treatment is introduced when complications occur. An international prognostic score prognosis depends on age, presence or not of anaemia, serum LDH and disease burden as measured by size and extent of lymph node and bone marrow involvement. At the current time, chemotherapy is not a curative option. Therapy is usually based on rituximab, either alone or in combination with chemotherapy such as bendamustine (B-R), cyclophosphamide, vincristine and prednisolone (R-CVP), with an anthracycline added for more aggressive cases (R-CHOP). Ibrutinib is also active and when combined with rituximab results in deep, durable remissions. As with CLL, ibrutinib is moving to first-line therapy. The combination of

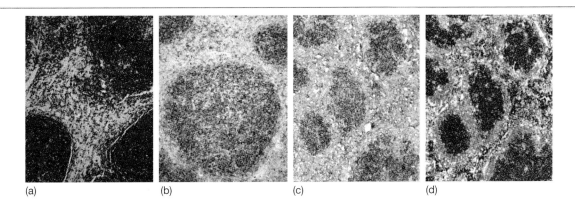

Figure 20.12 Follicular lymphoma: immunostains. **(a)** The neoplastic cells are diffusely positive for B-cell markers (CD20). **(b)** The neoplastic cells are diffusely positive for CD10, a germinal centre marker, and are located in the follicular and interfollicular areas. **(c)** The neoplastic cells are positive for BCL-6, a germinal centre marker. **(d)** The neoplastic cells are positive for BCL-2.

lenalidomide with rituximab has been found to be as effective as chemotherapy in some studies. Chlorambucil is active, but is now rare given all the other active agents. CAR-T cells are being introduced for refractory patients.

The first-line regimens can provide clinical responses in up to 90% of patients and usually achieve a remission of several years. Following remission, rituximab infusions are often given as maintenance therapy, usually every 2–3 months for at least 2 years. Maintenance therapy prolongs remission time, but does not increase overall survival.

Disease relapse for stage II–IV disease is almost inevitable (but may not occur for many years after initial therapy) and is usually treated initially with similar chemotherapy regimens followed by rituximab maintenance. Over time the disease may become increasingly difficult to control with, for example, acquisition of TP53 mutations. More intensive chemotherapy or radiolabelled anti-CD20 antibody therapy is

then considered. Autologous SCT may be valuable in patients with a history of at least one relapse and allogeneic SCT using reduced-intensity protocols offers the prospect of cure for some patients. The BCL2 inhibitor ventoclax, PI3K inhibitors idelalisib, duvelisib and copanlisib, and BTK inhibitors ibrutinib and acalabrutinib are also active agents for relapsed disease (see Fig. 9.4).

Mantle cell lymphoma

Mantle cell lymphoma (MCL) is derived from pre-germinal centre cells localized in the primary follicles or in the mantle region of secondary follicles. WHO 2016 recognizes two major subtypes: one classical involving lymph nodes and extranodal sites and the other a leukaemic, non-nodal subtype. The cells usually show angular nuclei in histological sections (Fig. 20.13) and often circulate in the blood (Fig. 20.5). MCL has a characteristic phenotype of CD19$^+$ and CD5$^+$ (like CLL) but,

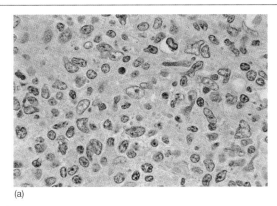

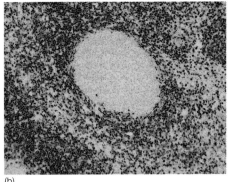

Figure 20.13 (a) Mantle cell lymphoma: showing characteristic deformed pattern of small lymphocytes with angular nuclei ('centrocytes'). **(b)** Mantle cell lymphoma: expression of cyclin D1 shown by immunohistochemistry. Source: E. Campo, S.A. Pileri. In A.V. Hoffbrand *et al.* (eds) (2016) *Postgraduate Haematology*, 7th edn. Reproduced by permission of John Wiley & Sons.

in contrast to CLL, is CD22$^+$ and CD23$^-$. A specific t(11;14) translocation juxtaposes the cyclin D1 gene *CCND1* to the immunoglobulin heavy-chain gene, and leads to **increased expression of cyclin D1** (Fig. 20.13b), which alters cell cycle behaviour. Presence of this translocation is required for diagnosis. Other mutations are usually present (Table 20.4).

Clinical presentation of the classical type of MCL is with lymphadenopathy and the leukaemic type with systemic symptoms and blood bone marrow and splenic disease. The Mantle Cell International Prognostic Index (MIPI), based on age, performance status, serum LDH and leucocyte count, is useful. The nodal disease tends to be more aggressive, with high expression of Ki67 and with acquisition of additional genetic abnormalities. Of the patients with the leukaemic subtype, some show an indolent course similar to that of CLL. They may be diagnosed when a blood test is performed for other purposes. In both subtypes, patients with TP53 deletions or mutations have an inferior outcome.

Current treatment regimens include:

1 Chemotherapy, such as R-CHOP (as for DLBCL) or bendamustine-rituximab combinations for older (>65 years) patients. For younger, fitter patients more intensive regimens may be used, such as R-CHOP/high-dose methotrexate or cytosine arabinoside/cisplatin.
2 Ibrutinib and acalabrutinib are effective and are being increasingly used in various combinations for both initial therapy and relapsed disease.
3 Autologous or allogeneic haemopoietic SCT.
4 Maintenance with rituximab is given for patients in remission following chemotherapy, with or without autologous SCT, and delays relapse.

The prognosis of mantle cell lymphoma historically has been quite poor, but may improve with the addition of newer agents such as ibrutinib, acalabrutinib, ventoclax and CAR-T cell therapy.

High-grade NHL

Diffuse large B-cell lymphomas

DLBCL are a heterogeneous group of disorders representing the classic 'high-grade' lymphomas. Histologically the biopsy shows large neoplastic cells with prominent nucleoli. They are subdivided into 'germinal centre' (GCB) and 'activated B cell' (ACB) subtypes, which stain with antibodies to BCL6 and CD19 or MUM1 respectively (Table 20.3; Fig. 20.14).

The clinical presentation is usually with rapidly progressive lymphadenopathy, which may also involve the bone marrow, gastrointestinal tract, brain (Fig. 20.15), spinal cord, kidneys or other organs.

A variety of clinical and laboratory findings are relevant to the outcome of therapy. According to the **International Prognostic Index (IPI)** these include age, performance status, stage, number of extranodal sites and serum LDH (Table 20.5). Bulky disease (major mass >5 cm diameter), prior history of low-grade disease or HIV infection, and ABC compared to GCB type are also associated with a poorer prognosis, but are not included in the IPI. There is a variety of histological patterns including centroblastic, immunoblastic and anaplastic. The most common cytogenetic changes involve the IGH locus on chromosome 14 and the *BCL6* gene at chromosome 3q27, and translocation of the *BCL2* gene occurs in 20%. Somatic mutations are frequent in all types (Table 20.4). **Double expressor or 'double hit' DLBCL** aberrantly express both MYC and either BCL-2 or

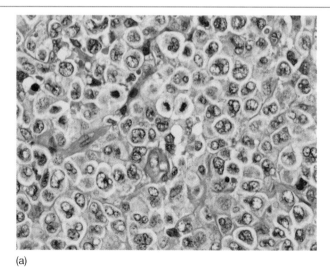
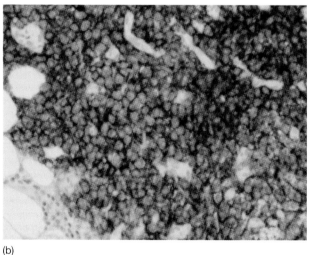

(a)

(b)

Figure 20.14 (a) Diffuse large B-cell lymphoma. **(b)** The cells stain positive for CD10. This suggests a germinal centre cell origin in this case. Source: E. Campo, S.A. Pileri. In A.V. Hoffbrand *et al.* (eds) (2016) *Postgraduate Haematology*, 7th edn. Reproduced by permission of John Wiley & Sons.

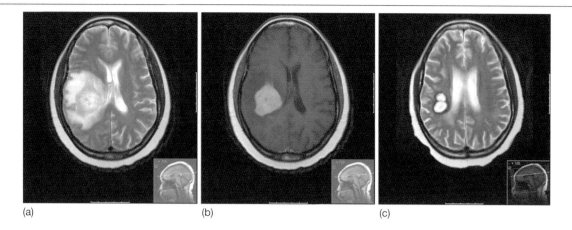

Figure 20.15 Cerebral lymphoma in HIV infection; magnetic resonance imaging (MRI). **(a)** T2-weighted magnetic resonance brain scan showing heterogeneous mass and adjacent oedema in right inferior frontoparietal region. There is compression of the right lateral ventricle and displacement of midline structures. Biopsy showed diffuse large B-cell lymphoma. **(b)** The mass enhances after intravenous gadolinium injection. **(c)** Enhanced image after chemotherapy showing regression of the mass. Source: Courtesy of the Department of Radiology, Royal Free Hospital, London.

BCL-6 proteins due to mutations/rearrangements in the corresponding genes (Table 20.1). They have an inferior prognosis.

The mainstay of treatment is rituximab in combination with CHOP – cyclophosphamide, hyroxodaunorubicin (doxorubicin), vincristine (Oncovin) and prednisolone – given in 3-weekly cycles, typically for six to eight courses, although four courses are adequate for younger lower-risk patients. More intensive regimens have been used for younger poor-risk patients, but these are not established to improve their overall survival.

For localized disease, combined radiotherapy and chemotherapy (e.g. three courses of R-CHOP) may be optimal. Prophylactic therapy to prevent central nervous system (CNS) disease, such as intrathecal or high-dose systemic methotrexate, should be considered for patients with high-risk disease, particularly those with bone marrow involvement. The response to treatment is monitored by repeat CT or PET/CT scans midway through chemotherapy and then following completion.

For patients who relapse, high-dose chemotherapy with drug regimens such as R-ICE (rituximab, ifosfamide, carboplatin and etoposide) or gemcitabine- or platinum-based regimens can be effective. For CD30+ cases addition of brentuximab may be beneficial, while ventoclax and polatuzumab vedotin, an antibody–drug conjugate targeting CD79b, also show promise, combined with other chemotherapy for relapsed and refractory DLBCL. In those patients who respond to these treatments, autologous SCT is often used. Anti-CD19 CAR-T cells are active and have achieved regulatory approval, and are now increasingly used for relapsed/resistant patients. Reduced-intensity allogeneic SCT has also been shown to be effective. However, for those with primary refractory or chemoresistant disease, the outlook is poor.

Primary central nervous system lymphoma

This is a rare diffuse large B-cell lymphoma, more common in older patients and those with HIV infection. Mutations of *MYD88*, *CD79b* and *CDKN2A* underlie the tumour. Diagnosis is made by stereotactic biopsy and tumour cells may also be found in the cerebrospinal fluid. Contrast-enhanced magnetic resonance imaging (MRI) is recommended for initial imaging and for response assessment. Patients are treated with cycles of high-dose methotrexate with partner cytotoxic agents, e.g. high-dose cytosine arabinoside and rituximab. Anti-HIV therapy is added if the patient is HIV positive. Whole brain radiotherapy is considered for consolidation, but subsequent long-term cognitive dysfunction can then be a major problem. Chemotherapy consolidation is also being studied. For relapsed or refractory disease, chemotherapy with drugs such as ifosphamide or thiotepa with or without autologous SCT may improve survival in a minority.

Primary mediastinal B-cell lymphoma

This is a rare type of NHL arising in the thymus, presenting mainly in adolescents and young adults. The histology resembles nodular sclerosing Hodgkin lymphoma, but in contrast to Hodgkin lymphoma, in mediastinal lymphoma CD30 expression is weak and CD15 negative, even though cells resembling Reed–Sternberg cells can be present. PAX5 and BCL-6 are expressed in most cases, as are B-cell antigens (CD19, CD20, CD22, CD79b). Half of cases have amplification of the *REL* gene on chromosome 2q16, and tumour suppressor *SOCS1* is mutated or deleted in a similar proportion of cases. The tumour invades locally. Treatment is with R-CHOP or more intensive regimens with or without subsequent local radiotherapy or autologous transplant.

Burkitt lymphoma

Burkitt lymphoma occurs in endemic or sporadic forms.
Endemic (African) Burkitt lymphoma is seen in areas with chronic malaria exposure and is associated with Epstein–Barr virus (EBV) infection. In virtually all cases the *MYC* oncogene is overexpressed because it is translocated to an immunoglobulin gene, usually the heavy-chain locus t(8;14) (Fig. 11.11) and less commonly to one of the light chains. As a result, the gene is expressed in parts of the cell cycle during which it should normally be switched off.

Typically the patient, usually a child, presents with massive lymphadenopathy, often of the jaw (Fig. 20.16), which is initially very responsive to chemotherapy, although long-term cure is uncommon. Sporadic Burkitt lymphoma may occur anywhere in the world and EBV infection is seen in 20% of cases. There is an increased incidence in HIV infection. The histological picture is distinctive, with a very high proliferative index of over 95% (Fig. 20.17). The prognosis is excellent using chemotherapy regimens which include high doses of methotrexate, cytosine arabinoside and cyclophosphamide, e.g.

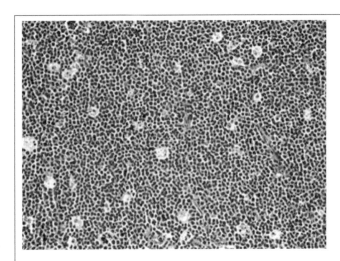

Figure 20.17 Burkitt lymphoma: histological section of lymph node showing sheets of lymphoblasts and 'starry sky' tingible body macrophages.

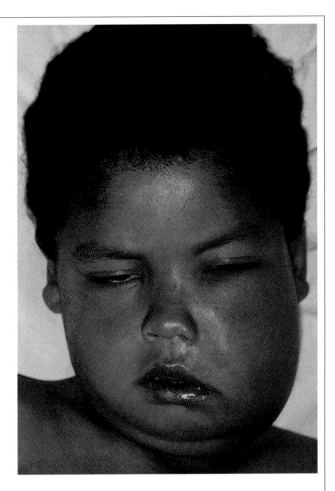

Figure 20.16 Burkitt lymphoma: characteristic facial swelling caused by extensive tumour involvement of the mandible and surrounding soft tissues.

CODOX-M/IVAC (which also includes doxorubicin, ifosphamide and etoposide). Intrathecal chemotherapy is also given.

Primary central nervous system lymphoma

These are rare tumours, more common in older patients and those with HIV infection. Patients are treated with high-dose methotrexate and cytosine arabinoside, and with anti-HIV therapy if they are HIV positive. Whole brain radiotherapy is also considered, but subsequent long-term cognitive dysfunction can then be a major problem.

Lymphoblastic lymphomas

Lymphoblastic lymphomas (B or T cell) occur mainly in children and young adults and these conditions merge clinically and morphologically with acute lymphoblastic leukaemia (ALL). The cells, like those in ALL, are terminal deoxynucleotide transferase positive (Chapter 17), whereas this test is negative in all the other B- and T-cell lymphomas. They are treated as ALL using similar protocols.

T-cell lymphomas

T-cell lymphomas are a heterogeneous group of rare tumours that present with lymphadenopathy or with extranodal disease. They comprise about 15% of NHL in Western countries, but more in Asia, and are usually of CD4⁺ phenotype. Several variants of T-cell lymphomas are recognized (Fig 20.18).

Peripheral T-cell non-Hodgkin lymphoma, unspecified

These derive from T cells at various stages of differentiation. They are treated with combined chemotherapy (e.g. CHOP).

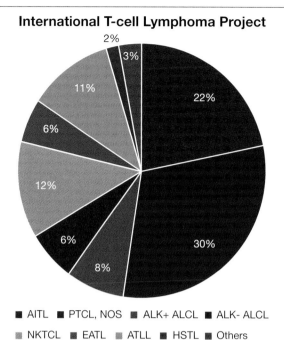

International T-cell Lymphoma Project

- AITL
- PTCL, NOS
- ALK+ ALCL
- ALK- ALCL
- NKTCL
- EATL
- ATLL
- HSTL
- Others

Figure 20.18 The relative frequencies of T-cell non-Hodgkin lymphomas. AITL, angioimmunoblastic T-cell lymphoma; ALCL, anaplastic large cell lymphoma; ALK⁺ or ALK⁻, anaplastic lymphoma tyrosine kinase; ATLL, adult T-cell leukaemia/lymphoma; EATL, enteropathy-associated T-cell lymphoma; HSTL, hepatosplenic T-cell lymphoma; NKTCL, natural killer/T-cell lymphoma; NOS, not otherwise specified; PTCL, peripheral T-cell lymphoma. Source: N. Schmitz et al. (2018) *Blood* 132: 246.

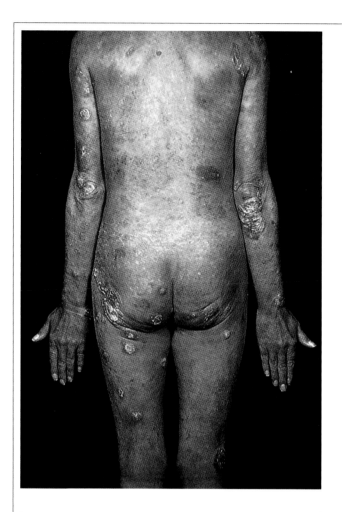

Figure 20.19 Mycosis fungoides.

Brentuximab may be useful in CD30⁺ cases of this and the other T-cell lymphomas. The prognosis is poor. Autografting for patients with chemosensitive disease is often performed. CAR-T cells are in development for T-cell lymphomas, but difficulty distinguishing between CAR-T cells, endogenous T cells and neoplastic T cells has made assessment of effectiveness difficult.

Angioimmunoblastic lymphadenopathy

Angioimmunoblastic lymphadenopathy usually occurs in elderly patients with lymphadenopathy, hepatosplenomegaly, skin rashes and a polyclonal increase in serum IgG. Patients are treated with chemotherapy or histone deacetylase inhibitors.

Mycosis fungoides

Mycosis fungoides is a chronic cutaneous T-cell lymphoma that presents with severe pruritus and psoriasis-like eczematoid skin lesions that can later become plaques and ulcerated tumours (Fig. 20.19). In contrast to Sézary syndrome, tumour cells do not circulate in the blood. Ultimately, deeper organs are affected, particularly lymph nodes, spleen, liver and bone marrow. Treatment is with phototherapy or chemotherapy (e.g. CHOP). Histone deacetylase inhibitors vorinistat and romidepsin are approved for treatment of relapsed and progressive cutaneous T-cell lymphomas. Brentuximab is also useful in CD30⁺ patients.

Sézary syndrome

In Sézary syndrome, there is dermatitis and generalized erythroderma, but also lymphadenopathy and circulating T-lymphoma cells. The cells are usually CD4⁺ and have a folded or cerebriform nuclear chromatin. Initial treatment is by local irradiation, topical chemotherapy or photochemotherapy with psoralen and ultraviolet light (PUVA). Chemotherapy as used for mycosis fungoides may be needed, but is rarely effective for long.

Adult T-cell leukaemia/lymphoma

This is associated with human T-cell leukaemia/lymphoma virus type 1 (HTLV-1) infection (Chapter 18).

Enteropathy-associated T-cell lymphomas

Enteropathy-associated T-cell lymphomas are associated with gluten-induced enteropathy and have a poor response to treatment. Trials using brentuximab, immunotherapy and autografts are in progress.

Anaplastic large cell lymphoma

Anaplastic large cell lymphoma is particularly common in children and is usually of T-cell phenotype. The disease is CD30$^+$ and is usually associated with the t(2;5) (p23;q35) translocation. This leads to overexpression of ALK. It has an aggressive course, characterized by systemic symptoms and extranodal involvement. ALK-negative cases occur and have a worse prognosis. Crizotinib is a specific inhibitor of ALK activity and is a valuable treatment. The anti-CD30 antibody brentuximab is also active. Some cases are seen in association with breast implants.

Extranodal NK/T cell lymphoma

This disease occurs mainly in Asia and Central and South America. It is associated with EBV infection and usually affects the nose ('nasal-type'). The peak age is around 50 years. The disease causes local destruction. It is treated by chemotherapy, usually with local radiotherapy.

Histiocytic and dendritic cell neoplasms

These are rare diseases including dendritic and macrophage-derived sarcomas, which may be localized or disseminated. They usually present as tumours at extranodal sites, especially the intestinal tract, skin and soft tissues. Systemic symptoms are present. The outlook is poor, except for those with small localized tumours who may do well. Langerhans cell histocytosis, a clonal disease of histiocytes, is discussed on page 107.

Castleman disease

This is a rare lymphoproliferative disease that may in some subtypes progress to a B-cell lymphoma. It occurs in localized or multicentric forms, most frequently affecting thoracic or abdominal nodes. **The multicentric form, which is usually associated with systemic symptoms, is most common in subjects with HIV infection** when the cells contain the human herpesvirus-8 (HHV8). Microscopically the localized form usually shows a hyaline vascular appearance, and the multicentric form usually shows proliferation of plasma cell types. Mixed and plasmablastic forms also occur. The localized form may be treated by surgery, the multicentric form by corticosteroids, chemotherapy or immunotherapy.

SUMMARY

- Non-Hodgkin lymphomas are a large group of clonal lymphoid neoplasms. Approximately 85% are of B-cell origin and 15% derive from T or NK cells.
- Their clinical presentation and natural history are more variable than Hodgkin lymphoma and can range from a very indolent disease to rapidly progressive subtypes that need urgent treatment.
- The NHL are divided into low-grade and high-grade disease. Low-grade disorders are typically slowly progressive, respond well to chemotherapy, but are difficult to cure, whereas high-grade lymphomas are aggressive and need urgent treatment, but are more often curable.
- Investigation is with lymph node biopsy, blood tests and imaging, usually by PET/CT. Immunohistochemistry of the lymph node is essential and cytogenetic or gene mutation analysis is helpful in many cases.
- Clinical staging is performed as for Hodgkin lymphoma.
- Some of the more common subtypes are as follows:
  - *Small lymphocytic lymphoma* is the lymphoma equivalent of chronic lymphocytic leukaemia.
  - *Lymphoplasmacytic lymphoma* usually produces an IgM paraprotein, when it is also known as Waldenström macroglobulinaemia, and often leads to anaemia and hyperviscosity.
  - *Marginal zone lymphomas* arise from marginal zone B cells of lymphoid follicles and can occur as mucosa associated (MALT) lymphoma, most frequent in the stomach.
- *Follicular lymphoma* represents 25% of all NHL and is associated with the t(14;18) translocation. Treatment usually achieves disease remission, but the only curative option is allogeneic stem cell transplantation.
- *Mantle cell lymphoma* is associated with increased expression of the cyclin D1 gene and has clinical features of an 'intermediate grade' lymphoma with nodal and leukaemic subtypes.
- *Diffuse large B-cell lymphoma* is a common subtype and is an aggressive disease which needs urgent treatment. There is a wide variety of subtypes. Over 50% of cases are cured.
- *Burkitt lymphoma* is one of the most highly proliferative subtypes of neoplasm. Endemic cases in Africa are associated with EBV infection. Treatment is with aggressive chemotherapy regimens.
- T-cell lymphomas are less common and include *mycosis fungoides*, *peripheral T-cell lymphomas* and *anaplastic large cell lymphoma*.
- Treatments for NHL are based on a variety of chemotherapy regimens. Anti-CD20 antibodies are used in most cases of B-cell lymphomas and have markedly improved the prognosis. Ibrutinib, acalabrutinib and ventoclax are entering front-line regimens, and CAR-T cells directed against CD19 are being increasingly prescribed for relapsed/refractory patients.

 Now visit **www.wileyessential.com/haematology** to test yourself on this chapter.

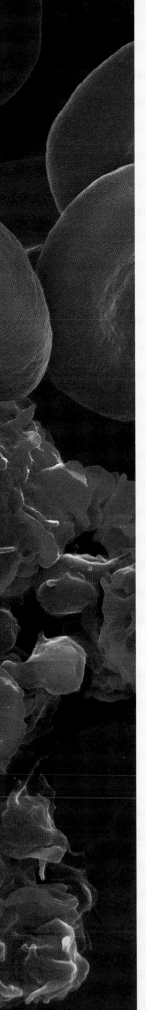

CHAPTER 21
Multiple myeloma and related plasma cell neoplasms

Key topics

Hoffbrand's Essential Haematology, Eighth Edition. By A. Victor Hoffbrand and David P. Steensma.
© 2020 John Wiley & Sons Ltd. Published 2020 by John Wiley & Sons Ltd.
Companion website: www.wileyessential.com/haematology

Paraproteinaemia

Normally, serum immunoglobulins are polyclonal and represent the combined output from billions of different plasma cells making antibodies with diverse antigen specificities. A monoclonal immunoglobulin band (M-protein), or **paraprotein**, reflects the increased synthesis of a specific type of immunoglobulin from a single expanded clone of plasma cells (Fig. 21.1). When a monoclonal immunoglobulin is detected in the blood, it is called **paraproteinaemia**. This may occur as a primary neoplastic disease, or secondary to an underlying benign or neoplastic disease affecting the immune system (Table 21.1).

Usually the monoclonal protein produced by a plasma cell neoplasm is an intact immunoglobulin, but in some cases clonal plasma cells produce only a light chain or heavy chain. A **free light chain** is an immunoglobulin light chain circulating in plasma in a free, unbound state or excreted as such in the urine.

Multiple myeloma

Multiple myeloma, also termed plasma cell myeloma, is a neoplastic disease characterized by plasma cell accumulation in the bone marrow (Fig. 21.2), the presence of monoclonal protein in the serum or urine or both and, in symptomatic patients, related tissue damage (Table 21.2; Fig. 21.3). Other plasma cell neoplasms are listed in Table 21.3.

Almost all cases of myeloma occur over the age of 40 years, with a peak incidence between 65 and 70 years. The disease is twice as common in individuals of African compared to those of European or Asian origin.

Table 21.1 Diseases associated with monoclonal immunoglobulins.

Neoplastic
Multiple myeloma
Solitary plasmacytoma
Monoclonal gammopathy of undetermined significance (MGUS)
Osteosclerotic myeloma and POEMS (polyneuropathy, organomegaly, endocrinopathy, monoclonal protein, skin changes) syndrome
Waldenström's macroglobulinaemia
Non-Hodgkin lymphoma
Chronic lymphocytic leukaemia
Primary (light-chain, AL) amyloidosis
Heavy-chain disease
Cryoglobulinemia (some forms may have polyclonal immunoglobulins, or a mixture of polyclonal and monoclonal)

Non-neoplastic
Chronic cold haemagglutinin disease
Transient (e.g. with infections)
HIV infection
Gaucher disease

Pathogenesis

The myeloma neoplastic cell is a post-germinal centre plasma cell that has undergone immunoglobulin class switching and somatic hypermutation and secretes the paraprotein that is present in serum. Normal plasma cells are located primarily within the bone marrow and this feature is retained by the neoplastic cell.

Myeloma neoplastic cells contain an average of 35 somatic mutations at the time of diagnosis, more than the median number of mutations for leukaemias (Fig. 11.3). Immunoglobulin heavy and light chain genes are recurrently clonally rearranged, with translocations involving the heavy chain on chromosome 14q being the most frequent finding. Neoplastic cells accumulate complex genetic changes, with chromosomal aneuploidy present in almost all cases. Dysregulated or increased expression of the cyclin D1, D2 or D3 genes, either directly through translocations or indirectly via mutations, is an early unifying genetic event. Later genetic events include secondary translocations, e.g. of *MYC*, point mutations, e.g. of *RAS* or *TP53*, deletions, e.g. *TP53*, or epigenetic abnormalities.

Analysis of stored serum samples has shown that **almost all cases of myeloma develop from a pre-existing monoclonal gammopathy of undetermined significance (MGUS)**, described further below (Table 21.2; Fig. 21.3). Like myeloma, MGUS is also more common in persons of African descent. Most of the early plasma cell genetic changes characteristic of myeloma are present at the MGUS stage, but the size of the clone is considerably smaller (Fig. 21.3).

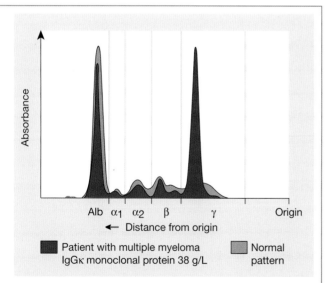

Figure 21.1 Serum protein electrophoresis in multiple myeloma showing an abnormal paraprotein in the γ-globulin region with reduced levels of background β- and γ-globulins.

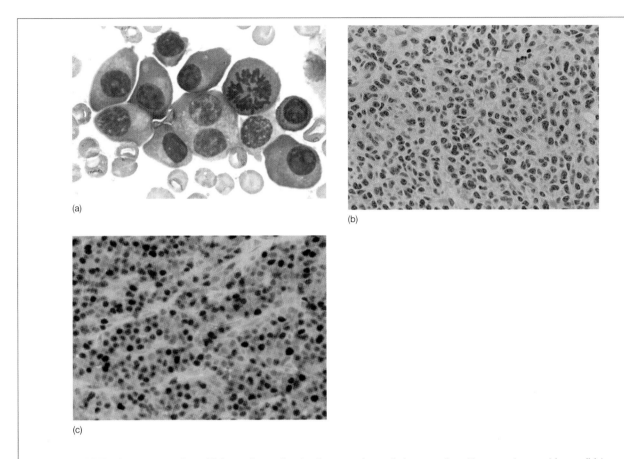

(a)

(b)

(c)

Figure 21.2 (a) The bone marrow in multiple myeloma showing large numbers of plasma cells, with many abnormal forms. **(b)** Low-power view showing sheets of plasma cells replacing normal haemopoietic tissue. **(c)** Immunohistochemical staining of the bone marrow in myeloma with antibody to CD138 revealing extensive numbers of plasma cells.

Table 21.2 The clinical and laboratory features of monoclonal gammopathy of uncertain significance (MGUS), smouldering myeloma and symptomatic myeloma.

	MGUS	Smouldering myeloma	Symptomatic myeloma
Marrow plasma cells	<10%	≥10%	≥10%
Paraprotein	<30 g/L	≥30 g/L	≥30 g/L
Normal immunoglobulins	Normal	Reduced	Reduced
Free light chain ratio	Normal or abnormal	Abnormal	Abnormal
Clinical features	Usually none (see p. 266)	None	Hypercalcaemia C
			Renal failure R
			Anaemia A
			Bone lesions B*
Progression to symptomatic multiple myeloma	1%/year	10%/year	N/A

*Magnetic resonance imaging (MRI) or positron emission tomography (PET) scan needed to exclude bone lesions, especially of the spine, which may not be detected on plain radiographs. Other clinical features include amyloid, hyperviscosity, recurrent infections, peripheral neuropathy and deep vein thrombosis.

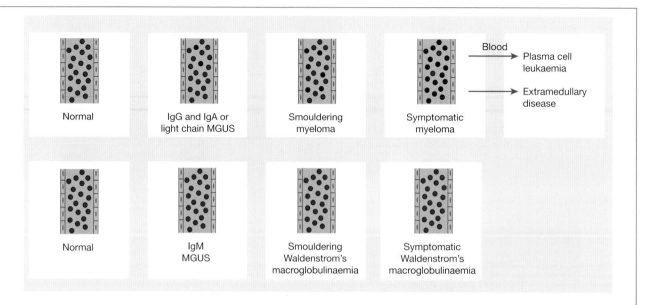

Figure 21.3 The degree of involvement of bone marrow by clonal neoplastic cells in: **(a)** monoclonal gammopathy of undetermined significance (MGUS), smouldering and symptomatic myeloma and plasma cell leukaemia associated with a serum immunoglobin (Ig) G or IgA paraprotein; **(b)** MGUS and Waldenström's macroglobulinaemia (lymphoplasmacytic lymphoma) associated with a serum IgM paraprotein.

Table 21.3 Plasma cell neoplasms (World Health Organization, 2016).

Monoclonal gammopathy of undetermined significance (MGUS), IgM

Monoclonal gammopathy of undetermined significance (MGUS), IgG/IgA
Plasma cell myeloma
Variants:
  Asymptomatic (smouldering) myeloma
  Non-secretory myeloma
  Plasma cell leukaemia

Solitary plasmacytoma of bone
Extraosseous (extramedullary) plasmacytoma
Monoclonal immunoglobulin deposition diseases
Heavy chain deposition diseases (μ heavy-chain disease, γ heavy-chain disease, α heavy-chain disease)

Ig, immunoglobin.

Myeloma cells adhere to bone marrow stromal cells and extracellular matrix through a variety of adhesion molecules. This inhibits their apoptosis and stimulates a cascade of cytokine release. Osteolytic lesions are caused by osteoclast activation resulting from high serum levels of receptor activator of nuclear factor-κB (NF-κB) ligand (RANKL), produced by plasma cells and bone marrow stroma, which binds to activating RANK receptors on the osteoclast surface.

Smouldering myeloma

The term **asymptomatic** or **smouldering myeloma** is used for cases with similar laboratory findings to multiple myeloma, but no organ or tissue damage causing clinical features (Table 21.2). There is about a 10% chance each year of these cases becoming symptomatic and requiring therapy. The risk is greater if there are more than 60% plasma cells in the marrow, circulating plasma cells, a greatly unbalanced free light chain ratio (see below), focal lesions on spinal magnetic resonance imaging (MRI), or certain unfavourable cytogenetic abnormalities. Treatment as for symptomatic myeloma is usually begun if there are more than 60% plasma cells in the marrow, since such patients are at high risk of progression and tissue damage. Clinical trials are assessing whether early therapy of other smouldering or asymptomatic myeloma can improve outcome.

Diagnosis

Symptomatic myeloma is diagnosed if there is:

1 Monoclonal protein in serum, urine, or both (Fig. 21.1);
2 Increased clonal plasma cells in the bone marrow (Fig. 21.2); and
3 Disease-related organ or tissue impairment.

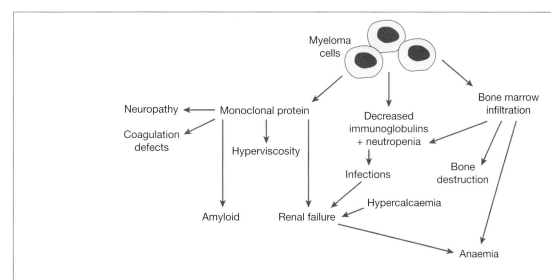

Figure 21.4 The pathogenesis of the clinical features of myeloma.

A useful acronym for myeloma-associated tissue damage is CRAB (hyper**c**alaemia, **r**enal impairment, **a**naemia, **b**one disease; Table 21.2). Amyloidosis, serum hyperviscosity, recurrent infections, peripheral neuropathy and deep vein thrombosis are other clinical complications of myeloma, which are less frequently presenting features (Fig. 21.4).

Clinical features

1 **Bone pain** (especially backache) resulting from vertebral collapse and pathological fractures (Fig. 21.5).
2 Features of **anaemia**, such as lethargy or dyspnea.
3 **Recurrent infections** related to deficient antibody production, abnormal cell-mediated immunity and neutropenia.
4 Features of **renal failure** or hypercalcaemia: polydipsia, polyuria, anorexia, vomiting, constipation and mental disturbance.
5 Abnormal **bleeding** tendency: myeloma protein may interfere with platelet function and coagulation factors; thrombocytopenia occurs in advanced disease.
6 **Amyloidosis** (light chain) occurs in 5% with features such as macroglossia, carpal tunnel syndrome, heart failure, periorbital purpura and diarrhoea.
7 In approximately 2% of cases there is a **hyperviscosity syndrome**, with purpura, haemorrhages, visual changes, central nervous system (CNS) symptoms, neuropathies and heart failure.

Laboratory diagnosis

1 **Presence of a paraprotein.** Serum and urine should be screened by immunoglobulin electrophoresis. The paraprotein is immunoglobulin (Ig) G in 60% of cases, IgA in 20% and light chain only in almost all the rest. Fewer than 1% have IgD or IgE paraprotein, and a similar number are non-secretory, where neither intact immunoglobulin nor light chain can be found in the serum or urine. Mass spectrometry is a new sensitive method of measuring paraproteins and free light chains.

2 **Elevated serum immunoglobulin free light chains.** Immunoglobulin free light chains (FLC) are κ or λ light chain proteins, synthesized by plasma cells, that have not been paired with heavy chain (Fig. 21.6). They are normally made in small quantities and filtered from the serum into the urine by the kidney, but can be measured in serum. Free light chains are produced by almost all malignant plasma cells and so the **serum free light chain** assay is useful in diagnosis and monitoring of myeloma and other forms of malignant paraproteinaemia. Typically in myeloma there is an increase in either the κ or λ serum free light chain value. The normal κ:λ serum free light chain ratio of 0.6 (range 0.26–1.65) is skewed with an excess of either κ or λ chains. Light chain assays have largely replaced the need for analysis of urine paraproteinaemia. Since free light chains are excreted in the urine, their total levels will increase in the presence of renal insufficiency, but the ratio in the absence of a plasma cell neoplasm will usually remain close to normal.

3 Normal serum immunoglobulin levels (IgG, IgA and IgM) are reduced, a feature known as **immunoparesis**. The urine contains free light chains, **Bence Jones protein**, in two-thirds of cases. Rare cases of myeloma are non-secretory and therefore not associated with a paraprotein or Bence Jones proteinuria, although some will still show a disturbed free light chain ratio in the serum.

4 There is usually a normochromic normocytic or macrocytic anaemia. Rouleaux formation is marked in many

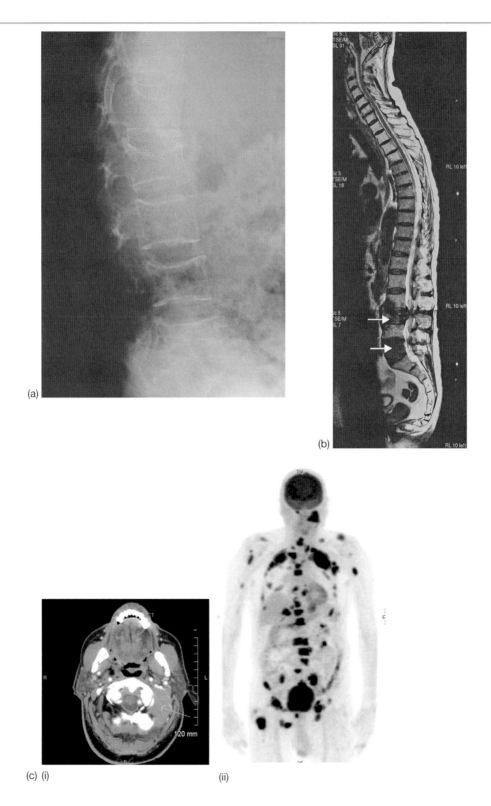

Figure 21.5 (a) Multiple myeloma: X-ray of lumbar spine showing severe demineralization with partial collapse of L_3. **(b)** Magnetic resonance imaging (MRI) of spine: T_2-weighted study. There is infiltration and destruction of L_3 and L_5 with bulging of the posterior part of the body of L_3 into the spinal canal compressing the corda equina (arrowed). Radiotherapy has caused a marrow signal change in vertebrae C_2–D_4 because of replacement of normal red marrow by fat (bright white signal). Source: Courtesy of Dr A. Platts. **(c)** (i) Computed tomography (CT) scan of base of skull showing paravertebral soft tissue extramedullary plasmacytoma (white arrow). (ii) Positron emission tomography (PET) scan of the same patient showing extensive medullary and extramedullary involvement. Source: T. Sher *et al*. (2010) *Br. J. Haematol.* 150(4): 418–27. Reproduced by permission of John Wiley & Sons.

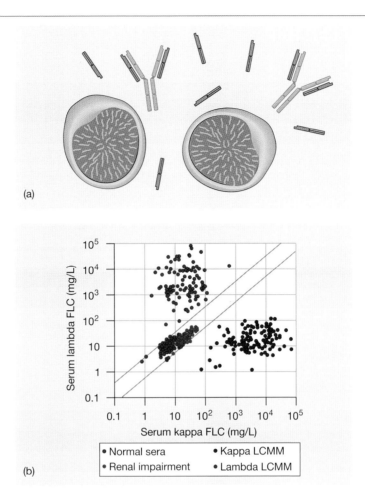

Figure 21.6 The value of serum immunoglobulin free light chain (FLC) measurement in multiple myeloma. **(a)** Serum free light chains are immunoglobulin light chains that are synthesized by plasma cells but not paired with heavy chains before they are released into the blood. Low levels are found in normal individuals and these are increased in patients with myeloma. **(b)** Profile of serum free light chains in healthy controls, patients with renal impairment and those with κ or λ light chain multiple myeloma (LCMM). As light chains are normally filtered by the kidney, their levels rise in patients with renal impairment, although the κ:λ ratio remains normal. Source: Adapted from C. Hutchison (2008) *BMC Nephrology* 9, 11–19 and A.R. Bradwell (2003) *Lancet* 361, 489–91.

cases (Fig. 21.7). Neutropenia and thrombocytopenia occur in advanced disease. Abnormal plasma cells appear in the blood film in 15% of patients and can be detected by sensitive flow cytometry in over 50%.

5 There is a high erythrocyte sedimentation rate (ESR), due to reduction in the normal red cell–repelling 'zeta potential' by immunoglobulin coating of erythrocyte surfaces.

6 There are increased plasma cells in the bone marrow (usually more than 20%), often with abnormal forms (Fig. 21.2). The characteristic **immunophenotype** of malignant plasma cells is CD38^{high}, CD138^{high} and CD45^{low}. Anti-CD138 is used to measure the number of plasma cells in the marrow biopsy (Fig. 21.2).

7 Radiological investigation of the skeleton reveals bone lesions such as osteolytic areas without evidence of surrounding

osteoblastic reaction or sclerosis in 60% of patients (Fig. 21.8) or generalized osteoporosis in 20% (Fig. 21.5). In addition, pathological fractures or vertebral collapse (Fig. 21.5) are common. Skeletal survey X-rays do not detect small lesions. **MRI of the spine** is needed in cases considered as smouldering myeloma in order to detect potential early bone lesions. Positron emission tomography (PET) scan is also a sensitive imaging technique to detect bone damage (Fig. 21.5). Cross-sectional imaging by MRI is best for follow-up of bone disease.

8 Serum calcium elevation occurs in ~45% of patients. Typically, the serum alkaline phosphatase is normal, except following pathological fractures.

9 The serum creatinine is raised in >20% of cases. Proteinaceous deposits from light chain proteinuria, glomerular

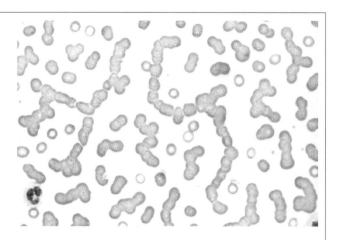

Figure 21.7 The peripheral blood film in multiple myeloma showing rouleaux formations. Rouleaux differ from agglutination in that the former are more linear, the latter typically clumped.

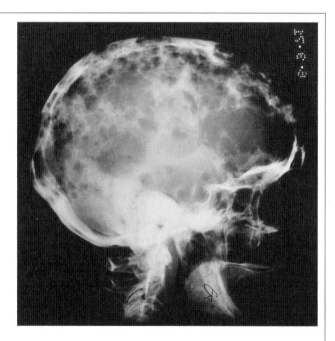

Figure 21.8 Skull X-ray in multiple myeloma showing many 'punched-out' lesions.

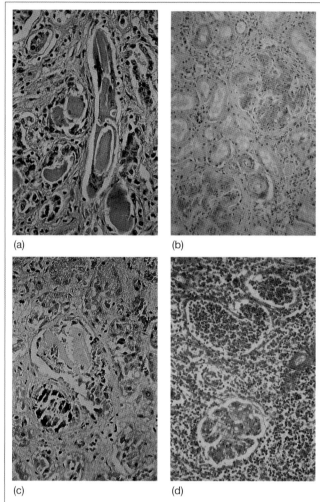

(a) (b)

(c) (d)

Figure 21.9 The kidney in multiple myeloma. **(a)** Myeloma kidney: the renal tubules are distended with hyaline protein (precipitated light chains or Bence–Jones protein). Giant cells are prominent in the surrounding cellular reaction. **(b)** Amyloid deposition: both glomeruli and several of the small blood vessels contain an amorphous pink-staining deposit characteristic of amyloid (Congo red stain). **(c)** Nephrocalcinosis: calcium deposition (dark 'fractured' material) in the renal parenchyma. **(d)** Pyelonephritis: destruction of renal parenchyma and infiltration by acute inflammatory cells.

injury, hypercalcaemia, uric acid, amyloid and pyelone-phritis may all contribute to renal failure (Fig. 21.9).

10 Serum lactate dehydrogenase (LDH) elevation occurs in advanced disease (Table 21.4).

11 A low serum albumin occurs with advanced disease and is a useful indicator of prognosis (Table 21.4).

12 Serum β_2-microglobulin is often raised and is a useful indicator of prognosis (Table 21.4), with higher levels correlating with poorer outcomes.

An International Staging System (ISS) divides patients into three groups, calculated by whether the serum albumin is $\geq$35 g/L or <35 g/L; and whether the serum β_2-microglobulin is <3.5 mg/L, 3.5–5.5 mg/L or >5.5 mg/L. A revised system (R-ISS) also includes chromosome abnormalities and serum LDH (Table 21.4)

Routine karyotype analysis in myeloma is often normal, since plasma cells do not divide rapidly in standard cytogenetic assays. However, interphase fluorescent *in situ* hybridization (FISH) shows that aneuploidy (more or fewer than 46 chromosomes) is almost universal, usually involving odd numbering chromosomes. There is also a high incidence of translocations involving the immunoglobulin heavy-chain gene (*IGH*)

Table 21.4 Standard risk factors for multiple myeloma: the Revised International Staging System (R-ISS).

Prognostic Factor	Criteria
ISS Stage	
■ I	■ Serum β_2-microglobulin <3.5 mg/L, serum albumin ≥35 g/L
■ II	■ Not ISS stage I or III
■ III	■ Serum β_2-microglobulin ≥5.5 mg/L
Chromosome abnormalities (CA) by iFISH	
■ High risk	■ Presence of del(17p) or translocation t(4;14) or t(14;16)
■ Standard risk	■ No high-risk chromosome abnormalities
LDH	
■ Normal	■ Serum LDH ≤ the upper limit of normal
■ High	■ Serum LDH > the upper limit of normal
R-ISS stage	
■ I	■ ISS stage I and standard risk CA by iFISH and normal LDH
■ II	■ Not R-ISS stage I or III
■ III	■ ISS stage III and either high-risk CA by iFISH or high LDH

CA, chromosome abnormalities; iFISH, interphase fluorescent *in situ* hybridization; ISS, International Staging System; LDH, lactate dehydrogenase; R-ISS, revised ISS.
Median overall survival of R-ISS I in a series of 3060 patients was not yet reached at >10 years, while that for R-ISS II was 83 months, and for R-ISS III 43 months.
Source: A. Palumbo *et al.* (2015) *J. Clin. Oncol.* 33: 2863–69. Reproduced with permission of the American Society of Clinical Oncology.

on chromosome 14. The D-cyclin genes are often involved in the translocations. Later-stage cases often have complex cytogenetic findings, as well as more point mutations relevant to progression. These genetic changes may be used (alone or with serum β_2-microglobulin, albumin and LDH) to classify the disease into standard, intermediate and high risk (see Table 21.4 and annotation to Fig. 21.10).

Treatment

This may be divided into specific and supportive (Fig. 21.10; Table 21.5).

Specific

The life expectancy of patients with myeloma has improved markedly in recent years with the introduction of new drugs such as proteasome inhibitors and immunomodulatory agents. The major initial treatment decision is between the use of **intensive combination chemotherapy** (mostly for patients aged less than 70 years, who may be candidates for autologous stem cell transplant, SCT) or **non-intensive therapy** for older patients. Alkylating agents such as melphalan must be avoided in patients who are potential SCT candidates because prolonged use makes stem cells more difficult to harvest.

Intensive therapy
Intensive therapy involves four to six courses of therapy to reduce the tumour burden, usually followed by stem cell collection and either maintenance drug therapy or autologous SCT after high-dose chemotherapy. The initial chemotherapy is given as repeated intravenous or oral chemotherapy cycles combining three drugs with distinct mechanisms of action against tumour cells: bortezomib or one of the newer proteasome inhibitors, lenalidomide or another immunomodulatory agent, and dexamethasone (Table 21.5).

Some commonly used combination therapies for patients who are transplant candidates include:
- VRD or RVD – bortezomib (Velcade), lenalidomide (Revlimid) and dexamethasone.
- KRD – carfilzomib (Kyprolis), lenalidomide and dexamethasone.
- IRD – ixazomib, lenalidomide and dexamethasone.

Other drugs including thalidomide and cyclophosphamide are also effective and still used as cheaper options in poorer countries. Alkylating agents such as melphalan are generally avoided, since their use makes subsequent collection of stem cells difficult.

Trials incorporating newer drugs already found to be effective in relapsed patients – pomalidomide, the anti-CD38 antibody daratumumab and others – are in progress, and these are being incorporated into initial therapy combinations. A four-drug combination in which daratumumab is added to one of the above three-drug regimens is promising with a high rate of complete response, but is very costly.

After several courses of treatment, when the number of tumour cells has been reduced, the patient usually undergoes an autologous SCT. Peripheral blood stem cells are usually collected after mobilization using a combination of chemotherapy and granulocyte colony-stimulating factor (G-CSF). High-dose melphalan is the typical conditioning regimen for SCT. Two consecutive autologous transplants are used in some centres for selected patients. For those who show no

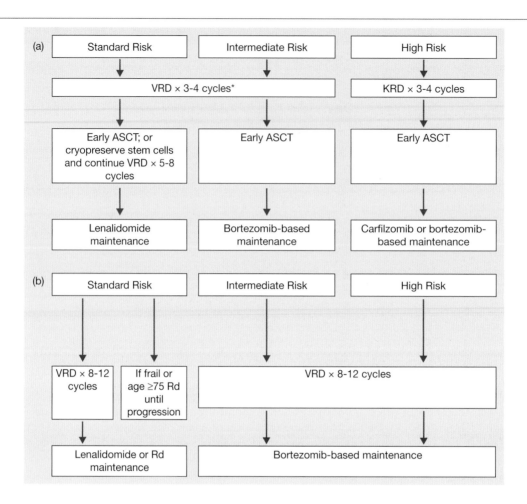

Figure 21.10 Algorithm of potential approaches to the management of multiple myeloma. Treatment approach to the patient with newly diagnosed multiple myeloma who is **(a)** transplant eligible or **(b)** transplant ineligible. Standard risk includes t(11;14), trisomies and t(6;14) and represents about 75% of newly diagnosed patients. Intermediate risk includes t(4;14) or gain of chromosome 1q and includes about 10% of patients. High risk includes t(14;16), t(14;20) and del(17p). Trials of four drug combinations as initial therapy, primarily by adding daratumumab to the triplet therapies listed, are in progress. ASCT, autologous stem cell transplantation; CR, complete response (no measurable disease); KRD, carfilzomib, lenalidomide, dexamethasone; Rd, lenalidomide plus dexamethasone; VGPR, very good partial response (i.e. marked improvement, but minimal disease still detectable); VRD, bortezomib, lenalidomide, dexamethasone. Source: S.V. Rajkumar (2018) *Am. J. Hematol.* 93: 1091–110.

evidence of disease in the marrow by sensitive molecular and immunological tests after the initial courses of chemotherapy, autologous SCT in first remission may have limited or no benefit.

Trials of post-transplant consolidation chemotherapy, especially in high-risk patients, are in progress. Maintenance treatment after autologous SCT with lenalidomide or bortezomib is usual, with combining lenalidomide and bortezomib or carfilzomib for higher-risk patients based on cytogenetics. Thalidomide is a cheaper option for post-transplant maintenance, but with more side effects.

About 10% of patients who have undergone intensive therapy and autologous SCT appear to be cured. The median life expectancy for myeloma has increased from 2–3 years in the 1990s to 8 years or more.

Although **allogeneic stem cell transplantation** may cure the disease, it carries a high procedure-related mortality, so is rarely undertaken. Moreover, patients frequently relapse after the procedure. It is only used in highly selected, multiply relapsed patients.

Non-intensive therapy

Typical options for patients who are not SCT candidates include courses of the oral alkylating agent melphalan in combination with prednisolone and lenalidomide or bortezomib; regimes omitting melphalan are increasingly used. Thalidomide is substituted for lenalidomide in resource-poor countries. Daratumumab may be added. Alternatively, combinations of agents similar to those used in the intensive regimes, such as VCD/ CyBorD (bortezomib, cyclophosphamide and dexamethasone) or RD (lenalidomide and dexamethasone) may be used,

Table 21.5 Treatment of myeloma.

Modality	Examples or indications
Corticosteroids	Dexamethasone, prednisolone, prednisone
Alkylating agents	Cyclophosphamide, melphalan
Proteasome inhibitors	Bortezomib (injectable), carfilzomib (injectable), ixazomib (oral)
Immunomodulators	Lenalidomide, pomalidomide, thalidomide
Monoclonal antibodies	Daratumumab (anti-CD38), elotuzumab (anti-SLAM7); others in development
Histone deacetylase inhibitor	Panobinostat
Cell therapy	Autologous SCT CAR-T cells, anti-BCMA or other myeloma antigens
Radiotherapy	External beam therapy used for painful local lytic lesions or spinal cord/nerve root compression; unstable lesions at risk for fracture (e.g. femoral neck) may also require orthopaedic surgery
Plasmapheresis	Used for acute treatment of hyperviscosity, and for monoclonal gammopathies with clinical consequences (e.g. acquired coagulation factor inhibitors, severe neuropathy)
Supportive care	Biphosphonates (e.g. pamidronate, zoledronic acid) Denusomab (RANKL inhibitor) Intravenous immunoglobulin (for patients with low gamma globulins and recurrent infection) Haemodialysis for severe renal failure

BCL, B cell lymphoma; BCMA, B cell maturation antigen; CAR-T, chimeric antigen receptor T cells; RANKL, receptor activator of nuclear factor κB ligand; SCT, stem cell transplant; SLAM, signalling lymphocytic activation molecule.

even for patients who are not SCT candidates. These protocols are normally given monthly, depending on response, for at least 12–18 months. Typically, paraprotein levels fall after treatment, bone lesions show improvement and blood counts may improve. When treatment is stopped, the patient is seen at regular intervals in the outpatient clinic, and treatment resumed when the M-protein begins to rise.

Relapsed patients

After a variable period of time the disease is likely to progress with rising paraprotein levels and return of symptoms. Further chemotherapy may be given with the above drugs, although the disease becomes increasingly difficult to control. After relapse on lenalidomide maintenance, pomalidomide or carfilzomib may still be effective. In young patients who have relapsed after multiple regimens, allo-SCT can be considered. Local radiotherapy to painful bone lesions can be given where needed. Bendamustine appears to be effective in some relapsed cases, as are the new drugs described above plus the histone deacetylase inhibitor panobinostat. The monoclonal antibodies anti-CD38 (daratumumab) and anti-SLAMF7 (elotuzumab) are also approved for relapsed cases.

The B cell maturation antigen (BCMA) is a transmembrane glycoprotein receptor involved in maturation of B lymphocytes into plasma cells. Antibody–drug conjugates against BCMA show promise. Chimeric antigen receptor (CAR)-T cells (see Chapters 9 and 12) targeted against BCMA and other antigens on myeloma cells may also be highly effective.

Notes on some specific drugs used in myeloma

Thalidomide was the first immune-modulator drug to be used in myeloma. It has a number of side-effects such as sedation, constipation, embryo toxicity, neuropathy, myelosuppression and venous thrombosis (Table 21.2). The addition of dexamethasone increases the response rate, but venous thrombosis becomes a major concern and prophylactic anticoagulation with low molecular weight heparin, a direct oral anticoagulant, warfarin or aspirin is needed if this combination is used. **Lenalidomide** is an analogue of thalidomide and is highly active in the management of myeloma. It is used widely for first-line therapy and for relapsed disease. It is also associated with myelosuppression and increased risk of thrombosis, but causes neuropathy less frequently than thalidomide (Table 21.2). **Pomalidomide** is the most recent addition to this class of drugs and shows a high level of activity against relapsed disease. Like lenalidomide it causes less neuropathy than thalidomide. All of these drugs work by binding to cereblon, a component of the E3 ubiquitin ligase complex, and increasing ubiquitin-mediated proteasome degradation of Ikaros family zinc finger proteins that are important survival factors for plasma cells.

Bortezomib inhibits the cellular proteasome and NF-κB activation. It is highly active in first-line treatment and relapsed disease. Its main side-effect is a neuropathy. **Carfilzomib** is a more recently introduced proteasome inhibitor which is less likely to cause a neuropathy. **Ixazomib** is similar and orally effective.

Monoclonal antibodies include **daratumumab** (anti-CD38) and **elotuzumab** (anti-SLAMF7. They bind to plasma cell-associated antigens and induce killing of tumour cells.

Panobinostat inhibits histone deacetylase and alters the folding of histone-associated chromatin (Fig. 16.1). It changes expression of a variety of genes in plasma cells that may decrease their survival.

Chimeric antigen receptor (CAR)-T cells are also being designed to target myeloma cell-specific antigens such as B-cell maturation antigen (BCMA).

Radiotherapy is useful in treating the symptomatic bone disease in myeloma. It is used for areas of bone pain or spinal cord compression.

Supportive care

Renal impairment It is advisable for patients to drink at least 2–3 L of fluid each day throughout the course of their disease in order to limit the accumulation of paraprotein within the kidney. Some patients present with renal failure and treatment should include rehydration and treatment of contributing factors, such as hypercalcaemia or hyperuricaemia (Fig. 21.9). Dialysis is generally well tolerated if required. Assessment of renal function is important in choosing which drugs to use initially and their doses.

Bone disease and hypercalcaemia Bisphosphonates, such as pamidronate or zoledronic acid, are effective in reducing the progression of bone disease and may also improve overall survival. Denusomab is an inhibitor of RANKL that may be useful in patients who cannot tolerate bisphosphonates due to renal insufficiency. Acute hypercalcaemia is treated with rehydration using isotonic saline, a diuretic and corticosteroids followed by a bisphosphonate.

Compression paraplegia Surgical decompression laminectomy or irradiation are treatments of choice. Chemotherapy and corticosteroid treatment are usually also given.

Anaemia Transfusion or an erythropoiesis-stimulating agent may be used.

Bleeding Bleeding caused by paraprotein interference with coagulation and hyperviscosity syndrome may be treated by repeated plasmapheresis. More durable remission can be obtained with treatment of the underlying disorder.

Infections Rapid treatment of any infection is essential. Prophylactic infusions of immunoglobulin concentrates together with oral broad-spectrum antibiotics and antifungal agents may be needed for recurrent infections in patients with hypogammaglobulinaemia.

Prognosis

The outlook for patients with myeloma is improving markedly. The overall median survival is now 7–10 years and in younger (less than 50 years) patients it is over 10 years with optimum therapy. Patients with high serum β_2-microglobulin ($\geq$5.5 mg/mL), low albumin, raised LDH, extramedullary disease or plasma cell leukaemia, high plasma cell labelling index (now a rarely used test) and certain higher-risk genetic abnormalities – e.g. t(4;14),

1q21 amplification, deletion of 1p or 17p, t(14;16) – tend to have poorer outcomes and therapy is risk-stratified (Fig. 21.10). The achievement of negativity for minimal residual disease (<1 tumour plasma cell in 10×6 bone marrow cells by next generation sequencing) after induction chemotherapy with or without autologous SCT, at the start of maintenance therapy, predicts for excellent progression-free and overall survival.

Other plasma cell neoplasms

Solitary plasmacytoma

These are isolated plasma cell neoplasms, usually involving bones (where they arise from underlying bone marrow) or soft tissue such as the mucosa of the upper respiratory and gastrointestinal tracts or the skin. An associated paraprotein, if present, disappears following radiotherapy to the primary lesion. Many patients will never develop myeloma.

Plasma cell leukaemia

This rare disease is characterized by a high number of circulating malignant plasma cells (Fig. 21.3). The clinical features tend to be a combination of those found in acute leukaemia (pancytopenia and organomegaly) with features of myeloma (hypercalcaemia, renal involvement and bone disease). Treatment is with supportive care and systemic chemotherapy, but prognosis is poor.

Osteosclerotic myeloma (POEMS syndrome)

Osteosclerotic myeloma and POEMS (polyneuropathy, organomegaly, endocrinopathy, monoclonal protein, skin changes) syndrome is a rare condition in which a polyneuropathy is associated with a monoclonal plasma cell disorder and osteosclerotic bone lesions. Elevated levels of vascular endothelial growth factor (VEGF) are present and there are often clinical features such as splenomegaly, hepatomegaly or lymphadenopathy, extravascular fluid overload, endocrine abnormalities, skin changes or Castleman disease.

Monoclonal gammopathy of undetermined significance

Transient or persistent paraproteins can occur in many other conditions as well as in multiple myeloma (Table 21.1). A persistent serum paraprotein may be sometimes be detected without any evidence of myeloma or other underlying disease and is termed **monoclonal gammopathy of undetermined significance (MGUS)**. It is increasingly common with age, being present in 3–4% of persons older than 50 years and more than 10% by age 80 years.

MGUS was formerly called 'benign monoclonal gammopathy', but the recognition of a disease progression risk as well as an increase in incidence of venous and arterial thrombosis, infections, osteoporosis, kidney and skin diseases and bone fractures compared to controls led to adoption of the MGUS term. Rarely, paraneoplastic changes including acquired haemophilia or neuropathy will result from monoclonal proteins with specific antigen binding properties.

The proportion of plasma cells in the marrow in MGUS is normal (less than 4%) or slightly raised (less than 10%; Table 21.2; Fig. 21.3). The concentration of monoclonal immunoglobulin in serum is less than 30 g/L and other serum immunoglobulins are not depressed. The κ or λ light chain is increased in serum in one-third of patients; the greater the imbalance, the more the risk of transformation.

No treatment is needed for most patients unless a complication such as neuropathy or nephropathy occurs. Patients with IgG or IgA MGUS develop overt myeloma at a rate of 1% each year and so are usually followed up regularly in the outpatient clinic. Patients with IgM MGUS are classified separately, as their risk is for development of lymphoplasmacytic lymphoma rather than myeloma, and their risk of progression is higher (Fig. 21.11a). The survival of patients with MGUS is modestly reduced compared with control populations and this effect increases with duration of follow-up and age (Fig. 21.11b).

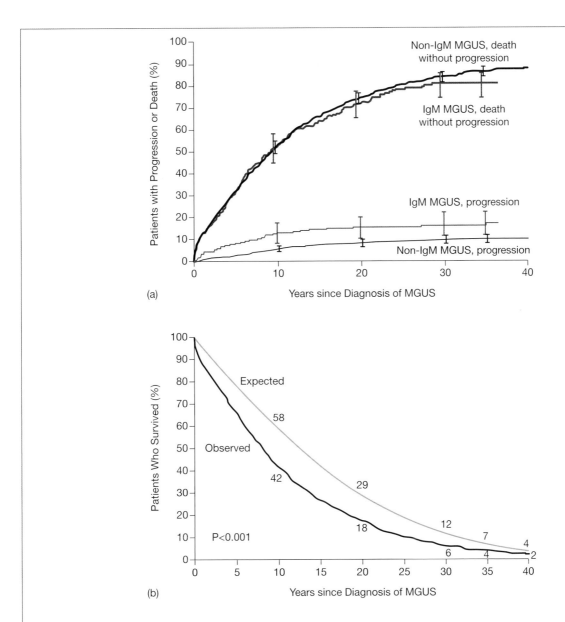

Figure 21.11 (a and b) Survival of patients with monoclonal gammopathy of undetermined significance (MGUS) (*n* = 1384) is reduced compared to the control population; median 8.1 vs 12.4 years, respectively (*p* < 0.001). Among the subset of patients with immunoglobin (Ig) M MGUS, adverse risk factors for progression included an abnormal serum free light-chain ratio and higher serum M protein level (≥1.5 g/dL). Both risk factors were associated with a risk of progression at 20 years of 55%, compared to 41% among patients with one risk factor and 19% among patients with neither risk factor. Source: R.A. Kyle *et al.* (2018) *N. Engl. J. Med.* 378: 241–49. Reproduced with permission of the Massachusetts Medical Society.

Table 21.6 Classification of amyloidosis: types, structure and organ involvement.

Type	Chemical nature	Organs involved
Systemic AL amyloidosis Associated with myeloma, Waldenström's macroglobulinaemia or MGUS May also occur on its own as primary amyloidosis (associated with an occult plasma cell proliferation) May also occur in localized form with local 'immunocyte' proliferation	Immunoglobulin light chains (AL)	Tongue Skin Heart Nerves Connective tissue Kidneys Liver Spleen
Reactive systemic AA amyloidosis Rheumatoid arthritis, tuberculosis, bronchiectasis, chronic osteomyelitis, inflammatory bowel disease, Hodgkin lymphoma, carcinomas, familial Mediterranean fever	Protein A (AA)	Liver Spleen Kidneys Bone marrow
Familial amyloidosis	e.g. Transthyretin abnormalities (many varieties exist)	Nerves Heart Eyes
Localized amyloidosis Central nervous system Endocrine Senile	β-Amyloid protein Peptic hormones Various	Alzheimer's disease Endocrine tumours Heart, brain, joints, prostate, etc.

MGUS, monoclonal gammopathy of undetermined significance.

Amyloidosis

The amyloidoses are a heterogeneous group of disorders characterized by the extracellular deposition of protein in an abnormal fibrillar form (Table 21.6). Amyloidosis may be hereditary or acquired, and deposits may be focal, localized or systemic in distribution. Whereas in reactive systemic AA amyloid the dominant organs involved are the liver, spleen, kidneys and bone marrow, in systemic amyloid light chain (AL) amyloidosis and in the inherited amyloidoses, as well as these organs (Fig. 21.12), the heart, nerves, tongue (Fig. 21.13), skin and eyes are often involved and cardiac amyloid is most frequently the dominant cause of morbidity and death. The amyloid is made from different amyloid fibril precursor proteins in each type of disease. Except for intracerebral amyloid plaques, all amyloid deposits contain a non-fibrillary glycoprotein amyloid P, which is derived from a normal serum precursor structurally related to C-reactive protein (CRP). The classic diagnostic histological test is red–green birefringence after staining with Congo red and viewing under polarized light (Fig. 21.14).

Systemic amyloid light chain amyloidosis

Systemic AL amyloidosis is caused by deposition of monoclonal light chains produced from a clonal plasma cell proliferation. The mutational landscape of the clonal plasma cells is similar to that of myeloma. The level of paraprotein may be very low and is not always detectable in serum or urine, but the serum free light chain ratio is usually abnormal (Fig. 21.6). The clinical features are caused by involvement of the heart in more than 50% of patients, usually with a restrictive cardiomyopathy, kidneys in 30% (Figure 21.9), tongue (Fig. 21.13), gastrointestinal tract, peripheral nerves and autonomic nervous system (Fig. 21.9). The patient may present with non-specific symptoms such as fatigue, anorexia or weight loss, or with heart failure, renal failure including the nephrotic syndrome, macroglossia, peripheral neuropathy or carpal tunnel syndrome. Cardiac MRI is used to detect and monitor cardiac amyloid, often showing asymmetric left ventricular hypertrophy. A serum amyloid P (SAP) scan (Fig. 21.14) can be used to determine the extent and severity of disease.

Four prognostic stages are based on the levels in serum of N-terminal prohormone of brain natriuretic peptide (NT-proBNP), cardiac troponin and the difference between the involved and the uninvolved free light chains. In Stage 0, none of these is abnormal (as defined for the staging), though the exact level of NT-proBNP still has prognostic value. In Stage 4, with the poorest prognosis, all three are abnormal.

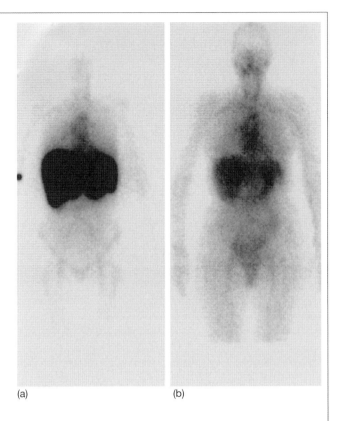

(a)   (b)

Figure 21.12 Serial anterior whole body ^{123}I-labelled serum amyloid P component (SAP) scans of a 52-year-old woman who presented with renal failure resulting from systemic AL amyloidosis. **(a)** The initial scan demonstrates a large amyloid load with hepatic, splenic, renal and bone marrow deposits. The underlying plasma cell dyscrasia responded to high-dose melphalan followed by autologous stem cell rescue. **(b)** Follow-up SAP scintigraphy 3 years after chemotherapy showed greatly reduced uptake of tracer, indicating substantial regression of her amyloid deposits. Source: Courtesy of Professor P.N. Hawkins, National Amyloidosis Centre, Royal Free Hospital, London.

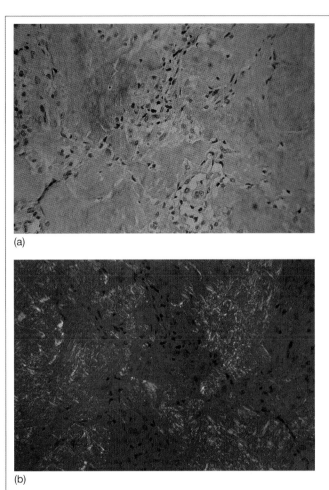

(a)

(b)

Figure 21.14 Amyloidosis. **(a)** Congo red staining and **(b)** blue–green birefringence under polarized light.

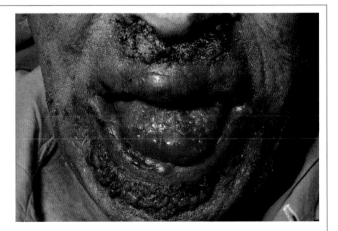

Figure 21.13 Multiple myeloma: the tongue and lips are enlarged because of nodular and waxy deposits of amyloid.

The more widely available brain natriuretic protein test may be substituted for NT-proBNP. Treatment is with combination chemotherapy similar to that used in myeloma, possibly with autologous SCT, which may improve prognosis. Patients are, however, more at risk of serious side-effects than those with myeloma, especially if there is cardiac or renal involvement.

Hyperviscosity syndrome

Hyperviscosity may occur in patients with myeloma or Waldenström macroglobulinaemia or in polycythaemia. A related condition, hyperleucocytosis, can affect patients with chronic myeloid or acute leukaemias associated with very high white cell counts. The clinical features of the hyperviscosity syndrome include visual disturbances, lethargy, confusion, muscle weakness, nervous system symptoms and signs, and congestive heart failure. The retina may show a variety of changes: engorged veins sometimes with

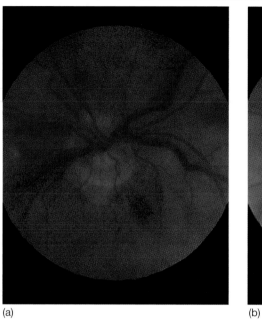
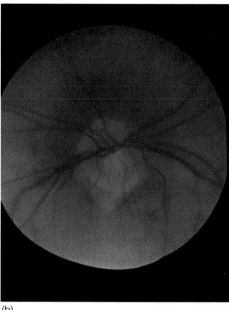

(a) (b)

Figure 21.15 Hyperviscosity syndrome in Waldenström's macroglobulinaemia. **(a)** The retina before plasmapheresis shows distension of retinal vessels, particularly the veins, which show bulging and constriction (the 'linked sausage' effect) and areas of haemorrhage. **(b)** Following plasmapheresis the vessels have returned to normal and the areas of haemorrhage have cleared.

sausage-like changes, haemorrhages, exudates and a blurred disc (Fig. 21.15).

Emergency treatment varies with the cause:

1 Correct dehydration in all patients, but do not transfuse unless absolutely necessary.

2 Venesection or isovolaemic exchange with a plasma substitute for red cells in a polycythaemic patient.

3 Plasmapheresis in myeloma, Waldenström's disease or hyperfibrinogenaemia.

4 Leucopheresis or chemotherapy in leukaemias associated with high white cell counts.

The long-term treatment depends on control of the primary disease with specific therapy.

SUMMARY

- The term *paraproteinaemia* refers to the presence of a monoclonal immunoglobulin band in serum, and reflects the synthesis of immunoglobulin or portion of an immunoglobulin from a single clone of plasma cells.
- Multiple myeloma is a neoplasm of plasma cells that accumulate usually to >20% of cells in the bone marrow, in >98% of cases release a paraprotein and/or an excess kappa or lambda immunoglobulin light chain which can cause tissue damage. The disease has a peak incidence in the seventh decade.
- Almost all cases of myeloma develop from a pre-existing *monoclonal gammopathy of undetermined significance* (MGUS) in which there is low-level paraprotein and no evidence of tissue damage. Approximately 1% of cases progress to myeloma each year.
- A useful reminder for the spectrum of tissue damage in symptomatic myeloma is *CRAB* – hyper**c**alaemia, **r**enal impairment, **a**naemia, **b**one disease (lytic lesions or osteoporosis).

- *Smouldering myeloma* describes patients with bone marrow and protein findings of myeloma but without CRAB or other clinical symptoms or findings.
- In patients younger than 70 years, symptomatic myeloma is usually treated by intensive chemotherapy with a three-drug combination followed by an autologous stem cell transplant, using stem cells harvested from the patient.
- In older patients chemotherapy without autologous SCT is used.
- Immunomodulatory drugs (thalidomide, lenalidomide, pomalidomide) and proteasome inhibitory drugs (bortezomib, ixazomib, carfilzomib), usually used in combination with dexamethasone, are improving the outlook for patients and median survival is now 7–10 years. Monoclonal antibodies including daratumumab (anti-CD38) and elotuzumab (anti-SLAM7) and the histone deacetylase inhibitor panbinostat are also approved. CAR-T cells against BCMA or other plasma cell-associated antigens are highly active.

■ A *plasmacytoma* is a localized mass of malignant plasma cells and is usually treated with radiotherapy. Many cases progress to myeloma.

■ *Amyloidoses* are caused by extracellular deposition of protein in an abnormal fibrillar form. Systemic AL amyloid disease is caused by monoclonal light chains produced from a clonal plasma cell proliferation and may cause heart failure, macroglossia, peripheral neuropathy or renal failure.

■ *Hyperviscosity syndrome* may occur in paraproteinaemia or in patients with a very high red cell count. Clinical features include visual disturbances, confusion and heart failure. Venesection, plasma exchange or chemotherapy may be required.

Now visit **www.wileyessential.com/haematology** to test yourself on this chapter.

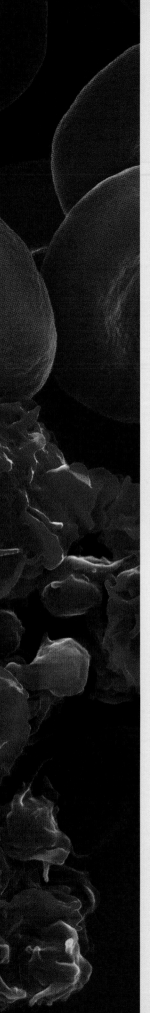

CHAPTER 22
Aplastic anaemia and bone marrow failure

Key topics

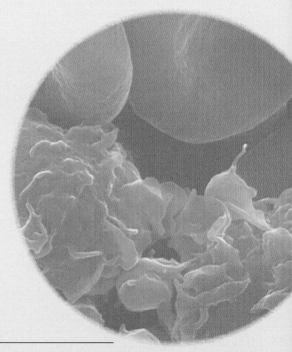

Hoffbrand's Essential Haematology, Eighth Edition. By A. Victor Hoffbrand and David P. Steensma.
© 2020 John Wiley & Sons Ltd. Published 2020 by John Wiley & Sons Ltd.
Companion website: www.wileyessential.com/haematology

Pancytopenia

Pancytopenia is a reduction in the blood count of all the major cell lines – red cells, white cells and platelets. Pancytopenia has several causes (Table 22.1), which can be broadly divided into decreased bone marrow production or increased peripheral destruction of blood cells. One cell line may be affected to a greater degree than the others.

Aplastic anaemia

Aplastic (hypoplastic) anaemia is defined as pancytopenia resulting from hypoplasia of the bone marrow (Fig. 22.1). It can be classified into primary (congenital or acquired) or secondary types (Table 22.2).

Pathogenesis

The underlying defect in all cases appears to be a substantial reduction in the number of haemopoietic pluripotential stem cells, and a fault in the remaining stem cells or an immune reaction against them, which makes them unable to divide and differentiate sufficiently to populate the bone marrow and blood.

Congenital marrow failure syndromes: Fanconi anaemia

Fanconi anaemia (FA) usually has an autosomal recessive pattern of inheritance and is often associated with growth retardation and congenital defects of the skeleton (e.g. microcephaly, absent radii or thumbs), of the renal tract (e.g. pelvic or horseshoe kidney; Fig. 22.2) or skin (areas of hyper- and hypopigmentation). Sometimes there is learning disability, but most often intelligence is normal. **The syndrome is genetically heterogeneous with at least 16 different genes involved:** *FANC A–Q*. *FANCD1* is identical to *BRCA2*, the breast cancer susceptibility gene. The proteins coded for by these genes cooperate in a common

Table 22.1 Causes of pancytopenia.
Decreased bone marrow function (but marrow still cellular), e.g. during an acute infection
Aplastic anaemia
Acute leukaemia, myelodysplastic syndromes
Infiltration with lymphoma, myeloma, metastatic solid tumours, tuberculosis
Megaloblastic anaemia
Paroxysmal nocturnal haemoglobinuria
Myelofibrosis, both primary (myeloproliferative neoplasm) and reactive
Haemophagocytic lymphohistiocytosis
Increased peripheral destruction (e.g. due to a microangiopathic process)
Splenomegaly

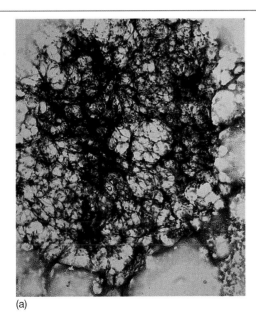
(a)

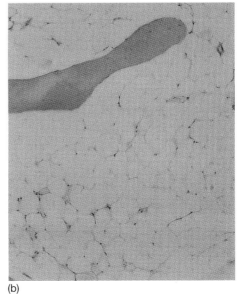
(b)

Figure 22.1 Aplastic anaemia: low power views of bone marrow show severe reduction of haemopoietic cells with an increase in fat spaces. **(a)** Aspirated fragment showing primarily stromal elements with absent haemopoietic cells. **(b)** Trephine biopsy.

Table 22.2 Causes of aplastic anaemia.

Primary	Secondary
Congenital (Fanconi anaemia, other inborn marrow failure syndromes)	*Ionizing radiation*: accidental exposure (radiotherapy, radioactive isotopes)
Idiopathic acquired, usually with an autoimmune pathophysiology	*Chemicals*: benzene, organophosphates and other organic solvents, DDT and other pesticides, recreational drugs (ecstasy) *Drugs*: Those that regularly cause marrow depression (e.g. busulphan, melphalan, cyclophosphamide, anthracyclines, nitrosoureas) Those that occasionally or rarely cause marrow depression (e.g. chloramphenicol, sulphonamides, gold, anti-inflammatory, antithyroid, psychotrophic, anticonvulsant/antidepressant drugs)
	Viruses: viral hepatitis (non-A, non-B, non-C, and non-G in most cases), EBV, other undefined viruses
	Autoimmune diseases: systemic lupus erythematosus
	Transfusion associated GVHD (see Chapter 23)
	Thymoma (this is more usually associated with red cell aplasia)

DDT, dichlorodiphenyltrichloroethane; EBV, Epstein–Barr virus; GVHD, graft-versus-host disease.

cellular pathway which results in ubiquitination of the FAN-CD2:FANCI dimer, which is important for normal DNA repair and protects cells against genetic damage. **Cells from FA patients show an abnormally high frequency of spontaneous chromosomal breakage**, and the diagnostic test is elevated breakage after incubation of peripheral blood lymphocytes with a DNA cross-linking agent such as diepoxybutane (DEB test) or mitomycin C.

The usual age of presentation of FA is 3–14 years, but some patients present in adulthood. Approximately 10% of patients develop myelodysplastic syndromes (MDS) or acute myeloid leukaemia (AML). Treatment is usually with androgens or stem cell transplantation (SCT).

The blood count usually improves with androgens, but side-effects, especially in children, can be distressing, including virilization and liver abnormalities; remission

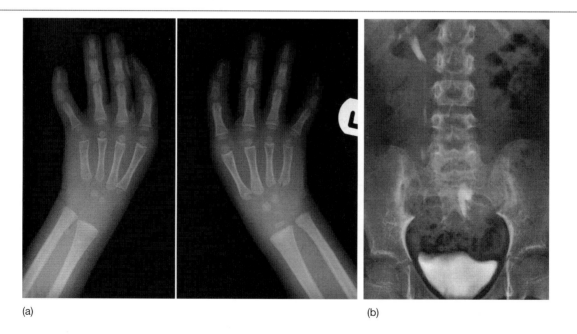

(a) (b)

Figure 22.2 (a) X-rays showing absent thumbs in a patient with Fanconi anaemia (FA). **(b)** Intravenous pyelogram in a patient with FA showing a normal right kidney but a left kidney abnormally placed in the pelvis.

with androgens rarely lasts more than 2 years. SCT may cure the patient of the marrow failure, but the risk for epithelial cancers continues to be increased and growth retardation and other congenital defects are not influenced. Because of the sensitivity of the patient's cells to DNA damage, conditioning regimes for SCT in FA patients are mild and irradiation is avoided.

Dyskeratosis congenita

Dyskeratosis congenita (DKC) is a rare disorder characterized by **a classic triad of nail dystrophy, lacy reticular pigmentation of the upper chest and neck, and oral leukoplakia.** There is a high risk of pulmonary fibrosis, cirrhosis, osteoporosis, marrow failure and epithelial cancer (e.g. oral, oesophageal, uterine cervix).

It is associated with mutations in the *DKC1* (dyskerin), *TERC* (telomerase reverse transcriptase RNA template), *TERT* or other genes encoding components of telomerase, an enzyme complex which is involved in the maintenance of telomere length. Milder forms of telomere shortening can result in components of the syndrome without the characteristic nail and skin findings.

Diagnosis is by measuring length of lymphocyte telomeres (granulocyte telomeres can also shorten in acquired marrow failure syndromes) and by genetic testing for mutations in telomere complex genes. Androgens can be helpful in improving blood counts and may lengthen telomeres. SCT can cure the marrow failure, but transplanted patients are still at risk for epithelial cancer and cirrhosis or pulmonary fibrosis.

Shwachman–Diamond syndrome

Shwachman–Diamond syndrome (SDS) is a rare autosomal recessive syndrome characterized by varying degrees of cytopenia, especially neutropenia with a propensity to transform to MDS or AML. Exocrine pancreatic dysfunction is a common feature, while skeletal abnormalities, hepatic impairment and short stature are frequent. The disorder results from inherited mutations in the gene *SBDS*, involved in ribosome assembly (see Fig. 22.6).

Other congenital marrow failure syndromes

Germline mutations of the *GATA2* transcription factor can cause pancytopenia, a hypoplastic marrow and predisposition to MDS or AML. *GATA2* mutations are also associated with warts, monocytopenia and lymphoedema; this syndrome's presentation is highly variable. Mutations of the gene for cytotoxic T-lymphocyte-associated antigen (*CTLA4*) also cause marrow failure and immune dysregulation. Germline mutations of the thrombopoietin gene (*MPL*) have been found more recently to cause bone marrow failure.

Other inherited bone marrow failure syndromes include Diamond–Blackfan anaemia (DBA; p. 278), severe congenital neutropenia (p. 104), amegakaryocytic thrombocytopenia

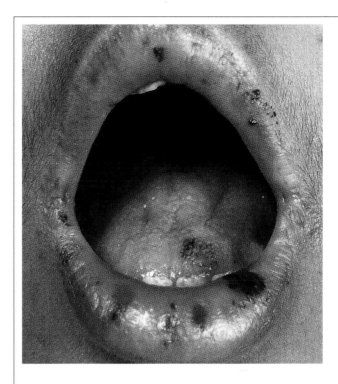

Figure 22.3 Aplastic anaemia: spontaneous mucosal haemorrhages in a 10-year-old boy with severe Fanconi anaemia. Platelet count <5×10⁹/L. Source: A.V. Hoffbrand *et al.* (2019) *Color Atlas of Clinical Hematology*, 5th edn. Reproduced by permission of John Wiley & Sons.

(p. 315) and thrombocytopenia with absent radii (p. 315). In DBA and SDS there are genetic defects in ribosomal biosynthesis and function (Fig. 22.3).

Idiopathic acquired aplastic anaemia

This is the dominant type of aplastic anaemia, accounting for at least two-thirds of acquired cases. In most, haemopoietic tissue is the target of an autoimmune process with oligoclonal expression of cytotoxic CD8⁺ T cells, possibly initiated by an infection or an acquired mutation in the STAT3 signalling pathway. Clonal haemopoiesis occurs in 50% of cases with somatic mutations of genes including *PIGA*, *BCOR*, *BCORL1*, *ASXL1*, *RUNX1* or *DNMT3A*, or loss of human leukocyte antigen (HLA) class I expression. This clonal haemopoiesis presumably arises by selection for survival of pre-existing clones in a failed marrow.

The disease may be difficult to distinguish from a late onset of a congenital form of aplastic anaemia and from hypoplastic MDS. Mutations of the telomere repair complex and short telomeres may be present, apparently as acquired abnormalities. The favourable responses to anti-lymphocyte globulin (ALG)/ anti-thymocyte globulin (ATG) and ciclosporin support the concept of an autoimmune disorder.

Secondary causes

Aplastic anaemia may also be caused by direct damage to the haemopoietic marrow by radiation or cytotoxic drugs. The antimetabolite drugs (e.g. methotrexate) and mitotic inhibitors (e.g. daunorubicin) cause only temporary aplasia, but the alkylating agents, particularly busulphan, may cause a more prolonged aplasia closely resembling idiopathic aplastic anaemia. **Some individuals develop aplastic anaemia as a rare idiosyncratic side-effect of drugs such as chloramphenicol or gold (Table 22.2).**

Patients may also develop the disease during or within a few months of **viral hepatitis** (most frequently negative for all known hepatitis viruses). Because the incidence of marrow toxicity is particularly high for chloramphenicol, this drug should be reserved for treatment of infections that are life-threatening and for which it is the optimum antibiotic (e.g. typhoid). **Chemicals** such as benzene may be implicated and, rarely, aplastic anaemia may be a presenting feature of acute lymphoblastic or myeloid leukaemia, especially in childhood. MDS (see Chapter 15) may also present with a hypoplastic marrow, and distinction of hypoplastic MDS from aplastic anaemia may be difficult, especially given the presence of clonal mutations in many patients with aplastic anaemia and occasional responses to immunosuppressive therapy in MDS.

Clinical features

The onset is at any age, with bimodal peak incidences around 10–25 and over 60 years. It is more frequent in Asia, e.g. China or Vietnam, than in Europe or the Americas. It can be insidious or acute, with symptoms and signs resulting from anaemia, neutropenia or thrombocytopenia. Bruising, bleeding gums, epistaxes and menorrhagia are the most frequent haemorrhagic manifestations and the usual presenting features (Fig. 22.3), often with symptoms of anaemia. Retinal haemorrhage may impair vision. Infections, particularly of the mouth and throat, are common and generalized infections are frequently life threatening. The lymph nodes, liver and spleen are not enlarged. A careful history and examination, e.g. for bone deformities, are needed at all ages to exclude inherited forms.

Laboratory findings

1 In aplastic anaemia, there must be at least two of the following:
   - **Anaemia (haemoglobin <100 g/L).** This is normochromic, normocytic or macrocytic, with mean cell volume (MCV) often 95–110 fL. The reticulocyte count is usually extremely low in relation to the degree of anaemia.
   - **Neutrophil count <1.5 × 10⁹/L.**
   - **Platelet count <50 × 10⁹/L.**
   Severe cases are defined by neutrophils <0.5 × 10⁹/L and platelets <20 × 10⁹/L, reticulocytes <20 × 10⁹/L and marrow cellularity <25%. Very severe cases also show neutrophils <0.2 × 10⁹/L.

2 **There are no abnormal cells in the peripheral blood that would indicate leukaemia.**
3 **The bone marrow shows hypoplasia**, with loss of haemopoietic tissue and replacement by fat which comprises over 75% of the marrow. Trephine biopsy may show patchy cellular areas in a hypocellular background. The main cells present are lymphocytes and plasma cells; megakaryocytes in particular are severely reduced or absent.
4 Cytogenetic and, more recently, molecular analysis is performed to exclude inherited forms or MDS. Aplastic anaemia cases may occasionally exhibit numerical chromosomal abnormalities such as monosomy 7 or trisomy 8, but usually the karyotype is normal. *PIGA*, *BCOR* and *BCORL1* mutations predict for a better prognosis and higher likelihood of response to immunosuppressive therapy, while mutations of *ASXL1*, *RUNX1* and splicing factor genes and short leucocyte telomeres predict lower response rates and higher likelihood of progression to MDS/AML.

Diagnosis

The disease must be distinguished from other causes of pancytopenia (Table 22.1). The assessment of disease severity is also important in treatment decisions and prognosis.

Paroxysmal nocturnal haemoglobinuria (PNH), discussed further below, must be excluded by flow cytometry testing. Large granular lymphocytic leukaemia (Chapter 18) may also be associated with pancytopenia and a hypoplastic marrow.

Treatment

This is best carried out in a specialized centre.

General

If a primary cause such as a drug has been identified, this is removed. Initial management consists largely of supportive care with blood transfusions, platelet concentrates, and treatment and prevention of infection. All blood products should be leucodepleted, to reduce the risk of alloimmunization, and irradiated, to prevent grafting of live donor lymphocytes. An antifibrinolytic agent (e.g. tranexamic acid) may be used to reduce haemorrhage in patients with severe prolonged thrombocytopenia. If a patient is a transplant candidate, transfusions prior to transplant should be minimized. Granulocyte transfusions are rarely used, but may be given to patients with severe bacterial or fungal infections not responding to antibiotics. Oral antibacterial and antifungal drugs may be used to reduce infections.

Specific

This must be tailored to the severity of the illness as well as the age of the patient and availability of stem cell donors. Severe cases have a high mortality in the first 6–12 months unless they respond to specific therapy. Less severe cases may have an acute transient course or a chronic course with ultimate recovery, although the platelet count often remains subnormal for many years. Relapses, sometimes severe and occasionally fatal, may also occur and rarely the disease transforms into MDS, AML or PNH (see below).

The following 'specific' treatments are used with varying success:

1 ***Anti-thymocyte globulin*** (ATG), also called anti-lymphocyte globulin (ALG). This is prepared by immunizing animals (usually horse or rabbit in the West, pig in China) with human thymocytes and alone is of benefit in approximately 50–60% of acquired cases. It is usually given with ciclosporin. Eltrombopag may improve the rate of response. Corticosteroids are given short term to reduce the immediate allergic effects and the incidence and severity of serum sickness (fever, rash and joint pains) which may occur approximately 7 days after administration. The platelet count should be maintained $>10 \times 10^9/L$. If there is no response to ATG after 3–4 months a second course may be tried, prepared from the same or another species. Overall, up to 80% of patients respond to combined ATG and ciclosporin. A randomized trial showed superiority of horse ATG to rabbit ATG, most likely because the latter is more lympho-depleting and increases infection risk. Patients with certain clonal mutations (*PIGA, BCOR, BCORL1*) are more likely to respond to ATG-based therapy, while those with other mutations (*DNMT3A*, other myeloid neoplasia-associated variants) are less likely to respond.

2 ***Ciclosporin*** This is an effective agent which appears particularly valuable in combination with ATG. In older subjects it is sometimes used alone. Some centres substitute tacrolimus, which may have fewer adverse events.

3 ***Eltrombopag*** This is a thrombomimetic (see Chapter 25) which stimulates platelet production, but may also result in a durable improvement in red cell and neutrophil counts. It is useful in some ATG-resistant cases. Eltrombopag in combination with ATG and ciclosporin may lead to more rapid improvement of blood counts, so this three-drug combination is likely to become the preferred first-line treatment for most severe cases.

4 ***Alemtuzumab*** (anti-CD52 antibody) This has proved effective in about 50% of patients in small studies, but is toxic and so is only used if at all, after ATG and other therapies have failed.

5 ***Androgens*** These are beneficial in improving blood counts in some patients, but do not improve survival. Side-effects from chronic use are marked, including virilization, salt retention and liver damage with cholestatic jaundice or rarely hepatocellular carcinoma. If there is no response in 4–6 months, androgens should be stopped. If there is a response, the drug should be withdrawn gradually.

6 ***Stem cell transplantation*** (SCT) Allogeneic SCT offers the chance of permanent cure in selected patients. It is the only cure for constitutional bone marrow failure syndromes. Conditioning in idiopathic aplastic anaemia is typically with cyclophosphamide without irradiation, and ciclosporin is used to reduce the risks of graft failure and graft-versus-host disease (GVHD; see Fig. 23.4). The relative role of SCT versus immunosuppressive therapy in individuals with acquired aplastic anaemia is under constant review. In general, SCT is favoured in patients less than 35 years old with severe aplastic anaemia and an HLA matching sibling donor. Cure rates of more than 90% in young children and more than 80% in adolescents are obtained, but with a survival rate of about 50% in those older than 40 years. Marrow rather than peripheral blood is the preferred source of stem cells, since the risk of GVHD is lower with marrow grafts.

Non-myeloablative transplants (p. 285) are used in congenital aplastic anaemia and for selected patients with acquired idiopathic aplastic anaemia over the age of 40 years. SCT using umbilical cord blood, unrelated volunteer donors and haplo-identical family members is used in carefully selected patients. *In vivo* T cell depletion and high-dose cyclophosphamide a few days after the stem cell infusion reduce the risk of severe GVHD. In older subjects and those with less severe disease, immunosuppression is tried first and SCT reserved for cases of immunosuppression failure.

7 ***Haemopoietic growth factors*** Granulocyte colony-stimulating factor (G-CSF) may produce minor responses, but does not lead to sustained improvement. Other growth factors besides eltrombopag have not proved helpful.

8 ***Iron chelation therapy*** This may be needed in patients who require regular red cell transfusion.

Paroxysmal nocturnal haemoglobinuria

Paroxysmal nocturnal haemoglobinuria (PNH) is a rare, acquired, clonal disorder of marrow stem cells in which there is deficient synthesis of the glycosylphosphatidylinositol (GPI) anchor, a structure that attaches several surface proteins to the cell membrane. This deficiency results in the clinical triad of chronic intravascular haemolysis, venous thrombosis and bone marrow failure. PNH results from acquired mutations in the X chromosome gene coding for phosphatidylinositol glycan protein class A (*PIGA*), which is essential for the formation of the GPI anchor (Fig. 22.4). The net result is that GPI-linked proteins (such as CD55 and CD59) are absent from the cell surface of all the cells derived from the abnormal stem cell (Fig. 22.4), including white cells and platelets. The lack of the surface molecules decay-activating factor (DAF, CD55) and membrane inhibitor of reactive lysis (MIRL, CD59) renders red cells sensitive to lysis by complement, which is normally cleared from the surface of cells by these factors, and the result is **chronic intravascular haemolysis**.

Haemosiderinuria is a constant feature of PNH and can give rise to iron deficiency, which may exacerbate the anaemia. The haemolysis is typically continuous and rarely paroxysmal or limited to the nocturnal period, despite the name of the condition. Haptoglobins are absent; free haemoglobin may damage the kidney and it removes nitric oxide from smooth muscle, causing oesophageal spasm and dysphagia, erectile dysfunction and pulmonary hypertension.

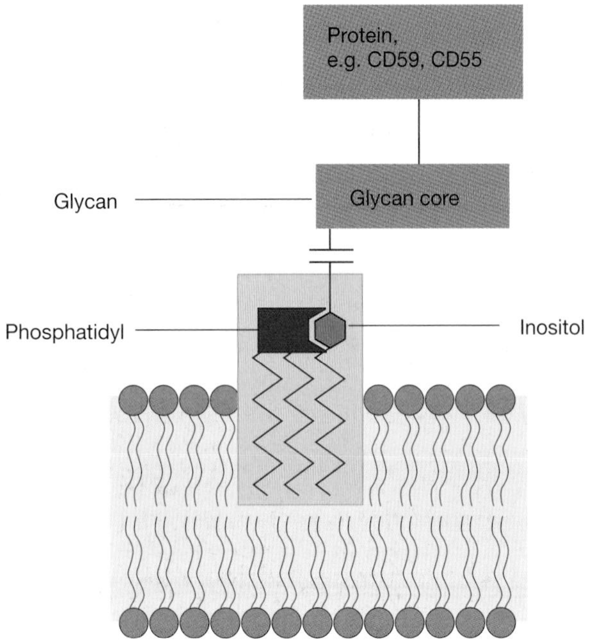

Protein,
e.g. CD59, CD55

Glycan

Glycan core

Phosphatidyl

Inositol

Figure 22.4 Schematic representation of the phosphatidylinositol glycan which anchors many different proteins to the cell membrane, e.g. CD59 (MIRL, membrane inhibitor of reactive lysis).

The other main clinical problem in PNH is of **venous thrombosis**. Patients may develop recurrent thromboses in any venous distribution including large vessels, such as the portal, hepatic and mesenteric veins and dural sinuses. Arterial thrombosis, such as strokes or myocardial infarction, can also occur. Intermittent abdominal pain due to mesenteric vein thrombosis is a common feature.

PNH is almost invariably associated with some form of bone marrow hypoplasia and there may even be complete aplastic anaemia. The PNH clone may expand as a result of a selective pressure, possibly immunologically mediated, against cells that have normal GPI-linked membrane proteins.

PNH is diagnosed by flow cytometry, which shows loss of expression of the GPI-linked proteins CD55 and CD59 or the fluorescent aerolysin (FLAER), this dye binding to normal but not to PNH cells.

Eculizumab and Ravulizumab are humanized antibody against complement C5 which inhibit the activation of terminal

components of complement and reduce haemolysis, transfusion requirements and the incidence of thrombosis. Ravulizumab is longer-acting and is given only once in eight weeks, whereas eculizumab, with which there is much longer experience, is given every fortnight. Orally bioavailable complement inhibitors are in development. Iron therapy is used for iron deficiency and long-term anticoagulation with warfarin may be needed. Immunosuppression can be useful and allogeneic SCT is a definitive treatment. The disease occasionally remits spontaneously. The median survival is over 10 years. As for aplastic anaemia, transformation to MDS or AML may occur.

Red cell aplasia

This is a rare group of syndromes characterized by anaemia with normal leucocytes and platelets and grossly reduced or absent erythroblasts in the marrow (Fig. 22.5).

Chronic forms

A congenital form of red cell aplasia is known as **Diamond–Blackfan anaemia** (Table 22.3) and is inherited as a recessive condition. It is associated with a varying number of somatic abnormalities (e.g. of the face or heart) and is typically diagnosed in the first 2 years of life. Mutation of one of several genes that encode ribosomal proteins underlies most cases (Fig. 22.6). Corticosteroids are the first line of treatment and SCT may be curative. Androgens

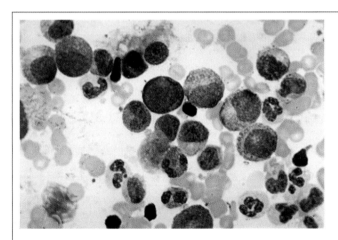

Figure 22.5 The bone marrow in red cell aplasia. There is selective loss of erythropoiesis.

Table 22.3 Classification of red cell aplasia.		
Acute, transient	**Chronic congenital**	**Chronic acquired**
Parvovirus infection Infancy and childhood Drugs (e.g. azathioprine, co-trimoxazole)	Diamond–Blackfan anaemia	Idiopathic Associated with thymoma, systemic lupus erythematosus, rheumatoid arthritis, lymphoma, chronic lymphocytic leukaemia, T-cell large granular lymphocytosis, myelodysplastic syndromes, viral infection, drugs

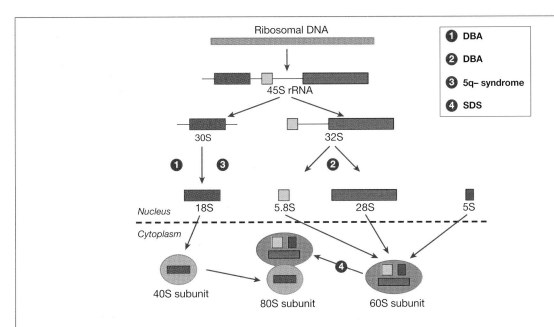

Figure 22.6 Ribosomal RNA processing and the sites of disruption in bone marrow failure syndromes. The different RNA species have roles in cell stress response, proliferation and apoptosis. Source: Courtesy of Professor I. Dokal. DBA, Diamond–Blackfan anaemia; SDS, Shwachman–Diamond syndrome.

may also produce improvement, but side-effects on growth can be severe. Iron chelation is needed after multiple transfusions.

The acquired chronic form can occur without any obvious associated disease or precipitating factor (idiopathic), or may be seen with autoimmune diseases (especially systemic lupus erythematosus), with a thymoma, lymphoma or chronic lymphocytic leukaemia. Monoclonal antibodies, such as rituximab (anti-CD20), are being used increasingly in treatment of refractory acquired red cell aplasia and other autoimmune cytopenias. In some cases, other immunosuppressive drugs can be helpful.

If regular blood transfusions are needed, iron chelation therapy will also be necessary. SCT has been carried out in some severe cases.

Transient form

Parvovirus B19 infects red cell precursors via the P antigen and causes a transient (5–10 days) red cell aplasia. This can result in rapid onset of severe anaemia in patients with pre-existing shortened red cell survival, such as those with sickle cell disease or hereditary spherocytosis (Fig. 22.7). Transient red cell aplasia with anaemia may also occur in association with drug therapy (Table 22.3) and in normal infants or children, often with a history of a viral infection in the preceding 3 months.

Congenital dyserythropoietic anaemias

Congenital dyserythropoietic anaemias (CDAs) are a group of **hereditary refractory anaemias characterized by ineffective erythropoiesis and often erythroblast multinuclearity**.

The patient may be jaundiced, with bone marrow expansion. The white cell and platelet counts are normal. The reticulocyte count is low for the degree of anaemia, despite increased marrow cellularity. The anaemia is of variable severity and is usually first noted in infancy or childhood. Iron overload may develop and splenomegaly is common.

The CDAs have been classified into several types based on the degree to which megaloblastic changes, giant erythroblasts and dyserythropoietic changes are present. CDA type 1 is due to mutation of the gene *CDAN1*, active during the S phase of the cell cycle. Somatic abnormalities are common. CDA Type 2 is known as HEMPAS (hereditary erythroblast multinuclearity with a positive acidified serum lysis test). The test is positive with some sera, but not with the patient's serum. The basic lesion in HEMPAS is a defect in the gene *SEC23B* coding for a protein involved in synthesis of endoplasmic reticulum-derived vesicles destined for the Golgi component. α-Interferon has induced remission in some cases. The other types of CDA are very rare.

Osteopetrosis

This is a rare heterogeneous group of disorders due to **failure of bone resorption by osteoclasts**. Inheritance may be recessive or dominant. The bones are dense but brittle and fractures are common. The marrow space is reduced and a leucoerythroblastic anaemia occurs. The liver and spleen are enlarged. Early death from the consequences of bone marrow failure is usual. SCT offers a chance of cure.

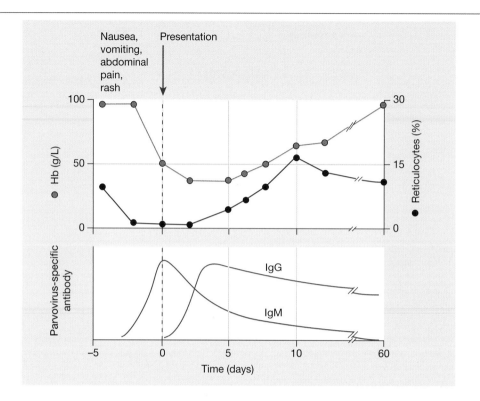

Figure 22.7 Parvovirus infection: flow chart showing transient fall in haemoglobin and reticulocytes in a patient with hereditary spherocytosis.

SUMMARY

- Aplastic anaemia presents as pancytopenia (subnormal haemoglobin, neutrophils and platelets) associated with a hypoplastic bone marrow.
- Marrow failure syndromes may be congenital (e.g. Fanconi anaemia, dyskeratosis congenital, Shwachman–Diamond syndrome) or acquired (idiopathic or due to drugs, viral infection or toxins).
- Fanconi anaemia is usually autosomal recessive, associated with congenital skeletal, skin or renal abnormalities. It is caused by inherited mutations of genes involved in DNA repair.
- Dyskeratosis congenita is due to short telomeres resulting from inherited mutations of genes encoding parts of the telomerase complex. It is associated with nail dysplasia, oral leukoplakia and skin abnormalities.
- Acquired aplastic anaemia is treated with immunosuppressive drugs (e.g. anti-thymocyte globulin, ciclosporin with eltrombopag) or by stem cell transplantation.
- Paroxysmal nocturnal haemoglobinuria is an acquired clonal haemolytic anaemia associated with pancytopenia arising in a hypoplastic marrow. There is defective synthesis of the glycosylphosphatidylinositol anchor for many membrane proteins. It is treated with complement inhibitors and often anticoagulation.
- Red cell aplasia causes anaemia with normal white cell and platelet counts. It may be transient, usually caused by parvovirus infection, or chronic. Chronic red cell aplasia may be congenital (Diamond–Blackfan anaemia) or acquired, e.g. associated with systemic lupus erythematosus, lymphoma or chronic lymphocytic leukaemia.
- Congenital dyserythropoietic anaemias are a group of rare inherited disorders of erythropoiesis.

Now visit **www.wileyessential.com/haematology** to test yourself on this chapter.

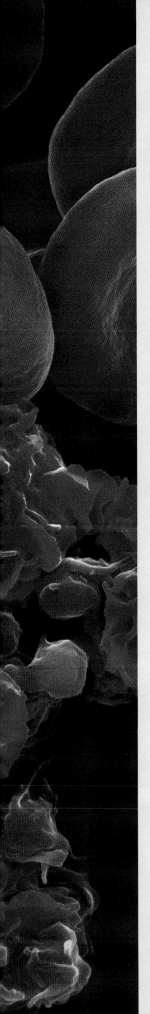

CHAPTER 23
Haemopoietic stem cell transplantation

Key topics

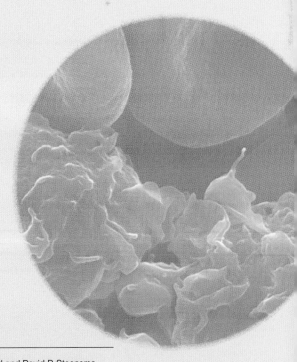

Hoffbrand's Essential Haematology, Eighth Edition. By A. Victor Hoffbrand and David P. Steensma.
© 2020 John Wiley & Sons Ltd. Published 2020 by John Wiley & Sons Ltd.
Companion website: www.wileyessential.com/haematology

Principles of stem cell transplantation

Haemopoietic stem cell transplantation (SCT) involves replacing the patient's haemopoietic and immune system with stem cells either from another individual or with a previously harvested portion of the patient's own haemopoietic stem cells (Fig. 23.1). Depending on the source of the stem cells, the term includes **bone marrow transplantation** (BMT), **peripheral blood stem cell** (PBSC) transplantation and **umbilical cord blood** transplantation. Depending on the type of donor and source of stem cells, SCT may be **syngeneic** (identical twin), **allogeneic** (family member or unrelated person) or **autologous** (self) (Table 23.1).

The principal diseases for which SCT is performed are listed in Table 23.2. However, the exact role of SCT in the management of each disease is complex and depends on factors such as disease severity and subtype, remission status, patient age and co-morbid conditions, and, for allogeneic transplantation, availability of a donor.

Collection of stem cells

Stem cells can be collected from the peripheral blood, bone marrow or umbilical cord blood. Regardless of source, the collection typically includes harvest of not just true pluripotential stem cells, but other more differentiated progenitor cells that may be important in facilitating early post-transplant engraftment and haemopoietic recovery.

Peripheral blood stem cell collection

This is currently the most commonly used source of stem cells for both autologous and allogeneic transplantation. PBSCs are obtained using a cell-separator machine connected to the patient or donor via peripheral venous cannulae (Fig. 23.2). Blood is taken through one cannula and pumped around the machine, where mononuclear cells (the circulating cell population enriched for stem cells) are collected by centrifugation, before the red cells and plasma are returned to the donor. This

Table 23.1 Haemopoietic stem cell transplantation: potential donors.

Donor	Type of transplant
HLA-matching sibling Unrelated fully HLA-matching or nearly fully HLA-matching volunteer Haploidentical (half HLA-matching) family member Umbilical cord blood	Allogeneic
Identical twin	Syngeneic
Self	Autologous

HLA, human leucocyte antigen.

Table 23.2 Haemopoietic stem cell transplantation: indications.

Allogeneic (or syngeneic)	Autologous
Acquired disorders: acute lymphoblastic or myeloid leukaemia. Other malignant disorders of the marrow (e.g. myelodysplastic syndromes, myeloproliferative neoplasms). Severe aplastic anaemia or refractory pure red cell aplasia.	Acquired disorders: Hodgkin and non-Hodgkin lymphoma, multiple myeloma, primary amyloidosis
Inherited disorders: thalassaemia major, sickle cell anaemia, immune deficiencies, congenital marrow failure syndromes, inborn errors of metabolism in the haemopoietic and mesenchymal system (e.g. osteopetrosis)	Inherited disorders: with *ex vivo* genetic manipulation, for 'gene therapy' of inherited diseases such as beta-thalassaemia major or immunodeficiency states

continuous process may take a few hours before enough mononuclear cells are collected.

Peripheral blood normally contains too few haemopoietic stem cells to allow collection of sufficient numbers for transplantation, so stem cells must be 'mobilized' into the blood in greater numbers to facilitate collection. Growth factors can increase the number of circulating stem cells by around 10–100 times. Granulocyte colony-stimulating factor (G-CSF) is given to patients (for autologous transplantation) or donors (for syngeneic or allogeneic transplant) as a course of injections until the white cell count starts to rise. Plerixafor, an inhibitor of stem cell adhesion in the bone marrow, is also given if mobilization is likely to be inadequate. For autologous transplant, cytotoxic chemotherapy may also be used to both reduce malignant cells and mobilize stem cells, since during recovery after chemotherapy the circulating stem cell numbers transiently increase.

After mobilization, PBSC collections are then taken and, depending on the efficiency of stem cell mobilization, repeated collections may be needed for up to 4 days. A typical outpatient protocol is G-CSF on days 1–4 and harvests on days 5 and 6. The adequacy of the collection is assessed by CD34$^+$ cell count, as CD34 is a marker of stem and progenitor cells. Generally greater than 2.0×10^6 CD34$^+$ cells per kilogram of the recipient weight are needed for successful engraftment.

Bone marrow collection

For this type of stem cell collection, mobilization is not necessary. The donor is given a general anaesthetic and 500–1200 mL of marrow are harvested from the pelvis. The marrow is anticoagulated and a mononuclear cell count is taken periodically

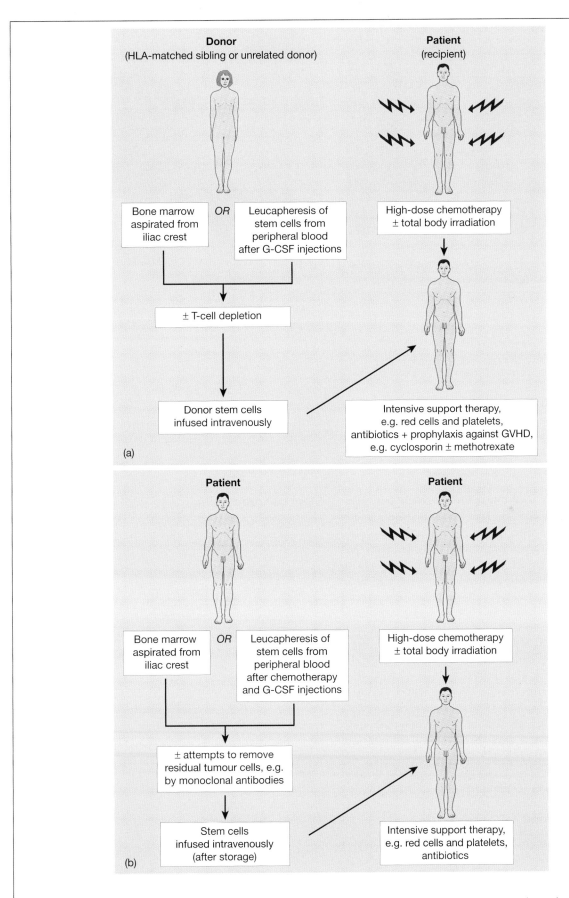

Figure 23.1 Procedures for **(a)** allogeneic, and **(b)** autologous stem cell transplantation. G-CSF, granulocyte colony-stimulating factor; GVHD, graft-versus-host disease.

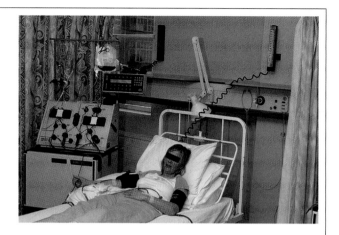

Figure 23.2 Peripheral blood stem cell (PBSC) collection: a donor undergoing collection of PBSCs on a cell separator.

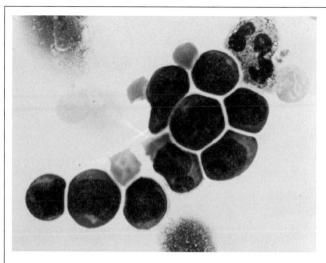

Figure 23.3 Peripheral blood stem cell collection: enriched CD34⁺ cells stained by May–Grünwald–Giemsa stain. The cells have the appearance of small and medium-sized lymphocytes.

while marrow is being obtained, in order to assess the yield, which should be approximately $2-4 \times 10^8$ nucleated cells/kg body weight of the recipient.

Compared to PBSCs, bone marrow reduces the risk of graft failure, but increases the risk of chronic graft-versus-host disease (GVHD). The risk of relapse of the primary disease and of acute GVHD is similar between stem cell sources.

Choice of donor

The most frequently used donor for allogeneic transplant is a fully human leucocyte antigen (HLA)-matching family member (brother or sister). (The HLA system is described further below.) Multiparous female donors are more likely than male donors to result in GVHD in the recipient due to alloimmunization to paternal antigens during prior pregnancies. An identical twin can also be used as donor, but there is no graft versus leukaemia/lymphoma effect from a syngeneic donor, so relapse of the original disease is more likely.

An HLA-matching unrelated donor may be sought from international volunteer donor panels, but new protocols are also enabling mismatched and one-half HLA-matching 'haploidentical' donors – i.e. father, mother, child or sibling donors – to be safely used. **For haploidentical transplants, a large dose of cyclophosphamide is given alone or with other immunosuppressive drugs 3 or 4 days after the stem cell infusion.** This protocol reduces the risk of donor T cells proliferating and causing severe GVHD, and is now also employed in identical sibling and fully matched transplants.

Umbilical cord blood

Fetal blood is a rich source of haemopoietic stem cells, which may be collected from cord blood at the time of delivery. Because of the relatively small numbers of stem cells collected from a single cord, they are most useful for children who do

not have a fully matching sibling or unrelated donor. Less stringent HLA matching is needed due to the immunological naïveté of the stem cells, resulting in less GVHD. Double cord donations may be needed to obtain sufficient stem cells for adult recipients. Immune reconstitution is slower after cord blood transplantation.

Stem cell processing

CD34⁺ stem cells may be selected from both types of harvest (Fig. 23.3). After collection, the stem cell harvest is processed with removal of red cells and concentration of the mononuclear cells. In some protocols, antibodies to remove T lymphocytes are used *in vitro*. This reduces the risk of GVHD, but increases the risk of non-engraftment, viral infections and, if the transplant is being done for malignant disease, relapse. Autologous collections may also be 'purged' by chemotherapy or antibodies in an attempt to remove residual malignant cells.

Conditioning

Prior to infusion of haemopoietic stem cells, patients receive chemotherapy, sometimes in combination with total body irradiation (TBI; Fig. 23.1) in a procedure called conditioning. The primary goal of conditioning is to induce a state of immunosuppression so that the recipient's body does not immediately reject the donor cells. In the case of malignant disease, the conditioning regimen may also cytoreduce or even eliminate any remaining neoplastic cells.

Myeloablative conditioning regimens

These regimens aim at irreversibly destroying the haemopoietic function of the bone marrow with high doses of chemotherapy, with or without TBI. The conditioning is also aimed at destroying the patient's immune system and any malignant cells in the bone marrow. TBI is usually used in patients with malignant disease and is most frequently administered over several days (**fractionated**). The most commonly used chemotherapy drug is cyclophosphamide, but the alkylating agents busulphan, melphalan, treosulfan or other drugs are given in some protocols. Alemtuzumab (anti-CD52) or anti-thymocyte globulin (ATG) is also employed as a T cell-depleting agent *in vivo* in some protocols. At least 36 hours are typically allowed for the elimination of the drugs from the circulation following the last dose of conditioning chemotherapy before donor stem cells are infused. Conditioning is often complicated by mucositis, and patients must be scrupulous about oral hygiene and sometimes need parenteral nutrition. Early mortality after the procedure exceeds 10%.

Before autologous transplantation, high-dose melphalan is given for myeloma and a combination regimen, e.g. 'BEAM' – carmustine (BCNU), etoposide, cytarabine (Ara-C) and melphalan – is given for lymphoma.

Reduced-intensity (non-myeloablative) conditioning regimens

Reduced-intensity regimens are used to reduce the morbidity and mortality of allogeneic transplantation. **These regimens do not completely destroy the host bone marrow as myeloablative conditioning does**. Instead, the aim in reduced-intensity transplants is to use enough immunosuppression to allow donor stem cells to engraft without completely eradicating host marrow stem cells.

Such regimens extend the age range of feasibility for transplant to above 70 years, and increase the treatment indications for allogeneic transplantation. Conditioning agents commonly employed in such regimens include fludarabine, low doses of busulphan or cyclophosphamide, low-dose irradiation, and ATG, alemtuzumab or other antibodies that deplete T cells.

Donor leucocyte infusions (DLI) are commonly used at a later stage after reduced-intensity allografting in order to encourage complete donor engraftment or to enhance a graft-versus-leukaemia (GVL) or -lymphoma effect. They can also be used in the event of loss of chimerism or relapse of malignant disease post-allografting, including after myeloablative transplant.

Prevention of graft-versus-host disease

Immune-suppressing drugs, usually methotrexate or rapamycin with either ciclosporin or tacrolimus, are given post-transplantation to reduce the risk of GVHD. As discussed above, a high dose of cyclophosphamide given 3 or 4 days after the stem cell infusion reduces the risk of GVHD without causing graft rejection or loss of the GVL effect, and is commonly used, particularly in haploidentical transplants.

In vivo T cell depletion of the donor stem cells with anti-thymocyte immunoglobulin (ATG) or anti-CD52 reduces the risk of GVHD, but in most studies has increased the risk of graft failure, infections, relapse of malignant disease (if malignant disease was the indication for transplant) and of post-transplantation lymphoproliferative disease. *In vitro* T cell depletion of harvested stem cells also reduces the risk of GVHD, but similarly results in increased graft failure and rejection, relapse and viral infections.

Post-transplant engraftment and immunity

After a period of typically 1–3 weeks of severe pancytopenia, the first signs of successful engraftment are monocytes and neutrophils in the blood, with a subsequent increase in platelet count (Fig. 23.4). G-CSF may be used to reduce the period of severe neutropenia. Engraftment is usually a few days faster following PBSC transplantation compared with BMT.

The marrow cellularity gradually returns towards normal, but the marrow reserve remains impaired for 1–2 years and in some cases is impaired permanently. There is profound T cell immunodeficiency for 3–12 months with a low level of CD4 helper cells. Immune recovery is quicker after autologous and syngeneic SCT than following allogeneic HSCT. The patient's blood group changes to that of the donor, and antigen-specific immunity becomes that of the donor (including predisposition to allergic reactions) after approximately 60 days. Revaccination against common childhood viruses is usually carried out beginning at 9–12 months post-transplant.

Autologous stem cell transplantation

Stem cells are harvested from the patient and stored before a high-intensity treatment is given and are then reinfused to rescue the patient from the myeloablative effects of the treatment (Fig. 23.1). This allows the delivery of a higher dose of myelotoxic chemotherapy, with or without radiotherapy, which otherwise would result in prolonged bone marrow aplasia and severe infection risk.

A limitation of the autologous procedure is that, in the setting of neoplastic disease, malignant cells contaminating the stem cell harvest may be reintroduced into the patient. Nevertheless, autografting has a major role in the treatment of haematological diseases such as lymphoma and myeloma. Autografting is also used in gene therapy for inherited bone marrow diseases by eliminating with chemotherapy stem cells carrying the genetic disease, and replacing them with the patient's harvested stem cells that have had the gene defect corrected *in vitro*.

The major problem associated with autografting is recurrence of the original disease, especially if the indication for transplant was a neoplasm (Fig. 23.5). GVHD is not an issue. Other complications depend on the conditioning regimen and may include intestinal, lung, mucous membrane, liver or cardiac damage. Procedure-related mortality is generally well below 5%.

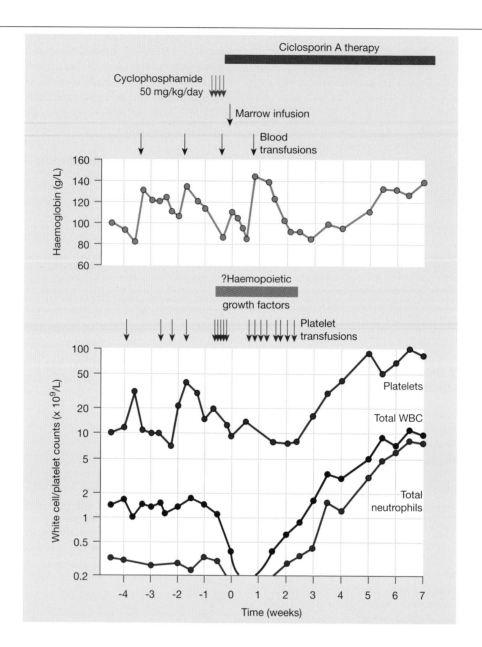

Figure 23.4 Typical haematological chart of a patient undergoing allogeneic marrow transplantation for aplastic anaemia. WBC, white blood cells.

The human leucocyte antigen system

One of the major reasons for failure of allogeneic transplantation is the immunological incompatibility between donor and patient despite matching of the HLAs. This mismatch may manifest as immunodeficiency, GVHD or graft failure (Fig. 23.5). There is also a beneficial GVL or graft-versus-lymphoma effect in which donor immune cells identify remaining neoplastic cells in the recipient and destroy them. This underlies much of the success of the procedure.

Allografting would be impossible without the ability to perform HLA typing. **The short arm of chromosome 6 contains a cluster of genes known as the major histocompatibility complex (MHC) or the HLA region (Fig. 23.6a).** Genes in this region encode the HLA antigens and many other molecules, including complement components, tumour necrosis factor (TNF) and proteins associated with antigen processing.

HLA molecules are of two types: class I and II (Table 23.3). Their role is to bind intracellular peptides and 'present' these to

T lymphocytes for antigen recognition (see Chapter 9). Class I HLA molecules (HLA-A, -B and -C) present antigens such as virus peptide fragments to CD8⁺ T cells, resulting in destruction of the infected cell. Class II molecules (HLA-DR, -DQ and -DP) present antigens to CD4⁺ T cells, which results in proliferation of these T cells and of B cells which make antibodies to the relevant antigen (Fig. 23.6b).

As there are 12 antigen-presenting HLA molecules, each highly polymorphic, the chances of two unrelated individuals matching at all 12 loci, even in the same ethnic group (since specific HLA markers generally cluster within ethnic groups),

Autologous

Other 15%
Infection 8%
IPn 1%
Organ toxicity 6%
Relapse 70%

HLA-identical sibling

GVHD 13%
Other 16%
Relapse 41%
Infection 17%
IPn 3%
Organ toxicity 10%

Unrelated donor

GVHD 14%
Other 16%
Relapse 34%
Infection 20%
IPn 6%
Organ toxicity 10%

Figure 23.5 The causes of death following autologous, HLA-matched sibling and unrelated allogeneic transplantation. IPn, interstitial pneumonitis. Source: C. Craddock, R. Chakraverty. In A.V. Hoffbrand *et al.* (eds) (2016) *Postgraduate Haematology*, 7th edn. Reproduced by permission of John Wiley & Sons.

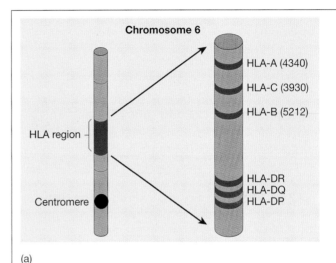

(a)

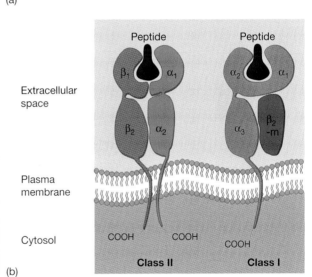

(b)

Figure 23.6 (a) The human leucocyte antigen (HLA) complex. The number of allele variants at each locus identified to date is shown. **(b)** HLA class I and II molecules showing protein domains and bound peptide. Class I alpha chains are encoded by genes HLA-A, HLA-B or HLA-C. Class II alpha DR chains are encoded by gene HLA-DRA, and beta chains by genes HLA-DRB1, -DRB3, -DRB4 or -DRB5. DRB2 is a non-protein coding pseudogene. Class II DP alpha chains are encoded by gene HLA-DPA, while beta chains are encoded by HLA-DPB. Class II DQ alpha chains are encoded by gene HLA-DQA, while beta chains are encoded by HLA-DQB.

Table 23.3 The human leucocyte antigens (HLA).

	Class I	Class II
Antigens	HLA-A, B, C	HLA-DR, -DP, -DQ
Distribution	All nucleated cells, platelets	B lymphocytes Monocytes Macrophages Activated T cells
Structure	Large polypeptide chain) and a β_2-microglobulin	Two polypeptide chains (α and β)
Interacts with	CD8 lymphocytes	CD4 lymphocytes

is very unlikely. Allelic diversity among HLA markers is greater in some ethnic groups, such as those of African or South Asian descent, than others such as Northern Europeans. Overall there are more than 18 000 HLA alleles, of which more than 13 000 are class I and more than 5000 class II (Figure 23.6a).

Class I HLA molecules are present on most nucleated cells and on the cell surface they are associated with β_2-microglobulin. The α chain is encoded on chromosome 6, whereas β_2-microglobulin is encoded on chromosome 15. **Class II HLA molecules** have a more restricted tissue distribution. These comprise α and β chains, both encoded by genes on chromosome 6 in the HLA region (Fig. 23.6a).

The inheritance of the HLA loci is closely linked: one set of loci is inherited from each parent, so that there is approximately a one in four chance of two full siblings having identical HLA antigens (Fig. 23.7a). Crossing-over of genes during meiosis and non-paternity accounts for occasional unexpected disparities. The inheritance of HLA molecules is independent of sex or blood group.

Human leucocyte antigen and transplantation

The natural role of HLA molecules is in directing T-lymphocyte responses and the greater the HLA mismatch, the more severe is the immune response between transplanted cells and host tissues. HLA typing is critical in donor selection for allogeneic SCT.

Minor histocompatibility antigens, e.g. HA-1, HA-2 and Hy, are peptides that are presented by HLA molecules and are able to act as antigens in SCT, either because they are polymorphic in the population or because they are encoded on the Y chromosome and therefore represent novel antigens to a female immune system that has engrafted in a male. They are likely to be important antigens in GVHD and the GVL reaction (see below).

HLA typing may be carried out by serological or molecular techniques. The nomenclature for *HLA* alleles is standardized. A single antigenic specificity defined by serological typing (e.g. HLA-A2) can be divided into different alleles by DNA sequencing. Each allele is given in numerical designation. The gene name is followed by an asterisk. The first field of digits indicates the allele group. The second field of digits lists subtypes, which differ in the protein sequence. Subsequent digits indicate minor differences in non-coding regions. As an example, alleles at the *HLA-A* loci are written as *HLA-A*01:01* to *HLA-A*80:01*. The nomenclature for the class II genes is similar, but complicated by the fact that there may be more than one *HLA-DRB* gene on each chromosome (Fig. 23.7b).

When searching for an unrelated donor, the aim is to match HLA-A, -B –C and DRB1 and –DQB1 between recipient and donor, and this is then called a 10/10 match. An exception is when a donor with only a single HLA haplotype match, usually a parent or sibling, is used in a **haploidentical SCT**. There are many millions of volunteer donors registered on international registries, and the chance of identifying a matched unrelated donor for a patient lacking an HLA identical sibling (depending on the ethnic group) is greater than 70% in populations of European descent.

Chimerism analysis

Following allogeneic SCT, the recipient's blood shows the presence of both donor and recipient cells (chimerism). This admixture can be detected by fluorescence *in situ* hybridization (FISH) analysis (see Chapter 11) of the proportion of Y chromosome-containing cells if there is a sex mismatch, or by DNA analysis techniques regardless of donor and recipient sex. Following successful engraftment, loss of donor chimerism may be a harbinger of impending graft failure or relapse of a malignant disease.

Complications (Table 23.4)

The causes of death following SCT are shown in Figure 23.5. The overall rate from the procedure itself is lowest (less than 5%) for autologous SCT and highest in unrelated and haploidentical SCT.

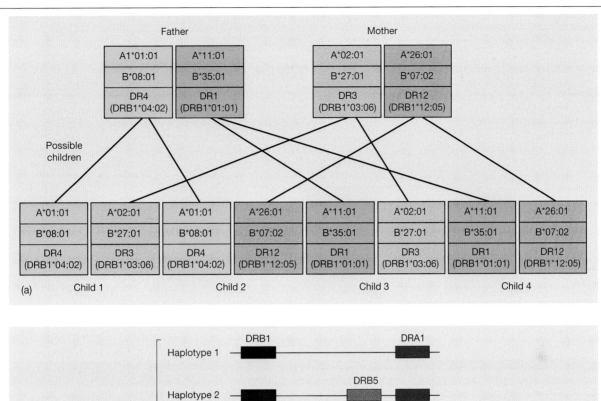

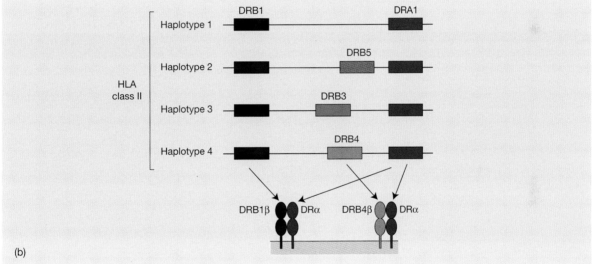

Figure 23.7 (a) An example of the possible pattern of inheritance of the A, B and DR (*DRB1*) series alleles of the human leucocyte antigen (HLA) complex. **(b)** Molecular genetics of the HLA class II gene complex. There are four major haplotypes of MHC class II genes in the population and each individual may have up to two (one on each chromosome). The *DRA1* gene codes for the DRα protein and the *DRB1*, *DRB3*, *DRB4* and *DRB5* genes encode DRβ chains. Expression from the *DRB1* gene is higher than from the other genes. The number of alleles at each gene is shown in Figure 23.6a. Alleles at each locus have a standard nomenclature (e.g. the alleles at the *DRB1* gene are termed *DRB1*0101* to *DRB1*1608*).

Graft-versus-host disease

GVHD is caused by donor-derived immune cells, particularly T lymphocytes, reacting against recipient tissues. Its incidence increases with increasing age of donor and recipient and the degree of HLA mismatch between them. Donor alloimmunization, e.g. a female who has had multiple pregnancies, and, in the recipient, viral infection (e.g. cytomegalovirus, CMV), liver, inflammatory bowel or rheumatological disease and use of PBSC also increase the risk of acute GVHD. GVHD prophylaxis is usually given as ciclosporin (or tacrolimus) with methotrexate. Sirolimus, rapamycin or mycophenolate mofetil is also used in some protocols. With time, these prophylactic medications can be tapered off in patients without active GVHD.

Table 23.4 Complications of stem cell transplantation.

Early (usually <100 days)	Late (usually >100 days)
Infections, especially bacterial, fungal, herpes simplex virus, CMV, BK polyoma virus	Infections, especially varicella-zoster, capsulate bacteria
Haemorrhage	Chronic-pattern GVHD (arthritis, malabsorption, hepatitis, scleroderma, sicca syndrome, lichen planus, pulmonary disease including bronchiolitis obliterans, serous effusions); acute GVHD may also persist beyond 100 days
Acute-pattern GVHD (skin, liver, gut)	Chronic pulmonary disease
Graft failure	Autoimmune disorders
Haemorrhagic cystitis	Cataract
Interstitial pneumonitis	Infertility
Others: veno-occlusive disease, cardiac failure	Second malignancies, lymphoproliferative diseases

CMV, cytomegalovirus; GVHD, graft-versus-host disease.

Table 23.5 Acute pattern graft-versus-host disease: clinical staging (Glucksberg system).

Stage	Skin	Liver (bilirubin, μmol/L)	Gut (diarrhoea, L/day)
I	Rash <25% body surface	34–51	0.5–1.0 or persistent nausea
II	Rash 25–50% body surface	52–101	1.0–1.5
III	Generalized erythroderma	102–255	>1.5
IV	Bullae, desquamation	>255	Severe pain, ileus

In **acute GVHD**, usually occurring in the first 100 days but often persisting beyond that time frame, the skin, gastrointestinal tract or liver is affected (Table 23.5). The skin rash typically affects the face, palms, soles and ears, but may, in severe cases, affect the whole body (Fig. 23.8). Diarrhoea may lead to fluid and electrolyte depletion. Typically, bilirubin and alkaline phosphatase are raised, but the other hepatic enzymes are relatively normal. Acute GVHD is usually treated by high doses of corticosteroids, which are effective in the majority of cases. Trials of other agents including sirolimus are in progress. Second-line drugs include sirolimus, JAK1/2 inhibitors such as ruxolitinib, various monoclonal antibodies and faecal microbiota transplants.

In **chronic pattern GVHD**, which usually occurs after 100 days and may evolve from acute GVHD, these tissues are involved, but also the joints and other serosal surfaces, the oral mucosa and lacrimal glands. Features of autoimmune disease with scleroderma, Sjögren's syndrome, myositis and lichen planus may develop. The immune system is impaired

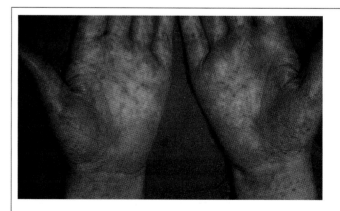

Figure 23.8 Widespread erythematous skin rash in acute graft-versus-host disease following allogeneic stem cell transplantation.

(including hyposplenism) with risk of infection. Malabsorption and pulmonary abnormalities, e.g. bronchiolitis obliterans, are frequent. Corticosteroids are tried together with second-line drugs, including ibrutinib, JAK1/2 inhibitors, ciclosporin, rituximab, sirolimus, mycophenolate mofetil or extracorporeal photopheresis. The response may be poor.

Infections

In the early post-transplant period, bacterial or fungal infections are frequent (Fig. 23.9). These may be reduced by reverse barrier nursing with laminar or positive-pressure air flow and the use of skin and mouth antiseptics. Prophylactic therapy with aciclovir, antifungal agents and oral antibiotics is often given. If a fever or other evidence of an infection occurs, broad-spectrum intravenous antibiotics are commenced immediately after blood cultures and other appropriate microbiological specimens have been taken. Failure of response to antibacterial agents is usually an indication to commence systemic antifungal therapy with amphotericin, caspofungin, micafungin, voriconazole, posaconazole or isavucanozium. Fungal infections, especially *Candida* and *Aspergillus* species (see Chapter 12), are a particular problem because of the prolonged neutropenia.

Viral infections, particularly with the herpes group of viruses, are frequent with herpes simplex, CMV and varicella zoster virus (VZV) occurring at different peak intervals (Fig. 23.9). CMV presents a particular threat and is associated with a potentially fatal interstitial pneumonitis (Fig. 23.10), as well as with hepatitis and falling blood counts. The infection may be caused by reactivation of CMV in the recipient or a new infection transmitted by the donor. In CMV-seronegative patients with CMV-seronegative donors, CMV-negative, leucodepleted blood products must be given. Aciclovir may be useful in prophylaxis. Patients are screened regularly (usually weekly in the first few months after transplant) for evidence of CMV reactivation following allogeneic transplantation. If these tests become positive, ganciclovir may suppress the virus before clinical complications occur. Ganciclovir, foscarnet, cidofovir and CMV immunoglobulin may be tried for established CMV infection.

VZV infection is also frequent post-SCT but occurs later, with a median onset at 4–5 months. Rarely, disseminated VZV infection occurs. Intravenous aciclovir is indicated for this complication. Antivirals are also helpful in Epstein–Barr virus (EBV) infections and EBV-associated lymphoproliferative disease (see Fig. 23.13). In refractory viral infections,

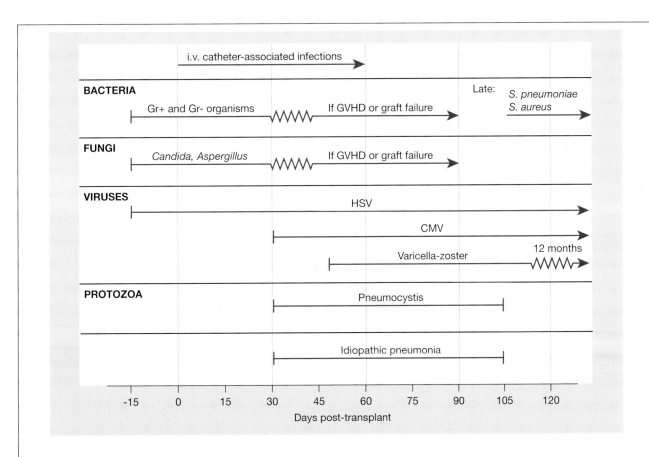

Figure 23.9 Time sequence for development of different types of infection following allogeneic stem cell transplantation. CMV, cytomegalovirus; Gr+, Gr–, Gram-positive or -negative; GVHD, graft-versus-host disease; HSV, herpes simplex virus.

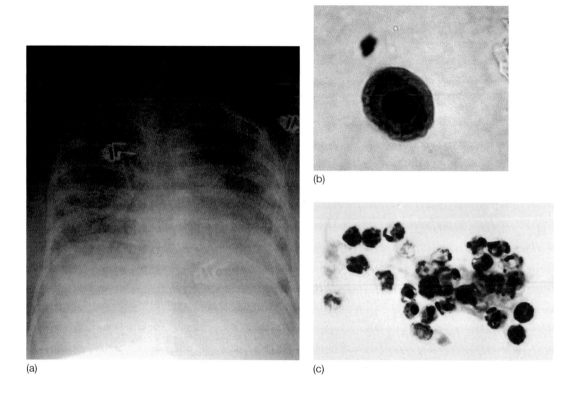

Figure 23.10 (a) Chest radiograph showing interstitial pneumonitis following bone marrow transplantation. Widespread diffuse mottling can be seen. The patient had received total body irradiation and had grade III graft-versus-host disease. No infective cause of the pneumonitis was identified. Possible causes include pneumocystis, cytomegalovirus, herpes zoster, fungal infection or a combination of these. **(b)** Sputum cytology: intranuclear cytomegalovirus inclusion body in a pulmonary cell. Papanicolaou stain. **(c)** *Pneumocystis jirovecii* in bronchial washings, Gram–Weigert stain.

T cells with specificity for these organisms can be selectively harvested from donors and administered to patients.

Pneumocystis jirovecii (Fig 23.10) is a cause of pneumonitis that may be prevented by prophylactic co-trimoxazole or atovaquone.

Interstitial pneumonitis

This is one of the most frequent causes of death post-SCT (Fig. 23.10). CMV is a frequent agent, but other herpes viruses and *P. carinii* account for other cases; in most cases, however, no specific cause other than the previous radiation and chemotherapy can be implicated. Diffuse alveolar haemorrhage may also occur. Trans-bronchoscopic biopsy or open lung biopsy may be needed to establish the diagnosis. High-dose corticosteroids are usually administered.

Blood product support

Platelets and blood transfusions given in the post-transplant period must be irradiated prior to administration in order to kill any passenger live lymphocytes that might cause GVHD. Platelet concentrates are given to maintain a count of 10×10^9/L or more.

Other complications of allogeneic transplantation

Graft failure

The risk of graft failure is increased if the patient has aplastic anaemia, if T cell depletion of donor marrow is used as GVHD prophylaxis, or if peripheral blood is used as a stem cell source. This suggests that donor T cells are needed to overcome host resistance to engraftment of stem cells. Occasionally, even after myeloablative regimens, the patient's own marrow will eventually recover after several months. Graft failure often requires additional stem cells to be administered for haemopoiesis to recover. It is commonly fatal.

Haemorrhagic cystitis

This can be caused by the cyclophosphamide metabolite acrolein. Mesna is given in an attempt to prevent this. Certain viruses (e.g. adenovirus or the BK polyomavirus) may also cause this complication. Therapy is typically supportive care, since specific antivirals are not available.

Other complications

Veno-occlusive disease (VOD) of the liver, also called sinusoidal obstruction syndrome (SOS), manifests as jaundice, hepatomegaly and ascites or weight gain. Patients who have received TBI are at increased risk, as are those who have received calicheamicin-containing antibody–drug conjugates such as gemtuzumab or inotuzumab prior to transplant. Defibrotide, a mixture of single-stranded oligonucleotides derived from pig mucosa, is approved for treatment of VOD/SOS, though the mechanism of action is incompletely understood.

Cardiac failure may develop as a result of the conditioning regime (especially high doses of cyclophosphamide) and previous chemotherapy on the heart. Haemolysis because of ABO incompatibility between donor and recipient may cause problems in the first weeks. Microangiopathic haemolytic anaemia may also occur due to endothelial injury from the conditioning regimen. It responds poorly to plasma exchange.

Late complications

For patients undergoing transplant for neoplastic disorders, relapse of the original disease (e.g. myelodysplasia or acute or chronic leukaemia) is the leading cause of post-transplant death (Fig. 23.5). Bacterial infections remain frequent even after neutrophil recovery, especially with encapsulated organisms affecting the respiratory tract. Oral antibiotics and immune globulin infusions are often given prophylactically to reduce this risk. VZV, HSV and fungal infections are also frequent. The use of prophylactic co-trimoxazole or atovaquone, and oral aciclovir or valaciclovir, for at least 3–6 months reduces the risk of *Pneumocystis* and herpes infections, respectively. Antifungal prophylaxis varies from centre to centre based on local microbiological epidemiology.

Delayed pulmonary complications include restrictive pneumonitis and bronchiolitis obliterans. Endocrine complications include hypothyroidism, growth failure in children, impaired sexual development and infertility. These endocrine problems are more marked if TBI has been used. Clinically apparent autoimmune disorders are infrequent and include myasthenia, rheumatoid arthritis, anaemia, thrombocytopenia or neutropenia. Autoantibodies are frequently detected in the absence of symptoms. Second malignancies (especially non-Hodgkin lymphoma) occur with a six- or seven-fold incidence compared with controls. Central nervous system complications include neuropathies and eye problems caused by chronic GVHD (sicca syndrome) or cataracts.

Iron overload may be present due to repeated red cell transfusions before and after transplantation. This can be treated by iron chelation or, when there is adequate red cell recovery, venesections. It is not necessary to 'de-iron' before the transplant procedure; there is usually not time for adequate chelation and it has not been proven to be of benefit.

Graft-versus-leukaemia effect and donor leucocyte infusions

After allogeneic transplantation, the donor immune system helps to eradicate the patient's leukaemia, a phenomenon known as the **graft-versus-leukaemia** effect. Graft-versus-lymphoma and -myeloma effects also exist, though these terms are rarely used. Evidence for GVL includes the decreased relapse rate in patients who have GVHD (the GVHD provides evidence of immunocompetence of the graft), the increased relapse rate in identical twins who are usually entirely immunophenotypically identical even for minor antigens, and, most convincingly, the ability of DLI to cure relapsed leukaemia in some patients. The principle of DLI is that peripheral blood mononuclear cells including T cells are collected from the original allograft donor and directly infused into the patient at the time of leukaemia relapse, detected by molecular or cytogenetic techniques or morphologically (Fig. 23.11).

There is a large difference in the outcome of different diseases treated by DLI. Chronic myeloid leukaemia (CML) is most sensitive (although transplant is now rarely necessary for chronic-phase CML given the availability of multiple highly effective tyrosine kinase inhibitors), whereas acute lymphoblastic leukaemia (ALL) rarely responds. Polymerase chain reaction (PCR) can be used to monitor serial blood samples for evidence of recurrence of the *BCR-ABL1* transcript or other known molecular abnormality of the original disease before karyotypic or clinical relapse occurs (Fig. 23.11). In the case of ALL, flow cytometry is often used to monitor for early relapse. The response to DLI may take several weeks, but can result in a permanent cure. The mechanism is incompletely understood, but a T-cell-mediated alloreactive immune response is likely to be a major component.

Positron emission tomography (PET) scans can be used to detect residual disease in cases of lymphoma and to guide the requirement for DLI and determining the disease response (Fig. 23.12).

Post-transplant lymphoproliferative disease (PTLD)

These are polyclonal or monoclonal, usually B-cell lymphoid proliferations that occur in recipients of stem cell or more frequently solid organ allografts, as a result of the intensive immunosuppression. The polyclonal lymphocytosis or lymphoma is usually EBV driven, especially for solid organ in recipients who were EBV seronegative before the transplant and develop primary infection subsequently while still on immunosuppressive therapy. This explains why PTLD is common in children than adults.

The incidence of non-Hodgkin lymphoma in solid-organ transplant recipients is about 10 times normal and of Hodgkin lymphoma about 4 times depending mainly on which organ is being transplanted. For recipients of allogeneic haemopoietic stem cell transplants, the overall incidence of lymphoma is about 3%. This depends mainly on the degree of HLA matching and the use of T cell depletion protocols. The highest incidence is in haploidentical transplants, but this may diminish with the increased use of high-dose cyclophosphamide after SCT instead of T cell depletion to prevent GVHD. The lymphoma is derived from EBV-infected donor lymphocytes and usually occurs in the first year post-transplantation.

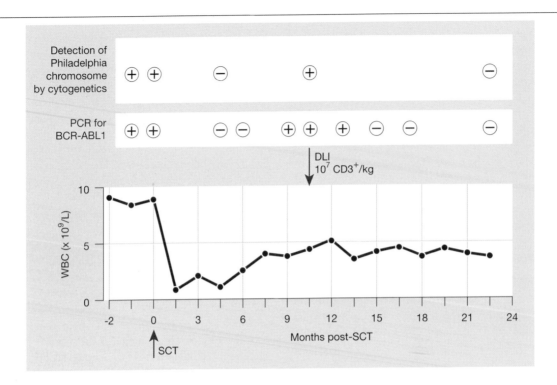

Figure 23.11 Donor leucocyte infusions. Example of donor leucocyte infusion (DLI) in the treatment of chronic myeloid leukaemia (CML) which relapsed following allogeneic stem cell transplantation (SCT). Polymerase chain reaction (PCR) analysis of the blood for the *BCR-ABL1* transcript shows that there was transient loss of the transcript, but molecular and cytogenetic relapse occurred at 10 months. One infusion of donor leucocytes led to re-establishment of a durable complete remission.

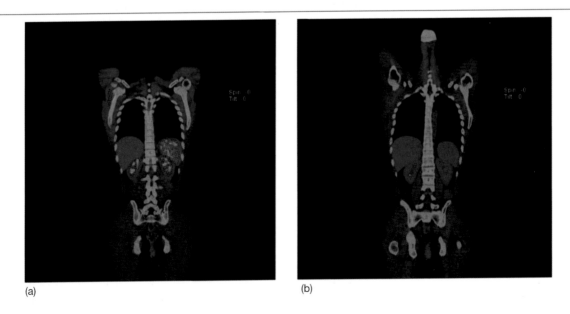

(a)   (b)

Figure 23.12 Example of disease control following administration of a donor leucocyte infusion (DLI) after stem cell transplantation. **(a)** A positron emission tomography (PET) scan revealed residual disease activity in a patient at 6 months following allogeneic transplantation for non-Hodgkin lymphoma. The bright signals reflect the metabolic activity of malignant cells in the spleen and axillary lymph nodes. Donor leucocyte infusion was then given and after 3 months a repeat PET scan **(b)** revealed no evidence of residual disease. Source: Courtesy of Professor Nigel Russell.

There is often extranodal involvement of bowel, lung, brain or bone marrow (Fig. 23.13). EBV– cases resemble closely diffuse large B cell non-Hodgkin lymphoma (DLBCL), with many of the same genomic aberrations, whereas EBV+ cases have fewer genomic abnormalities. Treatment is by withdrawing immunosuppression (if feasible), anti-CD20 antibodies such as rituximab, and chemotherapy, local radiotherapy or surgery for selected cases. Newer strategies involve therapy with ibrutinib, phosphoinositide 3-kinase (PI3K) inhibitors (see p. 225) and proteasome inhibitors.

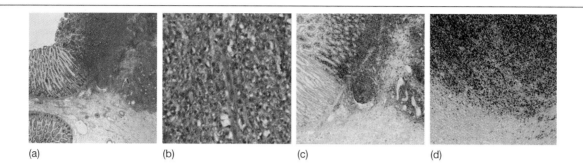

(a) (b) (c) (d)

Figure 23.13 Post-transplantation lymphoproliferative diseases: 17-year-old male 5 months after renal transplantation had small bowel perforation caused by diffuse large B-cell lymphoma. **(a)** Low-power view of lymphoid mass invading small bowel. **(b)** High-power view of lymphoid mass. **(c)** Immunostaining for CD20. **(d)** EBV-ISH (*in situ* hybridization) stain showing the tumour cells are positive for Epstein–Barr virus. Source: Courtesy of Professor P. Amrolia and Dr N. Sebire.

SUMMARY

- Haemopoietic stem cell transplantation (SCT) involves replacing the haemopoietic and immune systems by stem cells from either the same subject (autologous) or another individual (allogeneic). The donor stem cells can be harvested from bone marrow, peripheral or umbilical cord blood.

- Autologous SCT is most frequently performed for lymphomas or myeloma. It is also used in gene therapy protocols for inherited bone marrow diseases.

- For allogeneic SCT the recipient's own haemopoietic and immune systems are either eliminated by myeloablative conditioning by chemotherapy, radiotherapy and monoclonal antibody 'conditioning', or partly eliminated by reduced-intensity (non-myeloablative) conditioning.

- Allogeneic SCT requires a tissue (HLA) matching sibling, a matching unrelated or an haploidentical family member donor. The human leucocyte antigens (HLAs, class I or II) are coded for by genes on chromosome 6. They are extremely polymorphic and are involved in presentation of antigens to T lymphocytes.

- Allogeneic HSCT is indicated in selected cases of acute leukaemia, other malignant bone marrow diseases, and severe acquired or genetic marrow diseases (e.g. aplastic anaemia, thalassaemia major).

- Reduced-intensity conditioning SCT is preferred in older subjects.

- Donor leucocyte infusions may be given to treat relapse of leukaemia post-allogeneic SCT, by a 'graft-versus-leukaemia' effect.

- Early (first 100 days) complications of allogeneic SCT include acute graft-versus-host disease, infections, graft failure and veno-occlusive disease. Long-term complications include relapse of the original disease, chronic GVHD, damage to many different organs (e.g. skin, heart, lungs and liver) and post-transplant lymphoproliferative disease.

Now visit **www.wileyessential.com/haematology** to test yourself on this chapter.

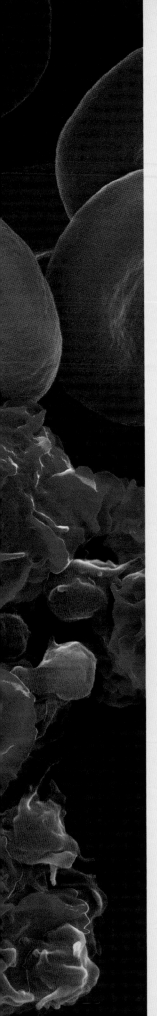

CHAPTER 24
Platelets, blood coagulation and haemostasis

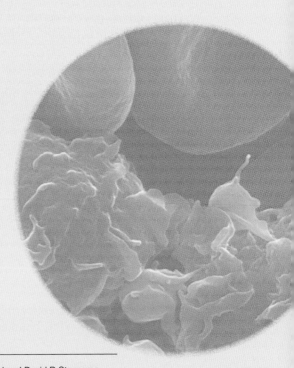

Hoffbrand's Essential Haematology, Eighth Edition. By A. Victor Hoffbrand and David P. Steensma.
© 2020 John Wiley & Sons Ltd. Published 2020 by John Wiley & Sons Ltd.
Companion website: www.wileyessential.com/haematology

The normal haemostatic response to vascular damage depends on a closely linked interaction between the blood vessel wall, circulating platelets and blood coagulation factors (Fig. 24.1).

An efficient and rapid mechanism for stopping bleeding from sites of blood vessel injury is clearly essential for survival. Nevertheless, such a response needs to be tightly controlled to prevent extensive clots developing and to be able to break down such clots once damage is repaired. The haemostatic system thus represents a delicate balance between procoagulant and anticoagulant mechanisms allied to a process for fibrinolysis. The five major components involved are platelets, coagulation factors, coagulation inhibitors, fibrinolysis and blood vessels.

Platelets

Platelet production

Platelets are produced in the bone marrow by fragmentation of the cytoplasm of megakaryocytes, one of the largest cells in the body. The precursor of the megakaryocyte – the megakaryoblast – arises by a process of differentiation from the haemopoietic stem cell (see Fig. 1.2). The megakaryocyte matures by endomitotic synchronous replication (i.e. DNA replication in the absence of nuclear or cytoplasmic division) enlarging the cytoplasmic volume as the number of nuclear lobes increases in multiples of two (Fig. 24.2). Early on invaginations of plasma membrane are seen, called the demarcation membrane, which evolves through the development of the megakaryocyte into a highly branched network. At a variable stage in development the cytoplasm becomes granular. Mature megakaryocytes are extremely large, with an eccentrically placed single lobulated nucleus and a low nuclear : cytoplasmic ratio (Fig. 24.3). Platelets form by fragmentation from the tips of cytoplasmic extensions of megakaryocyte cytoplasm, each megakaryocyte giving rise approximately to 1000–5000 platelets (Fig. 24.3c, d). The platelets are released through the endothelium of the vascular niches of the marrow where megakaryocytes reside. The time interval from differentiation of the human stem cell to the production of platelets averages 10 days.

Thrombopoietin (TPO) is the major regulator of platelet formation and 95% is produced by the liver. Approximately 50% is produced constitutively, the plasma level depending on its removal from plasma by binding to c-MPL receptors on platelets and megakaryocytes (Fig. 24.4a). Therefore, levels are high in thrombocytopenia as a result of marrow aplasia, but

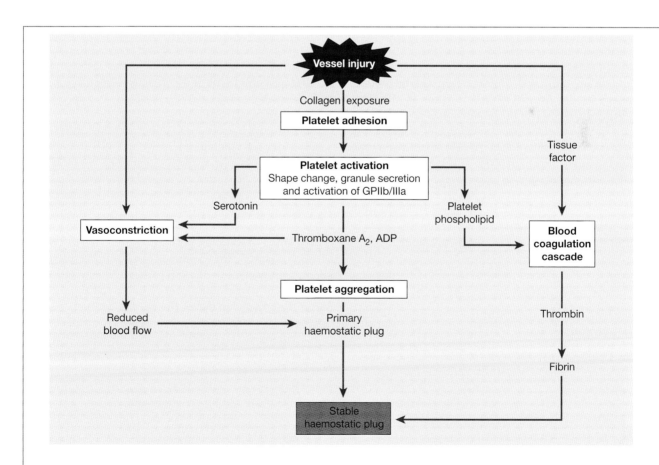

Figure 24.1 The involvement of blood vessels, platelets and blood coagulation in haemostasis. ADP, adenosine diphosphate.

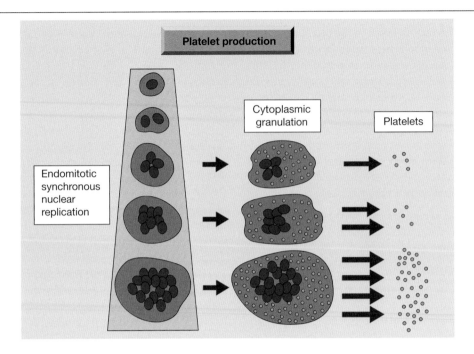

Figure 24.2 Simplified diagram to illustrate platelet production from megakaryocytes.

low in patients with raised platelet counts. The other 50% is regulated in response to platelet destruction. **As platelets age they lose surface sialic acid. This exposes galactose residues that attach to the Ashwell–Morell receptor in the liver. This attachment signals for the production of new TPO (Fig 24.4b).** TPO increases the number and rate of maturation of megakaryocytes via c-MPL receptors. Platelet levels start to rise 6 days after the start of therapy. Although TPO itself is not available for clinical use, thrombomimetic agents which bind to c-MPL are now used clinically to increase the platelet count (see p. 316).

The normal platelet count is approximately 250×10^9/L (range $150–400 \times 10^9$/L) and the normal platelet lifespan is 10 days. This is determined by the ratio of the apoptotic BAX and anti-apoptotic BCL-2 proteins in the cell. Up to one-third of the marrow output of platelets may be trapped at any one time in the normal spleen, but this rises to 90% in cases of massive splenomegaly (see Fig. 25.9).

Platelet structure

Platelets are extremely small and discoid, $3.0 \times 0.5\,\mu m$ in diameter. The ultrastructure of platelets is represented in Fig. 24.5. The glycoproteins (GPs) of the surface coat are particularly important in the platelet reactions of adhesion and aggregation, which are the initial events leading to platelet plug formation during haemostasis (Fig. 24.6).
- **Glycoprotein Ib** (defective in Bernard–Soulier syndrome), which forms a macromolecular complex with GPs V and IX, is important in the initial attachment of platelets to

von Willebrand factor (VWF) and hence to vascular sub-endothelium (Fig. 24.6).
- **Glycoproteins Ia–IIa and VI** facilitate adhesion to exposed collagen of the vessel wall (Fig. 24.7).
- **Glycoprotein IIb/IIIa** (also called integrin αIIb and β3 and defective in Glanzman's thrombasthenia) is important for additional binding of platelets to VWF and for facilitating platelet–platelet aggregation, both by binding to VWF and to fibrinogen, which is also involved in platelet–platelet aggregation.

The plasma membrane invaginates into the platelet interior to form an open membrane (canalicular) system, which provides a large reactive surface to which the plasma coagulation proteins may be selectively adsorbed. **The membrane phospholipids (previously known as platelet factor 3) are of particular importance in the conversion of coagulation factor X to Xa and prothrombin (factor II) to thrombin (factor IIa) (see Fig. 24.9).**

The platelet contains three types of storage granules: dense, α and lysosomes (Fig. 24.5). The more frequent specific α granules contain clotting factors, VWF, platelet-derived growth factor (PDGF) and other proteins. Dense granules are less common and contain adenosine diphosphate (ADP), adenosine triphosphate (ATP), serotonin and calcium. Lysosomes contain hydrolytic enzymes. Platelets are also rich in signalling and cytoskeletal proteins, which support the rapid switch from quiescence to activation that follows vessel damage. During the release reaction described below, the contents of the granules are discharged into the open canalicular system.

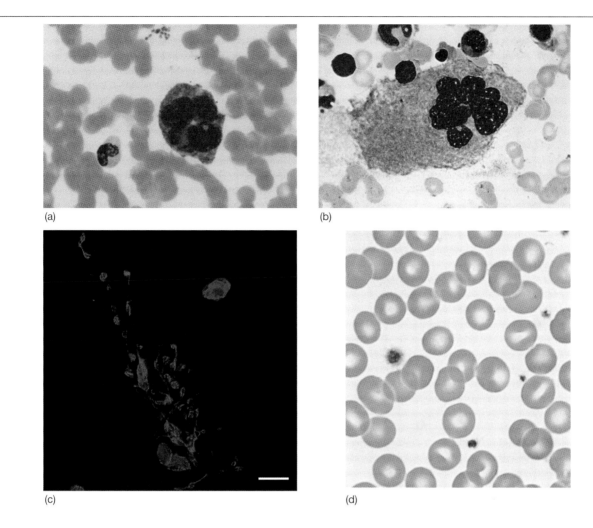

Figure 24.3 Megakaryocytes: **(a)** immature form with basophilic cytoplasm; **(b)** mature form with many nuclear lobes and pronounced granulation of the cytoplasm. **(c)** Megakaryocyte in culture, stained for α-tubulin (green). Proplatelets can be seen budding from the tips of megakaryocyte cytoplasm. **(d)** Normal red cells are mean 8 μm in diameter with minor variations in size and shape. The majority show a central pale area of diminished staining. Platelets, 1–3 μm across, are also evident. Source: (a)–(c) A. Pecci *et al*. (2009) *Thromb. Haemost.* 109: 90–96. (d) A.V. Hoffbrand *et al*. (2019) *Color Atlas of Clinical Hematology*, 5th edn. Reproduced by permission of John Wiley & Sons.

Platelet antigens

Several platelet surface proteins have been found to be important antigens in platelet-specific autoimmunity and they have been termed human platelet antigens (HPA). In most cases, two different alleles exist, termed a or b alleles (e.g. HPA-1a). Platelets also express ABO and human leucocyte antigen (HLA) class I but not class II antigens.

Platelet function

The main function of platelets is the formation of mechanical plugs during the haemostatic response to vascular injury. In the absence of platelets, spontaneous leakage of blood through small vessels may occur. There are three major platelet functions: **adhesion, aggregation** and **release reactions and amplification.** The immobilization of platelets at the sites of vascular injury requires specific platelet–vessel wall (adhesion) and platelet–platelet (aggregation) interactions, both partly mediated through VWF (Figs 24.6, 24.7).

Von Willebrand factor

VWF is involved in shear-dependent platelet adhesion to the vessel wall and to other platelets (aggregation; Figs 24.6, 24.7). It also carries factor VIII (Fig 26.7). It is a large glycoprotein, with multimers made up on average of 2–50 dimeric subunits. Damage to the vessel wall exposes subendothelial collagen, which normally binds large VWF

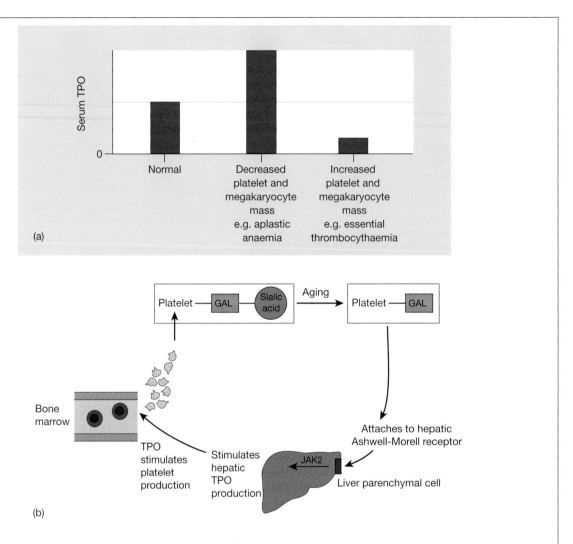

Figure 24.4 (a) Thrombopoietin (TPO) binds to the MPL receptor on the surface of megakaryocytes and platelets and is not recycled. Plasma levels of TPO, constitutively produced by the liver, are therefore affected by platelet and megakaryocyte MPL mass, the levels being high if this mass is low, as in aplastic anaemia, and low if this mass is high, as in essential thrombocythaemia. **(b)** The regulation of platelet production through hepatic clearance of de-sialylated platelets which attach to the Ashwell–Morell hepatic receptor. This initiates a signal via JAK2 for further TPO and hence platelet production. GAL, galactose.

multimers. Shear stress unfolds these large molecular weight multimers, exposing the platelet binding site, allowing capture of platelets via their GP1b-V-IX and then IIb/IIIa binding sites (Figs 24.6, 24.7).

VWF is synthesized in both endothelial cells and megakaryocytes, and stored in Weibel–Palade bodies and platelet α granules, respectively. Plasma VWF is almost entirely derived from endothelial cells, with two distinct pathways of secretion. The majority is continuously secreted and a minority is stored in Weibel–Palade bodies. The stored VWF can raise the plasma levels when released under the influence of several secretagogues, such as stress, exercise, adrenaline and infusion of desmopressin (1-diamino-8-D-arginine vasopressin; DDAVP). The VWF released from Weibel–Palade bodies is in the form of

large and ultra-large multimers, the most adhesive and reactive form of VWF. They are in turn cleaved in plasma to smaller multimers and monomeric VWF by the specific plasma metalloprotease ADAMTS13 (see Fig. 25.7).

Platelet aggregation

This is characterized by cross-linking of platelets through active GPIIb/IIIa receptors via VWF or fibrinogen bridges. A resting platelet has GPIIb/IIIa receptors which do not bind fibrinogen, VWF or other ligands. Stimulation of a platelet leads to a conformational change in GPIIb/IIIa and an increase in surface GPIIb/IIIa molecules, enabling platelet cross-linking via VWF and fibrinogen bridges (Fig. 24.7).

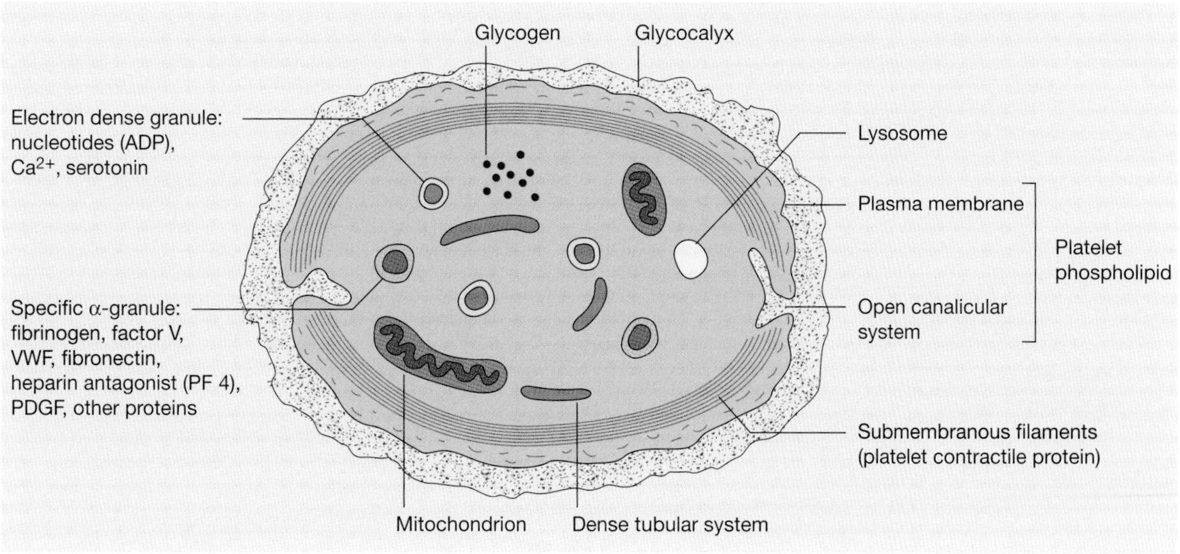

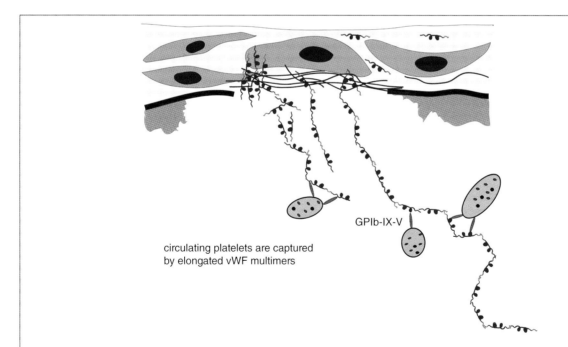

Figure 24.5 The ultrastructure of platelets. ADP, adenosine diphosphate; PDGF, platelet-derived growth factor; PF, platelet factor; VWF, von Willebrand factor.

GPIb-IX-V

circulating platelets are captured
by elongated vWF multimers

Figure 24.6 The interaction of platelets with the endothelium via von Willebrand factor (VWF). Disruption of the endothelial layer unravels the high molecular weight VWF, exposing the binding sites for collagen and platelets. The key platelet receptor for VWF is GPIb-IX-V. Source: A.V. Hoffbrand *et al.* (2019) *Color Atlas of Clinical Hematology*, 5th edn. Reproduced by permission of John Wiley & Sons.

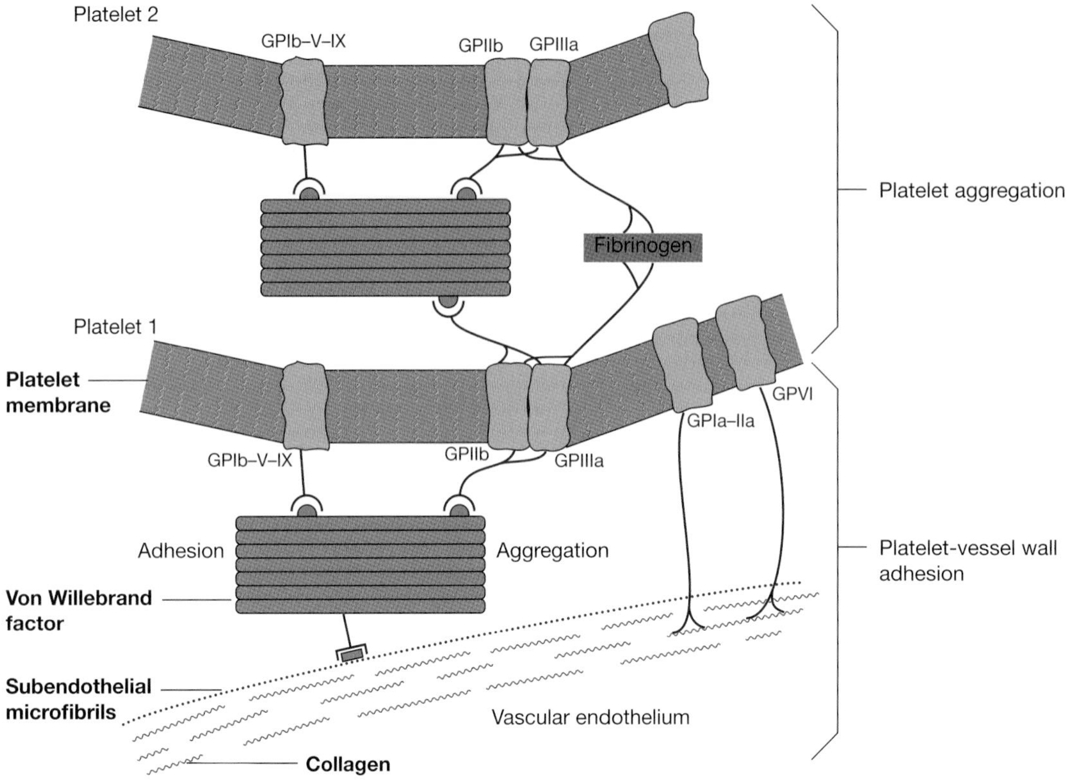

Figure 24.7 Platelet adhesion to the damaged blood vessel wall and to each other (aggregation). The binding of the platelet glycoprotein GPIb, which forms a complex with GPV and GPIX to exposed long multimers of von Willebrand factor (VWF), leads to platelet adhesion to the subendothelium. It also exposes the GPIIb/IIIa binding sites, leading to further binding to VWF and so further platelet adhesion to the subendothelium. The GPI-IIa and -VI sites form direct attachments to exposed subendothelial collagen. Platelets also attach to each other (platelet aggregation) via binding to VWF and to fibrinogen by the GPIIb/IIIa receptors.

Platelet release reaction and amplification

Primary activation by various agonists induces intracellular signalling, leading to the release of α granule contents. These have an important role in platelet aggregate formation and stabilization and, in addition, the ADP released from dense granules has a major positive feedback role in promoting platelet activation.

Thromboxane A$_2$ (TXA2) is important in secondary amplification of platelet activation to form a stable platelet aggregate. It is formed *de novo* upon activation of cytosolic phospholipase A$_2$ (PL$_{A2}$; Fig. 24.8). TXA2 lowers platelet cyclic adenosine monophosphate (cAMP) levels and initiates the release reaction (Fig. 24.7). TXA2 not only potentiates platelet aggregation, but also has powerful vasoconstrictive activity. The release reaction is inhibited by substances that increase the level of platelet cAMP. One such substance is prostacyclin (PGI$_2$), which is synthesized by vascular endothelial cells. It is a potent inhibitor of platelet aggregation and prevents their deposition on normal vascular endothelium.

Platelet procoagulant activity

After platelet aggregation and release, the exposed membrane phospholipid (platelet factor 3) is available for two reactions in the coagulation cascade. Both phospholipid-mediated reactions are calcium-ion dependent. The first (tenase) involves factors IXa, VIIIa and X in the formation of factor Xa (Fig. 24.9). The second (prothrombinase) results in the formation of thrombin from the interaction of factors Xa, Va and prothrombin (II). The phospholipid surface forms an ideal template for the crucial concentration and orientation of these proteins.

Growth factor

PDGF found in the α granules of platelets stimulates vascular smooth muscle cells to multiply and this may hasten vascular healing following injury.

Natural inhibitors of platelet function

Nitric oxide (NO) is constitutively released from endothelial cells (Fig. 24.10) and also from macrophages and platelets. It

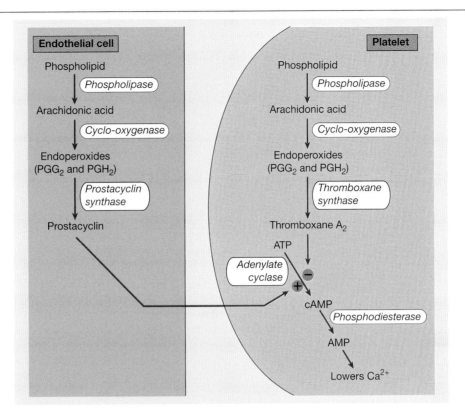

Figure 24.8 The synthesis of prostacyclin and thromboxane A$_2$. The opposing effects of these agents are mediated by changes in the concentration of cyclic adenosine monophosphate (cAMP) in platelets via stimulation or inhibition of the enzyme adenylate cyclase. cAMP controls the concentration of free calcium ions in the platelet, which are important in the processes that cause adhesion and aggregation. High levels of cAMP lead to low free calcium ion concentrations and prevent aggregation and adhesion. ATP, adenosine triphosphate; Ca, calcium; PG, prostaglandin (G$_2$ and H$_2$).

inhibits platelet activation and promotes vasodilatation. Prostacyclin synthesized by endothelial cells also inhibits platelet function (Fig. 24.10) and causes vasodilatation by raising cyclic guanosine monophosphate (GMP) levels. An ectonucleotidase (CD39) acts as an ADPase and helps prevent platelet aggregation in the intact vessel wall.

Blood coagulation

The coagulation cascade

Blood coagulation in vivo involves initiation by activation of clotting factor VII by tissue factor released and exposed by damaged blood vessels (Fig. 24.9). Then there is a biological amplification phase initiated by small amounts of thrombin (factor IIa) generated in the initiation phase. Relatively few initiation substances sequentially activate by proteolysis a cascade of circulating precursor proteins (the coagulation factor enzymes; Table 24.1), which culminates in the generation of larger amounts of thrombin; this, in turn, converts soluble plasma fibrinogen into fibrin (Fig. 24.11). Fibrin enmeshes the platelet aggregates at the sites

of vascular injury and converts the unstable primary platelet plugs to firm, definitive and stable haemostatic plugs.

Surface-mediated reactions occur on exposed collagen, platelet phospholipid and tissue factor. With the exception of fibrinogen, which is the fibrin clot subunit, the coagulation factors are either enzyme precursors or cofactors (Table 24.1). All the enzymes, except factor XIII, are serine proteases (i.e. their ability to hydrolyse peptide bonds depends upon the amino acid serine at their active centre). The operation of this enzyme cascade requires local concentration of circulating coagulation factors at the site of injury.

The scale of amplification achieved in this system is dramatic (e.g. 1 mol of activated factor XI through sequential activation of factors IX, X and prothrombin may generate up to 2×10^8 mol of fibrin).

Coagulation *in vivo*

The generation of thrombin *in vivo* is a complex network of amplification and negative feedback loops to ensure a localized and limited production. **The generation of large amounts of thrombin is dependent on three enzyme complexes, each**

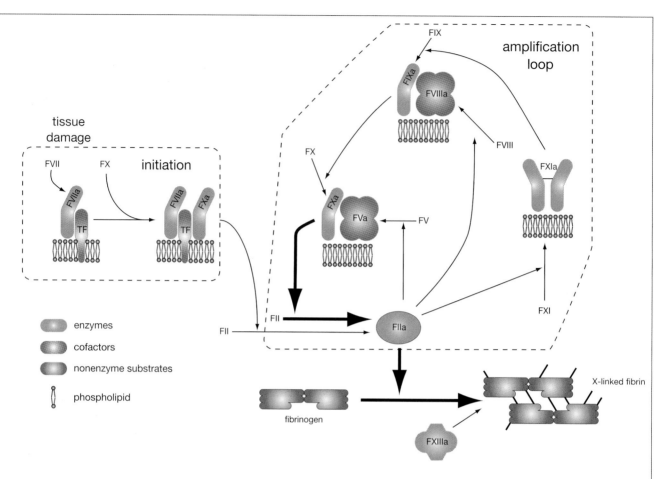

Figure 24.9 Fibrin clot formation is initiated *in vivo* by tissue damage exposing tissue factor to factor VII. A small amount of thrombin is formed that is not sufficient to form fibrin clot, but activates the amplification loop containing the rest of the coagulation factors. This leads to a large burst of thrombin formation (shown by thick arrows) that converts soluble fibrinogen into insoluble fibrin. Coagulation enzymes are shown as blue shapes and cofactors are in red. The negatively charged phospholipid membrane on which these reactions occur is mostly provided by activated platelets. Source: A.V. Hoffbrand *et al.* (2019) *Color Atlas of Clinical Hematology*, 5th edn. Reproduced by permission of John Wiley & Sons.

consisting of protease, cofactor, phospholipids (PL) and calcium (Fig. 24.9). They are: (i) extrinsic Xase (VIIa, TF, PL, Ca^{2+}), generating FXa; (ii) intrinsic Xase (IXa, VIIIa, PL, Ca^{2+}), also generating FXa; and (iii) prothrombinase complex (Xa, Va, PL, Ca^{2+}), generating thrombin. The generation of thrombin following vascular injury occurs in two waves of very different magnitude. During the initial phase only small amounts of thrombin are generated (picomolar concentrations) by activated factor X. This thrombin leads to a second million times larger burst of thrombin production (Fig. 24.9). These phases of coagulation are described in further detail next.

Initiation

Coagulation is initiated after vascular injury by the interaction of the membrane bound tissue factor (TF), exposed and activated by vascular injury, with plasma factor VII. TF is expressed on fibroblasts and small muscles of the vessel

wall and in the bloodstream on microparticles, and on other non-vascular cells. The factor VIIa–tissue factor (extrinsic factor Xase) complex activates both factor IX and factor XI. Factor Xa, in the absence of its cofactor, forms only small amounts of thrombin from prothrombin. This is insufficient to initiate significant fibrin polymerization. Amplification is needed.

Amplification

The initiation pathway or extrinsic Xase is rapidly inactivated by tissue factor pathway inhibitor (TFPI). Thrombin generation is now dependent on the traditional intrinsic pathway (Figs 24.9 and 24.12). In this pathway factor VIII and V are converted to VIIIa and Va by the small amounts of thrombin generated during initiation. In this amplification phase the intrinsic Xase, formed by IXa and VIIIa on phospholipid surface in the presence of Ca^{2+}, activates sufficient Xa, which then, in combination with Va, PL and Ca^{2+}, forms the prothrombinase complex

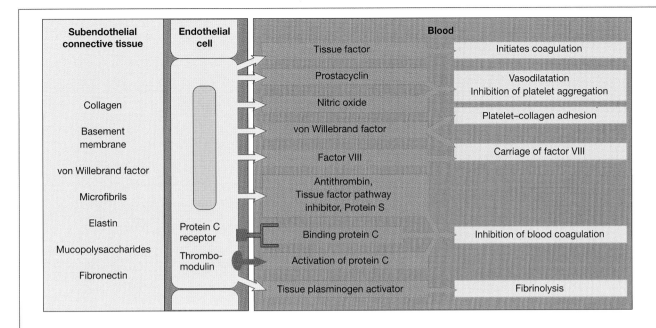

Figure 24.10 The endothelial cell forms a barrier between platelets and plasma clotting factors and the subendothelial connective tissues. Endothelial cells produce substances that can initiate coagulation, cause vasodilatation, inhibit platelet aggregation or haemostasis, or activate fibrinolysis.

Table 24.1 The coagulation factors.

Factor number	Descriptive name	Active form
I	Fibrinogen	Fibrin subunit
II	Prothrombin	Serine protease
III	Tissue factor	Receptor/cofactor*
V	Labile factor	Cofactor
VII	Proconvertin	Serine protease
VIII	Antihaemophilic factor	Cofactor
IX	Christmas factor	Serine protease
X	Stuart–Prower factor	Serine protease
XI	Plasma thromboplastin antecedent	Serine protease
XII	Hageman (contact) factor	Serine protease
XIII	Fibrin-stabilizing factor Prekallikrein (Fletcher factor)	Transglutaminase serine protease
	HMWK (Fitzgerald factor)	Cofactor*

*Active without proteolytic modification.
HMWK, high molecular weight kininogen.

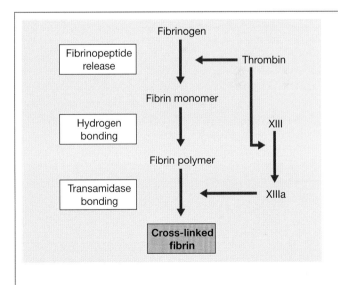

Figure 24.11 The formation and stabilization of fibrin.

and results in the explosive generation of thrombin which acts on fibrinogen to form the fibrin clot.

Factor XI does not seem to have a role in the physiological initiation of coagulation except during contact activation of the intrinsic coagulation pathway, especially in the setting of artificial surfaces such as catheters, heart valves, during

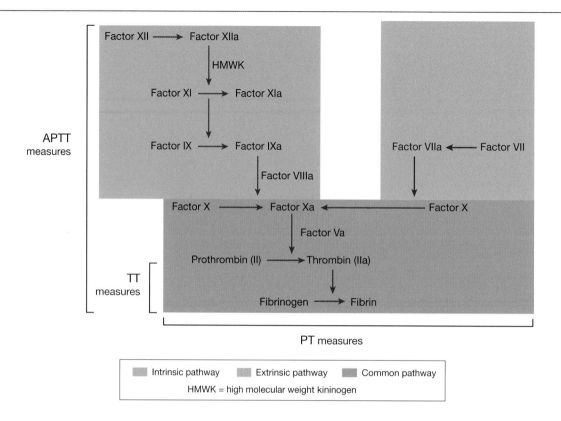

Figure 24.12 The intrinsic (contact), extrinsic and common pathways of blood coagulation. The APPT tests the intrinsic and common pathways, the PT the extrinsic and common pathways and the TT tests for thrombin inhibitors and deficiency or abnormality of fibrinogen. APTT, activated partial thromboplastin time; HMWK, high molecular weight kininogen; PT, prothrombin time; TT, thrombin time.

extracorporeal membrane oxygenation (ECMO) and other similar exposures. It has a supplementary role in the activation of factor IX (see above) and may be important at major sites of trauma or at operations, in which situations factor XI-deficient individuals tend to bleed excessively.

Thrombin hydrolyses fibrinogen, releasing fibrinopeptides A and B to form fibrin monomers (Fig. 24.11). Fibrin monomers link spontaneously by hydrogen bonds to form a loose insoluble fibrin polymer. Factor XIII is also activated by thrombin and stabilizes the fibrin polymers with the formation of covalent bond cross-links.

Fibrinogen consists of two identical subunits, each containing three dissimilar polypeptide chains (α, β and γ) which are linked by disulphide bonds. After cleavage by thrombin of small fibrinopeptides A and B from the α and β chains, fibrin monomer consists of three paired α, β and γ chains which rapidly polymerize.

Some of the properties of the coagulation factors are listed in Table 24.2. The activity of factors II, VII, IX and X is dependent upon vitamin K, which is responsible for carboxylation of a number of terminal glutamic acid residues on each of these molecules (see Fig. 26.8).

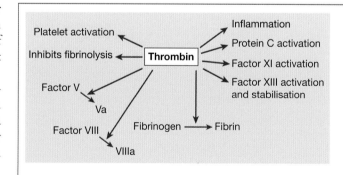

Figure 24.13 The actions of thrombin in the coagulation pathway. It also activates platelets and inflammation.

Although factor VIII and V cofactors are not protease enzymes, they circulate in a precursor form that requires limited cleavage by thrombin for expression of full cofactor activity (Fig. 24.13).

Table 24.2 The coagulation factors.

Factor	Plasma half-life (h)	Plasma concentration (mg/L)	Comments
II	65	100	Prothrombin group: vitamin K needed for synthesis; require Ca^{2+} for activation
VII	5	0.5	
IX	25	5	
X	40	10	
I	90	3000	Thrombin interacts with them; increase in inflammation, pregnancy, oral contraceptives
V	15	10	
VIII	10	0.1	
XI	45	5	
XIII	200	30	

Endothelial cells

The endothelial cell has an active role in the maintenance of vascular integrity. This cell provides the basement membrane that normally separates collagen, elastin and fibronectin of the subendothelial connective tissue from the circulating blood (Fig. 24.10). Loss of or damage to the endothelium results in both haemorrhage and activation of the haemostatic mechanism. The endothelial cell also has a potent inhibitory influence on the haemostatic response, largely through the synthesis of prostaglandin, NO and the ectonucleotidase CD39, which have vasodilatory properties and inhibit platelet aggregation.

Synthesis of tissue factor that initiates haemostasis only occurs in endothelial cells following activation, when its natural inhibitor, TFPI, is also synthesized. Endothelial synthesis of prostacyclin, VWF, factor VIII, plasminogen activator, antithrombin and thrombomodulin, the surface protein responsible for activation of protein C, provides agents that are vital to both platelet reactions and blood coagulation (Fig. 24.10).

Haemostatic response (Fig. 24.1)

The different components required for a haemostatic response to injury have been described above. The sequence of events *in vivo* and how the response is limited to the site of injury are described next.

Vasoconstriction

Immediate vasoconstriction of the injured vessel and reflex constriction of adjacent small arteries and arterioles is responsible for an initial slowing of blood flow to the area of injury. When there is widespread damage, this vascular reaction prevents exsanguination. The reduced blood flow allows contact activation of platelets and coagulation factors. The vasoactive amines and TXA2 liberated from platelets (Fig. 24.8), and the fibrinopeptides liberated during fibrin formation (Fig. 24.11), also have vasoconstrictive activity.

Platelet reactions and primary haemostatic plug formation

Following a break in the endothelial lining, there is an initial adherence of platelets (via GP1b-V-IX receptor to high molecular weight VWF multimers and via GP 1a-IIa and GPVI to exposed collagen; Fig 24.7). Under conditions of high shear stress (e.g. arterioles), the exposed subendothelial matrix is initially coated with VWF that also binds to exposed collagen. Collagen exposure and thrombin generated through activation of tissue factor produced at the site of injury cause the adherent platelets to release their granule contents and also activate platelet prostaglandin synthesis, leading to the formation of TXA2. Released ADP causes platelets to swell and aggregate.

Platelet rolling in the direction of blood flow over exposed VWF with activation of GPIIb/IIIa receptors results in firmer binding and in platelet aggregation. Additional platelets from the circulating blood are drawn to the area of injury. This continuing platelet aggregation, also facilitated by fibrinogen binding, promotes the growth of the haemostatic plug, which soon covers the exposed connective tissue. The unstable primary haemostatic plug produced by these platelet reactions in the first minute or so following injury is usually sufficient to provide temporary control of bleeding. The highly localized enhancement of platelet activation by ADP and TXA2 results in a platelet mass large enough to plug the area of endothelial injury.

Stabilization of the platelet plug by fibrin

Definitive haemostasis is achieved when fibrin monomers, formed by cleavage of fibrinogen by thrombin, are cross-linked by factor XIII, condensing the platelet mass and resulting in clot retraction/compaction.

Following vascular injury, the formation of extrinsic Xase (VIIa, TF, PL and Ca^{2+}) initiates the coagulation cascade. Platelet aggregation and release reactions accelerate the coagulation process by providing abundant membrane phospholipid. The much larger amount of thrombin generated by the secondary intrinsic Xase at the injury site converts soluble plasma fibrinogen into fibrin, potentiates platelet aggregation and secretion and also activates factor XI and XIII and cofactors V and VIII. The fibrin component of the haemostatic plug increases as the fused platelets completely degranulate and autolyse, and after a few hours the entire haemostatic plug is transformed into a solid mass of cross-linked fibrin (Fig. 24.11). Clot retraction occurs, which is mediated by GPIIb/IIIa receptors which link the cytoplasmic actin filaments to surface-bound fibrin polymers. Nevertheless, because of the incorporation of plasminogen and TPA (see p. 309), this plug begins to autodigest during the same time frame.

Physiological limitation of blood coagulation

Unchecked, blood coagulation would lead to dangerous occlusion of blood vessels (thrombosis) if the protective mechanisms of coagulation factor inhibitors, blood flow and fibrinolysis were not in operation.

Coagulation factor inhibitors

It is important that the effect of thrombin is limited to the site of injury. The first inhibitor to act is TFPI, which is synthesized in endothelial cells, is present in plasma and platelets, and accumulates at the site of injury caused by local platelet activation. TFPI inhibits Xa and VIIa and tissue factor to limit the main *in vivo* pathway. There is also direct inactivation of thrombin and other serine protease factors by other circulating inhibitors, of which antithrombin is the most potent. It inactivates serine proteases (see Fig. 28.3). Heparin potentiates its action markedly. Another protein, heparin cofactor II, also inhibits thrombin. α_2-Macroglobulins, α_2-antiplasmin, C_1 esterase inhibitor and α_1- antitrypsin also exert inhibitory effects on circulating serine proteases.

Protein C and protein S

These are inhibitors of coagulation cofactors V and VIII. Thrombin binds to an endothelial cell surface receptor, thrombomodulin. The resulting complex activates the vitamin K-dependent serine protease, protein C, which is able to destroy activated factors V and VIII, thus preventing further thrombin generation. The action of protein C is enhanced by another vitamin K-dependent protein, S, which binds protein C to the platelet surface (Fig. 24.14). An endothelial protein C receptor localizes protein C to the endothelial surface, promoting protein C activation by the thrombin–thrombomodulin complex. In addition, activated protein C enhances fibrinolysis (Fig. 24.14).

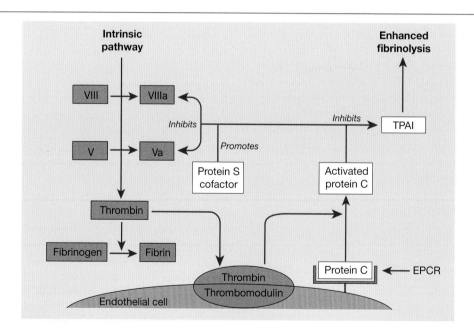

Figure 24.14 Activation and action of protein C by thrombin which has bound to thrombomodulin on the endothelial cell surface. Protein S is a cofactor that facilitates binding of activated protein C to the platelet surface. The inactivation of factors Va and VIIIa results in the inhibition of blood coagulation. The inactivation of tissue plasminogen activator inhibitor (TPAI) enhances fibrinolysis. EPCR, endothelial protein C receptor.

As with other serine proteases, activated protein C is subject to inactivation by serum protease inactivators (serpins), e.g. antithrombin.

Blood flow

At the periphery of a damaged area of tissue, blood flow rapidly achieves dilution and dispersal of activated factors before fibrin formation has occurred. Activated factors are destroyed by liver parenchymal cells and particulate matter is removed by liver Kupffer cells and other reticuloendothelial cells.

Fibrinolysis

Fibrinolysis (like coagulation) is a normal haemostatic response to vascular injury. Plasminogen, a proenzyme in blood and tissue fluid, is converted to the serine protease plasmin by thrombin and activators either from the vessel wall (intrinsic activation) or from the tissues (extrinsic activation) (Fig. 24.15). **The most important route follows the release of tissue plasminogen activator (TPA) from endothelial cells.** TPA is a serine protease that binds to fibrin. This enhances its capacity to convert thrombus-bound plasminogen into plasmin. This fibrin dependence of TPA action strongly localizes plasmin generation by TPA to the fibrin clot. Release of TPA occurs after such stimuli as trauma, exercise or emotional stress. Activated protein C stimulates fibrinolysis by destroying plasma inhibitors of TPA (Fig. 24.14).

Plasmin generation at the site of injury limits the extent of the evolving thrombus. The split products of fibrinolysis are also competitive inhibitors of thrombin and fibrin polymerization. Normally, α_2-antiplasmin inhibits any local free plasmin.

Fibrinolytic agents are widely used in clinical practice (see p. 357). Recombinant TPA, the bacterial agent, streptokinase and urokinase, initially isolated from human urine, are available. Anti-fibrinolytic agents such as epsilon aminocaproic acid and tranexamic acid are used to prevent fibrinolysis, such as in trauma or post-partum haemorrhage.

Plasmin is capable of digesting fibrinogen, fibrin, factors V and VIII and many other proteins. Cleavage of peptide bonds in fibrin and fibrinogen produces a variety of split (degradation) products (Fig. 24.11). Large amounts of the smallest fragments can be detected in the plasma of patients with disseminated intravascular coagulation (see p. 333).

Inactivation of plasmin

Tissue plasminogen activator is inactivated by plasminogen activator inhibitor (PAI). Circulating plasmin is inactivated by the potent inhibitors α_2-antiplasmin and α_2-macroglobulin.

Tests of haemostatic function

Defective haemostasis with abnormal bleeding may result from:
1. A vascular disorder;
2. Thrombocytopenia or a disorder of platelet function; or
3. Defective blood coagulation.

A number of simple tests are employed to assess the platelet, vessel wall and coagulation components of haemostasis.

Blood count and blood film examination

As thrombocytopenia is a common cause of abnormal bleeding, patients with suspected bleeding disorders should initially have a blood count, including platelet count and blood film examination. In addition to establishing the presence of thrombocytopenia, the cause may be obvious (e.g. acute leukaemia). Modern counters measure platelet volume, but this parameter is not used routinely in clinical practice for diagnosis of platelet disorders. The absolute count of immature platelets (which contain RNA) correlates with increased platelet production, e.g. after haemorrhage, but again is not routinely measured or used clinically.

Screening tests of blood coagulation

Screening tests provide an assessment of the 'extrinsic' and 'intrinsic' systems of blood coagulation and also the central conversion of fibrinogen to fibrin (Fig. 24.12; Table 24.3).

The **prothrombin time (PT)** measures factors VII, X, V, prothrombin and fibrinogen. Tissue thromboplastin (a brain extract) or (synthetic) tissue factor with lipids and calcium is added to citrated plasma. The normal time for clotting is 10–14 s. It may be expressed as the international normalized ratio (INR; p. 353).

The **activated partial thromboplastin time (APTT)** measures factors VIII, IX, XI and XII in addition to factors X, V, prothrombin and fibrinogen. Three substances – phospholipid, a surface activator (e.g. kaolin) and calcium – are added to citrated plasma. The normal time for clotting is approximately 30–40 s.

Prolonged clotting times in the PT and APTT because of factor deficiency are corrected by the addition of normal

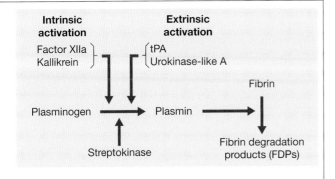

Figure 24.15 The fibrinolytic system. Thrombin activates a fibrinolysis inhibitor. tPA, tissue plasminogen activator.

Table 24.3 Screening tests used in the diagnosis of coagulation disorders (see also Fig. 24.12).

Screening tests	Abnormalities indicated by prolongation	Most common cause of coagulation disorder
Thrombin time (TT)	Deficiency or abnormality of fibrinogen or inhibition of thrombin by heparin or FDPs	DIC, heparin therapy
Prothrombin time (PT)	Deficiency or inhibition of one or more of the following coagulation factors: VII, X, V, II, fibrinogen	Liver disease, warfarin therapy, DIC
Activated partial thromboplastin time (APTT or PTTK)	Deficiency or inhibition of one or more of the following coagulation factors: XII, XI, IX (Christmas disease), VIII (haemophilia), X, V, II, fibrinogen	Haemophilia, Christmas disease (+ conditions above)
Fibrinogen quantitation	Fibrinogen deficiency	DIC, liver disease

N.B. Platelet count and the tests of platelet function are also used in screening patients with a bleeding disorder (p. 322).
DIC, disseminated intravascular coagulation; FDPs, fibrin degradation products.

plasma to the test plasma (50:50 mix). If there is no correction or incomplete correction with normal plasma, the presence of an inhibitor of coagulation is suspected.

The **thrombin (clotting) time (TT)** is sensitive to a deficiency of fibrinogen or inhibition of thrombin. Diluted bovine thrombin is added to citrated plasma at a concentration giving a clotting time of 14–16 s with normal subjects.

Specific assays of coagulation factors

Most factor assays are based on an APTT or PT in which all factors except the one to be measured are present in the substrate plasma. This usually requires a supply of plasma from patients with hereditary deficiency of the factor in question or artificially produced factor-deficient plasma. The corrective effect of the unknown plasma on the prolonged clotting time of the deficient substrate plasma is then compared with the corrective effect of normal plasma. Results are expressed as a percentage of normal activity.

A number of chemical, chromogenic and immunological methods are available for quantification of other proteins such as fibrinogen, VWF, factor Xa and factor VIII.

Tests of platelet function

Conventional **platelet aggregometry** measures the fall in light absorbance in platelet-rich plasma as platelets aggregate. Initial (primary) aggregation is caused by an external agent; the secondary response is caused by aggregating agents released from the platelets themselves. The five external aggregating agents most commonly used are ADP, collagen, ristocetin, arachidonic acid and adrenaline. The pattern of response to each agent helps to make the diagnosis (see Fig. 25.10). Flow cytometry is now increasingly used in routine practice to identify platelet glycoprotein defects.

In the **PFA-100 test**, citrated blood is aspirated through a capillary tube onto a membrane coated with collagen/ADP or collagen/adrenaline. Blood flow is maintained. Platelets begin to adhere and aggregate, primarily via VWF interactions with GPIb and GPIIb/IIIa, resulting in occlusion of the aperture. The PFA-100 is prolonged in VW disease and with other defects of platelet function. The analysis may give false-negative results with relatively common platelet defects. Full platelet aggregation tests and VWF screening may be required to exclude abnormal platelet function, even if the PFA-100 test is normal.

Tests of fibrinolysis

Testing for hyperfibrinolysis by traditional tests, such as the euglobulin clot lysis times, is rarely performed. A clinically significant hyperfibrinolytic state, e.g. during liver transplantation, can be detected by viscoelastic measurement of clot stability using **thromboelastography** (**TEG**) or **thromboelastometry** (**ROTEM**; see Fig. 26.10). Treatment with tranexamic acid reduces hyperfibrinolysis and reduces bleeding.

D-dimer is a measurement of fibrin degradation products and is an indication of sequential thrombin and then plasmin activity. The test can be performed on citrated plasma samples along with simple coagulation tests. There are many causes of a high D-dimer, including infection, cancer and pregnancy, as well as venous thromboembolism. Plasma levels are very high in patients with disseminated intravascular coagulation (DIC).

SUMMARY

- Normal haemostasis requires vasoconstriction, platelet aggregation and blood coagulation. The intact endothelial cell separates collagen and other subendothelial connective tissues that would stimulate platelet aggregation from circulating blood. The endothelial cells also produce prostacyclin, nitric oxide and an ectonucleotidase, which inhibit platelet aggregation.

- Platelets are produced from megakaryocytes in the bone marrow stimulated by thrombopoietin. They have surface glycoproteins which facilitate adherence to subendothelial tissues via von Willebrand factor, to collagen, to other platelets (aggregation) and to fibrinogen. Platelets contain different types of storage granules which are released after platelet activation.

- Blood coagulation *in vivo* in response to vascular injury commences with tissue factor binding to clotting factor VII and this initiates a cascade which results in thrombin generation. The small amounts of thrombin then activate cofactors VIII and V and factor XI, which greatly amplify the coagulation pathway resulting in a fibrin clot.

- Coagulation factor inhibitors include antithrombin, protein C and protein S.

- Dissolution of fibrin clots (fibrinolysis) occurs by activation of plasminogen to plasmin.

- Tests of haemostatic function include the thrombin time (TT), prothrombin time (PT), activated partial thromboplastin time (APTT) as well as individual coagulation factor assays and assay of von Willebrand factor. Tests of platelet function include the PFA-100 and platelet aggregation tests.

Now visit **www.wileyessential.com/haematology** to test yourself on this chapter.

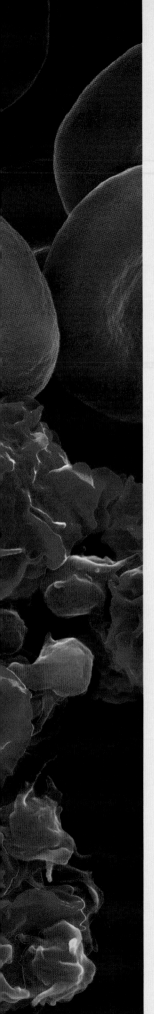

CHAPTER 25

Bleeding disorders caused by vascular and platelet abnormalities

Key topics

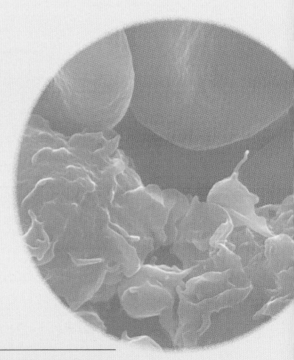

Hoffbrand's Essential Haematology, Eighth Edition. By A. Victor Hoffbrand and David P. Steensma.
© 2020 John Wiley & Sons Ltd. Published 2020 by John Wiley & Sons Ltd.
Companion website: www.wileyessential.com/haematology

Abnormal bleeding

This may result from:

1 Vascular disorders;
2 Thrombocytopenia;
3 Defective platelet function; or
4 Defective coagulation.

The pattern of bleeding is relatively predictable depending on the aetiology. Vascular and platelet disorders tend to be associated with bleeding from mucous membranes and into the skin, whereas in coagulation disorders the bleeding is often into joints or soft tissue (Table 25.1). Table 25.2 shows the World Health Organization grades of bleeding.

The first three categories are discussed in this chapter and the disorders of blood coagulation follow in Chapter 26.

Vascular bleeding disorders

The vascular disorders are a heterogeneous group of conditions characterized by easy bruising and spontaneous bleeding from the small vessels. The underlying abnormality is either in the vessels themselves or in the perivascular connective tissues. Most cases of bleeding caused by vascular defects alone are not severe. Frequently, the bleeding is mainly in the skin, causing petechiae, ecchymoses or both. In some disorders there is also bleeding from mucous membranes. In these conditions the standard screening tests are normal. The bleeding time is usually normal and the other tests of haemostasis are also normal. Vascular defects may be inherited or acquired.

Inherited vascular disorders

Hereditary haemorrhagic telangiectasia

This uncommon disease is transmitted as an autosomal dominant trait. Various genetic defects underlie the disease, such as mutations of the endothelial protein, endoglin. There are dilated microvascular swellings which appear during childhood and become more numerous in adult life. These telangiectasia develop in the skin, mucous membranes (Fig. 25.1a) and internal organs. Pulmonary, hepatic, splenic and cerebral arteriovenous shunts are seen in a minority of cases and may need local treatment. All patients are screened for pulmonary arteriovenous shunts. Recurrent epistaxes are frequent and recurrent gastrointestinal tract haemorrhage may cause chronic iron deficiency anaemia. Treatment is with embolization, laser treatment, oestrogens, tranexamic acid and iron supplementation. Thalidomide, lenalidomide, danazole, epsilon-aminocaproic acid and bevacizumab (anti-vascular endothelial growth factor) have been used to try to reduce gastrointestinal bleeding and bleeding at other sites in severe cases.

Connective tissue disorders

In the Ehlers–Danlos syndromes there are hereditary collagen abnormalities with purpura resulting from defective platelet adhesion, hyperextensibility of joints and hyperelastic friable skin. Pseudoxanthoma elasticum is associated with arterial haemorrhage and thrombosis. Patients may present with superficial bruising and purpura following minor trauma or after the application of a tourniquet. Bleeding and poor wound healing after surgery may be a problem.

Giant cavernous haemangioma

These congenital malformations occasionally cause chronic activation of coagulation, leading to laboratory features of consumptive coagulopathy similar to disseminated intravascular coagulation (DIC), including in some cases thrombocytopenia.

Acquired vascular defects

1 **Simple easy bruising** is a common benign disorder which occurs in otherwise healthy women, especially those of child-bearing age.
2 **Senile purpura** caused by atrophy of the supporting tissues of cutaneous blood vessels is seen mainly on dorsal aspects of the forearms and hands (Fig. 25.1b).

Table 25.1 Clinical differences between diseases of platelets/vessel wall and of coagulation factors.

	Platelets/vessel wall diseases	Coagulation diseases
Mucosal bleeding	Common	Rare
Petechiae	Common	Rare
Deep haematomas	Rare	Characteristic
Bleeding from skin cuts	Persistent	Minimal
Sex of patient	Equal	>80% male

Table 25.2 World Health Organization bleeding grades.

Grade 0	None
Grade 1	Petechiae, ecchymoses, occult blood loss, mild spotting
Grade 2	Gross bleeding, i.e. epistaxis, haematuria, haematemesis not requiring transfusion
Grade 3	Haemorrhage requiring transfusion
Grade 4	Haemorrhage with haemodynamic compromise, retinal haemorrhage with visual impairment, CNS haemorrhage, fatal at any location

CNS, central nervous system.

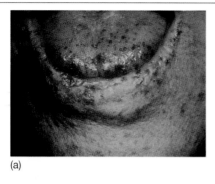

(a)

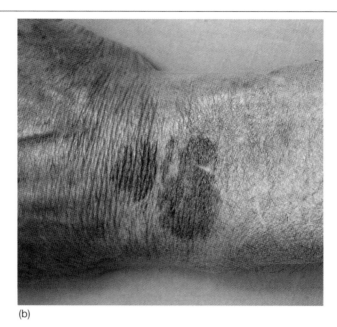

(b)

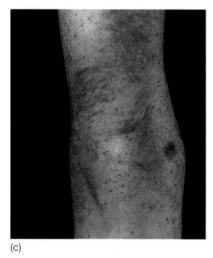

(c)

Figure 25.1 **(a)** Hereditary haemorrhagic telangiectasia: the characteristic small vascular lesions are obvious on the lips and tongue. **(b)** Senile purpura. **(c)** Characteristic perifollicular petechiae in vitamin C deficiency (scurvy).

3 Purpura associated with infections, mainly of bacterial, viral or rickettsial origin, may cause purpura from vascular damage by the organism, from DIC or as a result of immune complex formation (e.g. measles, dengue fever or meningococcal septicaemia).

4 The **Henoch–Schönlein syndrome** is usually seen in children and often follows an acute upper respiratory tract infection. It is an immunoglobulin (Ig) A-mediated vasculitis. The characteristic purpuric rash accompanied by localized oedema and itching is usually most prominent on the buttocks and extensor surfaces of the lower legs and elbows (Fig. 25.2). Painful joint swelling, haematuria and abdominal pain may also occur. It is usually a self-limiting condition but occasional patients develop renal failure.

5 **Scurvy.** In vitamin C deficiency defective collagen may cause perifollicular petechiae, bruising and mucosal haemorrhage (Fig. 25.1c).

6 **Steroid purpura.** The purpura, which is associated with long-term steroid therapy or Cushing's syndrome, is caused by defective vascular supportive tissue.

Tranexamic acid and aminocaproic acid are useful antifibrinolytic drugs that may reduce bleeding resulting from vascular disorders or thrombocytopenia, but are relatively contraindicated in the presence of haematuria because they might lead to clots obstructing the renal tract.

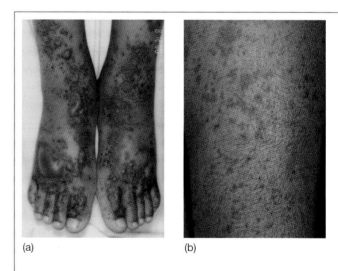

(a)

(b)

Figure 25.2 Henoch–Schönlein purpura: **(a)** unusually severe purpura on legs with bulla formation in a 6-year-old child; and **(b)** early urticarial lesions.

Thrombocytopenia

Abnormal bleeding associated with thrombocytopenia or abnormal platelet function is characterized by spontaneous skin purpura (Fig. 25.3) and mucosal haemorrhage and prolonged bleeding after trauma (Table 25.1). The main causes of thrombocytopenia are listed in Tables 25.3 and 25.4.

Failure of platelet production

This is the most common cause of thrombocytopenia and is usually part of a generalized bone marrow failure (Table 25.3). Selective megakaryocyte depression may result from drug toxicity or viral infection. Rarely it is congenital as a result of mutation of the *c-MPL* thrombopoietin receptor or of the *RBM8A* gene in association with absent radii. It is also seen in the MYH9-related disorders, which are the result of mutations in the *MYH9* gene resulting in thrombocytopenia, including the May–Hegglin anomaly with large inclusions in granulocytes as

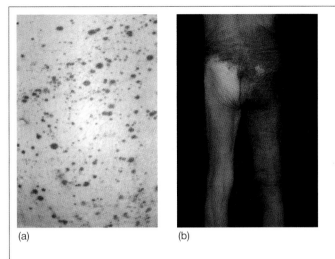

(a) (b)

Figure 25.3 (a) Typical purpura; and **(b)** massive subcutaneous haemorrhage in a patient with drug-induced thrombocytopenia.

well as in in Wiskott–Aldrich syndrome (WAS) with eczema and immune deficiency (see Chapter 8). WAS is caused by mutation of the *WASP* gene, the protein being a regulator of signalling in haemopoietic cells. Diagnosis of these causes of thrombocytopenia is made from the clinical history, peripheral blood count, the blood film and bone marrow examination.

Chronic liver disease can also be associated with thrombocytopenia, either due to splenic sequestration of platelets if the liver disease is associated with splenomegaly, or due to decreased production of thrombopoeitin. A specific TPO-mimetic, avatrombopag, has been approved for preoperative use to increase the platelet count in patients with chronic liver disease who require surgery.

Table 25.3 Causes of thrombocytopenia.

Failure of platelet production
Selective megakaryocyte depression
 Rare congenital defects (see text)
 Drugs, chemicals, viral infections
Part of general bone marrow failure
 Cytotoxic drugs
 Radiotherapy
 Aplastic anaemia
 Leukaemia
 Myelodysplastic syndromes
 Myelofibrosis
 Marrow infiltration (e.g. carcinoma, lymphoma, Gaucher's disease)
 Multiple myeloma
 Megaloblastic anaemia
 HIV infection

Increased consumption of platelets
Immune
 Autoimmune
 Idiopathic
 Associated with systemic lupus erythematosus, chronic lymphocytic leukaemia or lymphoma
 Infections: *Helicobacter pylori*, HIV, other viruses, malaria
 Drug-induced, e.g. heparin
 Post-transfusional purpura
 Feto-maternal alloimmune thrombocytopenia
Disseminated intravascular coagulation
Thrombotic thrombocytopenic purpura

Abnormal distribution of platelets
Splenomegaly (e.g. liver disease)

Dilutional loss
Massive transfusion of stored blood to bleeding patients

HIV, human immunodeficiency virus.

Table 25.4 Thrombocytopenia as a result of drugs or toxins.

Bone marrow suppression
Predictable (dose-related)
 Ionizing radiation, cytotoxic drugs, ethanol
Occasional
 Chloramphenicol, co-trimoxazole, idoxuridine, penicillamine, organic arsenicals, benzene, etc.

Immune mechanisms (proven or probable)
Analgesics, anti-inflammatory drugs
 Gold salts
Antimicrobials
 Penicillins, rifamycin, sulphonamides, trimethoprim, para-aminosalicylate, vancomycin, cephalosporins
Sedatives, anticonvulsants
 Diazepam, sodium valproate, carbamazepine
Diuretics
 Acetazolamide, chlorathiazides, furosemide
Antidiabetics
 Chlorpropamide, tolbutamide
Others
 Digitoxin, heparin, methyldopa, oxyprenolol, quinine, quinidine

Increased destruction of platelets

Autoimmune (idiopathic) thrombocytopenic purpura

Autoimmune (idiopathic) thrombocytopenic purpura may be divided into chronic and acute forms.

Chronic idiopathic thrombocytopenic purpura (ITP)

This is a relatively common disorder. The highest incidence has been considered to be in women aged 15–50 years, although some reports suggest an increasing incidence with age. **It is the most common cause of thrombocytopenia without anaemia or neutropenia**. It is usually idiopathic, but may be seen in association with other diseases such as systemic lupus erythematosus (SLE), human immunodeficiency virus (HIV) infection, hepatitis C virus (HCV), *Helicobacter pylori* infection, chronic lymphocytic leukaemia (CLL), Hodgkin lymphoma or autoimmune haemolytic anaemia (Table 25.3).

Pathogenesis

Platelet autoantibodies, usually IgG, result in the premature removal of platelets from the circulation by macrophages of the reticuloendothelial system, especially the spleen (Fig. 25.4). In many cases, the antibody is directed against the glycoprotein (GP) IIb/IIIa or Ib complex. The normal lifespan of a platelet is 10 days, but in ITP this is reduced to a few hours. Total megakaryocyte mass and platelet turnover are increased in parallel to approximately five times normal.

Clinical features

The onset is often insidious with petechial haemorrhage, easy bruising and, in women, menorrhagia. Mucosal bleeding (e.g. epistaxes or gum bleeding) occurs in severe cases, but fortunately intracranial haemorrhage is rare. The severity of bleeding in ITP is usually less than that seen in patients with comparable degrees of thrombocytopenia from bone marrow failure; this is attributed to the circulation of predominantly young, larger

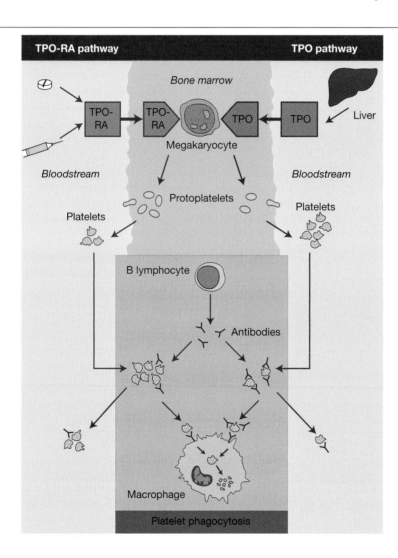

Figure 25.4 The pathogenesis of thrombocytopenia in autoimmune thrombocytopenic purpura. Platelets coated by antibodies are phagocytosed by macrophages. The actions of thrombopoietin (TPO) and thrombopoietin receptor agonists (TPO-RA; thrombomimetics) are shown. These are orally active or given by injection and act to increase platelet production.

sized and functionally superior platelets in ITP. Chronic ITP tends to relapse and remit spontaneously, so the course may be difficult to predict. Many asymptomatic cases are discovered by a routine blood count. The spleen is not palpable unless there is an associated disease causing splenomegaly.

Diagnosis

1 The platelet count is usually $10–100 \times 10^9$/L. The haemoglobin concentration and white cell count are typically normal unless there is iron deficiency anaemia because of blood loss.
2 The blood film shows reduced numbers of platelets, those present often being large. There are no morphological abnormalities in the other cell lines.
3 The bone marrow shows normal or increased numbers of megakaryocytes.
4 Sensitive tests are able to demonstrate specific anti-glyco-protein GPIIb/IIIa or GPIb antibodies on the platelet surface or in the serum in most patients. Platelet-associated IgG assays are less specific. These tests are not usually used in clinical practice.

Treatment

As this is a chronic disease, the aim of treatment should be to maintain a platelet count above the level at which spontaneous bruising or bleeding occurs with the minimum of intervention. In general, a platelet count above 20×10^9/L without symptoms does not require treatment.

1 *Corticosteroids* High-dose corticosteroid therapy is considered first-line therapy, on which 80% of patients remit. Dexamethasone at 40 mg a day for 4 days and then reduced can be used, as can prednisolone 1 mg/kg/day in adults, with the dosage gradually reduced after 10–14 days. In poor responders the dosage is reduced more slowly, but alternative immunosuppression or splenectomy is considered.
2 *High-dose intravenous immunoglobulin therapy* This is able to produce a rapid rise in platelet count in the majority of patients. A regimen of 400 mg/kg/day for 5 days or 1 g/kg/day for 2 days is used. It is particularly useful in patients with life-threatening haemorrhage, in steroid-refractory ITP, during pregnancy or prior to surgery. The mechanism of action may be blockage of Fc receptors on macrophages or modification of autoantibody production.
3 *Monoclonal antibody* Rituximab (anti-CD20) produces responses in approximately 80% of patients, which are often durable, and it is now usually tried before splenectomy.
4 *Thrombopoietin-receptor agonists* Romiplostim (subcutaneously), eltrombopag and avatrombopag (orally) are active non-peptide thrombopoietin-receptor agonists (thrombomimetics; Fig. 25.4). They stimulate thrombopoiesis (Fig. 25.5) and are indicated for patients in whom steroids are contraindicated or who are refractory to steroids. Small trials of their use as initial therapy in combination with corticosteroids or rituximab have yielded good responses with no increased toxicity. Increased reticulin and fibrosis in the bone marrow may occur with prolonged treatment, but are reversible on stopping the therapy. Extended duration of therapy trials has revealed no long-term adverse events in over 5 years of continuous use.

5 *Splenectomy* With the increase in number of alternative drugs, splenectomy is now performed less frequently for ITP than previously. Good results occur in most patients, with durable response in 60–80%, but in those with ITP refractory to steroids, immunoglobulin or rituximab there may be little benefit. Splenunculi must be removed, otherwise subsequent relapse of ITP can occur.
6 *Immunosuppressive drugs* These (e.g. vincristine, cyclophosphamide, bortezomib, mycophenolate mofetil or ciclosporin alone or in combination) are usually reserved for those patients who do not respond sufficiently to the above treatments. Fostamatinib is also licensed for this indication. It inhibits the protein product of the *SYK* gene, which is involved in signal transduction in B and other cells of the immune system.
7 *Other treatments* Alternatives that may elicit a remission include danazol (an androgen which may cause virilization in women) and intravenous anti-D immunoglobulin. It is often necessary to combine two drugs (e.g. danazol and an immunosuppressive agent). *Helicobacter pylori* infection should be treated, as there are some reports that this may improve the platelet count, particularly in countries where the incidence of the infection is common. Hepatitis C should also be treated, if present.
8 *Platelet transfusions* Platelet concentrates are beneficial in patients with acute life-threatening bleeding, but their benefit will only last for a few hours.
9 *Stem cell transplantation* This has cured some severe cases.

Acute idiopathic thrombocytopenic purpura

This is most common in children. In approximately 75% of patients the episode follows vaccination or an infection such as chickenpox or infectious mononucleosis. Most cases are caused by non-specific immune complex attachments to platelets. Spontaneous remissions are usual, but in 5–10% of cases the disease becomes chronic, lasting more than 6 months. Fortunately, morbidity and mortality in acute ITP are very low. The main risk is of cerebral haemorrhage, fortunately rare. Most children do not have any bleeding even with platelet counts $<10 \times 10^9$/L, but need to avoid trauma such as contact sports.

The diagnosis is one of exclusion. If the platelet count is over 30×10^9/L no treatment is necessary unless the bleeding is severe. Indeed, many doctors do not treat even with platelet counts $<10 \times 10^9$/L if there is no haemorrhage. The main risk is of cerebral haemorrhage. Treatment is with steroids and/or intravenous (IV) immunoglobulin, especially if there is significant bleeding. First-line treatment with IV Ig results in less bleeding and faster recovery, but not in a lower incidence of chronic ITP.

Infections

It seems likely that the thrombocytopenia associated with many viral and protozoal infections is immune-mediated. In HIV infection, reduced platelet production is also involved (see p. 367).

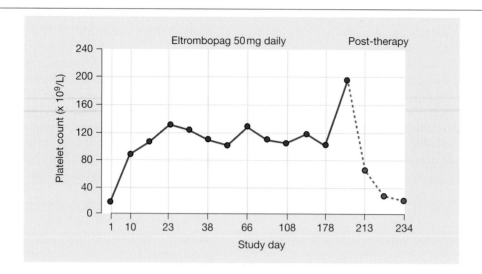

Figure 25.5 Response to eltrombopag in chronic immune thrombocytopenic purpura in a female aged 75 after failure of response to prednisolone. Source: Courtesy of Professor A. Newland.

Drug-induced immune thrombocytopenia

An immunological mechanism has been demonstrated as the cause of many drug-induced thrombocytopenias (Fig. 25.6). Quinine (including that in tonic water), quinidine and heparin are particularly common causes (Table 25.4).

The platelet count is often less than 10×10^9/L, and the bone marrow shows normal or increased numbers of megakaryocytes. Drug-dependent antibodies against platelets may be demonstrated in the sera of some patients. The immediate treatment is to stop all suspected drugs, but platelet concentrates should be given to patients with dangerous bleeding.

Post-transfusion purpura

This occurs as thrombocytopenia approximately 10 days after a blood transfusion, and has been attributed to antibodies in the recipient developing against human platelet antigen-1a (HPA-1a) on the transfused platelets (see p. 299). Although autologous platelets are also destroyed, the mechanism for autologous

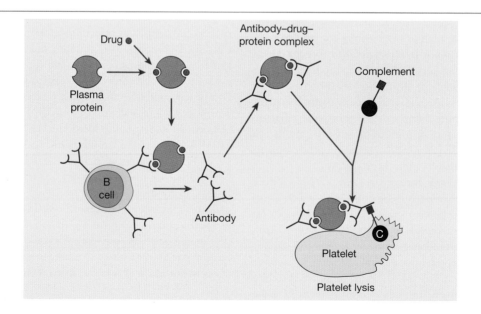

Figure 25.6 Usual type of platelet damage caused by drugs in which an antibody–drug–protein complex is deposited on the platelet surface. If complement is attached and the sequence goes to completion, the platelet may be lysed directly. Otherwise it is removed by reticuloendothelial cells because of opsonization with immunoglobulin and/or the C3 component of complement.

platelet destruction is not fully understood. Treatment with high-dose IV IgG and transfusion of HPA-1a-negative platelets may be necessary.

Thrombotic thrombocytopenic purpura and haemolytic uraemic syndrome

Thrombotic thrombocytopenic purpura (TTP) occurs in familial or acquired forms. There is deficiency of the ADAMTS13 metalloprotease which breaks down ultra-large von Willebrand factor multimers (ULVWF; Fig. 25.7). In the familial forms more than 50 ADAMTS13 mutations have been reported, whereas the acquired forms follow the development of an inhibitory IgG autoantibody, the presence of which may be stimulated by infection (including HIV), autoimmune/connective tissue disease, pregnancy, certain drugs, cancer, stem cell transplantation or cardiac surgery. The lack of ADAMTS13 activity results in the anchoring of ULVWF multimeric 'strings' secreted from Weibel–Palade bodies to the endothelial cells. Passing platelets adhere via their GPIb

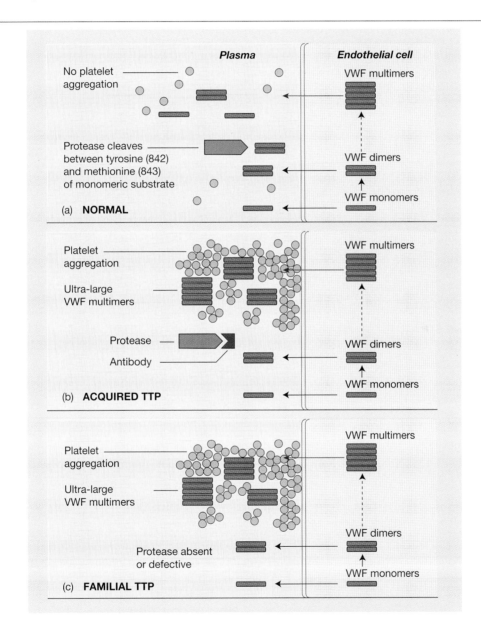

Figure 25.7 Pathogenesis of thrombotic thrombocytopenic purpura (TTP). Von Willebrand factor (VWF) consists of a series of VWF multimers each of molecular weight (MW) 250 kDa which are covalently linked. **(a)** Under physiological circumstances a metalloprotease ADAMTS13 cleaves high molecular weight multimers at a Tyr-842–Met-843 bond and the resulting VWF has an MW of 500–20 000 kDa. **(b)** In non-familial TTP, an antibody develops to the metalloprotease and so blocks cleavage of VWF multimers. **(c)** In congenital forms of TTP, the protease appears to be absent. In both cases, the resultant ultra-large VWF multimers can bind platelets under high shear stress conditions and lead to platelet aggregation.

receptors. Increasing platelet aggregation onto the ULVWF multimeric strings has the potential to form large occlusive platelet thrombi. These strings are capable of embolizing to microvessels downstream and contributing to organ ischemia (Fig. 25.8). In the closely related clinical syndrome haemolytic uraemic syndrome (HUS), ADAMTS13 levels are normal.

TTP has traditionally been described as a pentad of **thrombocytopenia, microangiopathic haemolytic anaemia, neurological abnormalities, renal failure and fever**. The microvascular thrombosis causes variable degrees of tissue ischaemia and infarction and is responsible for the microangiopathic haemolytic anaemia and thrombocytopenia (Fig. 25.8). Thrombocytopenia, schistocytes in the blood film and an impressively elevated serum lactate dehydrogenase (LDH) value are sufficient to suggest the diagnosis. The serum LDH is derived both from ischaemic or necrotic tissue cells and lysed red cells. Coagulation tests are normal, in contrast to the findings in DIC (see

Fig. 26.9). ADAMTS13 is absent or severely reduced in plasma and an anti-ADAMTS13 antibody is present, but the turnaround time to get test results for these can be days, so that treatment must be initiated before results are available.

Treatment is with plasma exchange, using fresh frozen plasma (FFP) or cryosupernatant. This removes the large molecular weight VWF multimers and the antibody and provides ADAMTS13. The platelet count and serum LDH are useful for monitoring the response to treatment. Rituximab (anti-CD20) is also effective, used in conjunction with plasma infusions or with plasma exchange, and subsequently for reducing the risk of relapse. Caplacizumab, an anti-VWF antibody that inhibits binding of platelets to ultra-large VWF multimers, promotes faster resolution of acute TTP. In refractory cases and chronic relapsing cases, high-dose corticosteroids, vincristine, intravenous immunoglobulin, rituximab and immunosuppressive therapy with cyclosporine, cyclophosphamide or bortezomib have been used. In untreated cases mortality may approach 90%. If the ADAMTS13 level falls to <10% during follow-up, pre-emptive rituximab therapy can reduce substantially relapse of TTP.

HUS in children has many common features, but organ damage is limited to the kidneys. There is also usually diarrhoea and epileptic seizures may occur. Many cases are associated with *Escherichia coli* infection with the verotoxin 0157 strain or with other organisms, especially *Shigella*. Supportive renal dialysis and control of hypertension are the mainstays of treatment. Platelet transfusions are contraindicated in HUS and TTP. Mutations in complement regulatory proteins (factor H, factor I or membrane cofactor protein) are present in many patients with atypical HUS. For atypical HUS, treatment is as for renal failure, but eculizumab (see p. 278) may be added to inhibit complement activation.

Disseminated intravascular coagulation (see p. 333)

In this disorder thrombocytopenia may result from a high rate of platelet destruction due to increased levels of consumption.

Increased splenic pooling

The major factor responsible for thrombocytopenia in splenomegaly is platelet 'pooling' by the spleen. In splenomegaly, up to 90% of platelets may be sequestered in the spleen, whereas normally this accounts for approximately one-third of the total platelet mass (Fig. 25.9). Platelet lifespan is normal and, in the absence of additional haemostatic defects, the thrombocytopenia of splenomegaly is not usually associated with bleeding.

Massive transfusion (see p. 335)

Platelets are unstable in blood stored at 4°C and the platelet count rapidly falls in blood stored for more than 24 hours. Patients transfused with massive amounts of stored blood, such as more than 10 units over a 24-hour period, frequently show abnormal clotting and thrombocytopenia. These should be corrected by the use of platelet transfusions and FFP.

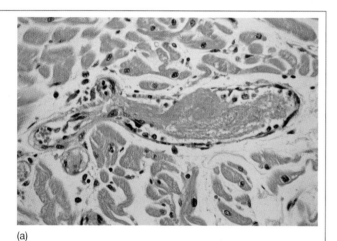
(a)

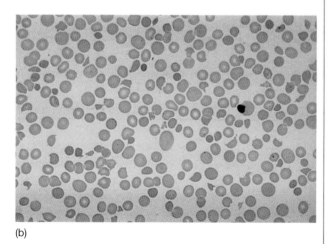
(b)

Figure 25.8 Thrombotic thrombocytopenic purpura. **(a)** Platelet thrombus in a small cardiac vessel with minor endothelial and inflammatory reaction. Source: Courtesy of Dr J.E. McLaughlin. **(b)** Peripheral blood film showing red cell fragmentation.

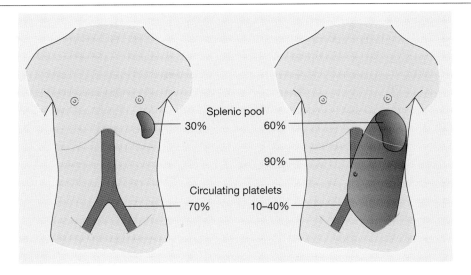

Figure 25.9 The platelet distribution between the circulation and spleen in normal individuals (left), and in patients with moderate or massive splenomegaly (right).

Disorders of platelet function

Disorders of platelet function are suspected in patients who show skin and mucosal haemorrhage despite a normal platelet count and normal levels of VWF. These disorders may be hereditary or acquired.

Hereditary disorders

Rare inherited disorders may produce defects at each of the different phases of the platelet reactions leading to the formation of the haemostatic platelet plug.

Thrombasthenia (Glanzmann's disease)

This autosomal recessive disorder leads to failure of primary platelet aggregation. It is caused by a variety of different mutations in the genes coding for GPIIb or IIIa (Fig. 24.6). It usually presents in the neonatal period and, characteristically, platelets fail to aggregate *in vitro* to any agonist except ristocetin.

Bernard–Soulier syndrome

In this autosomal recessive disease due to mutations in the GPIb gene, the platelets are larger than normal. There is defective binding to VWF, defective adherence to exposed subendothelial connective tissues and platelets do not aggregate with ristocetin. There is a variable degree of thrombocytopenia.

Storage pool diseases

A mutation in a growth factor independent gene (*GFI1B*) underlies the grey-platelet syndrome. The platelets are larger than normal, with virtual absence of alpha granules. In the more common delta-storage pool disease, there is deficiency of dense granules. Platelet-dependent haemostasis is abnormal in the much more common von Willebrand disease because of an inherited defect in VWF (see p. 329).

Acquired disorders

Antiplatelet drugs

Aspirin therapy is the most common cause of defective platelet function. It produces abnormal closure times in the platelet function analysis-100 (PFA-100) test and, although purpura may not be obvious, the defect may contribute to the associated gastrointestinal haemorrhage. The cause of the aspirin defect is inhibition of cyclo-oxygenase with impaired thromboxane A_2 synthesis (see Fig. 28.5). There is consequent impairment of the release reaction and aggregation (Fig. 25.10). After a single dose the defect lasts 10 days (i.e. the life of the platelet). While aspirin causes permanent inhibition of cyclo-oxygenase, other non-steroidal anti-inflammatory drugs (NSAIDs) cause a reversible inhibition and so can also be associated with defective platelet function leading to bruising and mucosal bleeding.

Dipyridamole inhibits platelet aggregation by blocking reuptake of adenosine and is usually used as an adjunct to aspirin. **Clopidogrel, prasugrel, ticagrelor and others** inhibit binding of ADP to its platelet receptor (Fig. 28.5), shown by impaired aggregation with ADP (Fig. 25.10). They are used mainly for prevention of thrombotic events (e.g. after coronary stenting or angioplasty) in patients with a history of symptomatic athero-sclerotic disease. The intravenous agents abciximab, eptifi-batide and tirofiban are inhibitors of GPIIb/IIIa receptor sites (Fig 28.5) and may be used in patients undergoing percutaneous coronary intervention, with unstable angina and acute coronary syndromes. There is a risk of transient thrombocytopenia with these agents.

See also Chapter 28.

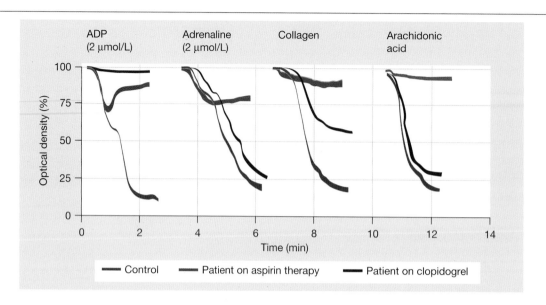

Figure 25.10 Defective platelet aggregation in patients on aspirin or clopidogrel therapy. With aspirin there is no secondary phase aggregation with adenosine diphosphate (ADP) and reduced responses to arachidonic acid, adrenaline and collagen. With clopidogrel the defect is mainly in ADP-induced aggregation.

Hyperglobulinaemia

Hyperglobulinaemia associated with multiple myeloma or Waldenström's disease may cause interference with platelet adherence, release and aggregation.

Myeloproliferative and myelodysplastic disorders

Intrinsic abnormalities of platelet function occur in many patients with essential thrombocythaemia, other myeloproliferative and myelodysplastic diseases and in paroxysmal nocturnal haemoglobinuria.

Uraemia

This is associated with various abnormalities of platelet function.

Diagnosis of platelet disorders

Patients with suspected platelet or blood vessel abnormalities should initially have a blood count and blood film examination (Fig. 25.11). Examination of the platelets on the peripheral blood film can give useful information. If platelets are clumped then the patient likely has pseudothrombocytopenia, an *in vitro* artifact due to the chelator EDTA. If so, repeat blood count in acid citrate dextrose or heparin will yield a normal platelet count. A low number of large platelets suggests ITP or a consumptive process. **Bone marrow examination is often needed in thrombocytopenic patients to determine whether or not there is a failure of platelet production.** The marrow may also reveal one of the conditions associated with defective production (Table 25.3). In children and young adults with isolated thrombocytopenia, the marrow test is often not performed.

In the elderly, marrow examination is needed particularly to exclude myelodysplasia. In patients with thrombocytopenia, normal haemoglobin and white cell counts, a negative drug history, normal or excessive numbers of marrow megakaryocytes and no other marrow abnormality or splenomegaly, ITP is the usual diagnosis. Screening tests for DIC are also useful, as are tests for an underlying disease such as SLE or HCV or HIV infection.

When the blood count, including platelet count and blood film examination, is normal, platelet aggregation tests and the PFA-100 can be used to detect abnormal platelet function. In most patients with abnormal platelet function demonstrated by the PFA-100 test the defect is acquired and associated either with systemic disease (e.g. uraemia) or with aspirin therapy. The rare hereditary defects of platelet function require more elaborate *in vitro* tests to define the specific abnormality. These include platelet aggregation studies (Fig. 25.10) and measurements of platelet nucleotide levels. If von Willebrand disease is suspected, assay of VWF and coagulation factor VIII are required (see p. 329).

Treatment of thrombocytopenia and platelet disorders

Thrombomimetics

These are drugs that increase platelet production by activating the thrombopoietin receptor on megakaryocytes. Three such drugs are **romiplostim**, given subcutaneously once weekly, and **eltrombopag** and **avatrombopag**, active orally and given daily. They are used in ITP (Fig. 25.5) and in other conditions, e.g. post-chemotherapy, myelodysplasia, aplastic anaemia and liver disease. They may cause disturbed liver function. Their long-term use may cause increased marrow reticulin and fibrosis, which is reversible

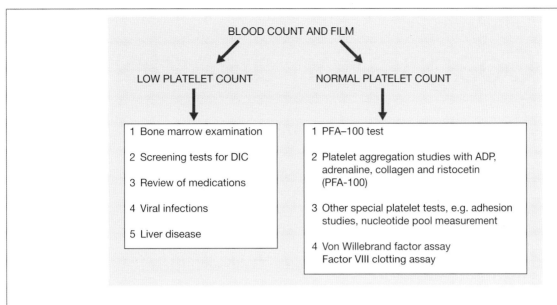

Figure 25.11 Laboratory tests for platelet disorders. N.B. Some intrinsic platelet functional disorders are associated with thrombocytopenia (e.g. Bernard–Soulier syndrome). ADP, adenosine diphosphate; DIC, disseminated intravascular coagulation.

by stopping the drug. Avatrombopag has been approved in the USA for thrombocytopenia associated with chronic liver disease to increase the platelet count prior to surgery or procedures.

Platelet transfusions

Transfusion of platelet concentrates is indicated in the following circumstances:

1 Thrombocytopenia or abnormal platelet function when bleeding or before invasive procedures and where there is no alternative therapy available (e.g. steroids, high-dose immunoglobulin or thrombomimetic agents). The platelet count should be above 50×10^9/L before, for example, liver biopsy or lumbar puncture.

2 Prophylactically in patients with platelet counts of less than $5–10 \times 10^9$/L. If there is infection, potential bleeding sites or coagulopathy, the count should be kept above 20×10^9/L. The indications for transfusion of platelet concentrates are discussed further on page 384. These indications may change with the wider use of thrombomimetic drugs.

SUMMARY

- Vascular bleeding disorders may be congenital, including hereditary haemorrhagic telangiectasia and the Ehlers–Danlos syndrome.
- Acquired vascular disorders include fragile capillaries in healthy women, senile purpura, purpura associated with infections, Henoch–Schönlein syndrome, scurvy and steroid therapy.
- Thrombocytopenia, if severe, also causes skin and mucous membrane bleeding. It has a wide range of causes including (i) failure of platelet production from a congenital cause, drugs or viral infection or a general bone marrow failure; (ii) increased consumption of platelets. This may be acute or chronic autoimmune, drug-induced, caused by disseminated intravascular coagulation or thrombotic thrombocytopenic purpura.

- Chronic autoimmune thrombocytopenia is treated with corticosteroids, rituximab, high-dose immunoglobulin, thrombomimetics, splenectomy or immunosuppression, e.g. with cyclophosphamide, bortezomib or ciclosporine.
- The platelet count may be raised by platelet transfusion as well as by the thrombomimetic drugs romiplostim, eltrombopag or avatrombopag.
- Disorders of platelet function may be hereditary, as in von Willebrand disease, Glanzmann's thrombasthenia and Bernard–Soulier syndrome, or acquired, most frequently caused by drugs (e.g. aspirin, clopidogrel and dipyridamole), but also by NSAIDs.
- Platelet function analysis (PFA-100), platelet aggregation studies and VWF assays may be needed to diagnose platelet functional defects.

 Now visit **www.wileyessential.com/haematology** to test yourself on this chapter.

CHAPTER 26
Coagulation disorders

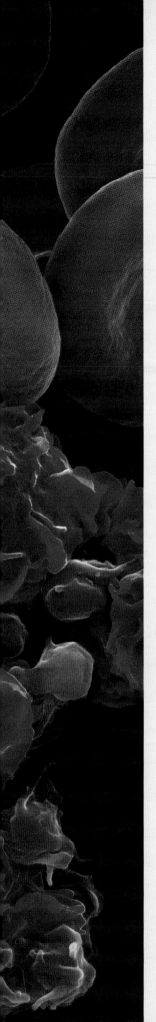

Key topics

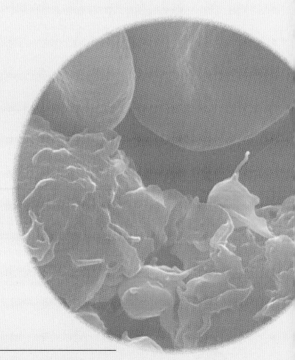

Hoffbrand's Essential Haematology, Eighth Edition. By A. Victor Hoffbrand and David P. Steensma.
© 2020 John Wiley & Sons Ltd. Published 2020 by John Wiley & Sons Ltd.
Companion website: www.wileyessential.com/haematology

Hereditary coagulation disorders

Hereditary deficiencies of each of the coagulation factors have been described. Haemophilia A (factor VIII deficiency), haemophilia B (Christmas disease, factor IX deficiency) and von Willebrand disease (VWD) are the most frequent; the others are rarer.

Haemophilia A

Haemophilia A is the most common of the hereditary clotting factor deficiencies. The prevalence is of the order of 30–100 per million population. The inheritance is sex-linked (Fig. 26.1), but up to one-third of patients have no family history and these cases result from recent mutation.

Molecular genetics

The factor VIII gene is situated near the tip of the long arm of the X chromosome. It is extremely large and consists of 26 exons. The factor VIII protein includes a triplicated region $A_1A_2A_3$, a duplicated region C_1C_2 and a heavily glycosylated B domain which is removed when factor VIII is activated by thrombin. The protein is synthesized in endothelial cells.

The defect is an absence or low level of plasma factor VIII. Approximately half of the patients have missense or frameshift mutations or deletions in the factor VIII gene. In others a characteristic 'flip-tip' inversion is seen, in which the factor VIII gene is broken by an inversion at the end of the X chromosome (Fig. 26.2). This mutation leads to a severe haemophilia A.

Clinical features

Infants may develop profuse post-circumcision haemorrhage or joint and soft tissue bleeds and excessive bruising when they start to be active. **Recurrent painful haemarthroses and muscle haematomas dominate the clinical course of severely affected patients and, if inadequately treated, lead to progressive joint deformity and disability** (Figs 26.3, 26.4, 26.5 and 26.6). Local pressure can cause entrapment neuropathy or ischaemic necrosis. Prolonged bleeding occurs after dental extractions. Spontaneous haematuria and gastrointestinal haemorrhage, sometimes with obstruction resulting from intramucosal bleeding, can also occur. **The clinical severity of the disease correlates inversely with the factor VIII level (Table 26.1).** Operative and post-traumatic haemorrhage are life-threatening in both severely and mildly affected patients. Although not common, spontaneous intracerebral haemorrhage occurs more frequently than in the general population and is an important cause of death in patients with severe disease.

Haemophilic pseudotumours are large encapsulated haematomas with progressive cystic swelling from repeated haemorrhage. They are best visualized by magnetic resonance imaging (MRI; Fig. 26.5b). They may occur in fascial and muscle planes, in large muscle groups and in the long bones, pelvis and cranium. In the bones they result from repeated subperiosteal haemorrhages with bone destruction and new bone formation.

As a result of human immunodeficiency virus (HIV) present in concentrates made from human plasma during the early 1980s, over 50% of haemophiliacs treated in the USA or Western Europe became infected with HIV. AIDS was a significant cause of death until the introduction of effective anti-viral therapy.

Many patients were infected with hepatitis C virus before testing of donors and blood products became possible. This has resulted in chronic hepatitis, cirrhosis and hepatoma. Hepatitis B transmission may also be a risk. Liver transplantation cures the haemophilia.

Laboratory findings

See Table 26.2. The following tests are abnormal:
1 Activated partial thromboplastin time (APTT).
2 Factor VIII clotting assay.
The platelet function analysis-100 (PFA-100) and prothrombin time (PT) are normal.

Carrier detection and antenatal diagnosis

Carriers are detected with DNA probes. A known specific mutation can be identified or restriction fragment length polymorphisms within or close to the factor VIII gene allow the mutant allele to be tracked. Chorionic biopsies at 8–10 weeks' gestation provide sufficient fetal DNA for analysis. Antenatal diagnosis is also possible following the demonstration of low levels of factor VIII in fetal blood obtained at 16–20 weeks' gestation from the umbilical vein. This method is only used if DNA analysis is uninformative (1% of carriers).

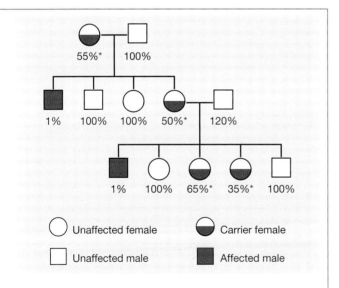

Figure 26.1 A typical family tree in a family with haemophilia. Note the variable levels of factor VIII activity in carriers (*) because of random inactivation of X chromosome (Lyonization). The percentages show the degree of factor VIII activity as a percentage of normal.

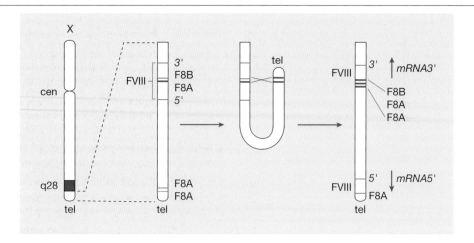

Figure 26.2 The mechanism of the flip-tip inversion leading to disruption of the factor VIII gene. **(Left)** The orientation of the factor VIII gene is shown with the three copies of gene A (F8A) in this region (one within an intron 22 and two near the telomere). **(Middle)** During spermatogenesis at meiosis, the single X pairs with the Y chromosome in the homologous regions. The X chromosome is longer than the Y and there is nothing to pair with most of the long arm of X. The chromosome undergoes homologous recombination between the A genes. **(Right)** The final result is that the factor VIII gene is disrupted. cen, centromeric end; tel, telomere; the arrows indicate the direction of transcription from the A gene.

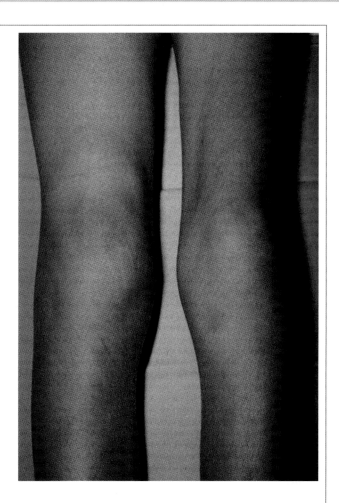

Figure 26.3 Haemophilia A: acute haemarthrosis of the right knee joint with swelling of the suprapatellar region. There is wasting of the quadriceps muscles, particularly on the left.

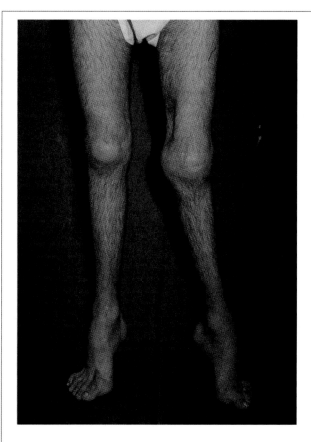

Figure 26.4 Haemophilia A showing severe disability. The left knee is swollen with posterior subluxation of the tibia on the femur. The ankles and feet show residual deformities of talipes equinus, with some cavus and associated toe clawing. There is generalized muscle wasting. The scar on the medial side of the left lower thigh is the site of a previously excised pseudotumour.

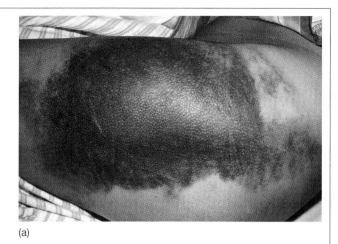

(a)

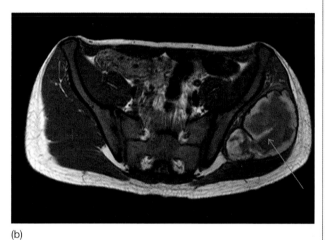

(b)

Figure 26.5 **(a)** Haemophilia A: massive haemorrhage in the area of the right buttock. **(b)** 15-year-old boy with sudden left hip pain and haemophilia A. Magnetic resonance imaging (MRI) axial image, T2-weighted, revealing large left spontaneous haematoma (yellow arrow) in left gluteus maximus muscle compared with normal right side (red cross). Source: Courtesy of Dr P. Wylie.

Treatment

Most patients in developed countries attend specialized haemophilia centres where there is a multidisciplinary team dedicated to their care. Advances in prophylactic treatment to maintain prolonged elevation of factor VIII coagulant activity are discussed below. **Nevertheless, spontaneous and trauma-induced bleeding still occurs. This is treated with factor VIII replacement therapy**, **and spontaneous bleeding is usually controlled if the patient's factor VIII level is raised to 30–50% of normal.** Guidelines exist for the plasma level to be achieved for different types of haemorrhage. For major surgery, serious post-traumatic bleeding or when haemorrhage is occurring at a dangerous site, the factor VIII level should be elevated to 100% and, when acute bleeding has stopped, maintained above 50% until healing has occurred. On average, factor VIII infusion produces a plasma increment of 20 U/L for each unit infused/kg body weight.

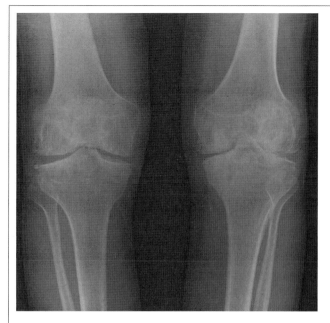

Figure 26.6 Haemophilia A: X-ray of the knee joints shows destruction and narrowing of the left joint space.

Recombinant factor VIII and plasma-derived purified factor VIII preparations, which are heat and solvent-detergent treated, are available for clinical use; they are preferred over plasma-derived sources..

1-Diamino-8-D-arginine vasopressin (DDAVP; desmopressin) provides an alternative means of increasing the plasma factor VIII level in milder haemophiliacs. Following the intravenous administration of this drug, there is a two- to fourfold rise maximum at 30–60 minutes in the patient's own factor

Table 26.1 Correlation of coagulation factor activity and disease severity in haemophilia A or B.

Coagulation factor activity (percentage of normal)	Clinical manifestations
<1	Severe disease
	Frequent spontaneous bleeding into joints, muscles, internal organs from early life
	Joint deformity and crippling if not adequately prevented or treated
1–5	Moderate disease
	Bleeding after minor trauma
	Occasional spontaneous episodes
>5	Mild disease
	Bleeding only after significant trauma, surgery

Table 26.2 Main clinical and laboratory findings in haemophilia A, factor IX deficiency (haemophilia B, Christmas disease) and von Willebrand disease.

	Haemophilia A	Factor IX deficiency	von Willebrand disease
Inheritance	Sex-linked	Sex-linked	Dominant (incomplete)
Main sites of haemorrhage	Muscle, joints, post-trauma or postoperative	Muscle, joints, post-trauma or postoperative	Mucous membranes, skin cuts, post-trauma or postoperative
Platelet count	Normal	Normal	Normal
PFA-100	Normal	Normal	Prolonged
Prothrombin time	Normal	Normal	Normal
Partial thromboplastin time	Prolonged	Prolonged	Prolonged or normal
Factor VIII	Low	Normal	May be moderately reduced
Factor IX	Normal	Low	Normal
Von Willebrand factor	Normal	Normal	Low antigen or abnormal function or both (see Table 26.3)
Ristocetin-induced platelet aggregation	Normal	Normal	Impaired

VIII by release of von Willebrand factor (VWF) from endothelial cells; VWF binds factor VIII and increases its circulating half-life. DDAVP may also be taken subcutaneously or nasally; this has been used as immediate treatment for mild haemophilia after accidental trauma or haemorrhage. DDAVP has an antidiuretic action and should be avoided in the elderly; fluid restriction is advised after its use.

Local supportive measures used in treating haemarthroses and haematomas include resting the affected part, application of ice and the prevention of further trauma.

Prophylactic treatment

The availability of factor VIII concentrates stored in domestic refrigerators has dramatically altered haemophilia treatment. At the earliest indication of bleeding, the haemophiliac child may be treated at home. This advance has reduced the occurrence of crippling haemarthroses and the need for in-patient care. Severely affected patients are now reaching adult life with little or no arthritis. After the first spontaneous joint bleed, most boys with severe haemophilia are started on prophylactic factor VIII three times a week, aiming to keep their factor VIII trough levels above 1%. This may require the placement of a vascular access device such as Port-a-Cath if venous access is difficult. **Regular prophylaxis is far superior to on-demand treatment.** The half-life of factor VIII is only 8–12 hours. Longer-acting derivatives of factor VIII and IX such as Fc-fusion and PEGylated proteins are now licensed. They reduce the frequency of replacement therapy by achieving more sustained elevation of factor levels.

Emicizumab represents a new approach with excellent success at sustaining coagulation activity and decreasing the frequency of major bleeds. Emicizumab is a bispecific monoclonal antibody that binds factors IX and X, resulting in activation of factor X. This leads to thrombin generation and by-passes the need for FVIII. Once steady state activity in the plasma is reached, it has a half-life of 4 weeks, allowing once a month dosing. Like prophylaxis with FVIII concentrates, it significantly decreases spontaneous and mild trauma-associated bleeds. Its use is associated with thrombotic microangiopathy and thrombosis when given with high doses of activated prothrombin complex concentrates, however, so careful management of bleeding is required.

Haemophilia patients are advised to have regular conservative dental care. Haemophilic children and their parents often require extensive help with social and psychological matters. With modern treatment the lifestyle of a haemophilic child can be almost normal, but certain activities such as extreme contact sports are to be avoided, or undertaken with extra prophylaxis.

Inhibitors

One of the most serious complications of haemophilia is the development of antibodies (inhibitors) to infused factor VIII which occurs in 30–40% of severely affected patients, especially with recombinant compared with plasma-derived factor VIII and usually within the first 50 days of exposure. This renders the patient refractory to further replacement therapy. Immunosuppression and immune tolerance regimens have been used in an attempt to eradicate the antibody with success (at great cost) in about two-thirds of cases. Activated prothrombin complex concentrates (FEIBA – factor VIII inhibitor bypassing activity) can be useful in the treatment of bleeding episodes.

Infused recombinant factor VIIa complexes with tissue factor exposed at the site of injury and produces local haemostasis. The process is independent of factor VIII or IX and is not affected by their inhibitors. Factor VIIa has a short half-life and therefore frequent doses may be needed. In the longer term, immunosuppression with cyclophosphamide, rituximab and intravenous immunoglobulin and high-dose factor VIII has also been successful.

Emicizumab has made the biggest impact in haemophilia A patients with inhibitors, since as discussed above emicizumab by-passes the need for FVIII for coagulant activity. Patients can be treated once a month after steady state levels have been achieved, significantly reducing bleeds, prolonged hospital stays and co-morbid conditions. Inhibitors of antithrombin and of tissue factor pathway inhibitor are also in trials for reducing bleeding in patients with inhibitors of factor IX or VIII.

Gene therapy

Gene-based therapy aimed at maintaining factor levels above 1% to prevent most of the mortality and morbidity of factor VIII or IX deficiency is now in clinical trials. Adeno-associated virus (AAV) is the vector of choice, but retroviral as well as non-viral vectors are being explored. Durable (more than 8 years after a single injection) increased levels of factor IX have been obtained with an adenoviral vector carrying the gene to the liver sufficient to obviate the need for replacement therapy except for trauma or surgery (Fig. 26.7). An immune-mediated transaminitis after the infusion of the construct in some patients is controlled by steroid therapy. The use of a mutant factor IX, FIX Padua, which is associated with production of elevated levels, results in even higher plasma concentrations than wild type. Trials of similar gene therapy for factor VIII deficiency are yielding similar results.

Factor IX deficiency (haemophilia B, Christmas disease)

The inheritance and clinical features of factor IX deficiency (Christmas disease, haemophilia B) are identical to those of haemophilia A. Indeed, the two disorders can only be distinguished by specific coagulation factor assays. The incidence is one-fifth that of haemophilia A. Factor IX is coded by a gene close to the gene for factor VIII near the tip of the long arm of the X chromosome. Its synthesis is vitamin K dependent. Carrier detection, antenatal diagnosis, replacement and gene therapy are similar to those of haemophilia A. Bleeding episodes are treated with high-purity or recombinant factor IX concentrates. Because of its longer biological half-life, infusions do not have to be given as frequently as do factor VIII concentrates in haemophilia A. Recombinant factor IX is preferred, but higher doses are needed than with plasma-derived factor IX to attain the same response. Longer-acting factor IX, PEGylated or Fc fused entail less frequent infusions. Gene therapy is discussed above.

Laboratory findings

See Table 26.2. The following tests are abnormal:
1 APTT;
2 Factor IX clotting assay. As in haemophilia A, the PFA-100 and PT tests are normal.

Von Willebrand disease

In this disorder there is either a reduced level or abnormal function of VWF resulting from a wide variety of mainly missense mutations in different parts of the gene. VWF is produced in endothelial cells and megakaryocytes. Figure 26.8 shows the various domains with their binding sites and site of cleavage by ADAMTS-13. It has two main roles (see Chapter 24). It promotes platelet adhesion to subendothelium and to each other at high shear rates and it is the carrier molecule for factor VIII, protecting it from premature destruction. The latter property explains the reduced factor VIII levels found in VWD. VWF has a half-life in plasma of about 24 hours, but this varies with blood type and is shorter in patients with type O blood.

Chronic elevation of VWF is part of the acute phase response to injury, inflammation, neoplasia or pregnancy. VWF is synthesized as a large 600 kDa protein which then forms high molecular weight multimers, which are the largest molecules in blood. Three types of VWD have been described (Table 26.3). Type 2 is divided into four subtypes depending on the type of functional defect. Type 1 accounts for 65–75% and type 2 for most of the remainder.

VWD is the most common inherited bleeding disorder. Usually, the inheritance is autosomal dominant. The severity of bleeding is highly variable, depending on mutation type and epigenetic effects, such as ABO blood group. Women are more severely affected than men at a given VWF level. Typically, there is mucous membrane bleeding (e.g. epistaxes, menorrhagia), excessive blood loss from superficial cuts and abrasions, and operative and post-traumatic haemorrhage. The severity is variable in the different types. Haemarthroses and muscle haematomas are rare, except in type 3 disease.

Laboratory findings

See Table 26.2.
1 The PFA-100 test (see p. 310) is abnormal. Factor VIII levels are often low. If low, a factor VIII/VWF binding assay is performed.
2 The APTT may be prolonged.
3 VWF antigen levels are usually low. The sites of the mutations underlying the four subtypes of VWD are shown in Fig. 26.8.
4 There is defective platelet aggregation by patient plasma in the presence of ristocetin (VWF: Rco). Aggregation to other agents – adenosine diphosphate (ADP), thrombin or adrenaline – is usually normal. Other types of assay for VWF platelet binding are more frequently being used to

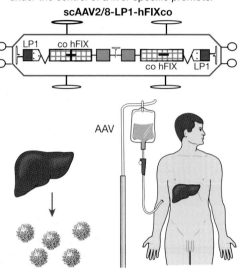

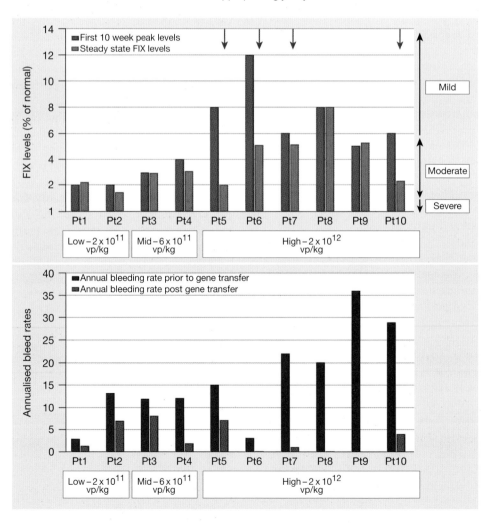

Figure 26.7 Gene therapy for factor IX deficiency. Pt, patient. Source: Courtesy of Professor Amit Nathwani, Department of Haematology, Royal Free Hospital, London, UK.

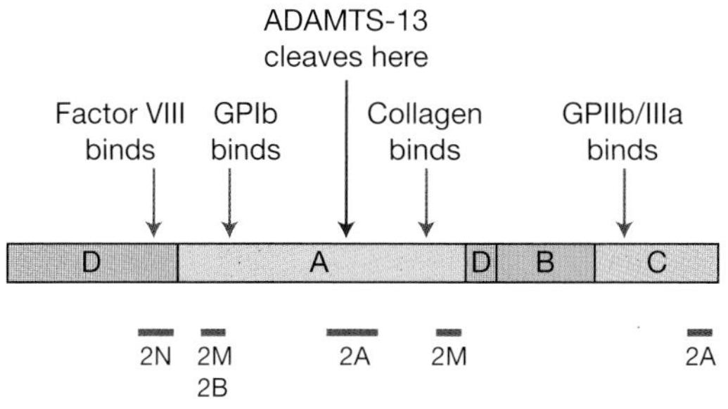

Figure 26.8 Von Willebrand factor monomer showing the A, B, C, D domains, the binding sites for key ligands and the site of cleavage by ADAMTS-13. The locations of variants associated with type 2 disease are shown as horizontal bars. Source: Adapted from A.V. Hoffbrand *et al.* (2019) *The Color Atlas of Clinical Hematology*, 5th edn. Reproduced by permission of John Wiley & Sons.

Table 26.3 Classification of von Willebrand disease.

Type 1	Quantitative partial deficiency
Type 2	Functional abnormality
Type 3	Complete deficiency

Secondary classification of type 2 VWD

Subtype	Platelet-associated function	Factor VIII binding capacity	High MW VWF multimers
2A	Decreased	Normal	Absent
2B	Increased affinity for GPIb	Normal	Usually reduced/absent
2M	Decreased binding to GPIb	Normal	Normal
2N	Normal	Reduced	Normal

GPIb, glycoprotein Ib; MW, molecular weight; VWD, von Willebrand disease; VWF, von Willebrand factor.

avoid the variability and labour intensive ristocetin cofactor assay and reported as VWF: Ac for VWF activity.

5 Collagen-binding function (VWF: CB) is usually reduced (but rarely measured).

6 Multimer analysis is useful for diagnosing different subtypes (Table 26.3).

7 The platelet count is normal except for type 2B disease (where it is low).

Treatment

Options are as follows:

1 Local measures and antifibrinolytic agent (e.g. tranexamic acid for mild bleeding).

2 DDAVP infusion for those with mild to moderate type 1 VWD. This releases VWF from endothelial cells 30 minutes after intravenous infusion.

3 High-purity VWF concentrates for patients with very low VWF levels. Plasma-derived factor VIII/VWF concentrates are used. Recombinant VWF is also available.

Hereditary deficiency of other coagulation factors

All of these disorders (deficiency of fibrinogen, prothrombin, factors V, VII, combined V and VIII, factors X, XI, XIII or mutation of thrombomodulin) are rare. In all the inheritance is autosomal recessive, except for factor XI deficiency where there is variable penetrance. Recombinant factor VIIa is available for therapy. Although a factor X concentrate is available, deficiency is rare. **Factor XI deficiency is seen mainly in Ashkenazi Jews and occurs in either sex. The bleeding risk shows incomplete correlation to the severity of the deficiency.** Bleeding only occurs after trauma such as surgery. Treatment is with fibrinolytic inhibitor, factor XI concentrate or fresh frozen plasma (FFP). Factor XIII deficiency produces a severe bleeding tendency, characteristically with umbilical stump bleeding. Plasma concentrates and recombinant preparations of factor XIII are available.

Acquired coagulation disorders

The acquired coagulation disorders (Table 26.4) are more common than the inherited disorders. Unlike the inherited disorders, multiple clotting factor deficiencies are usual.

Vitamin K deficiency

Fat-soluble vitamin K is obtained from green vegetables and bacterial synthesis in the gut. **Deficiency may present in the newborn (haemorrhagic disease of the newborn) or in later life.**

Deficiency of vitamin K is caused by an inadequate diet, malabsorption or inhibition of vitamin K by vitamin K antagonist drugs such as warfarin. **Warfarin is associated with a decrease in the functional activity of factors II, VII, IX and X and proteins C and S**, but immunological methods show normal levels of these factors. The non-functional proteins are called **PIVKA** (proteins formed in vitamin K absence). Conversion of PIVKA factors to their biologically active forms requires a post-translational event involving carboxylation of glutamic acid residues in the N-terminal region (Fig. 26.9). Gamma-carboxylated glutamic acid binds calcium ions, inducing a reversible shape change in the N-termini of vitamin K-dependent proteins. This exposes hydrophobic residues which bind to phospholipid. In the process of carboxylation, vitamin K is converted to vitamin K epoxide, which is cycled back to the reduced form by a reductase (VKORC-1). **Warfarin inhibits vitamin K epoxide reductase, leading to a functional vitamin K deficiency.**

Table 26.4 The acquired coagulation disorders.

Deficiency of vitamin K-dependent factors
Haemorrhagic disease of the newborn
Biliary obstruction
Malabsorption of vitamin K (e.g. tropical sprue, gluten-induced enteropathy)
Prolonged use of antibiotics
Vitamin K-antagonist therapy (e.g. coumarins, indandiones)
Liver disease – complex dysregulation with synthetic failure of pro- and anticoagulant factors
Disseminated intravascular coagulation – consumption of all clotting factors and platelets

Inhibition of coagulation
Specific inhibitors (e.g. antibodies against factor VIII)
Non-specific inhibitors (e.g. antibodies found in systemic lupus erythematosus or rheumatoid arthritis, which paradoxically cause thrombosis)

Miscellaneous
Diseases with M-protein production that interfere with haemostasis
L-asparaginase
Therapy with heparin, defibrinating agents or thrombolytics
Massive transfusion syndrome

Haemorrhagic disease of the newborn

Vitamin K-dependent factors are low at birth and fall further in breast-fed infants in the first few days of life. Liver cell immaturity, lack of gut bacterial synthesis of the vitamin and low quantities in breast milk may all contribute to a deficiency which causes haemorrhage, usually on the second to fourth day of life, but occasionally later during the first two months.

Diagnosis

The PT and APTT are both abnormal. The platelet count and fibrinogen are normal with absent fibrin degradation products.

Treatment

1 Prophylaxis. For many years vitamin K has been given to all newborn babies as a single intramuscular injection of 1 mg. This remains the most appropriate and safest treatment. Following epidemiological evidence suggesting a possible link between intramuscular vitamin K and an increased risk of childhood tumours (which has not been substantiated), some centres recommended an oral regimen, but this has never been subjected to randomized controlled trial.

2 In bleeding infants with vitamin K deficiency, vitamin K 1 mg intramuscularly is given every 6 hours with, initially, prothrombin complex concentrate if haemorrhage is severe.

Vitamin K deficiency in children or adults

Deficiency resulting from obstructive jaundice, pancreatic or small bowel disease occasionally causes a bleeding diathesis in children or adults.

Diagnosis

Both PT and APTT are prolonged. There are low plasma levels of factors II, VII, IX and X. FVII has the shortest half-life of 6 hours, so the increase in the PT/INR often precedes increase in the APTT.

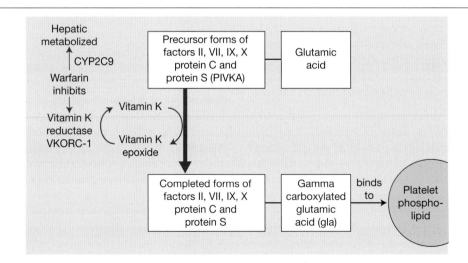

Figure 26.9 The action of vitamin K in γ-carboxylation of glutamic acid in coagulation factors, which are then able to bind Ca^{2+} and attach to the platelet phospholipid. Warfarin inhibits vitamin K reductase. It is metabolized in the liver and genetic variations in the reductase enzyme VKORC-1 and in the cytochrome CYP2C9 largely account for wide variations in the warfarin sensitivity of individuals.

Treatment

1 Prophylaxis: vitamin K 5 mg/day orally.
2 Active bleeding or prior to liver biopsy: vitamin K 10 mg slowly intravenously. Some correction of PT is usual within 6 hours. The dose should be repeated on the next 2 days, after which optimal correction is usual.
3 Rapid correction may be achieved by infusion of prothrombin complex concentrate.

Liver disease

Multiple haemostatic abnormalities contribute to a bleeding tendency and may exacerbate haemorrhage from oesophageal varices.

1 Biliary obstruction results in impaired absorption of vitamin K and therefore decreased synthesis of factors II, VII, IX and X by liver parenchymal cells.
2 With severe hepatocellular disease, in addition to a deficiency of these factors, there are often reduced levels of factor V and fibrinogen and increased amounts of plasminogen activator.
3 Functional abnormality of fibrinogen (dysfibrinogenaemia) is found in many patients.
4 Decreased thrombopoietin production from the liver contributes to thrombocytopenia.
5 Hypersplenism associated with portal hypertension frequently results in thrombocytopenia.
6 Disseminated intravascular coagulation (DIC; see below) may be related to release of thromboplastins from damaged liver cells and reduced concentrations of antithrombin, protein C and α_2-antiplasmin. In addition, there is impaired removal of activated clotting factors and increased fibrinolytic activity.
7 The net haemostatic imbalance in liver disease may be prothrombotic rather than haemorrhagic.

Disseminated intravascular coagulation

Widespread inappropriate intravascular deposition of fibrin with consumption of coagulation factors and platelets occurs as a consequence of many disorders that release procoagulant material into the circulation or cause widespread endothelial damage or platelet aggregation (Table 26.5). It may be associated with a fulminant haemorrhagic or thrombotic syndrome with organ dysfunction, or run a less severe and more chronic course. The main clinical presentation is with bleeding, but 5–10% of patients manifest thrombotic lesions (e.g. with gangrene of limbs).

Pathogenesis

The key event underlying DIC is increased activity of thrombin in the circulation that overwhelms its normal rate of removal by natural anticoagulants (Fig. 26.10). This can come from tissue factor (TF) release into the circulation from damaged tissues present on tumour cells, or from up-regulation of TF on circulating monocytes or endothelial cells in response to proinflammatory cytokines (e.g. interleukin-1, tumour necrosis factor, endotoxin).

Table 26.5 Causes of disseminated intravascular coagulation.

Infections
Gram-negative and meningococcal septicaemia
Clostridium welchii septicaemia
Severe falciparum malaria
Viral infection – varicella, HIV, hepatitis, cytomegalovirus

Malignancy
Widespread mucin-secreting adenocarcinoma
Acute promyelocytic leukaemia

Obstetric complications
Amniotic fluid embolism
Premature separation of placenta
Eclampsia; retained placenta
Septic abortion

Hypersensitivity reactions
Anaphylaxis
Incompatible blood transfusion

Widespread tissue damage
Following surgery or trauma
After severe burns

Vascular abnormalities
Kasabach–Merritt syndrome
Leaking prosthetic valves
Cardiac bypass surgery
Vascular aneurysms

Miscellaneous
Liver failure
Pancreatitis
Snake and invertebrate venoms
Hypothermia
Heat stroke
Acute hypoxia
Massive blood loss

1 DIC may be triggered by the entry of procoagulant material into the circulation in the following situations: severe trauma, amniotic fluid embolism, premature separation of the placenta, widespread mucin-secreting adenocarcinomas, acute promyelocytic leukaemia, liver disease, severe falciparum malaria, haemolytic transfusion reaction and some snake venoms.
2 DIC may also be initiated by widespread endothelial damage and collagen exposure (e.g. endotoxaemia, Gram-negative and meningococcal septicaemia, septic abortion), certain virus infections and severe burns or hypothermia. Proinflammatory cytokines and activation of monocytes by bacteria up-regulate tissue factor as well as releasing microparticles expressing tissue factor into the circulation.

In addition to its role in the deposition of fibrin in the microcirculation, intravascular thrombin formation produces large

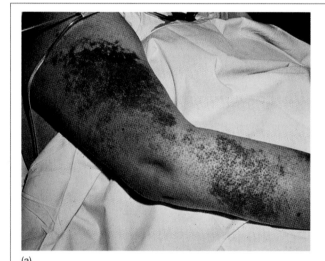

Figure 26.10 The pathogenesis of disseminated intravascular coagulation and the changes in clotting factors, platelets and fibrin degradation products (FDPs) that occur in this syndrome.

amounts of circulating fibrin monomers, which form complexes with fibrinogen and interfere with fibrin polymerization, thus contributing to the coagulation defect. Intense fibrinolysis is stimulated by thrombi on vascular walls and the release of split products interferes with fibrin polymerization, thus contributing to the coagulation defect. The combined action of thrombin and plasmin causes depletion of fibrinogen and all coagulation factors. Intravascular thrombin also causes widespread platelet aggregation in the vessels. The bleeding problems which may be a feature of DIC are compounded by thrombocytopenia caused by consumption of platelets.

Clinical features

These are usually dominated by bleeding, particularly from venepuncture sites or wounds (Fig. 26.11a). There may be generalized bleeding in the gastrointestinal tract, the oropharynx, into the lungs, urogenital tract and, in obstetric cases, vaginal bleeding may be particularly severe. Less frequently, microthrombi may cause skin lesions, renal failure, gangrene of the fingers or toes (Fig. 26.11b) or cerebral ischaemia. A microangiopathic haemolytic anaemia may also complicate the clinical picture.

Some patients may develop subacute or chronic DIC, especially with mucin-secreting adenocarcinoma.

Laboratory findings

See Table 26.6. In many acute syndromes the blood may fail to clot because of gross fibrinogen deficiency.

Tests of haemostasis:
1 The platelet count is low.
2 Fibrinogen concentration is low.
3 The thrombin time is prolonged.
4 High levels of fibrin degradation products such as D-dimers are found in serum and urine.
5 The PT and APTT are prolonged in the acute syndromes. Compensation by the liver in chronic DIC may render some of the coagulation tests normal.

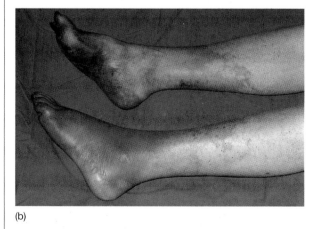

Figure 26.11 Clinical features of disseminated intravascular coagulation: **(a)** indurated and confluent purpura of the arm; **(b)** peripheral gangrene with swelling and discoloration of the skin of the feet in fulminant disease.

Table 26.6 Haemostasis tests: typical results in acquired bleeding disorders.

	Platelet count	Prothrombin time	Activated partial thromboplastin time	Thrombin time
Liver disease	Low	Prolonged	Prolonged	Normal (rarely prolonged)
DIC	Low	Prolonged	Prolonged	Grossly prolonged
Massive transfusion	Low	Prolonged	Prolonged	Normal
Coumarin anticoagulants	Normal	Grossly prolonged	Prolonged	Normal
Heparin	Normal (rarely low)	Mildly prolonged	Prolonged	Prolonged
Circulating anticoagulant	Normal	Normal or prolonged	Prolonged	Normal

DIC, disseminated intravascular coagulation.

Blood film examination

In many patients there is a haemolytic anaemia ('microangiopathic') and the red cells show prominent fragmentation because of damage caused when passing through fibrin strands in small vessels (see p. 76).

Treatment

Treatment of the underlying cause is most important. The management of patients who are bleeding differs from that of patients with thrombotic problems.

Bleeding
Supportive therapy with FFP (Table 26.7) and platelet concentrates is indicated in patients with dangerous or extensive bleeding. Cryoprecipitate or fibrinogen concentrates provide more concentrated fibrinogen; red cell transfusions may be required.

Thrombosis
The use of heparin or antiplatelet drugs to inhibit the coagulation process is considered in those with thrombotic problems such as skin ischaemia. Use of anticoagulants, however, has not been shown to affect mortality. Fibrinolytic inhibitors should not be used because of consequent failure to lyse thrombi in organs such as the kidney.

Coagulation deficiency caused by antibodies

Circulating antibodies to coagulation factors are occasionally seen, with an incidence of approximately 1 per million per year rising markedly with age. Alloantibodies to factor VIII occur in 5–10% of subjects with haemophilia. Factor VIII autoantibodies may result in a bleeding syndrome. These immunoglobulin G antibodies occur rarely post-partum, in certain immunological disorders (e.g. rheumatoid arthritis), in cancer and in old age. Treatment consists of a combination of immunosuppression and factor replacement, usually as human factor VIII, recombinant VIIa or activated prothrombin complex concentrate (FEIBA).

Another protein known as the **lupus anticoagulant** interferes with lipoprotein-dependent stages of coagulation and is usually detected by prolongation of the APTT test (Table 26.6). This *in vitro* inhibitor is detected in 10% of patients with systemic lupus erythematosus (SLE) and in patients with other autoimmune diseases who frequently have antibodies to other lipid-containing antigens (e.g. cardiolipin). The antibody is not associated with a bleeding tendency, but there is an increased risk of arterial or venous thrombosis and, as with other causes of thrombophilia, an association with recurrent miscarriage (see Chapter 27).

Massive transfusion syndrome (see also p. 385)

Many factors may contribute to a bleeding disorder following massive transfusion. Blood loss results in reduced levels of platelets, coagulation factors and inhibitors. Further dilution of these factors occurs during replacement with red cells.

Management

For women under the age of 50 of unknown blood group, type **O Rh− blood** is given until the blood group is known. For males, O Rh+ is considered initially. Red cell salvage is practised in some obstetric, trauma, cardiac and vascular centres. **Platelet concentrates are given to maintain a platelet count**

Table 26.7 Indications for the use of fresh frozen plasma (National Institutes of Health Consensus Guidelines).

Coagulation factor deficiency (PCC where specific or combined factor concentrate is not available)

Reversal of warfarin effect (only if PCC is unavailable)

Multiple coagulation defects (e.g. in patients with liver disease, DIC) – PCC are much better, plasma is virtually useless

Massive blood transfusion with coagulopathy and clinical bleeding

Thrombotic thrombocytopenic purpura

Some patients with immunodeficiency syndromes

DIC, disseminated intravascular coagulation; PCC, prothrombin complex concentrates.

above 50–75 × 109/L or 100 × 109/L in cerebral injury or after trauma. The PT and APTT should be kept to less than 1.5 times normal, with FFP given initially at 15 mL/kg. **It is usually necessary to give 4–6 units of FFP for every 6 units of red cells transfused**. FFP is started early with red cell transfusion. Some protocols include 1 : 1 : 1 for red cells, platelet packs and FFP. **Cryoprecipitate or fibrinogen concentrate** is given to keep fibrinogen above 1.5 g/L. Trials of fibrinogen concentrates have been performed in obstetric emergencies and perioperative bleeding during cardiac surgery, with good results. Tranexamic acid can be given intravenously if trauma is the cause of the bleeding. Monitoring by platelet count, PT and fibrinogen level is essential by near-patient testing every 30–60 minutes. Thromboelastography or ROTEM (see below) can also be used.

Thromboelastography: near-patient (point-of-care) testing

Thromboelastography (TEG) and thromboelastometry (ROTEM) are techniques for a global assessment of haemostatic function of a single blood sample, in which the reaction of platelets with the protein coagulation cascade is observed from the time of the initial platelet fibrin interaction through platelet aggregation, clot strengthening and fibrin cross-linkage to eventual clot lysis. It is suited as a monitor of haemostasis in surgery (e.g. of the liver or heart) associated with haemostatic defects. Freshly drawn blood is placed in a cuvette which is oscillated, the motion being transferred to a pin which transmits deflection as torsion to a photoelectric detector with computerized data capture. As fibrin strands form, the fibrin clot affects movement of the pin. The normal trace shows the rate of initial fibrin formation, the time to formation of a clot (coagulation time), strength of the fibrin clot, clot lysis index or retraction. It requires fresh whole blood samples and trained operators to get valid results.

Typical patterns showing results in fibrinolysis, hypercoagulability, haemophilia and thrombocytopenia are shown in Figure 26.12. The assays are helpful in managing major post-partum haemorrhage, in predicting bleeding in liver disease, and after liver transplantation, cardiac surgery and major trauma.

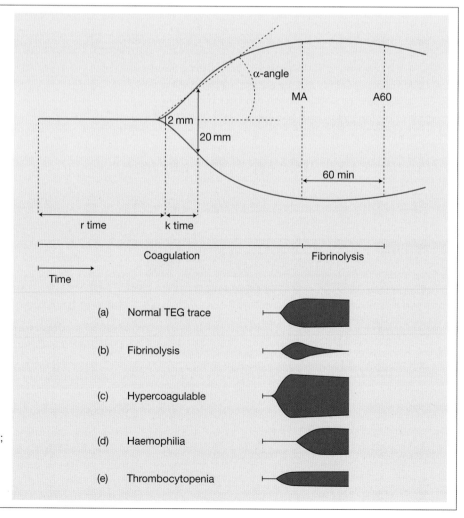

Figure 26.12 Thromboelastography (TEG): **(a–e)** normal trace and appearances in different pathological states. α-angle, speed of solid clot formation; A_{60}, measure of clot lysis or retraction at 60 min; k, clot formation time; MA, absolute strength of fibrin clot; r, rate of initial fibrin formation. Source: S.V. Mallett, D.J.A. Cox (1992) *Br. J. Anaesth.* 69: 307–13. Reproduced with permission of OUP.

SUMMARY

- Coagulation disorders may be inherited or acquired.
- Haemophilia A is the most common inherited deficiency of a clotting factor. It is severe if factor VIII activity in plasma is <1% of normal. It presents with excess bruising or prolonged bleeding after trauma and with spontaneous bleeding, usually into muscles and joints, which can result in joint deformity.
- Many older patients are infected with hepatitis C or HIV as a result of receiving contaminated blood products.
- The APTT is prolonged and PT normal.
- Antenatal diagnosis is usually carried out by polymerase chain reaction (PCR) techniques, the gene being carried on the X chromosome.
- Treatment is with recombinant or concentrates of factor VIII, or with drugs, e.g. DDAVP (desmopressin). New long-acting recombinant preparations are being introduced as well as emicizumab, which activates factor X and then thrombin without the need for factor VIII.
- Factor IX deficiency has a similar pattern of inheritance and clinical manifestations.
- Gene therapy for factor VIII and factor IX deficiencies is under trial.

- Von Willebrand disease is the most frequent inherited bleeding disorder. Haemorrhage occurs from mucous membranes, skin cuts and post-trauma. It usually has a dominant inheritance. Platelet function is abnormal and VWF levels usually low.
- DDAVP (vasopressin) is a useful treatment for mild VWD and for mild haemophilia A
- Acquired coagulation disorders include those caused by vitamin K deficiency (e.g. in the newborn or with malabsorption) or by vitamin K antagonist therapy (e.g. warfarin).
- Other common coagulation abnormalities are those in liver disease, mainly caused by reduced synthesis of coagulation factors, and in disseminated intravascular coagulation, which causes consumption of coagulation factors and platelets.
- Massive transfusion syndrome requires transfusion of red cells, platelets and coagulation factors in the correct proportions.
- Fresh frozen plasma is used in treatment of multiple coagulation defects, or specific defects if the appropriate concentrate is not available, and in therapy for thrombotic thrombocytopenic purpura.

Now visit **www.wileyessential.com/haematology** to test yourself on this chapter.

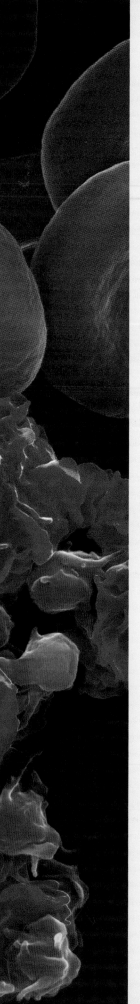

CHAPTER 27
Thrombosis 1: pathogenesis and diagnosis

Key topics

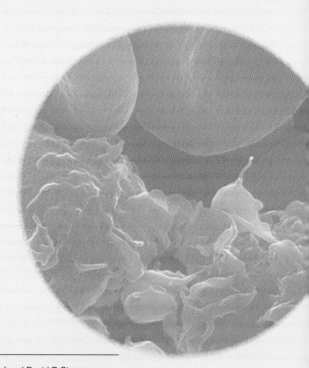

Hoffbrand's Essential Haematology, Eighth Edition. By A. Victor Hoffbrand and David P. Steensma.
© 2020 John Wiley & Sons Ltd. Published 2020 by John Wiley & Sons Ltd.
Companion website: www.wileyessential.com/haematology

Thrombi are solid masses or plugs formed in the circulation from blood constituents. Platelets and fibrin form the basic structure. Their clinical significance lies in the ischaemia that results from local vascular obstruction or distant embolization. Thrombi are involved in the pathogenesis of myocardial infarction, cerebrovascular disease, peripheral arterial disease, deep vein thrombosis (DVT) and pulmonary embolism (PE).

Thrombosis, both arterial and venous, is more common as age increases and is frequently associated with risk factors such as surgery or pregnancy. The term **thrombophilia** is used to describe inherited or acquired disorders of the haemostatic mechanism that predispose to thrombosis.

The role of inflammation in the development of both arterial and venous thrombosis is becoming more apparent. Not only does inflammation result in an increase in procoagulant clotting factors such as fibrinogen, FVIII and VWF, but there is also a drop in the level of the natural anticoagulant free protein S, due to binding of protein S by complement C4b binding protein. Neutrophil extra-cellular traps (NETs), which are mainly formed by decondensed nucleosomes and proteins derived from intracellular granules, such as neutrophil elastase (NE) and myeloperoxidase, can complex with platelets, resulting in platelet activation and formation of thrombi in arteries and veins.

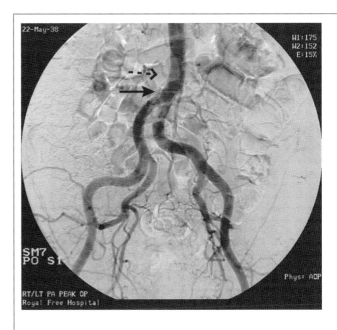

Figure 27.1 Arteriogram showing saddle embolus at the aortic bifurcation (dotted arrow) and embolus in the left common iliac artery (solid arrow).

Arterial thrombosis

Pathogenesis

Atherosclerosis of the arterial wall, plaque rupture and endothelial injury expose blood to subendothelial collagen and tissue factor. This initiates the formation of a platelet nidus on which platelets adhere and aggregate.

Platelet deposition and thrombus formation are important in the pathogenesis of atherosclerosis. Platelet-derived growth factor (PDGF) stimulates the migration and proliferation of smooth muscle cells and fibroblasts in the arterial intima. Regrowth of endothelium and repair at the site of arterial damage result in thickening of the vessel wall. The intrinsic pathway of fibrin formation (see Fig. 24.11) is involved in pathological thrombosis *in vivo* by contact activation on damaged blood vessels.

As well as blocking arteries locally, emboli of platelets and fibrin may break away from the primary thrombus to occlude distal arteries. Examples are carotid artery thrombi leading to cerebral thrombosis and transient ischaemic attacks, and heart valve and chamber thrombi leading to systemic emboli and infarcts (Fig. 27.1).

Clinical risk factors

The risk factors for arterial thrombosis are related to the development of atherosclerosis (Table 27.1). The identification of patients at risk is largely based on clinical assessment. A number of epidemiological studies have resulted in the construction of coronary artery thrombosis risk profiles based on gender, age, elevated blood pressure, high levels of serum cholesterol, glucose intolerance, cigarette smoking and electrocardiogram abnormalities. These profiles have allowed pre-symptomatic assessment of young and apparently fit subjects, and are valuable in counselling a change in lifestyle or for recommending medical therapy in individuals at risk. Cancer is also a risk factor, with increased incidence of arterial thromboembolic events in the months before the cancer is diagnosed.

Venous thrombosis

Pathogenesis and risk factors

Virchow's triad suggests that there are three components that are important in both arterial and venous thrombus formation:
1 **Slowing down of blood flow.**
2 **Hypercoagulability of the blood.**
3 **Vessel wall damage.**
For venous thrombosis, increased systemic coagulability and stasis are most important, with vessel wall damage being somewhat less important than in arterial thrombosis, although it may be important in patients with sepsis, in-dwelling catheters and sites of damage to veins by previous thrombosis. Stasis allows the completion of blood coagulation at the site of initiation of the thrombus (e.g. behind the valve pockets of the leg veins in immobile patients). Table 27.2 lists a number of recognized risk factors.

Table 27.1 Risk factors for arterial thrombosis (atherosclerosis).

Positive family history

Male sex

Hyperlipidaemia

Hypertension

Diabetes mellitus

Gout

Polycythaemia

Cancer

Hyperhomocysteinaemia

Cigarette smoking

ECG abnormalities

Elevated CRP, IL6, fibrinogen, lipoprotein-associated phospholipase A_2

Lupus anticoagulant

Collagen vascular diseases

Behçet's disease

Malignancy

CRP, C-reactive protein; ECG, electrocardiogram; IL, interleukin.

Table 27.2 Hereditary and acquired risk factors for venous thrombosis.

Hereditary haemostatic disorders
Factor V Leiden
Prothrombin G20210A variant
Protein C deficiency
Antithrombin deficiency
Protein S deficiency
Dysfibrinogenaemia
Non-O ABO blood group
Deep vein thrombosis in close relative (especially if unprovoked)

Hereditary or acquired haemostatic disorders
Raised plasma levels of factor VIII
Raised plasma levels of fibrinogen
Raised plasma levels of homocysteine (uncertain)

Acquired disorders
Lupus anticoagulant
Oestrogen therapy (oral contraceptive and hormone replacement therapy)
Heparin-induced thrombocytopenia
Pregnancy and puerperium
Surgery, especially abdominal, hip and knee surgery
Major trauma
Malignancy
Acutely ill hospitalized medical patients including cardiac or respiratory failure, infection, inflammatory bowel disorders
Myeloproliferative disease
Hyperviscosity, polycythaemia
Stroke
Pelvic obstruction
Nephrotic syndrome
Dehydration
Varicose veins
Previous superficial vein thrombosis
Age
Obesity
Paroxysmal nocturnal haemoglobinuria
Behçet's disease

Hereditary disorders of haemostasis

The prevalence of inherited disorders associated with increased risk of thrombosis is higher than that of hereditary bleeding disorders. **Approximately one-third of patients who suffer DVT or PE have an identifiable heritable risk factor such as rare deficiency of antithrombin, protein C or protein S, or common mutations affecting factor V (factor V Leiden) or prothrombin (Table 27.2).** Venous thromboembolism frequently results from gene–environment interaction, so additional risk factors (surgery, immobility, oestrogen exposure) are often present in patients with heritable thrombophilia when they develop thrombosis. Although heritable thrombophilia partly explains the gene–environment interaction leading to clinical expression of disease, testing for heritable thrombophilic defects has limited clinical utility, as a positive test result rarely predicts a higher risk of recurrence compared to patients without identifiable abnormalities. The history of a spontaneous DVT in a close relative increases an individual's risk of DVT even if no known genetic predisposition can be identified. However, testing for heritable thrombophilia can help clinical decision making in thrombosis-prone families.

Factor V Leiden (FVL) gene mutation

This is the most common inherited cause of an increased risk of venous thrombosis. It occurs in approximately 3–7% of factor V alleles in white people (Fig. 27.2). There is failure of activated protein C (APC) to prolong the activated partial thromboplastin time (APTT) test when added to plasma of patients with FVL, so the phenotype is sometimes referred to as 'activated protein C resistance'. Activated protein C normally breaks down activated factor V and so it should slow the clotting reaction and prolong the APTT. APC resistance is caused by a genetic polymorphism in the factor V gene, which makes factor V less susceptible to cleavage by APC (Fig. 27.3). The frequency of factor V Leiden in the general population in Western countries means that it is not a rare mutation, but

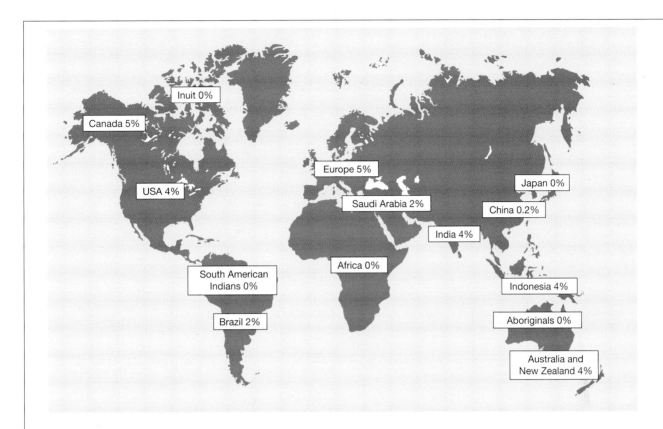

Figure 27.2 The incidence of carriers of factor V Leiden in different countries.

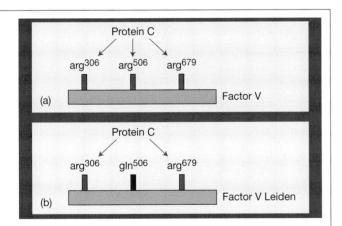

Figure 27.3 The genetic basis of factor V Leiden. **(a)** Activated protein C (APC) inactivates factor Va by proteolytic cleavage at three sites in the Va heavy chain. **(b)** In the factor V Leiden mutation the Arg506Gln polymorphism leads to glutamine at position 506, with less efficient inactivation of factor V by APC and increased risk of thrombosis.

instead is a genetic polymorphism that is maintained in the population (Fig. 27.2). Presumably, individuals with this allele have been 'selected', probably because of a reduced bleeding tendency (e.g. post-partum). It does not increase the risk of arterial thrombosis. A small minority of patients with APC resistance do not have factor V Leiden but have other mutations of factor V. Acquired APC resistance can occur when there is significant elevation of other clotting factors such as FVIII and fibrinogen, such as during pregnancy or prolonged inflammation.

Patients who are heterozygous for factor V Leiden are at an approximately five- to eight-fold increased risk of venous thrombosis compared to the general population, but only 10% of carriers develop thrombosis during their lifetime. Individuals who are homozygous have a 30–140-fold risk. Following venous thrombosis they have a slightly higher risk of re-thrombosis than individuals with DVT but normal factor V. **The incidence of factor V Leiden in patients with venous thrombosis is approximately 20–40%.** Genetic screening is relatively easy and is widely performed. **However, even if a person is a carrier of factor V Leiden, their absolute risk of thrombosis is still very low in the absence of other risk factors.** It is not recommended to start anticoagulation therapy in individuals with the Leiden mutation, even if homozygous, if they have no history of thrombosis. If they have a clearly provoked venous thrombosis, it is not recommended to continue anticoagulation indefinitely simply because of the presence of the FVL mutation.

Antithrombin deficiency

Inheritance is autosomal dominant. There are recurrent venous thromboses, usually starting in early adult life, and arterial thrombi may occur. Antithrombin concentrates are available and are occasionally used to prevent thrombosis during surgery or childbirth. Many molecular variants of antithrombin have been categorized and are associated with varying degrees of risk of thrombosis. Treatment with heparin, including low molecular weight heparin, is effective in the vast majority of patients, and treatment of DVT and PE is the same for patients with and without antithrombin deficiency.

Protein C deficiency

Inheritance is autosomal dominant with variable penetrance. Protein C levels in heterozygote individuals are approximately 50% of normal. Characteristically, many patients develop skin necrosis as a result of dermal vessel occlusion when treated with warfarin alone, thought to be caused by a further reduction of protein C levels in the first day or two of warfarin therapy. Rarely, infants may be born with homozygous deficiency and characteristically present with severe disseminated intravascular coagulation (DIC) or purpura fulminans in infancy.

Protein S deficiency

Protein S deficiency has been found in a number of families with a thrombotic tendency. It is a cofactor for protein C. The clinical features of protein S deficiency are similar to those of protein C deficiency, including a tendency to skin necrosis with unopposed warfarin therapy. The inheritance is autosomal dominant.

Prothrombin allele G20210A

G20210A is a mutation in the promoter region of the prothrombin gene that has a prevalence of 2–3% in the population. It leads to increased plasma prothrombin levels and increases thrombotic risk up to five-fold. It is probable that the cause of venous thrombosis with this mutation is that there is increased pre-mRNA stability, allowing continued translation of prothrombin even when signals for increased transcription are absent.

Hyperhomocysteinaemia

High levels of plasma homocysteine may be genetic or acquired. Increased levels were previously thought to be associated with an increased risk for venous thrombosis. However, large well-controlled trials have demonstrated that the risk for venous thrombosis is unrelated except in patients with deficiency of cystathione β-synthase (CBS), when patients can have levels five times higher than the upper limit of normal. Homocysteine is derived from dietary methionine and is removed by either remethylation to methionine (see Fig. 5.3) or conversion to cysteine via a *trans*-sulphuration pathway. Classic homocystinuria is a rare autosomal recessive disorder caused by deficiency of CBS, the enzyme responsible for *trans*-sulphuration. Vascular disease and thrombosis are major features of CBS deficiency and are accompanied by other manifestations, including cognitive abnormalities. Methylenetetrahydrofolate reductase is involved in the remethylation of tetrahydrofolate (THF), methylTHF being responsible for methylating homocysteine to methionine (see Fig. 5.5). A common thermolabile variant of the enzyme can be found in up to 25% of the global population, but is not associated with thrombosis.

Acquired risk factors for hyperhomocysteinaemia include deficiency of vitamin B_6, folate, drugs (e.g. ciclosporin), renal damage and smoking. The levels also increase with age and are higher in men and post-menopausal females. The role of elevated homocysteine in arterial events is unclear. There does appear to be a relationship between high levels of homocysteine and arterial damage; however, high doses of pyridoxine and folic acid, which lower homocysteine, levels do not decrease the risk for recurrent arterial events such as myocardial infarction.

Defects of fibrinogen

Defects of fibrinogen are usually clinically silent or cause excess bleeding. Thrombosis is a rare association and is seen with congenital dysfibrinogenemia and not hypofibrinogenemias.

ABO blood group

Non-O blood group carriers have a higher risk of venous thrombosis or embolism than O carriers. This is related to their higher plasma levels of von Willebrand factor and factor VIII.

Hereditary or acquired disorders of haemostasis

High plasma factor VIII or fibrinogen levels are also associated with venous thrombosis, although the association is weak. No genetic mechanisms for increased FVIII or fibrinogen levels have been found. The combination of multiple risk factors is associated with increased risk of thrombosis. If these are persistent they may represent a reason for extended anticoagulation.

Acquired risk factors

These may cause thrombosis in patients without another identifiable abnormality, but are more likely to do so if an inherited predisposing abnormality such as factor V Leiden is also present.

Hospital-acquired thrombosis

Hospital-acquired thrombosis (HAT) is responsible for up to 50% of cases of DVT and PE. Thrombosis may occur many weeks after discharge from hospital and HAT is now regularly defined as venous thromboembolism (VTE) occurring within 90 days of hospitalization. In many countries there are national strategies to reduce the incidence of HAT, such as through universal patient risk assessment on admission and administration of thromboprophylaxis to high-risk patients. Thromboprophylaxis is typically given for the duration of admission and is extended after discharge in very high-risk patients, such as those having had hip or knee replacement.

Postoperative venous thrombosis

This is more likely to occur in the elderly, obese, those with a previous or family history of venous thrombosis, and in those in whom major abdominal or hip operations are performed. Elasticated stockings, mechanical methods and pharmacological prophylaxis are used to reduce the risk of DVT (see Chpater 28).

Venous stasis and immobility

These factors are probably responsible for the high incidence of postoperative venous thrombosis and for venous thrombosis associated with congestive cardiac failure, myocardial infarction and varicose veins. In atrial fibrillation, thrombin generation from accumulation of activated clotting factors leads to a high risk of clot formation in the atrial appendage and consequent systemic embolization. The use of muscle relaxants during anaesthesia may also contribute to venous stasis. Venous thrombosis has a higher frequency after prolonged (>4 hours) aeroplane journeys.

Malignancy

Patients with carcinoma of the ovary, brain and pancreas have a particularly increased risk of venous thrombosis or its recurrence, but there is an increased risk with all cancers and myeloproliferative diseases. The tumours produce tissue factor and a procoagulant that directly activates factor X. Mucin-secreting adenocarcinomas may be associated with DIC. Direct compression of vessels by solid tumours and lymph nodes can also result in VTE.

Inflammation

This up-regulates procoagulant factors and down-regulates anticoagulant pathways, particularly protein C. Thrombosis is particularly likely in inflammatory bowel disease, Behçet's disease, systemic tuberculosis, systemic lupus erythematosus (SLE) and diabetes.

Superficial venous thrombosis

The risk of DVT is increased in those who have had a previous superficial venous thrombosis or thrombophlebitis, especially if there are additional risk factors.

Blood disorders

Increased viscosity, thrombocytosis and enhanced platelet functional responses are possible factors for the high incidence of thrombosis in patients with polycythaemia vera and essential thrombocythaemia. **Testing for the *JAK2 V617F* mutation may indicate an otherwise unsuspected myeloproliferative disease in patients with hepatic or portal vein thrombosis**. The *CALR* mutation is rarely associated with VTE (see p. 183). There is a high incidence of venous thrombosis in patients with paroxysmal nocturnal haemoglobinuria, including thrombi in large veins such as the hepatic vein. An increased tendency to venous thrombosis also occurs in patients with sickle cell disease, post-splenectomy, and in those with a paraprotein.

Oestrogen therapy

Oestrogen therapy, particularly high-dose therapy, is associated with increased plasma levels of factors II, VII, VIII, IX and X, and depressed levels of protein S and C and tissue plasminogen activator in the vessel wall. There is a high incidence of postoperative venous thrombosis in women on high-dose oestrogen therapy and full-dose oestrogen-containing oral contraceptives. The risk is much less with low-dose oestrogen contraceptive preparations. Hormone replacement therapy increases the risk of thrombosis, largely obviated by the use of low-oestrogen preparations. Some newer progestin formulations have also been associated with development of thrombosis.

Heparin-induced thrombocytopenia

This hypercoagulable state is discussed in Chapter 28.

The antiphospholipid syndrome

The antiphospholipid syndrome (APS) can be defined as the occurrence of venous or arterial thrombosis and/or recurrent miscarriage in association with laboratory evidence of persistent antiphospholipid antibody. One antiphospholipid is the **lupus anticoagulant (LA)**, which was initially detected in patients with SLE and is identified by a prolonged plasma APTT which does not correct with a 50:50 mixture with normal plasma. Paradoxically, in view of its name, the syndrome is associated with venous and arterial thrombosis. A second test dependent on limiting quantities of phospholipid (such as the dilute Russell's viper venom test) is also used in diagnosis. Whereas lupus anticoagulants are reactive in the fluid phase, other antiphospholipid antibodies, such as anti-cardiolipin antibodies and antibodies to β_2-GP (glycoprotein) I-1, are identified by solid phase immunoassay. Both solid phase assays and coagulation tests for LA should be used in the diagnosis of APS.

As well as in patients with SLE, antiphospholipid antibodies are found in other autoimmune disorders, particularly of connective tissues, as well as in lymphoproliferative diseases, post-viral infections, treatment with certain drugs including phenothiazines and as an 'idiopathic' phenomenon in otherwise healthy subjects. Arterial thrombosis may cause peripheral limb ischaemia, stroke or myocardial infarction. Venous thrombosis includes DVT, PE and thrombosis in vessels supplying the abdominal organs. As with other causes of thrombophilia, recurrent abortion caused by placental infarction is also an association (Table 27.3). Thrombocytopenia may be present and livedo reticularis is a frequent dermal manifestation.

Treatment is with anticoagulation where indicated. It is usual to maintain an international normalized ratio (INR) of between 2.0 and 3.0 with warfarin, but higher levels or alternative anticoagulants may be needed if previous arterial or major DVT has occurred or recurrence of thrombosis occurs on warfarin therapy. Low-dose heparin and aspirin may be useful in the management of recurrent miscarriage, although the data are conflicting.

Table 27.3 Clinical associations of lupus anticoagulant and anti-cardiolipin antibodies.

Venous thrombosis: deep venous thrombosis/pulmonary embolism, renal, hepatic, retinal veins
Arterial thrombosis
Recurrent fetal loss
Thrombocytopenia
Livedo reticularis
N.B. Recurrent fetal loss may also occur in other types of thrombophilia.

Collagen vascular diseases and Behçet's syndrome are also associated with arterial and venous thrombosis, whether or not the lupus anticoagulant is present.

It is important to remember that patients require both persistently positive laboratory tests at least 12 weeks apart (same tests positive) and a clinical event to make the diagnosis of antiphospholipid syndrome. Up to 5% of healthy blood donors will have the presence of an antiphospholipid antibody that has no clinical significance and does not appear to increase their risk for thrombosis.

Investigation of thrombophilia

Decisions regarding duration of anticoagulation, such as whether to continue it lifelong or for a defined period, should be made with reference to whether the first episode of venous thrombosis was provoked or not, other risk factors, and risk of anticoagulant therapy-related bleeding, regardless of whether a heritable thrombophilia is known (see Chapter 28). Testing for heritable thrombophilia may influence decisions regarding duration of anticoagulation and for family counselling. However, routine testing of all patients with an episode of VTE is not generally valuable.

Tests that should be performed in patients with a tendency to venous thrombosis include:

1 Blood count and erythrocyte sedimentation rate – to detect elevation in haematocrit, white cell count, platelet count, fibrinogen and globulins.
2 Blood film examination – may provide evidence of myeloproliferative disorder; leucoerythroblastic features may indicate malignant disease.
3 Prothrombin time (PT) and APTT – a shortened APPT is often seen in thrombotic states and may indicate the presence of activated clotting factors. A prolonged APTT test, not corrected by the addition of normal plasma, suggests an LA or an acquired inhibitor to a coagulation factor.
4 Anticardiolipin and anti-β_2-GPI antibodies.
5 Thrombin time (and reptilase time) – prolongation suggests an abnormal fibrinogen.

6 Fibrinogen assay.
7 DNA analysis for factor V Leiden.
8 Antithrombin – immunological and functional assays.
9 Protein C and protein S – immunological and functional assays.
10 Prothrombin gene analysis for the G20210A variant.
11 Test for CD59 and CD55 expression (paroxysmal nocturnal haemoglobinuria) by flow cytometry in red cells if paroxysmal nocturnal haemoglobinuria is suspected.
12 Test for *JAK2 V617F* mutation if portal or hepatic vein thrombosis.
13 Protein electrophoresis for paraprotein.

Diagnosis of venous thrombosis

Deep vein thrombosis

Clinical suspicion **of DVT is suspected in patients with a painful and/or swollen limb**. It is more common in those with previous DVT or superficial venous thrombosis, cancer or recent confinement to bed (Table 27.2). In the leg, unilateral thigh or calf swelling or tenderness, pitting oedema and the presence of collateral superficial non-varicose veins are important signs. Homan's sign (pain in the calf on flexing the ankle) is unreliable.

Plasma D-dimer concentration The concentration of these fibrin breakdown products is raised when there is a fresh thrombosis. It is a useful assay when venous thrombosis is suspected and the **Wells score** can be used to predict the pre-test probability of thrombosis (Table 27.4). A negative result in emergency departments can be used to exclude DVT or PE and avoid the need for radiological imaging. The test is useful when a new thrombus is suspected at a site of scarring from

Table 27.4 Deep vein thrombosis: clinical assessment – the Wells score.

	Points
Active cancer (treatment ongoing or within previous 6 months or palliative)	1
Paralysis, plaster	1
Bed more than 3 days, surgery within 4 weeks	1
Tenderness along veins	1
Entire leg swollen (calf circumference >3 cm compared with other leg)	1
Pitting oedema	1
Collateral veins	1
Alternative diagnosis likely	−2
Low probability 0–1	
High probability 2 or more	

a previous thrombosis and scanning gives equivocal findings. D-dimer elevation in cancer, inflammation, after surgery or trauma and during pregnancy limits its usefulness. It is also useful when ultrasound is not possible.

Compression ultrasound **This is a reliable and practical method for patients with first suspicion of DVT in the legs and other sites (Fig. 27.4a).** It can be combined with spectral, colour (Fig. 27.4a) or power Doppler (duplex) scanning, which improves accuracy by focusing on individual veins. It does not distinguish between acute and chronic thrombi. Persisting venous obstruction detected by ultrasonography at the completion of warfarin therapy is not typically associated with an increased risk of recurrent thrombosis, and scanning to detect residual vein occlusion (RVO) is not routine practice.

Contrast venography This test is now rarely performed. Iodinated contrast medium is injected into a vein peripheral to the suspected DVT. This permits direct demonstration by X-ray of the site, size and extent of the thrombus (Fig. 27.4b). However, it is a painful invasive technique, with a risk of contrast reaction and procedure-induced DVT.

Magnetic resonance imaging (MRI) This may also be used, but is expensive. It is indicated when ultrasound might be inaccurate or difficult, such as because of obesity or patients in a plaster cast.

Impedance plethysmography is less sensitive and accurate and is falling out of use.

Computed tomography (CT) or MRI angiogram/venogram may be needed to detect pelvic vein such as iliac or common iliac vein thrombosis.

Pulmonary embolus

This usually presents with shortness of breath and there may be pleuritic chest pain, tachycardia, cough, dizziness or lightheadedness. PE should be particularly suspected in patients with signs or previous history of DVT, immobilization for more than 2 days or recent (<4 weeks) surgery, haemoptysis or cancer. Recurrent PE may lead to pulmonary hypertension.

Chest X-ray This is often normal, but may show evidence of pulmonary infarction or pleural effusion.

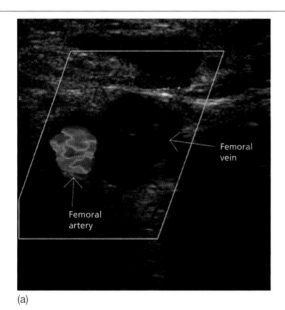

(a)

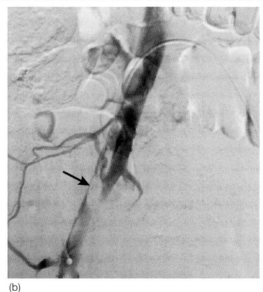

(b)

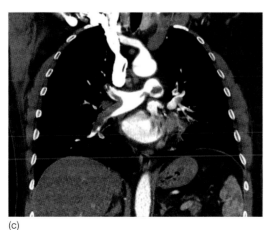

(c)

Figure 27.4 Diagnostic imaging of deep vein thrombosis (DVT) and pulmonary embolus (PE). **(a)** Colour power Doppler ultrasound of the right femoral vessels with compression shows normal flow in the femoral artery, but absent flow in the vein because of thrombus. A normal vein would collapse with compression of the probe. Source: Courtesy of Dr Tony Young. **(b)** Femoral venogram demonstrating extensive thrombus within the right external iliac vein. Source: Courtesy of Dr I.S. Francis and Dr A.F. Watkinson. **(c)** Computed tomography (CT) pulmonary angiography: a coronal image shows bilateral filling defects (green crosses) in the central pulmonary arteries, indicating pulmonary emboli. Source: Courtesy of Dr Tony Young.

Electrocardiogram This is performed to determine whether there is right heart 'strain', which occurs only in relatively severe cases.

Plasma D-dimer concentration D-dimer measurement using an appropriate assay has a similar negative predictive value in patients with PE as with DVT when used in conjunction with a clinical probability rule. As such, PE can be reliably excluded in a patient with a low pre-test probability score and a normal D-dimer test.

Ventilation perfusion (VQ) scintigraphy This detects areas of the lung being ventilated but not perfused.

CT pulmonary angiography Slices of the lung are scanned by spiral CT and timed to the phase of contrast flow so that filling defects in the pulmonary arteries are visualized (Fig. 27.4c).

Magnetic resonance pulmonary angiography Gadolinium-enhanced MRI is a relatively new and expensive but accurate technique.

Pulmonary angiography This is the traditional reference method, but is invasive with complications, albeit uncommon, such as arrhythmia or contrast reaction.

Post-thrombotic syndrome (PTS)

This occurs in up to a third of subjects months or years after a DVT of the lower limb. Venous thrombi that persist can destroy venous valves and venous return is then impaired. This leads to venous hypertension, which is responsible for fluid accumulation in the extravascular space. The syndrome is more common if inadequate anticoagulation has been given or after recurrent thrombosis in the same leg, or with persistent residual vein thrombosis impeding venous return. Symptoms include pain, cramps, heaviness, itching and paraesthesiae. These are worse at the end of the day and after standing for long periods. The lower leg shows redness, induration, patchy

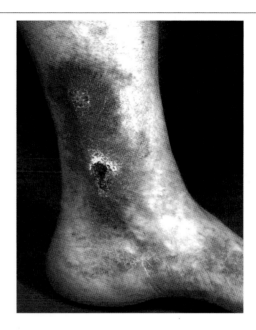

Figure 27.5 Post-thrombotic syndrome: a healing venous ulcer with surrounding pigmentation. Source: Courtesy of Professor G. Hamilton. A.V. Hoffbrand *et al.* (2019) *Color Atlas of Clinical Hematology*, 5th edn. Reproduced by permission of John Wiley & Sons.

hyperpigmentation, venous ectasia and in severe cases venous ulceration (Fig. 27.5). Compression stockings may reduce the discomfort, but there is doubt whether they reduce the incidence of PTS. There is no evidence that prolonged anticoagulation reduces the risk of PTS, but early walking and physical activity may do this. In severe cases prolonged anticoagulation may be indicated to prevent recurrent VTE events in the same leg.

SUMMARY

- Thrombosis is the formation of solid masses of platelets and fibrin in the circulation. It may be arterial or venous.
- Arterial thrombosis is mainly related to atherosclerosis of the vessel wall, with risk factors such as hypertension, hyperlipidaemia, smoking and diabetes.
- Venous thrombosis is related to genetic coagulation factor abnormalities (e.g. factor V Leiden, protein C deficiency), stasis of the circulation or to an acquired increase in coagulation factors (e.g. oestrogen therapy, postoperative, pregnancy, cancer) or to unknown factors (e.g. age or obesity).

- Myeloproliferative diseases predispose to both arterial and venous thrombosis.
- Diagnosis of deep vein thrombosis is with serial compression ultrasound combined with Doppler (duplex) scanning, contrast venography or MRI imaging. Plasma D-dimer concentration assay may help.
- Pulmonary embolus is diagnosed by chest X-ray, electrocardiogram, ventilation perfusion scintigraphy or CT angiography.
- Post-thrombotic syndrome occurs in up to a third of patients after a lower limb DVT.

Now visit **www.wileyessential.com/haematology** to test yourself on this chapter.

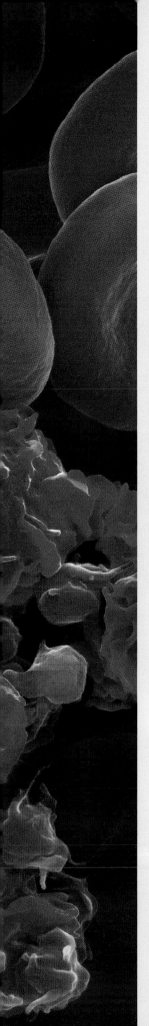

CHAPTER 28
Thrombosis 2: treatment

Key topics

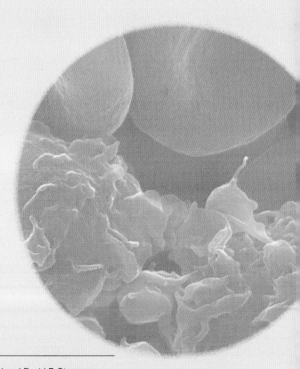

Hoffbrand's Essential Haematology, Eighth Edition. By A. Victor Hoffbrand and David P. Steensma.
© 2020 John Wiley & Sons Ltd. Published 2020 by John Wiley & Sons Ltd.
Companion website: www.wileyessential.com/haematology

Treatment overview

The treatment of thrombosis has evolved over the past 5–10 years with the availability of direct oral anticoagulants (DOACs), a major advance in anticoagulation therapy. Venous thromboembolism (VTE) management has changed as a result of the licensing of these anticoagulants. **DOACs are now used for the initial treatment of most cases of deep vein thrombosis (DVT) and for many with pulmonary embolism (PE). Data on the use of the DOACs have firmly established them as first-line agents for the prevention of** stroke and systemic embolism in patients with non-valvular atrial fibrillation (AF). Data are also accumulating for their use alone or in combination with antiplatelet drugs for other types of arterial thromboembolic events.

The wide range of oral and parenteral anticoagulants (Fig. 28.1) act either directly or indirectly at a specific site or at multiple sites in the coagulation cascade (Fig. 28.2) to prevent thrombus formation. The options for treatment of VTE now range from unfractionated heparin (UFH) administered by intravenous (IV) continuous infusion to outpatient oral DOACs that do not require monitoring.

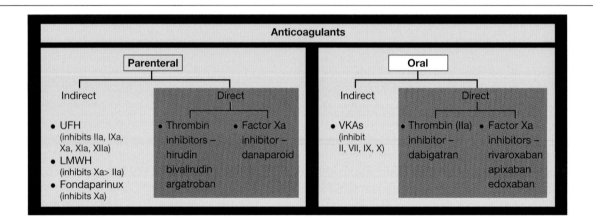

Figure 28.1 Classification of the anticoagulants based on their route of administration and mode of action. Source: Adapted from R. DeCaterina *et al.* (2013) *Thromb. Haemost.* 109: 4. LMWH, low molecular weight heparin; UFH, unfractionated heparin.

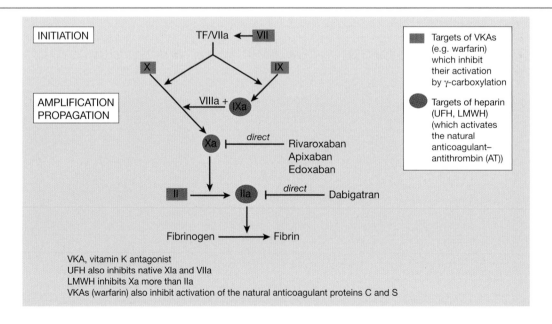

Figure 28.2 Sites of action of the more frequently used anticoagulants. Source: Adapted from R. DeCaterina *et al.* (2013) *Thromb. Haemost.* 109: 4.

Venous thromboembolism

Initial treatment

Patient-specific factors will determine whether a patient requires admission for treatment of a new PE or DVT. These factors also drive anticoagulant choice. For patients who are unstable due to haemodynamic compromise, limb-threatening oedema or ischaemia, increased bleeding risk, renal impairment or other factors requiring hospital admission, IV UFH or subcutaneous (SC) low molecular weight heparin (LMWH) is the initial agent of choice. Patients with PE or DVT with severe compromise may also require either systemic or catheter-directed thrombolysis. Transition to outpatient anticoagulants after hospitalization is also based on patient-specific factors. For patients with uncomplicated VTE who can be managed as outpatients, the DOACs are recommended as first-line therapy. Anticoagulation with warfarin is still important for patients with mechanical valves, antiphospholipid syndrome and severe renal failure, as the DOACs are inferior to warfarin for these indications.

Length of anticoagulation

It is important to treat an acute VTE with at least 3 months of full-intensity anticoagulation. If the VTE was provoked by a transient major predisposing event such as surgery or more than 3 days' immobilization, and is not extensive, 3 months' therapy alone is usually given. There are no specific guidelines for deciding between 3 versus 6 months of anticoagulation. The risk of recurrence is not changed if patients are treated for 3 or 6 months. Patients who presented with significant clot burden, life-threatening PE or other risk factors are most frequently treated for 6 months, sometimes longer depending on patient-specific additional VTE risks.

Longer-term (possibly indefinite) anticoagulation is usually needed for:
- Recurrent venous thrombosis, especially if unprovoked or with post-thrombotic syndrome.
- Patients with VTE and the antiphospholipid syndrome (APS).
- When VTE occurs at an unusual site, such as a mesenteric or cerebral vein.
- When the VTE is associated with persistent malignancy.
- Patients with severe deficiency of proteins C or S, or antithrombin.
- Patients with homozygous factor V Leiden or prothrombin gene mutations, or when compound heterozygotes for the two are detected and the patient has had recurrent or an unprovoked event.
- When a single VTE is unprovoked, the decision to continue anticoagulation after 3–6 months, apart from the indications listed above, is based on a number of variables, although definitive trials addressing these have not been performed. For patients with a first unprovoked VTE, the location of the clot, the presence of residual thrombosis or the post-thrombotic syndrome and other patient-specific factors (see below) are considered when determining how long to continue anticoagulation.

The risk of recurrent VTE is highest in the first two years following an unprovoked VTE, but the cumulative risk continues to increase over the ensuing years. Distal lower-extremity DVT, such as of a calf vein, has a lower risk of recurrence than more proximal DVT or than PE. Men, patients, subjects over 65 years, those who are obese, with the post-thrombotic syndrome or with a raised D-dimer concentration off anticoagulation are also at increased risk of recurrence, as are those with chronic medical diseases such as inflammatory bowel disease, auto-immune disorders, chronic obstructive airways disease and congestive heart failure, especially if the underlying disease remains active. Risk stratification scores based on clinical factors as well as D-dimer concentration, such as the Vienna prediction nomogram and the DASH score, are available to guide decision making regarding duration of anticoagulation.

Previously one of the biggest factors when trying to decide how long to continue anticoagulation when vitamin K antagonists (VKAs) were the only oral anticoagulants available was the balance between a patient's risk of recurrent VTE and risk of major bleeding. The DOACs, which are less burdensome than VKAs, have changed the approach to a longer duration of anticoagulation. The risks of bleeding with longer-duration anticoagulation with DOACs are lower than with warfarin, particularly with apixaban and rivaroxaban, for which prophylactic doses have been shown to have similar preventive efficacy as full dose with the same or even lower risk of bleeding. Prophylactic doses of rivaroxaban or apixaban have also been shown to be better than low-dose aspirin at preventing recurrent VTE in those at increased risk for recurrence after acute VTE treatment.

Arterial thrombosis

Arterial thrombotic events are considered to arise dominantly from different mechanisms than venous, with shear stress activation of platelets or adhesion to atherosclerotic lesions considered to be the primary aetiology. It is now recognized, however, that arterial and venous thrombosis involve some common pathways that activate coagulation.

Acute arterial thrombotic occlusion requires emergency treatment, especially for small-calibre arteries. For coronary artery occlusion, systemic anticoagulation with a parenteral anticoagulant, heparin or a direct thrombin inhibitor such as bivalirudin is given. Percutaneous interventions with thrombectomy and the placement of stents to maintain vessel patency in the setting of atherosclerotic plaque and thrombosis are also used to prevent or limit myocardial ischaemia and infarction (MI). For central nervous system (CNS) thromboembolic stroke, systemic thrombolysis is used unless there are contraindications (see Table 28.7), followed by a period of parenteral anticoagulation. After the emergency treatment, patients are discharged on antiplatelet agents, often aspirin plus a platelet ADP inhibitor such as clopidogrel (see

Fig. 28.6) if coronary artery stents are placed. Aspirin alone is given if the patient had a simple ischaemic CNS stroke. For arterial thrombosis in larger vessels such as in a lower extremity, acute interventional thrombectomy is often performed to prevent limb ischaemia, followed by systemic anticoagulation. The combination of aspirin and low-dose rivaroxaban appears to have significant benefit for patients with peripheral arterial disease, with the added benefit of reduction in other cardiovascular complications such as stroke and MI.

Parenteral anticoagulants

Heparin

This acidic unfractionated mucopolysaccharide of average molecular weight (MW) 15 000–18 000 is an inhibitor of blood coagulation by potentiating the activity of antithrombin (see below). As it is not absorbed it must be given by injection.

It is inactivated by the liver and excreted in the urine. The effective biological half-life is approximately 1 hour (Table 28.1).

Mode of action

Unfractionated heparin dramatically potentiates the formation of complexes between antithrombin and the activated serine protease coagulation factors, thrombin (IIa) and factors IXa, Xa and XIa (Fig. 28.3). This inactivates these factors irreversibly. In addition, unfractionated heparin impairs platelet function.

Low molecular weight heparin (LMWH) preparations (MW 2000–10 000) have a greater ability to inhibit factor Xa than to inhibit thrombin and interact less with platelets than standard heparin, and so have a lesser tendency to cause bleeding. They also have greater bioavailability and a more prolonged half-life in plasma, making once-daily administration feasible (Table 28.1).

Table 28.1 Comparison of unfractionated heparin with low molecular weight heparin and fondaparinux.

	Unfractionated heparin	Low molecular weight heparin	Fondaparinux
Mean molecular weight in kilodaltons (range)	15 (4–30)	4.5 (2–10)	1.5
Indications	■ Arterial and venous thromboembolism ■ ECMO ■ Cardiopulmonary bypass ■ DIC ■ Maintenance of in-dwelling arterial and venous catheters and lines	■ Arterial and venous thromboembolism ■ Cancer-associated VTE ■ VTE in pregnancy* ■ VTE prophylaxis for hospitalized patients and post- joint arthroplasty	■ Arterial and venous thromboembolism ■ HIT
Anti-Xa:anti-IIa	1:1	2:1 to 4:1	Anti-Xa only
Inhibits platelet function	Yes	No	No
Bioavailability	50%	100%	100%
Half-life			
intravenous	1 hour	2 hours	na
subcutaneous	2 hours	4 hours	17–20 hours
Elimination	Renal and hepatic	Renal	
Monitoring	APTT	Anti-Xa assay (usually not needed)	Anti-Xa assay (usually not needed)
Frequency of heparin-induced thrombocytopenia	High	Low	Can be used to treat HIT
Osteoporosis	Yes	Less frequent/unclear	

*Does not cross the placenta.
APTT, activated partial thromboplastin time; DIC, disseminated intravascular coagulation; ECMO, extracorporeal membrane oxygenation; HIT, heparin-induced thrombocytopenia; na, not available; VTE, venous thromboembolism.

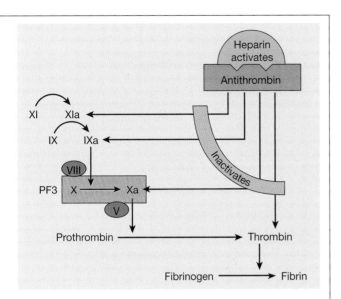

Figure 28.3 The action of heparin. This activates antithrombin, which then forms complexes with activated serine protease coagulation factors – thrombin (IIa), Xa, IXa and Xia – and so inactivates them.

Fondaparinux

This is a synthetic analogue of the antithrombin-binding pentasaccharide site of heparin. Its mechanism of action is similar to heparin, as it is an indirect factor Xa inhibitor which works through antithrombin. It is given subcutaneously, has a plasma half-life of 17 hours and, like the orally active factor Xa

inhibitors, does not require laboratory monitoring except in obese patients, those with renal failure and in children, when monitoring is by measuring factor anti-Xa levels.

Administration and laboratory control

Standard unfractionated heparin

Continuous intravenous infusion provides the smoothest control of UFH therapy and is the treatment of choice where rapid reversal of anticoagulation by protamine sulphate may be required (e.g. in surgical patients or late pregnancy). It has largely been replaced for treatment of acute PE and DVT by DOACs and LMWH. In an adult, 1000–2000 units/hour with a loading dose of 5000 units is usually satisfactory.

Therapy is monitored by maintaining the APTT at 1.5–2.5 times the ULN (upper limit of normal) value. Unfractionated heparin can also be monitored using the anti-Xa assay, which is a measure of the concentration of UFH in the blood, whereas the APTT is a pharmacodynamic assay of the impact of UFH on all of the relevant coagulation factors. It is usual to start warfarin early if warfarin will be used to treat the VTE and to discontinue heparin (UFH or LMWH) when the international normalized ratio (INR) has been above 2.0 on 2 successive days, with at least 5 days of overlap to allow for suppression of prothrombin (Fig. 28.4). If outpatient treatment will be with a DOAC, the switch is made simultaneously, with the IV UFH turned off and the DOAC given orally to allow continuation of therapeutic anticoagulation (Fig. 28.4). For acute coronary syndromes, both unfractionated heparin and LMWH are of benefit when used with aspirin in the prevention of mural thrombosis, systemic embolization and venous thrombosis.

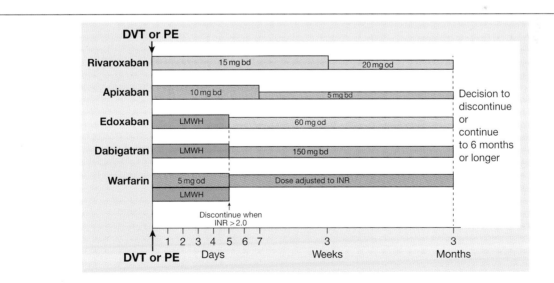

Figure 28.4 Drug regimens and doses for outpatient anticoagulant treatment of deep vein thrombosis (DVT) and pulmonary embolus (PE) of standard risk. Renal impairment, obesity, childhood or old age and other factors affect doses. **Recommended doses and protocols in National Formularies and Guidelines should be consulted for treating individual patients**.

Low molecular weight heparin

LMWH is given by subcutaneous injection and, as it has a longer half-life than UFH, it can be given once a day in prophylaxis, or once or twice daily for treatment (Table 28.1). There are many commercial preparations. Compared with unfractionated heparin, LMWH has a more predictable dose response which avoids the need for routine monitoring. **LMWH is the initial treatment of choice for DVT or PE in situations where DOACs cannot be used,** such as in patients at extremes of weight, with significant drug–drug interactions, poor gastrointestinal (GI) absorption, or GI tract lesions and concern for GI bleeding. LMWH is also given for the first 5 days if edoxaban or dabigatran is the DOAC to be used subsequently (Fig. 28.4). LMWH can be used for patients with renal impairment, as levels can be monitored using the anti-Xa level; there are no commercially available tests for monitoring DOACs.

LMWH is the preferred treatment of VTE in pregnancy because it does not cross the placenta. Although routine monitoring is not required, measurement of anti-Xa peak levels 4 hours after injection allows dose adjustment in selected patients (e.g. in pregnancy, renal impairment, gross obesity and in children). LMWH is also preferred for treatment of **catheter-related thrombosis**, as the bleeding risk with DOACs in this setting is still under study.

LMWH is used for the prevention of DVT in both medical and surgical patients. It is now mandatory in many hospitals to have a policy for prevention of DVT and PE for all hospitalized medical and surgical patients. LMWHs are the gold standard pharmaceutical agents for prophylaxis, but the DOACs are replacing LMWH in some situations such as after joint arthroplasty (see Table 28.5) and may replace LMWH for prophylaxis against recurrence of cancer-associated VTE.

Bleeding during heparin therapy

Bleeding may occur because of excessive prolonged anticoagulation or due to the antiplatelet functional effect of heparin. As intravenous heparin has a half-life of less than 1 hour, it is usually only necessary to stop the infusion. Protamine is able to inactivate heparin immediately. However, protamine itself may act as an anticoagulant when in excess and it may be associated with anaphylaxis and other allergic reactions.

Heparin-induced thrombocytopenia (HIT)

A mild lowering of the platelet count may occur in the first 24 hours as a result of platelet binding to heparin, which is of no clinical consequence. The important thrombocytopenia due to HIT occurs in up to 5% of patients treated with unfractionated heparin and paradoxically presents with thrombosis. It results from the binding of heparin to platelet factor 4 (PF4) followed by the generation of an immunoglobulin (Ig) G antibody to the heparin–PF4 complex, which leads to platelet activation, thrombocytopenia and, in many patients, thrombosis (Fig. 28.5). Typically, it presents as a fall of more than 50% in the platelet count 5 or more days after starting heparin, or earlier if heparin has been given previously. Diagnosis can be difficult, but assays have recently been developed for the detection of antibodies to immobilized heparin–PF4 complex and aid in the diagnosis. Heparin therapy must be discontinued as soon as HIT is suspected, as the mortality associated with unrecognized and untreated HIT can be 50%.

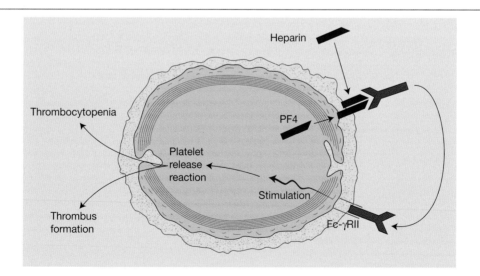

Figure 28.5 Mechanism of heparin-induced thrombocytopenia (HIT). Platelet factor 4 (PF4) is released from α granules and forms a complex on the platelet surface with heparin. Immunoglobulin G antibodies develop against this complex and can activate the platelet through the platelet immunoglobulin receptor Fc-γRII. This leads to platelet stimulation, further release of PF4 and the platelet release reaction, with consequent thrombocytopenia and thrombus development.

Argatroban, bivalirudin or fondaparinux is used in patients with HIT. DOACs are being investigated for the treatment of HIT and show promise in small studies. LMWH is less likely than unfractionated heparin to cause HIT. Warfarin therapy should not be started until normalization of the platelet count has been achieved, due to the initial decrease in protein S and C with risk of thrombosis or skin necrosis.

Osteoporosis

This can occur with long-term (more than 2 months) unfractionated heparin therapy, especially in pregnancy. The drug complexes minerals from bones, but the exact pathogenesis is unknown. It is much less frequent with LMWH therapy.

Direct-acting parenteral anticoagulants

Bivalirudin is used as an alternative to heparin in patients undergoing percutaneous coronary interventions. It is an intravenous direct thrombin inhibitor that can also be used to treat patients with HIT.

Argatroban is a small molecule direct inhibitor of thrombin given by continuous intravenous infusion. It is used to treat patients with HIT.

Oral anticoagulants

Vitamin K antagonists (warfarin)

The only available drugs for many years were derivatives of coumarin or phenindione. **Warfarin**, a coumarin, is the most widely used. Coumarins are vitamin K antagonists (see p. 332) and treatment results in decreased biological activity of the vitamin K-dependent factors II, VII, IX and X, and proteins C and S (Fig. 26.7). After warfarin is given, factor VII levels fall considerably within 24 hours, but prothrombin has a longer plasma half-life and only falls to 50% of normal at 3 days; only then is the patient fully anticoagulated. Although DOACs are endorsed as first-line treatment for both AF and VTE, there are a few clinical situations where warfarin is required. They include mechanical valves, antiphospholipid syndrome, and when precise measurement of anticoagulant effect is needed, as in severe renal failure.

Principles of oral anticoagulation with VKAs

A typical starting regimen for warfarin is 5 mg on days 1, 2 and 3 (Fig. 28.4). For treatment of VTE warfarin is usually commenced after 3 days of LMWH initial therapy, although it can be started simultaneously when it is clear that the patient will be treated with warfarin. LMWH is discontinued when the INR is >2.0 (Fig. 28.4). The daily dose should subsequently be monitored and adjusted by measurement of the INR (preferably by the patient 'at home'). Algorithms for this purpose are published. The initial dose can be 'tailor-made' using an algorithm based on clinical variables and genetic information on two genes involved in warfarin metabolism or action,

Table 28.2 Control tests for warfarin therapy: target levels recommended by the British Society for Haematology.

Target INR	Clinical state
2.5 (2.0–3.0)	Treatment of DVT, pulmonary embolism, atrial fibrillation, recurrent DVT off warfarin; symptomatic inherited thrombophilia, cardiomyopathy, mural thrombus, cardioversion
3.0 (2.5–3.5)	Recurrent DVT while on warfarin, mechanical prosthetic heart valves, antiphospholipid syndrome (some cases)

DVT, deep vein thrombosis; INR, international normalized ratio.

cytochrome p450 (*CYP2CP*) and vitamin K epoxide reductase (see Fig. 26.7). In practice few units do this, as it has not been shown to be a significant advantage for determining the long-term maintenance warfarin dose. This is usually 3–9 mg/day, but individual responses vary greatly. Lower loading dosage is recommended for the elderly or those with liver disease.

International normalized ratio

The effect of VKAs is monitored by the prothrombin time (PT). The INR is calculated from this and is based on the ratio of the patient's PT to a mean normal PT, with correction for the 'sensitivity' of the thromboplastin used. This is calibrated against a primary World Health Organization (WHO) standard thromboplastin. The indications and recommended ranges for INR with warfarin treatment are summarized in Table 28.2. Warfarin crosses the placenta and is teratogenic, so it is avoided in the early stages of pregnancy. Warfarin can be used after organogenesis is complete, but is usually only used for patients with mechanical valves; careful planning is then required for delivery.

Drug interactions

Approximately 97% of warfarin in the circulation is bound to albumin and only a small fraction of warfarin is free and can enter the liver parenchymal cells; it is this free fraction that is active. In the liver cells, warfarin is degraded in microsomes to an inactive water-soluble metabolite, which is conjugated and excreted in the bile and partially reabsorbed to be also excreted in urine. Drugs that affect the albumin binding or excretion of warfarin (or of other oral anticoagulants), or those that decrease the absorption of vitamin K, will interfere with the control of therapy (Table 28.3).

Management of warfarin overdose

If the INR is in excess of 4.5 without bleeding, warfarin should be stopped for 1 or 2 days and the dosage adjusted according

Table 28.3 Drugs and other factors that interfere with the control of coumarin (e.g. warfarin) therapy.

Potentiation of coumarin anticoagulants	Inhibition of coumarin anticoagulants
Drugs that increase the effect of coumarins	**Drugs that depress the action of coumarins**
Reduced coumarin binding to serum albumin	*Acceleration of hepatic microsomal degradation of coumarin*
Sulphonamides	Barbiturates
Inhibition of hepatic microsomal degradation of coumarin	Rifampicin
	Ribavirin
Amiodarone	*Enhanced synthesis of clotting factors*
Diltiazem	
Propanolol	Oral contraceptives
Antibiotics – ciprofloxacin, erythromycin, fluconazole	**Hereditary resistance to oral anticoagulants**
Alcohol	**Pregnancy**
Phenytoin	
Quinidine	
Allopurinol	
Tricyclic antidepressants	
Metronidazole	
Sulphonamides	
Alteration of hepatic receptor site for drug	
Thyroxine	
Quinidine	
Decreased synthesis of vitamin K factors	
High doses of salicylates	
Some cephalosporins, other antibiotics	
Liver disease	
Decreased synthesis of vitamin K factors	
Decreased absorption of vitamin K	
e.g. malabsorption, antibiotic therapy, laxatives	

N.B. Patients are also more likely to bleed if taking antiplatelet agents (e.g. non-steroidal anti-inflammatory drugs, dipyridamole or aspirin); alcohol in large amounts enhances warfarin action.

Table 28.4 Recommendations on the management of bleeding and excessive anticoagulation with warfarin.

INR 3.0–6.0 (target INR 2.5)	Reduce warfarin dose or stop
INR 4.0–6.0 (target INR 3.5)	Restart warfarin when INR <5.0
INR 6.0–8.0	Stop warfarin*
No bleeding or minor bleeding	Restart warfarin when INR <5.0
INR >9.0	Stop warfarin*
No bleeding or minor bleeding	Restart warfarin when INR <5.0
	If other risk factors for bleeding give 0.5–2.5 mg vitamin K orally
Major bleeding	Stop warfarin
	Give prothrombin complex concentrate (PCC) 50 units/kg, in preference
	FFP 15 mL/kg (if PCC not available)
	Give 5 mg vitamin K (IV)

*1 mg vitamin K may be given orally to rapidly reduce the INR to the therapeutic range within 24 hours in all patients with an INR above the therapeutic range and no bleeding.
FFP, fresh frozen plasma; INR, international normalized ratio; IV, intravenous.

to the INR. The long half-life of warfarin (40 hours) delays the full impact of dose changes for 4–5 days. If the INR is very high (e.g. >10) without bleeding, an oral dose of 0.5–2.5 mg vitamin K can be given. Mild bleeding usually only needs an INR assessment, drug withdrawal and subsequent dosage adjustment (Table 28.4). More serious bleeding needs cessation of therapy and vitamin K therapy or the infusion of PCC (prothrombin complex concentrate). Fresh frozen plasma rarely reverses the anticoagulant effect of vitamin K antagonists,

as it is not usually possible to give sufficient volume rapidly. Vitamin K is the specific antidote; an oral or intravenous dose of 2.5 mg is usually effective. However, it takes time to synthesize the coagulation factors. Higher doses of vitamin K result in resistance to further warfarin therapy for 2–3 weeks. Even larger doses, however, and for prolonged periods of weeks or months, are needed for those who have accidentally ingested coumarin-like rodenticides such as brodifacoum ('superwarfarins'), which are two logs more potent than warfarin and whose action lasts for weeks.

Management of surgery for patients receiving warfarin: bridging anticoagulation

For minor surgery (e.g. dental extraction), anticoagulation can be maintained and mouth rinses with tranexamic acid given. For patients with AF and no history of thrombosis, 'bridging' is not necessary when major surgery is being performed. In these patients warfarin can be stopped 5 days prior to surgery without the need for a heparin bridge. For major surgery in high-risk patients, e.g. those with a mechanical heart valve, warfarin should be stopped 5 days before surgery and LMWH is given until the day before surgery. As it takes several days for an anticoagulant effect to be re-established, LMWH as well as warfarin is recommenced postoperatively when haemostasis is secure. For these patients the LMWH is discontinued when the INR is in the therapeutic range. Prophylaxis against thrombosis, for example with low-dose LMWH, should be given postoperatively to patients previously receiving warfarin and at risk of hospital-acquired thrombosis if they are not using an LMWH bridge.

Direct oral anticoagulants

DOACs are inhibitors of coagulation factors Xa or IIa (thrombin) and offer improvement over VKAs (Tables 28.5 and 28.6) by virtue of:

- Rapid onset and offset of action.
- Predictable dose responses.
- No need for routine monitoring.
- Reduced need for dose adjustment.
- No food interactions.
- Few drug interactions.

The DOACs are now recommended as first-line treatment for AF and VTE. For both conditions the DOACs are non-inferior to VKAs for efficacy and in many situations have an improved safety profile, especially with a decreased risk of intracranial haemorrhage in patients with AF. They are also approved for post-joint replacement VTE prophylaxis.

DOACs have uniform bioavailability without the need for monitoring drug activity. Because of their shorter action, compliance with daily dosing is more important. Renal impairment requires lower doses, especially for dabigatran, and in severe renal failure LMWH and warfarin are preferred. However, commercial assays are being developed to assess drug concentration in those patients who develop bleeding or have specific characteristics that might affect DOAC concentration, such as renal impairment, extremes of body weight, children and where there is risk of drug–drug interaction. The assays can also be of benefit to assess levels before an invasive procedure and to assess compliance. For the direct Xa inhibitors, an anti-Xa

Table 28.5 The oral direct-acting anticoagulants compared with warfarin (see also Fig. 28.4).

	Xa inhibitor	Xa inhibitor	Xa inhibitor	Xa inhibitor	IIa (thrombin) inhibitor	Vitamin K antagonist
	Rivaroxaban	Apixaban	Edoxaban	betrixaban	Dabigatran	Warfarin
Daily	OD or BD* 10–20 mg	BD 2.5–10 mg	OD 30–60 mg*	OD	OD or BD* 75–150 mg*	OD
	Initial VTE treatment: 15 mg twice daily for 3 weeks followed by 20 mg once daily	Initial VTE treatment: 10 mg twice daily for 7 days followed by 5 mg twice daily	For VTE requires 5 days of parenteral agent before starting 60 mg once daily, 30 mg if decreased renal function	Loading dose 160 mg followed by 80 mg daily. For renal impairment loading dose 80 mg followed by 40 mg daily	For VTE treatment requires 5 days of parenteral agent before starting 150 mg twice daily in patients with normal renal function	
Half-life (h)	7–11	8–14	5–11	20	14–17	40
Renal excretion (%)	33	27	50		80	0
Peak effect	2–4 h	1–2 h	1–2 h	3-4 h	1–3 h	4–5 days
Laboratory test	Anti-Xa PT	Anti-Xa	Anti-Xa		Dilute thrombin time**	PT
Specific antidote	Andexanet alfa: recombinant decoy factor X molecule approved in the USA				Idarucizumab: monoclonal antibody that binds dabigatran	Vitamin K, prothrombin complex Fresh frozen plasma

*According to body weight.
**Rarely needed.
BD, twice daily; OD, once daily; PT, prothrombin time; VTE, venous thromboembolism.
N.B. All doses need adjusting if there is renal impairment. The doses given here are guides only and National Formularies and Guidelines should be consulted for dosing in individual patients.
Source: Adapted from C.H. Yeh *et al.* (2014) *Blood* 124: 1020–28.

Table 28.6 The advantages and disadvantages of the direct oral anticoagulant drugs compared to warfarin.

	Direct oral inhibitors	Warfarin
Advantages	Rapid onset of action Fixed dosing	Long experience
	No monitoring	Reversibility
	No food interactions	Safe in renal failure
	Few drug interactions	INR well validated
	Less major bleeding	Monitoring encourages compliance
	No requirement for parenteral heparins (rivaroxaban, apixaban) for VTE treatment	Less gastrointestinal bleeding
Disadvantages	Compliance more important because short action	Food and drug interactions
	Renal function effects	Narrow therapeutic range
	Avoid in liver dysfunction	Needs monitoring and variable dose
		Slow onset (need for heparin at initiation and bridging)
	Bleeding risk	Bleeding risk
	Not recommended for antiphospholipid syndrome, mechanical heart valves	Not recommended in pregnancy

INR, international normalized ratio; VTE, venous thromboembolism.

assay with specific drug calibrators to assess concentration is most promising, while for the direct thrombin inhibitor dabigatran a dilute thrombin assay with calibrators and an assay with ecarin, a snake venom that directly activates prothrombin, are being developed.

Drugs that are licensed for treatment of AF and VTE include dabigatran (a factor IIa inhibitor) and rivaroxaban, apixaban and edoxaban (all factor Xa inhibitors; Table 28.5). Betrixaban (a factor Xa inhibitor) has been approved in the USA for extended-duration VTE prophylaxis in the medically ill patient following hospitalization. Monitoring of dose is not needed, but specific laboratory tests for the degree of anticoagulation are in development for use if haemorrhage or thrombosis occurs. The initial doses of apixaban or rivaroxaban used for treatment of DVT or PE are higher at the beginning of treatment, as these DOACs can be used without a parenteral agent lead-in (Fig. 28.4); dabigatran and edoxaban require 5 days of a parenteral agent, either LMWH or UFH, before switching to the DOAC (Fig. 28.4).

Dabigatran

Dabigatran is an oral direct thrombin inhibitor with a short half-life. It is given once daily in prophylaxis, but twice daily in treatment of DVT or PE. Food has no significant effect on absorption. Aspirin and non-steroidal anti-inflammatory drugs (NSAIDs) should be avoided if possible. The monoclonal antibody idarucizumab is a specific reversal agent that is active against this factor II (thrombin) inhibitor (Table 28.5). The thrombin time can be used to exclude the presence of dabigatran activity until specific tests are available.

The 10% of patients who suffer indigestion and they should be given a proton pump inhibitor. The dose is reduced in those with impaired renal function and it should not be prescribed when the creatinine clearance is less than 30 mL/min.

Rivaroxaban, apixaban, edoxaban, betrixaban

These are direct factor Xa inhibitors (Table 28.5). Rivaroxaban is given once daily in prophylaxis and twice daily in the initial first three weeks of treatment of DVT or PE (Fig. 28.4). There are no interactions with dietary products. They must not be prescribed for patients with an estimated glomerular filtration rate (eGFR) of <15 mL/min for AF and <30 ml/min for VTE; the dose should be reduced for patients with an eGFR of 15–30 mL/min. In rare cases the PT can be used to assess the activity of rivaroxaban and edoxaban. However, an anti-Xa level calibrated for UFH/LMWH is very sensitive to the presence of the direct oral Xa inhibitors – a normal anti-Xa indicates that no anticoagulant activity is present. The assay can be used until specific tests are available. Reversal, if needed, can be achieved with andexanet alfa, a targeted reversal agent that is a recombinant decoy factor X molecule that lacks catalytic activity. It binds and sequesters all the oral Xa inhibitors and is also effective for reversal of LMWH and fondaparinux. It is approved for use in the USA to reverse the anticoagulant effects of apixaban and rivaroxaban and is undergoing review in the European Union. Prothrombin complex concentrate may also have some activity in reversing the Xa inhibitors. In view of their short half-lives, it may be sufficient to control local haemorrhage until the anticoagulation effect has worn off. Betrixaban is only approved for extended-duration VTE prophylaxis in hospitalized medically ill patients, and is only available in the USA.

Peri-procedure management of DOACs

Both the short onset of action and short half-lives of the DOACs make temporary interruption of anticoagulation for procedures not as cumbersome as for VKAs. For major bleeding risk procedures, the last dose can be given 48 hours prior to the procedure, although a longer interval such as 72 hours may be required for patients with renal impairment. For low bleeding risk procedures, omitting just 24 hours is sufficient. Resumption of anticoagulation post-procedure can begin when haemostasis is achieved, although the use of prophylactic-dose DOAC or LMWH may be required while in hospital with uncertain haemostatic status. Once it is clear that the patient can resume full-intensity anticoagulation, full-dose DOAC can be restarted.

Mechanical methods of prophylaxis of DVT and PE

Graduated compression stockings

These are often used postoperatively, post-partum and during long aeroplane flights to reduce the risk of DVT. After a DVT, they have been recommended to reduce the risk of the post-thrombotic syndrome, but their efficacy for this has been questioned. Knee-high stockings have been used in the vast majority of cases, using 30-40 mmHg graduated compression, and are worn except when the patient is recumbent.

Intermittent compression devices

Intermittent pneumatic compression and mechanical foot pumps are used in high-risk patients in whom bleeding as a result of LMWH is likely. They reduce the risk of thrombosis in both medical and surgical patients.

Inferior vena cava (IVC) filter

This can provide protection against pulmonary embolism when a DVT in the legs is diagnosed, but anticoagulation is contraindicated (e.g. ongoing or very recent intracranial or GI bleeding or where there is recurrent PE despite adequate anticoagulation). Over-use of IVC filters and lack of retrieval of temporary filters are currently being addressed.

Fibrinolytic drugs

Two fibrinolytic drugs, streptokinase and tissue plasminogen activator, are most frequently used to lyse fresh thrombi, although other drugs are available. These drugs may be used systemically for patients with acute myocardial infarction, thromboembolic stroke, major PE with haemodynamic decompensation or ilio-femoral thrombosis, and locally in patients with acute peripheral arterial occlusion. Catheter-directed use of thrombolytics for PE and proximal DVT is also thought to be of benefit, with potentially less risk of systemic side-effects due to localized use and lower systemic doses.

Administration of thrombolytic agents has been simplified with standardized dosage regimens. The therapy is most effective in the first 6 hours after symptoms begin, but is still of benefit up to 24 hours. Aspirin therapy is also given and the value of additional heparin therapy is under study. Laboratory tests for monitoring short-term thrombolytic therapy are unnecessary. However, certain clinical complications exclude the use of thrombolytic agents (Table 28.7).

Recombinant tissue plasminogen activator has a particularly high affinity for fibrin and this allows lysis of thrombi with less systemic activation of fibrinolysis.

Antiplatelet drugs

Antiplatelet agents are gaining an increasing role in clinical medicine. It is now clear that aspirin is valuable in the secondary prevention of vascular disease. Several other agents are being used for different indications (Table 28.8). The sites of action of the antiplatelet drugs are illustrated in Fig. 28.6.

Aspirin inhibits platelet cyclo-oxygenase irreversibly, thus reducing the production of platelet thromboxane A_2. Its action lasts for the whole of the lifespan of the platelet. Low-dose therapy (e.g. 75 mg/day) has a lesser risk of GI bleeding and is most commonly used in patients who have a history of

Table 28.7 Contraindications to thrombolytic therapy.

Absolute contraindications	Relative contraindications
Active gastrointestinal bleeding	Traumatic cardiopulmonary resuscitation
Aortic dissection	Major surgery in the past 10 days
Head injury or cerebrovascular accident in the past 2 months	Past history of gastrointestinal bleeding
	Recent obstetric delivery
	Prior arterial puncture
Neurosurgery in the past 2 months	Prior organ biopsy
	Serious trauma
Intracranial aneurysm or neoplasm	Severe arterial hypertension (systolic pressure >200 mmHg, diastolic pressure >110 mmHg)
Proliferative diabetic retinopathy	Bleeding diathesis

Table 28.8 Suggested regimens for antiplatelet therapy in patients with an acute coronary syndrome and in those undergoing percutaneous coronary intervention (PCI).

Drug	Target/patient group	Duration
Acute coronary syndrome		
Aspirin	All	Life-long
Clopidogrel	All	9–12 months
Glycoprotein IIb/IIIa inhibitors:		
Abciximab	None	–
Eptifibatide	High risk	48–72 hours
Tirofiban	High risk	48–72 hours
Patients undergoing PCI		
Aspirin	All	Life-long
Clopidogrel	All	9–12 months
Abciximab	High risk	12 hours after PCI
Eptifibatide	High risk	18–24 hours after PCI
Tirofiban	None	–

coronary artery or cerebrovascular disease. It is combined with clopidogrel for a year after coronary stenting or angioplasty. It may also be useful in preventing thrombosis in patients with thrombocytosis and has a mild action more generally in reducing the risk of DVT in subjects with normal platelet counts. Aspirin is contraindicated in patients with GI or genitourinary bleeding, retinal bleeding, peptic ulcer, haemophilia or uncontrollable hypertension.

P2Y12 inhibitors

P2Y12 is a G protein-coupled receptor that is involved in the ADP-stimulated activation of the IIb/IIIa receptor of platelets (Fig 28.6). Activation of IIb/IIIa results in enhanced platelet degranulation and thromboxane production, and prolonged platelet aggregation. Inhibition of P2Y12, often in combination with inhibition of cyclooxygenase by aspirin, is the mainstay of treatment of acute coronary syndromes, maintaining patency of coronary artery stents, and plays a role in the management of peripheral arterial vascular disease. The most commonly used P2Y12 inhibitors are listed below.

Clopidogrel is activated by cytochrome p450 in the liver and in some subjects this activation is reduced so that the level

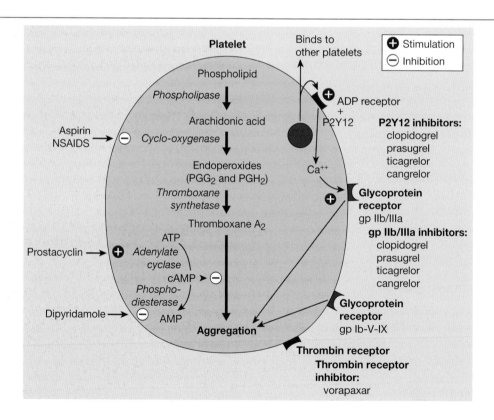

Figure 28.6 Sites of action of antiplatelet drugs. Aspirin acetylates the enzyme cyclo-oxygenase irreversibly. Sulphinpyrazone inhibits cyclo-oxygenase reversibly. Dipyridamole inhibits phosphodiesterase, increases cyclic adenosine monophosphate (cAMP) levels and inhibits aggregation. Clopidogrel and other P2Y12 inhibitors prevent signalling through the platelet ADP receptor, preventing direct activation of the platelet and activation via the IIb/IIIa glycoprotein (GP) receptor. Prostacyclin (epoprostenol) stimulates adenylatecyclase. The lipid-soluble β-blockers inhibit phospholipase. Calcium-channel antagonists block the influx of free calcium ions across the platelet membrane. Dextrans coat the surface, interfering with adhesion and aggregation.

of active drug is not effective. It is used at a dose of 75 mg daily for reduction of ischaemic events in patients with ischaemic stroke, myocardial infarction or peripheral vascular disease. It is used after coronary artery stenting or angioplasty and in patients requiring long-term antiplatelet therapy who are intolerant or allergic to aspirin.

Prasugrel, like clopidogrel, is a P2Y12 inhibitor that requires metabolism from prodrug to active drug form. It has more rapid onset of action, with significantly less patient to patient variability in conversion to active drug. It is more effective with a greater risk of bleeding.

Ticragelor inhibits platelet aggregation at a different site. It does not require hepatic activation and is an allosteric reversible inhibitor, which is an advantage if bleeding occurs or surgery is needed urgently. It needs to be given twice daily, which reduces compliance.

Cangrelor is a platelet ADP inhibitor that is given intravenously. It is the active compound and does not require metabolism to the active drug like clopidogrel, so is used most frequently when patients present acutely with acute coronary syndromes who are not already taking an ADP inhibitor.

Other platelet or vascular active drugs

Dipyridamole (Persantin®) is a phosphodiesterase inhibitor thought to elevate cyclic adenosine monophosphate levels in circulating platelets, which decreases their sensitivity to activating stimuli. Dipyridamole has been shown to reduce thromboembolic complications in patients with prosthetic heart valves and to improve the results in coronary bypass operations.

Glycoprotein IIb/IIIa inhibitors abciximab, eptifibatide and tirofiban are monoclonal antibodies that inhibit the platelet GPIIb/IIIa receptor. They are used in conjunction with heparin, aspirin and clopidogrel for the prevention of ischaemic complications in high-risk patients undergoing percutaneous transluminal coronary angioplasty. They can be used once only.

SUMMARY

- Anticoagulant drugs are used to prevent or treat venous or arterial thrombosis. They include parenteral and oral agents.
- Direct oral anticoagulants (DOACs) include the factor X_a inhibitors rivaroxaban, apixaban and edoxaban and the factor IIa (thrombin) inhibitor dabigatran. They have the advantage of fixed dosage, monitoring is not usually needed and compared with warfarin there are fewer drug and food interactions.
- DOACs are considered first-line treatment for patients with deep vein thrombosis (DVT) or pulmonary embolus (PE) or for stroke and systemic embolism prevention in patients with non-valvular atrial fibrillation.
- Heparin is given parenterally. It can be given in the unfractionated form. Much more frequently low molecular weight heparin is given subcutaneously. It is used e.g. if anticoagulation is needed in pregnancy, in prophylaxis of DVT and PE and as initial treatment for DVT or PE if warfarin or some of the DOACs are to be used subsequently.
- Warfarin is mainly used for high-risk patients, e.g. those with mechanical heart valves or antiphospholipid syndrome.
- The warfarin dose is usually aimed to raise the international normalized ratio (INR) to between 2.0 and 3.0. There are frequent drug and food interactions that affect the dose.
- Thrombi, if acute, may be dissolved by fibrinolytic agents (e.g. streptokinase) or recombinant tissue plasminogen activator.
- Antiplatelet drugs – aspirin, clopidogrel, prasugrel, ticragelor, cangrelor and dipyrimadole – are used to treat arterial disorders.

Now visit **www.wileyessential.com/haematology** to test yourself on this chapter.

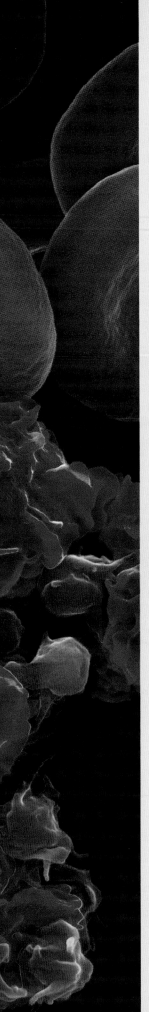

CHAPTER 29
Haematological changes in systemic diseases

Key topics

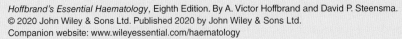

Hoffbrand's Essential Haematology, Eighth Edition. By A. Victor Hoffbrand and David P. Steensma.
© 2020 John Wiley & Sons Ltd. Published 2020 by John Wiley & Sons Ltd.
Companion website: www.wileyessential.com/haematology

Anaemia of chronic disorders

Many of the anaemias seen in clinical practice occur in patients with systemic disorders and are the result of a number of contributing factors. The anaemia of chronic disorders (ACD; also discussed on p. 38) can occur in patients with a variety of chronic inflammatory and malignant diseases (Table 29.1). **Usually, both the erythrocyte sedimentation rate (ESR) and C-reactive protein (CRP) are raised**, since inflammation contributes to suppression of erythropoiesis. ACD may be complicated by additional haematological changes due to the disease. The serum iron and total iron binding capacity (transferrin) are typically both low, while serum ferritin is normal or raised. The characteristic features and pathogenesis are described in Chapter 3.

ACD is corrected by the successful treatment of the underlying disease. It does not respond to iron therapy despite the low serum iron, since iron is typically present in the body in normal or elevated levels, but due to inflammation the developing erythroid cells cannot access it. Responses to recombinant erythropoietin therapy may be obtained, but ACD alone is not an approved indication. In many conditions ACD is complicated by concomitant anaemia from other causes (e.g. iron or folate deficiency, renal failure with decreased erythropoietin secretion, bone marrow infiltration by neoplastic cells, or hypersplenism).

Haematological problems in the elderly

Anaemia

The World Health Organization defines anaemia as a haemoglobin less than 130 g/L in adult men and less than 120 g/L in non-pregnant women. Using these criteria, the incidence of anaemia is substantial in the elderly, e.g. more than 25% in men and more than 20% in women over 85 years old. The incidence is higher in people of sub-Saharan African ancestry, increases with age and predicts for shorter survival. In the USA about 10% of subjects over 65 years old are anaemic and this is associated with increased hospitalization, disability and mortality.

Table 29.1 Causes of anaemia of chronic disorders.

Chronic inflammatory diseases

Infectious (e.g. pulmonary abscess, tuberculosis, osteomyelitis, pneumonia, bacterial endocarditis)

Non-infectious (e.g. rheumatoid arthritis, systemic lupus erythematosus and other connective tissue diseases, sarcoid, Crohn disease or ulcerative colitis)

Malignant disease

(e.g. carcinoma, lymphoma, sarcoma)

The three main causes of anaemia in the elderly are ACD, iron or B$_{12}$ deficiency and renal disease, but about a third of cases are unexplained after initial evaluation. Possibly some of the patients with unexplained anaemia have myelodysplastic syndromes. Clones with molecular mutations characteristic of myeloid neoplasms are increasingly present with advancing age in the bone marrow, without morphological changes, and their contribution to anaemia is often unclear (see Chapter 16).

The elderly also have reduced marrow reserve and develop more severe and prolonged anaemia (and neutropenia and thrombocytopenia) after chemotherapy than younger subjects.

Thrombosis

There is a greater incidence of arterial and venous thrombosis with advancing age. This is partly due to increase in plasma levels of some of the clotting factors as well as reduced fibrinolysis. Relative immobility due to degenerative arthritis and frailty may also contribute. For arterial thrombosis, atheromatous plaques are a major contributor. Elderly subjects tend to be more sensitive than younger patients to anticoagulants and need careful monitoring to avoid haemorrhage.

Malignant disease (other than primary bone marrow disease)

Anaemia

Contributing factors to anaemia in cancer include ACD, blood loss and iron deficiency (especially in uterine, gastric or colorectal tumours), marrow infiltration (Fig. 29.1), haemolysis and marrow suppression from radiotherapy or chemotherapy (Table 29.2). Marrow infiltration may be associated with a leuco-erythroblastic blood film (p. 103).

Microangiopathic haemolytic anaemia (p. 75) occurs with mucin-secreting adenocarcinoma (Fig. 29.2), particularly of the stomach, lung and breast. Less common forms of anaemia with malignant disease include autoimmune haemolytic anaemia with malignant lymphoma and rarely with other tumours; pure red cell aplasia with thymoma or lymphomas; and myelodysplastic syndromes secondary to chemotherapy. There is also an association of pernicious anaemia with carcinoma of the stomach.

The anaemia of malignant disease may respond partly to erythropoiesis-stimulating agents, but care must be taken not to accelerate tumour growth (see Chapter 2). Folic acid should only be given if there is definite megaloblastic anaemia caused by folate deficiency.

Polycythaemia

Secondary polycythaemia is occasionally associated with renal, hepatic, cerebellar and uterine tumours, which can secrete erythropoietin (see p. 14).

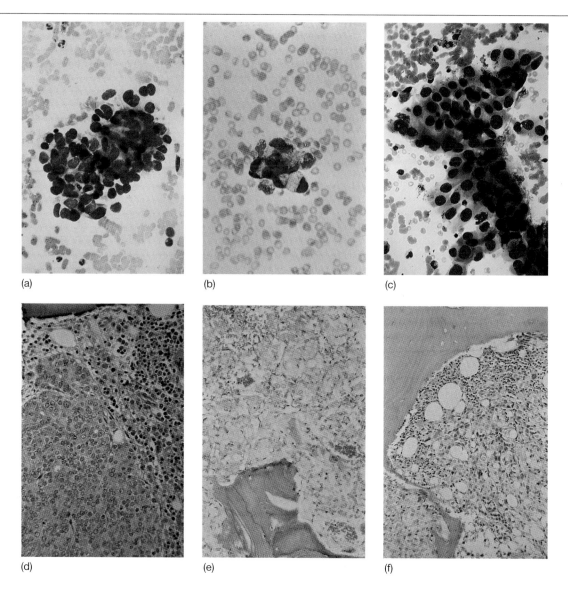

Figure 29.1 Metastatic carcinoma in bone marrow aspirates: **(a)** breast; **(b)** stomach; **(c)** colon; bone marrow trephine biopsies: **(d)** prostate; **(e)** stomach; **(f)** kidney.

White cell changes

Leukaemoid reactions (p. 103) may occur, with tumours showing widespread necrosis and inflammation. Use of granulocyte-colony stimulating factor (G-CSF) to prevent chemotherapy-induced neutropenia can also cause a leukaemoid reaction. Hodgkin lymphoma is associated with a variety of secondary white cell abnormalities, including eosinophilia, monocytosis and leucopenia. In non-Hodgkin lymphoma, malignant cells may circulate in the blood (see p. 241).

Platelet and blood coagulation abnormalities

Patients with malignant disease may show either thrombocytosis or thrombocytopenia. Disseminated tumours, particularly mucin-secreting adenocarcinomas, are associated with disseminated intravascular coagulation (DIC; see p. 333) and generalized haemostatic failure due to thrombocytopenia and consumption of coagulation factors. Activation of fibrinolysis occurs in some patients with carcinoma of the prostate or urinary bladder. Occasional patients with malignant disease have spontaneous bruising or bleeding caused by an acquired inhibitor of one or other coagulation factor, most frequently factor VIII.

Cancer patients have a high incidence (estimated at 15%) of venous thromboembolism. This risk is increased by surgery and by some drugs, e.g. thalidomide. Thrombosis is most common in ovarian, brain, pancreatic and colon cancers. Thrombosis may be difficult to manage with vitamin K antagonists because of bleeding, interruptions with chemotherapy

Table 29.2 Haematological abnormalities in malignant disease.

Haematological abnormality	Tumour or treatment associated
Pancytopenia	
Marrow hypoplasia	Chemotherapy, radiotherapy
Myelodysplasia	Chemotherapy, radiotherapy
Leucoerythroblastic	Metastases in marrow
Megaloblastic	Folate deficiency
	B_{12} deficiency (carcinoma of stomach)
Red cells	
Anaemia of chronic disorders	Most forms
Iron deficiency anaemia	Especially gastrointestinal, uterine
Pure red cell aplasia	Thymoma
Immune haemolytic anaemia	Lymphoma, ovary, other tumours
Microangiopathic haemolytic anaemia	Mucin-secreting carcinoma
Polycythaemia	Kidney, liver, cerebellum, uterus
White cells	
Neutrophil leucocytosis	Most forms
Leukaemoid reaction	Disseminated tumours, those with necrosis
Eosinophilia	Hodgkin lymphoma, others
Monocytosis	Various tumours
Platelets and coagulation	
Thrombocytosis	Gastrointestinal tumours with bleeding, others
Disseminated intravascular coagulation	Mucin-secreting carcinoma, prostate
Activation of fibrinolysis	Prostate
Acquired inhibitors of coagulation	Most forms
Paraprotein interfering with platelet function	Lymphomas, myeloma
Tumour cell procoagulants – tissue factor and cancer procoagulant (density activates factor X)	Especially ovarian, pancreas, brain, colon

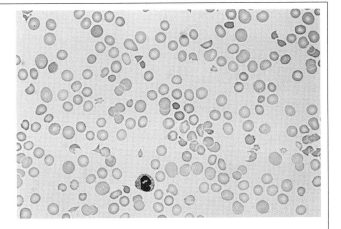

Figure 29.2 Peripheral blood film in metastatic mucin-secreting adenocarcinoma of the stomach showing red cell polychromasia and fragmentation and thrombocytopenia. The patient had disseminated intravascular coagulation.

and thrombocytopenia, anorexia or vomiting. Liver disease and drug interactions can cause further complications, so daily low molecular weight heparin injections is preferable and increasingly direct-acting oral anticoagulants are used.

Rheumatoid arthritis (and other connective tissue disorders)

In patients with rheumatoid arthritis, ACD is proportional to the activity and severity of the disease. Connective tissue disorders are complicated in some patients by iron deficiency caused by gastrointestinal bleeding related to therapy with salicylates, non-steroidal anti-inflammatory agents or corticosteroids. Bleeding into inflamed joints may also contribute to anaemia in rare cases. Marrow hypoplasia may follow therapy with gold salts.

In **Felty syndrome**, splenomegaly is associated with neutropenia and increased large granular lymphocyte numbers (Fig. 29.3). Anaemia and thrombocytopenia may also be present.

In systemic lupus erythematosus (SLE), 50% of patients are leucopenic with reduced neutrophil and lymphocyte counts, often associated with circulating immune complexes. Renal impairment and drug-induced gastrointestinal blood loss also contribute to the ACD. Autoimmune haemolytic anaemia – typically with immunoglobulin (Ig) G and complement (C3d) on the surface of the red cells – occurs in 5% of patients and may be the presenting feature of the syndrome. There may be autoimmune thrombocytopenia in 5% of patients.

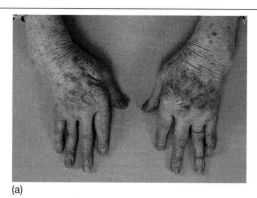

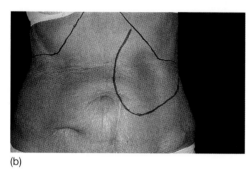

Figure 29.3 Felty syndrome: **(a)** the typical deformities of rheumatoid arthritis of the hand and **(b)** splenomegaly.

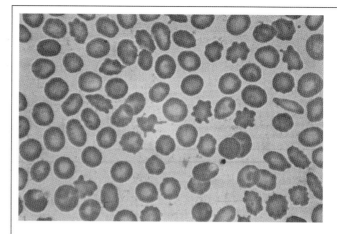

Figure 29.4 Peripheral blood film in chronic renal failure showing numerous 'burr' cells (echinocytes). With haemodialysis these typically are reduced in number, indicating their cause by a toxin normally cleared by the kidneys.

The lupus anticoagulant is described on page 343. This circulating anti-cardiolipin interferes with blood coagulation by altering the binding of coagulation factors to platelet phospholipid, and predisposes to both arterial and venous thrombosis and recurrent abortions. Tests for antinuclear antibodies (ANA) and anti-DNA antibodies are usually positive in SLE.

Patients with temporal arteritis and polymyalgia rheumatica have a markedly elevated ESR, pronounced red cell rouleaux in the blood film and a polyclonal immunoglobulin response. These and other vasculitides can also be associated with ACD.

Renal failure

Anaemia

A normochromic anaemia is present in most patients with chronic renal failure. Generally, there is a 20 g/L fall in haemoglobin level for every 10 mmol/L rise in blood urea, though there is wide variation. The dominant pathological mechanism is impaired red cell production as a result of defective erythropoietin secretion (see Fig. 2.6). Variable shortening of red cell lifespan also occurs and, in severe uraemia, the red cells show abnormalities including 'burr' cells (Fig. 29.4). Increased red cell 2,3-diphosphoglycerate (DPG) levels in response to the anaemia and hyperphosphataemia result in decreased oxygen affinity and a shift of the haemoglobin–oxygen dissociation curve to the right (see p. 17), which is augmented by uraemic acidosis. The patient's symptoms are therefore relatively mild for the degree of anaemia.

Other factors may complicate the anaemia of chronic renal failure (Table 29.3): ACD, iron deficiency from blood loss during dialysis or caused by bleeding because of defective platelet function, and folate deficiency in some chronic dialysis patients. Folic acid is usually given prophylactically.

Patients with polycystic kidneys usually have relatively retained erythropoietin production and have less severe anaemia for the degree of renal failure.

Table 29.3 Haematological abnormalities in renal failure.

Anaemia
Reduced erythropoietin production
Anaemia of chronic disorders
Iron deficiency
Blood loss (e.g. dialysis, venesection, defective platelet function)
Folate deficiency
Chronic haemodialysis without replacement therapy

Abnormal platelet function

Thrombocytopenia: immune complex-mediated (e.g. systemic lupus erythematosus, polyarteritis nodosa), acute nephritis, following allograft, haemolytic uraemic syndrome and thrombotic thrombocytopenic purpura

Thrombosis
Nephrotic syndrome

Polycythaemia
In renal allograft recipients
Rarely in renal cell carcinoma, cysts, arterial disease

Treatment

Recombinant erythropoietin corrects the anaemia in patients on dialysis or in chronic renal failure, providing that iron and folate deficiency have been corrected. The dosage of epoetin usually required is 50–150 units/kg three times a week, with a target haemoglobin of 120 g/L. Longer-acting preparations such as darbepoetin are increasingly used. Complications of therapy have included initial transient flu-like symptoms, hypertension and clotting of the dialysis lines.

A poor response to recombinant erythropoietin suggests iron or folate deficiency, infection or hyperparathyroidism. Intravenous iron is often needed to correct iron deficiency shown by low serum ferritin and percentage saturation of total iron-binding capacity (TIBC), and increased percentage of hypochromic red cells in the blood.

Platelet and coagulation abnormalities

A bleeding tendency with purpura, gastrointestinal or uterine bleeding occurs in 30–50% of patients with chronic renal failure and is marked in patients with acute renal failure. The bleeding may be out of proportion to the degree of thrombocytopenia and has been associated with abnormal platelet or vascular function, which can be reversed by dialysis. Correction of the anaemia with recombinant erythropoietin also improves the bleeding tendency.

Immune complex-mediated thrombocytopenia occurs in some patients with acute nephritis, SLE and polyarteritis nodosa and also following renal allografts. Renal allografts may also lead to polycythaemia in 10–15% of patients.

The haemolytic uraemic syndrome and thrombotic thrombocytopenic purpura are discussed on page 316. Patients with the nephrotic syndrome have an increased risk of venous thrombosis due to loss of anticoagulant proteins in the urine.

Congestive heart failure

Anaemia is present in 30–50% of patients with congestive heart failure due to chronic kidney disease, haemodilution and release of cytokines increasing hepcidin synthesis (reducing iron absorption and recycling of iron from macrophages) and reducing erythropoietin secretion. Treatment with oral or intravenous iron may improve left ventricular ejection fraction, lower CRP and brain natriuretic peptide (BNP) levels, reduce fatigue, and increase exercise capacity and quality of life, even in those without iron deficiency.

Liver disease

The haematological abnormalities in liver disease are listed in Table 29.4. Chronic liver disease can be associated with anaemia that is mildly macrocytic and often accompanied by target cells, mainly as a result of increased cholesterol in the membrane (Fig. 29.5a). Contributing factors to the anaemia may include blood loss (e.g. bleeding varices) with iron deficiency, dietary folate deficiency and direct suppression of haemopoiesis by alcohol.

Table 29.4 Haematological abnormalities in liver disease.

Liver failure ± obstructive jaundice ± portal hypertension

Refractory anaemia – usually mildly macrocytic, often with target cells; may be associated with:
Blood loss and iron deficiency
Alcohol (± ring sideroblastic change)
Folate deficiency
Haemolysis (e.g. Zieve syndrome, Wilson disease, immune, hypersplenism from portal hypertension)

Bleeding tendency
Deficiency of vitamin K-dependent factors; also of factor V and fibrinogen
Thrombocytopenia, immune platelet function defects
Functional abnormalities of fibrinogen
Increased fibrinolysis
Portal hypertension – haemorrhage from varices

Viral hepatitis
Aplastic anaemia

Hepatic tumours
Polycythaemia due to erythropoietin secretion by the cancer cells
Neutrophil leucocytosis and leukaemoid reactions

Haemolytic anaemia may occur in patients with alcohol intoxication (Zieve syndrome; Fig. 29.5b) and in Wilson disease (caused by copper oxidation of red cell membranes). Autoimmune haemolytic anaemia is found in some patients with chronic immune hepatitis. Haemolysis may also occur in end-stage liver disease because of abnormal red cell membranes resulting from lipid changes; 'spur' cells (acanthocytes) are common in advanced cirrhosis and are associated with a

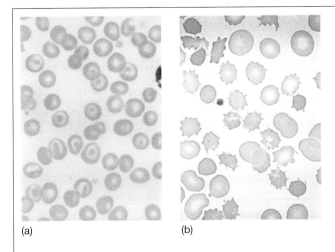

(a) (b)

Figure 29.5 Liver disease: peripheral blood film showing: **(a)** macrocytosis and target cells; and **(b)** marked acanthocytosis and echinocytosis in Zieve syndrome.

poor prognosis. Viral hepatitis can be associated with aplastic anaemia (see Chapter 22).

The acquired coagulation abnormalities associated with liver disease are described on page 333. There are deficiencies of vitamin K-dependent factors (II, VII, IX and X) and, in severe disease, of factor V and fibrinogen. Thrombocytopenia may occur from hypersplenism resulting from portal hypertension, or from immune complex-mediated platelet destruction. Abnormalities of platelet function may also be present. Dysfibrinogenaemia with abnormal fibrin polymerization may occur as a result of excess sialic acid in the fibrinogen molecules. A consumptive coagulopathy may be superimposed. These haemostatic defects may contribute to major blood loss from bleeding varices caused by portal hypertension.

Hypothyroidism

In mild hypothyroidism there are typically no haematological changes. In more severe hypothyroidism, a moderate anaemia is common, as triodothyronine (T3) and thyroxine (T4)

potentiate the action of erythropoietin. There is also a reduced oxygen need from the hypometabolic state and thus reduced erythropoietin secretion. The anaemia is often macrocytic and the mean corpuscular volume (MCV) falls with thyroxine replacement therapy.

Autoimmune thyroid disease, especially Hashimoto disease, is associated with pernicious anaemia. Iron deficiency may also be present, particularly in women with menorrhagia.

Infections

Haematological abnormalities are usually present in patients with infections of all types (Table 29.5). The effect of inflammation as a prothrombotic stimulus is also discussed on page 343.

Bacterial infections

Acute bacterial infections are the most common cause of neutrophil leucocytosis. Toxic granulation, Döhle bodies and

Table 29.5 Blood abnormalities associated with infections.

Haematological abnormality	Infection associated
Anaemia	
ACD	Chronic infections, especially tuberculosis
Aplastic anaemia	Viral hepatitis
Transient red cell aplasia	Human parvovirus
Marrow fibrosis	Tuberculosis
Immune haemolytic anaemia	Infectious mononucleosis, *Mycoplasma pneumoniae*
Direct red cell damage or microangiopathic	Bacterial septicaemia (associated DIC), *Clostridium perfringens*, malaria, bartonellosis
Hypersplenism	Viruses – haemolytic uraemic syndrome and TTP
	Chronic malaria, tropical splenomegaly syndrome, leishmaniasis, schistosomiasis
White cell changes	
Neutrophil leucocytosis	Acute bacterial infections
Leukaemoid reactions	Severe bacterial infections particularly in infants
Monocytosis	Tuberculosis
Eosinophilia	Parasitic diseases (e.g. hookworm, filariasis, strongyloidiasis, schistosomiasis, trichinosis)
Neutropenia	Recovery from acute infections
Lymphopenia	Chronic bacterial infections: tuberculosis, brucellosis, bacterial endocarditis, typhoid
Lymphocytosis	Viral infections – HIV, hepatitis, influenza
	Fulminant bacterial infections (e.g. typhoid, miliary tuberculosis)
	Infectious mononucleosis, toxoplasmosis, cytomegalovirus, rubella, viral hepatitis, pertussis, tuberculosis, brucellosis
	HIV infection
Thrombocytopenia	*Legionella pneumonophilia*
Megakaryocytic depression, immune complex mediated and direct interaction with platelets	Acute viral infections particularly in children (e.g. measles, varicella, rubella, malaria, severe bacterial infection)
Prothrombotic state	All with prolonged inflammation

ACD, anaemia of chronic disorders; DIC, disseminated intravascular coagulation; HIV, human immunodeficiency virus; TTP, thrombotic thrombocytopenic purpura.

metamyelocytes may be present in the blood (see Chapter 8). Leukaemoid reactions with a white cell count above 50×10^9/L and early granulocyte precursors in the blood may occur in severe infections, particularly in infants and young children. Mild anaemia is common if the infection is prolonged, such as in untreated tuberculosis. Severe haemolytic anaemia occurs in bacterial septicaemias, particularly those caused by Gram-negative organisms, where there is usually associated DIC (see p. 76).

DIC dominates the clinical picture in certain infections (e.g. bacterial meningitis). The acute phase response to infections is accompanied by a rise in coagulation factors and a fall in natural anticoagulants.

Clostridium perfringens organisms produce an α toxin, a lecithinase acting directly on the circulating red cells (Fig. 29.6). Haemolysis in bartonellosis (Oroya fever) is caused by direct red cell infection. *Mycoplasma pneumoniae* infections are associated with autoimmune haemolytic anaemia of the 'cold' type (see p. 74). With severe acute bacterial infections there may be thrombocytopenia. Chronic bacterial infections are associated with the ACD.

In tuberculosis, additional factors in the pathogenesis of anaemia include marrow replacement and fibrosis associated with miliary disease and reactions to antituberculous therapy (e.g. isoniazid is a pyridoxine antagonist and may cause sideroblastic anaemia). Disseminated tuberculosis is associated with leukaemoid reactions and patients with involvement of bone marrow may show leucoerythroblastic changes in the peripheral blood film (see Fig. 8.9).

Viral infections

Acute viral diseases are often associated with a mild anaemia. An immune haemolytic anaemia with an anti-i autoantibody is associated with infectious mononucleosis (see p. 75). Viral infections, as well as syphilis, have been associated with paroxysmal cold haemoglobinuria (see p. 75). Viruses have also been linked to the pathogenesis of the haemolytic uraemic syndrome, thrombotic thrombocytopenic purpura (see Chapter 24) and the haemophagocytic syndrome (see p. 107). Aplastic anaemia may occur with viral A hepatitis or more usually non-A, non-B, non-C hepatitis, due to an unknown virus. Transient red cell aplasia is associated with human parvovirus infection and this may result in severe anaemia in subjects with a haemolytic anaemia (see Chapter 6).

Acute thrombocytopenia is frequent in rubella and varicella infections, and in Dengue fever. Rubella, cytomegalovirus (CMV) and other viral infections may cause a reactive lymphocytosis similar to that found in infectious mononucleosis. CMV infections in infants are associated with massive hepatosplenomegaly. In haemopoietic stem cell transplant recipients or other immunosuppressed patients, CMV infections may cause pancytopenia as well as other severe disorders (see Chapter 23).

Human immunodeficiency virus (HIV) infection

HIV is associated with a wide range of haematological changes, which tend to be worse in more advanced disease. These are caused by marrow defects and immune cytopenias directly resulting from HIV infection, the effects of opportunistic infections or lymphoma, and the side-effects of drugs used to treat HIV itself or drugs for the complicating infection or lymphoma.

Anaemia is common and more severe as the disease progresses. It is usually multifactorial in origin: ACD, marrow dysplasia and drug therapy, especially zidovudine. Serum vitamin B_{12} is often low, most likely because of intestinal malabsorption, but the anaemia does not respond to vitamin B_{12} therapy. Blood transfusions or recombinant erythropoietin injections are needed.

Thrombocytopenia and neutropenia may be immune or secondary to marrow dysfunction. The marrow may be hypercellular with prominent plasma cells and lymphocytes, normocellular, hypocellular or fibrotic. Dysplastic features are common, with ineffective thrombopoiesis or granulocyte formation accounting at least in part for the cytopenia. The dysplastic marrow cells do not show the chromosome abnormalities found in myelodysplastic syndromes, however, and do not appear to be pre-leukaemic. Thrombocytopenia is treated if necessary by corticosteroids, high-dose gammaglobulin infusions or by other therapies for immune thrombocytopenia (see p. 317), or by anti-retroviral therapy.

Increased plasma cells in the marrow and polyclonal increase in immunoglobulins are frequent. A paraprotein is present in 5–10% of cases, but appears benign and usually resolves with highly active anti-retroviral therapy.

Non-Hodgkin lymphoma, in over 90% high grade, both systemically and in the central nervous system, occurs in HIV-infected individuals with over 100 times the frequency expected in the general population. Diffuse large B-cell lymphoma is the most common, with 20% confined to the central nervous system. A substantial minority are Burkitt lymphoma,

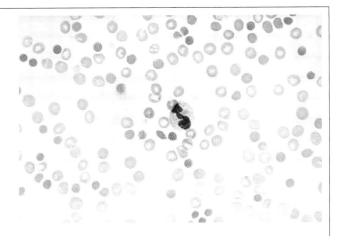

Figure 29.6 Peripheral blood film in a patient with haemolytic anaemia in clostridial septicaemia showing red cell contraction and spherocytosis.

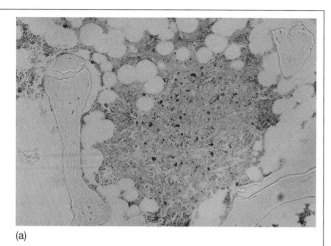

(a)

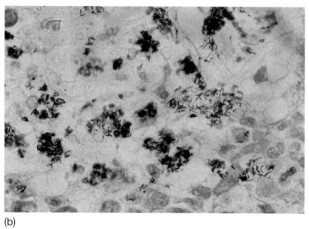

(b)

Figure 29.7 Human immunodeficiency virus (HIV) infection: bone marrow trephine biopsy. **(a)** Granuloma showing positivity with Ziehl-Nielsen stain. **(b)** Higher power shows large numbers of acid-fast bacilli.

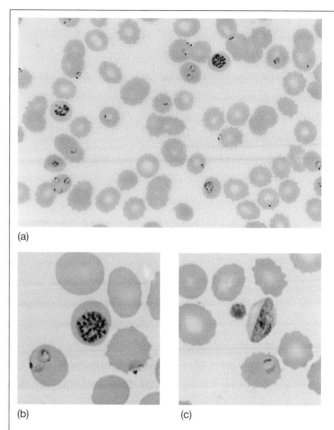

(a)

(b)   (c)

Figure 29.8 Malaria: peripheral blood in severe *Plasmodium falciparum* infection showing **(a)** many ring forms and a meront; and at higher magnification: **(b)** a meront; and **(c)** a gametocyte.

and HIV should always be sought in new cases of Burkitt and Burkitt-like lymphoma. Hodgkin lymphoma, usually of poor prognosis type, is also increased in frequency. EBV infection appears to underlie this as well as Burkitt lymphoma and multicentric Castleman's disease with HHV8 infection (see p. 254).

Treatment of lymphomas in the setting of HIV is with combination chemotherapy and immunotherapy (e.g. rituximab). Continuation of the necessary antiretroviral therapy exaggerates the tendency to cytopenia induced by chemotherapy, so prophylaxis against opportunistic infections is important. The bone marrow may indeed reveal the presence of opportunistic infection (Fig. 29.7).

Other infections

Malaria

Some degree of haemolysis is seen in all types of malarial infection (see Chapter 6). The most severe abnormalities are found in *Plasmodium falciparum* infections (Fig. 29.8). In the worst cases, DIC occurs and intravascular haemolysis is marked with haemoglobinuria. This may be associated with quinine therapy ('blackwater fever'). Thrombocytopenia is commonly found in acute malaria. Patients with chronic malaria have an anaemia of chronic disorders; hypersplenism may contribute to the anaemia and result in moderate thrombocytopenia and neutropenia. Tropical splenomegaly is probably a chronic immune reaction to malaria (see Chapter 10). Dyserythropoiesis in the marrow, folate deficiency and protein-calorie malnutrition may contribute to anaemia.

Toxoplasmosis

Toxoplasmosis in children and adults is associated with lymphadenopathy and large numbers of atypical lymphocytes in the blood. Congenital disease may cause a syndrome resembling hydrops fetalis with severe anaemia, a hydropic infant with gross hepatosplenomegaly and thrombocytopenia.

Kala-azar (visceral leishmaniasis)

The visceral form of leishmaniasis is associated with pancytopenia, hepatosplenomegaly and lymphadenopathy. Bone marrow

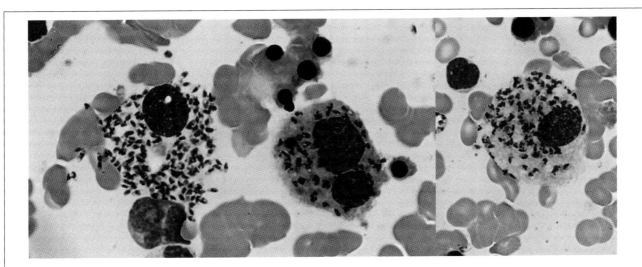

Figure 29.9 Kala-azar: bone marrow aspirates showing macrophages containing Leishman–Donovan bodies.

or splenic aspirates may show large numbers of parasitized macrophages (Fig. 29.9).

Other parasitic diseases

Chronic schistosomiasis (bilharzia) affects over 200 million people worldwide. It is one of the most frequent causes of iron deficiency due to bleeding from the bowel or bladder. Hypersplenism follows splenic enlargement associated with portal hypertension due to liver infestation. In the acute phase of both African and South American trypanosomiasis, organisms are found in the peripheral blood (Fig. 29.10). Microfilariae of bancroftian filariasis and loiasis are also detected during blood film examination (Fig. 29.11). In many parasitic diseases there is eosinophilia.

Non-specific monitoring of systemic disease

The inflammatory response to tissue injury includes changes in plasma concentrations of proteins known as acute phase proteins. These include fibrinogen, other clotting factors, complement components, CRP (p. 371), haptoglobin, serum amyloid A (SAA) protein, ferritin and others. The rise in these liver-derived proteins is part of a wider response, which includes fever, leucocytosis and increased immune reactivity. The acute phase response is mediated by cytokines (e.g. IL-1and TNF) released from macrophages and other cells (see Fig. 8.4). Quantitative measurements of acute phase proteins are valuable indicators of the presence and extent of inflammation and of its response to treatment. **When short-term (less than 24 hours) changes in the inflammatory response are expected, CRP is the test of choice (Table 29.6). Long-term changes in the acute-phase proteins are monitored by either the ESR or plasma**

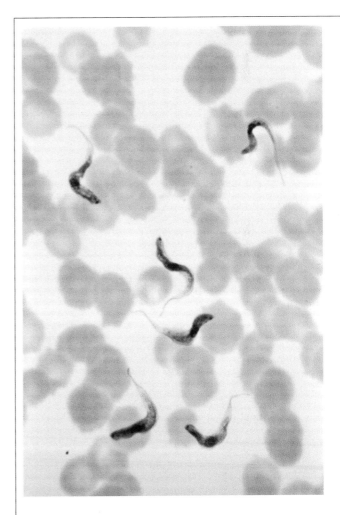

Figure 29.10 African trypanosomiasis: blood film showing *Trypanosoma brucei*.

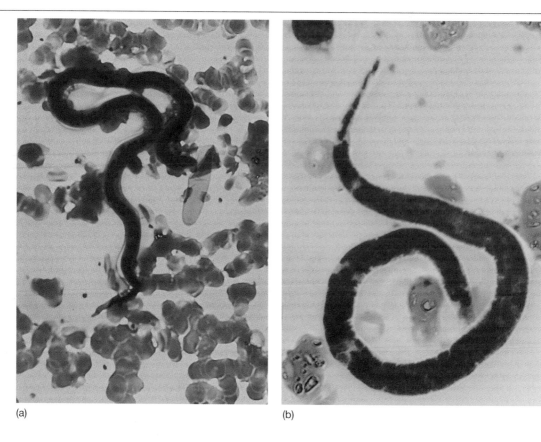

(a)   (b)

Figure 29.11 Peripheral blood films showing microfilariae of **(a)** *Wuchereria bancrofti*; and **(b)** *Loa loa*.

viscosity. These tests are influenced by plasma proteins, which are either slowly responding acute-phase reactants (e.g. fibrinogen) or are not acute-phase proteins (e.g. immunoglobulins).

Erythrocyte sedimentation rate

This commonly used but non-specific test measures the speed of sedimentation of red cells in plasma over a period of 1 hour. The speed is mainly dependent on the plasma concentration of large proteins (e.g. fibrinogen and immunoglobulins). The normal range in men is 1–5 mm/hour and in women 5–15 mm/hour, but there is a progressive increase with age. The ESR is raised in a wide variety of systemic inflammatory and neoplastic diseases and in pregnancy. It is useful for diagnosing and monitoring temporal arteritis and polymyalgia

Table 29.6 Advantages and disadvantages of the tests used to monitor the acute-phase response.

Advantages	Disadvantages
*CRP** Specific test of acute phase protein Fast response (6 hours) to change in disease activity High sensitivity – owing to large incremental change Can be measured on stored serum Small sample volumes Automated analysis	CRP is sensitive to interleukin-6 but less to other pro-inflammatory molecules Costly when assayed in small numbers Sophisticated equipment and antisera required
ESR and plasma viscosity Useful in chronic disease ESR inexpensive, easy, no electrical power required Plasma viscosity—result obtained quickly (15 min) Plasma viscosity not affected by anaemia	Not sensitive to acute changes (<24 hours) Not specific for acute phase response Slow to change with alteration in disease activity and insensitive to small changes in activity Fresh samples (<2 hours) required for ESR

* C-reactive protein (CRP) is normally present in plasma at low concentrations (<5 mg/L). Levels are not influenced by anaemia, pregnancy or heart failure. During severe acute infection the plasma concentration may rise 100-fold.
ESR, erythrocyte sedimentation rate.

rheumatica and for monitoring patients with Hodgkin lymphoma. High values (>100 mm/hour) have a 90% predictive value for serious disease, including infections, collagen vascular disease or malignancy, particularly myeloma. A raised ESR is associated with marked rouleaux formation of red cells in the peripheral blood film (see Fig. 21.7). Changes in the ESR can be used to monitor the response to therapy.

Lower than expected ESR readings occur in polycythaemia vera because of the high red cell concentration. Higher than expected values may occur in severe anaemia because of the low red cell concentration.

Plasma viscosity

Plasma viscosity is affected by the concentration of plasma proteins of large molecular size, especially those with pronounced axial asymmetry: fibrinogen and some immunoglobulins. Normal values at room temperature are usually in the range of 1.50– 1.70 mPa/s. Lower levels are found in neonates because of lower levels of proteins, particularly fibrinogen. Viscosity increases only slightly in the elderly as fibrinogen increases.

There is no difference in values between men and women. Other advantages over the ESR test include independence from the effects of anaemia and results that are available within 15 minutes.

C-reactive protein

Phylogenetically CRP is a crude 'early' immunoglobulin which initiates the inflammatory reaction. CRP–antigen complexes can substitute for antibody in the fixation of Clq and trigger the complement cascade, initiating the inflammatory response to antigens or tissue damage. Subsequent binding of C3b on the surface of microorganisms opsonizes them for phagocytosis.

After tissue injury, an increase in CRP, SAA protein and other acute phase reactants, synthesized in the liver, may be detected within 6–10 hours. Immunoassays of CRP are widely used for early detection of acute inflammation or tissue injury and for the monitoring of remission (e.g. response of infection to an antibiotic).

Table 29.6 lists the advantages and disadvantages of some of the tests used to assess the acute-phase response.

SUMMARY

- Chronic inflammation or malignant disorders cause anaemia with low serum iron and iron-binding capacity, normal or raised serum ferritin, an inadequate response to erythropoietin and reduced red cell lifespan. The degree of anaemia relates to the severity of the underlying disease. It does not respond to iron therapy.
- This anaemia may be complicated in systemic diseases by other causes of anaemia, e.g. iron or folate deficiencies, renal failure, bone marrow infiltration, haemolysis, hypersplenism.
- Polycythaemia is a much less frequent complication of systemic diseases, e.g. renal.
- White cell changes are also frequent in systemic diseases. These include neutrophil leucocytosis, especially in bacterial infections, leuco-erythroblastic or leukaemoid reactions, and, in viral and connective tissue diseases, neutropenia.
- Eosinophilia occurs with certain infections, particularly parasitic and allergic disease.
- Monocytosis is associated with chronic bacterial infections (e.g. tuberculosis, brucellosis).
- Lymphocytosis is a feature of viral infections and some bacterial infections, e.g. *Bordetella pertussis*.
- Platelets may be increased or low in malignant, infectious and other systemic diseases. Disseminated intravascular coagulation is a major cause of thrombocytopenia and a fall in coagulation factors in systemic diseases.
- C-reactive protein can be used for non-specific monitoring of systemic disease in the short term (hours or days) and erythrocyte sedimentation rate (or plasma viscosity) over weeks or months.

Now visit **www.wileyessential.com/haematology** to test yourself on this chapter.

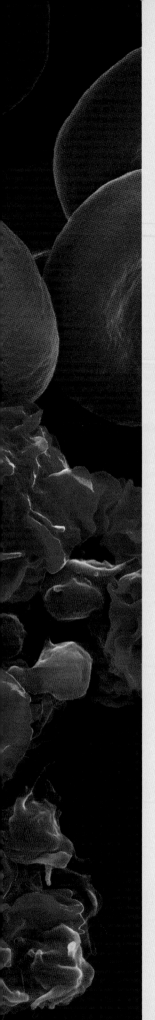

CHAPTER 30
Blood transfusion

Key topics

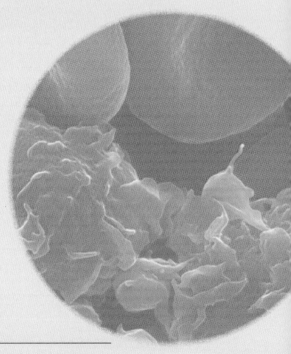

Hoffbrand's Essential Haematology, Eighth Edition. By A. Victor Hoffbrand and David P. Steensma.
© 2020 John Wiley & Sons Ltd. Published 2020 by John Wiley & Sons Ltd.
Companion website: www.wileyessential.com/haematology

Blood transfusion consists of the 'safe' transfer of blood components (Fig. 30.1) from a donor to a recipient. Blood product collection, processing and transfusion are tightly regulated. In the UK, for example, all blood banks are inspected by the Medicines and Healthcare Regulatory Agency (MHRA), while in the USA blood banks are under the jurisdiction of the Food and Drug Administration (FDA). MHRA and FDA inspect all blood facilities at least once every two years (more frequently if problems are detected) and quality standards are similar to those imposed on pharmaceutical manufacturers. All adverse events involving UK blood products must be reported to the online Serious Adverse Blood Reactions and Events (SABRE) scheme, and similar reporting mechanisms exist in other countries.

In the USA, more than 5 million individual patients receive blood products annually, with at least 15 million blood products dispensed. In England and north Wales, more than 500 000 patients receive a cumulative ~2 million blood products annually.

Blood donor selection

In most countries blood donors contribute on a voluntary basis and this is generally preferable in terms of product safety. The measures to protect donors and for donor selection are listed in Table 30.1. Prospective blood donors are asked a series of specific, direct questions about risk factors for infection with blood-transmissible diseases, and this screening is estimated to eliminate more than 90% of unsuitable donors.

Red cell antigens and blood group antibodies

The clinical significance of blood groups in blood transfusion is that individuals who lack a particular blood group antigen may have preformed antibodies or may produce antibodies reacting with that antigen, which may lead to a transfusion reaction. Approximately 400 red blood cell group antigens have been described. The different blood group antigens vary greatly in their clinical significance, with the ABO and Rh (formerly Rhesus) groups being the most important. Some other systems are listed in Table 30.2.

Blood group antibodies

The ABO blood group antigens are unusual in that naturally occurring antibodies – usually immunoglobulin M (IgM) and rarely IgG – occur in the plasma of subjects who lack the corresponding antigen, even if they have not been transfused or been pregnant (Tables 30.3 and 30.4). The origin of these antibodies is thought to be immunological recognition of bacterial cell wall glycoproteins in the gut that are similar to AB antigens and, consistent with this hypothesis, antibodies typically arise in the first few months of life as the bowel is colonised by normal bacterial flora. The most important of these natural antibodies are anti-A and anti-B. They are usually IgM, and react optimally at cold temperatures (4°C) so, although reactive at 37°C, they are called cold antibodies.

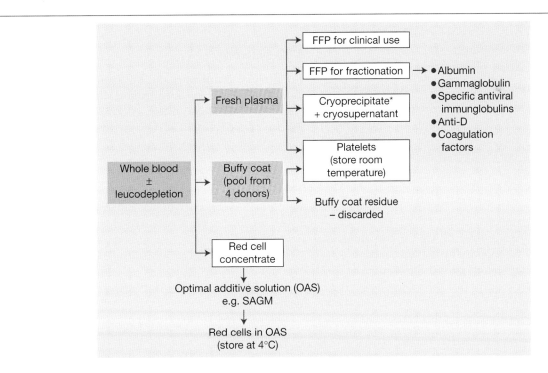

Figure 30.1 The preparation of blood components from whole blood. FFP, fresh frozen plasma; SAGM, saline-adenine-glucose-mannitol. *Cryoprecipitate is mainly a source of fibrinogen. Cryosupernatant is used for plasma exchange in thrombotic thrombocytopenic purpura. Leucodepletion – see text.

Table 30.1 Measures used to protect the donor and for donor selection.

Donor selection

Age 17–70 years (maximum 65 at first donation)

Weight above 50 kg (7 st 12 lb)

Haemoglobin >134 g/L for men, >120 g/L for women

Minimum donation interval of 12 weeks (16 weeks advised) and three donations per year maximum

Apheresis for platelets or plasma up to 24 times in 12 months

Pregnant and lactating women excluded because of high iron requirements; donation deferred for 9 months post pregnancy

Exclusion of those with:
Known cardiovascular disease, including hypertension
Significant respiratory disorders
Epilepsy and other CNS disorders
Gastrointestinal disorders with impaired absorption
Previous blood transfusions
Intravenous drug use
Insulin-dependent diabetes
Chronic renal disease
Cancer
Ongoing medical investigation or clinical trials

Exclusion of any donor returning within a short period to occupations such as driving a bus, plane or train, heavy machine or crane operator, mining, scaffolding, etc. because delayed faint would be dangerous

Defer for 12 months after body piercing or tattoo, paid sex or homosexual sex, after acupuncture

Defer for 2 months after live vaccinations such as measles, mumps

Defer if travel history suggests risk of infection

CNS, central nervous system.

Table 30.2 Donor testing in England and Wales.

1 Blood group, Rh status (D, C, E, c, e), K

2 Screen for red cell alloantibodies

3 *Microbiological tests*
Human immunodeficiency virus (HIV) 1 and 2; antibody and RNA
Hepatitis B virus (HBV) – antibody and RNA
Hepatitis C virus (HCV) – antibody and RNA
Human T-cell leukaemia viruses (HTLV) – antibody
Cytomegalovirus (CMV) – antibody, for immunosuppressed recipients
Malaria – antibody screening of potentially exposed donors
Chagas' disease – antibody screening of potentially exposed donors
Bacteria – all donations tested for antibody to syphilis (*Treponema pallidum*)

N.B. At the current time there is no reliable test for detecting prions in blood products. In the US, blood products are tested for eight microbial pathogen types: bacterial contamination (blood culture), hepatitis B (core antibody and surface antigen), hepatitis C (antibody and nucleic acid amplification testing), HIV-1 and HIV-2 (antibody testing for both, and nucleic acid testing for HIV-1), HTLV-I and HTLV-II (antibody testing for both), *Treponema pallidum* (anti-treponemal antibody testing) and West Nile Virus (nucleic acid testing); in 2018, universal testing for Zika virus (a nucleic acid test) was added. Although prions are not tested for, anyone who lived in the UK for at least 3 months between 1980 and 1996, or in Europe or Saudi Arabia for 5 years after 1980, is permanently barred from blood donation in the USA, because of a perceived risk of variant Creutzfeldt–Jacob disease.

Immune antibodies against non-ABO system antigens, in contrast, develop in response to the introduction – by transfusion or by transplacental passage during pregnancy – of red cells possessing antigens that the subject lacks. These antibodies are commonly IgG, although some IgM antibodies may also develop, usually in the early phase of an immune response. Immune antibodies react optimally at 37°C (warm antibodies). Only IgG antibodies are capable of transplacental passage from mother to fetus and the most important immune antibody is the Rh antibody, anti-D.

ABO system

The protein that defines the ABO antigens is a glycosyltransferase that is encoded from a single gene for which there are three major alleles, A, B and O. The A and B alleles catalyse the addition of different carbohydrate residues (*N*-acetyl galactosamine for group A and galactose for group B) to a basic antigenic glycoprotein or glycolipid with a terminal sugar l-fucose on the red cell, known as the H substance (Fig. 30.2). The O allele is non-functional and so does not modify the H substance. Although there are six common genotypes, the absence of a specific anti-H prevents the serological recognition of more than four phenotypes (Table 30.4). The A allele actually itself has two variants, A_1 and A_2, but these are of minor clinical significance. A_2 cells react more weakly than A_1 cells with anti-A, and patients who are A_2B can be wrongly grouped as B.

The A, B and H antigens are present on most body cells, including white cells and platelets. In the 80% of the population who possess **secretor genes**, these antigens are also found in soluble form in secretions and body fluids (e.g. plasma, saliva, semen and sweat).

Table 30.3 Clinically important blood group systems.

Systems	Frequency of antibodies	Cause of haemolytic transfusion reaction	Cause of haemolytic disease of newborn
ABO	Almost universal	Yes (common)	Yes (usually mild)
Rh	Common	Yes (common)	Yes
Kell	Occasional	Yes (occasional)	Anaemia not haemolysis
Duffy	Occasional	Yes (occasional)	Yes (occasional)
Kidd	Occasional	Yes (occasional)	Yes (occasional)
Lutheran	Rare	Yes (rare)	No
Lewis	Occasional	Yes (rare)	No
P	Occasional	Yes (rare)	Yes (rare)
MNS	Rare	Yes (rare)	Yes (rare)
Li	Rare	Unlikely	No

Table 30.4 The ABO blood group system.

Phenotype	Genotype	Antigens	Naturally occurring antibodies	Frequency (UK, %)
O	OO	O	Anti-A, anti-B	46
A	AA or AO	A	Anti-B	42
B	BB or BO	B	Anti-A	9
AB	AB	AB	None	3

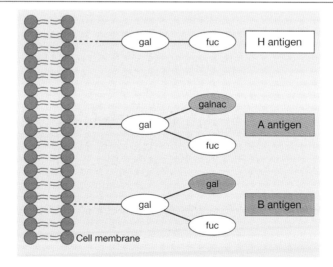

Figure 30.2 Structure of ABO blood group antigens. Each consists of a chain of sugars attached to lipids or proteins which are an integral part of the cell membrane. The H antigen of the O blood group has a terminal fucose (fuc). The A antigen has an additional *N*-acetyl galactosamine (galnac), and the B antigen has an additional galactose (gal). glu, glucose.

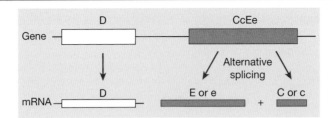

Figure 30.3 Molecular genetics of the Rh blood group. The locus consists of two closely linked genes, *RhD* and *RhCcEe*. The *RhD* gene codes for a single protein which contains the RhD antigen, whereas *RhCcEe* mRNA undergoes alternative splicing to three transcripts. One of these encodes the E or e antigen whereas the other two (only one is shown) contain the C or c epitope. A polymorphism at position 226 of the *RhCcEe* gene determines the Ee antigen status, whereas the C or c antigens are determined by a four amino acid allelic difference. Some individuals do not have an *RhD* gene and are therefore RhD−.

Rh system

The Rh blood group locus is composed of two related structural genes, *RhD* and *RhCE*, which encode the membrane proteins that carry the D, Cc and Ee antigens. The *RhD* gene may be either present or absent, giving the Rh D+ or Rh D− phenotype, respectively. Alternative RNA splicing from the *RhCE* gene generates two proteins, which encode the C or c and the E or e antigens (Fig. 30.3). A shortened nomenclature for the Rh phenotype is commonly used (Table 30.5).

Rh antibodies rarely occur naturally and are therefore immune antibodies that result from previous transfusion or pregnancy. Anti-D is responsible for most of the clinical problems associated with the system and a simple subdivision of subjects into Rh D+ and Rh D− using anti-D antibody is sufficient for routine clinical purposes. About 85% of the European population is Rh D+; some ethnic groups such as Basques have a lower proportion of Rh D+ persons. Anti-C, anti-c, anti-E and anti-e are occasionally seen and may cause both transfusion reactions and haemolytic disease of the newborn. Anti-D does not exist. Rh haemolytic disease of the newborn is described in Chapter 31.

Other blood group systems

Other blood group systems are less frequently of clinical importance. Although naturally occurring antibodies of the P, Lewis and MNS systems are not uncommon, they usually only react at low temperatures and hence are of no clinical consequence. Immune antibodies against antigens of these systems are detected infrequently. Many of the antigens are of low antigenicity and others (e.g. Kell), although comparatively immunogenic, are of relatively low frequency and therefore provide few opportunities for isoimmunization, except in multiply transfused patients.

Molecular techniques, including microarray technology and DNA sequencing, are now available for blood group testing and extended red cell genotyping. Molecular typing is particularly valuable for determining fetal blood group, e.g. if the pregnant woman has a blood group antibody likely to cause haemolysis in the fetus if the fetus has the corresponding antigen. Molecular typing is also useful in transfusion-dependent patients when serological tests are not possible, such as in patients with certain autoantibodies or patients treated with therapeutic antibodies that interfere with serological testing,

Table 30.5 The most common Rh genotypes in the UK population.			
CDE nomenclature	**Short symbol**	**Frequency in white people (%)**	**Rh D status**
cde/cde	rr	15	Negative
CDe/cde	R^{1}r	31	Positive
CDe/CDe	R^{1}R^1	16	Positive
cDE/cde	R^{2}r	13	Positive
CDe/cDE	R^{1}R^2	13	Positive
cDE/cDE	R^{2}R^2	3	Positive
Other genotypes		9	Positive (almost all)

such as daratumumab and CD47 antibodies, to determine the genotypes of clinically important blood groups so that appropriate matched blood can be given.

Hazards of allogeneic blood transfusion

A large number of measures are taken to protect the recipient (Table 30.6).

Infection

Donor selection and testing of all donations are designed to prevent transmission of diseases (Tables 30.1 and 30.2). The main risk is from viruses that have long incubation periods, especially where these are asymptomatic. Recent viral infections can be transmitted in the pre-symptomatic viraemic phase, if blood has been collected during that short period (Table 30.7).

Hepatitis

Donors with a history of hepatitis are deferred for 12 months. If there is a history of jaundice, they can be accepted if markers for HBV and HCV are negative and liver tests have normalized.

Human immunodeficiency virus (HIV)

This can be transmitted by cells or plasma. Men who have sex with men, intravenous drug users and sex workers are currently excluded from donation, as are their sexual partners and partners of haemophiliacs. Inhabitants of large areas of sub-Saharan Africa and South-East Asia where HIV infection is particularly

Table 30.6 Measures to protect recipient.
Donor selection (see Table 30.1)
Donor deferral/exclusion (see Table 30.1)
Stringent arm cleaning
Microbiological testing of donations (Table 30.2)
Immunohaematological testing of donations
Discarding the first 20–30 mL of blood collected from the donor in case of contamination by skin bacteria
Leucodepletion of cellular products
Post-collection viral inactivation of FFP
Monitoring and testing for bacterial contamination
Pathogen inactivation of cellular components
Safest possible sources of donor for plasma products
FFP, fresh frozen plasma.

common are also excluded in the UK, but not from donating in their home countries. Very rarely transmission may occur when the donor is incubating the infection but is not yet positive for the antigen–antibody test used ('window period transmission'), but this is extremely rare now that all blood is screened with nucleic acid testing for HIV-1.

Human T-cell leukaemia viruses

Human T-cell leukaemia virus type I (HTLV-I) is associated with adult T-cell leukaemia or tropical spastic paraparesis. Human T-cell leukaemia virus type II (HLTV II) has no known association with any clinical condition. Screening for both is mandatory in the UK and USA, despite the low prevalence of approximately 1 in 50 000 untested donors.

Cytomegalovirus

Post-infusion cytomegalovirus (CMV) infection is usually subclinical, but may cause an infectious mononucleosis syndrome. Immunosuppressed individuals are at risk of pneumonitis and a potentially fatal disease. These are premature babies (less than 1500 g), stem cell and other organ transplant recipients, patients who have received alemtuzumab (anti-CD52) and pregnant women (where the fetus is at risk). For such recipients, CMV-negative blood or blood components must be given, if they are CMV negative.

Other infections

Syphilis is more likely to be transmitted by platelets (stored at room temperature) than blood (stored at 4°C). However, all donations are tested. Malarial parasites are viable in blood stored at 4°C, so in endemic areas all recipients are given antimalarial drugs. In non-endemic areas, donors are carefully vetted for travel to tropical areas and in some centres tests for malarial antibodies are performed. Chagas' disease is a significant problem with blood transfusion in Latin America. Bacterial infections resulting from skin commensals are most frequently transmitted by platelets stored for more than 3 days. In the USA, all blood is now screened for Zika virus.

Prions

The risk of new variant Creuzfeldt–Jacob disease (nvCJD) is considered a threat to blood safety in the UK. Plasma for fractionation and fresh frozen plasma (FFP) for infants or children is obtained from the USA, where individuals who have lived in the UK for more than 3 months are excluded from donation by the FDA. It is unknown how many people could be infected with nvCJD. There are three rare reports of possible transmission by blood transfusion, so recipients of blood or blood components are now excluded as blood donors in the UK. No screening tests for prions are yet available.

Table 30.7 Infectious agents reported to have been transmitted by blood transfusion.

Viruses

Hepatitis viruses	Hepatitis A virus (HAV)
	Hepatitis B virus (HBV)
	Hepatitis C virus (HCV)
	Hepatitis D virus (HDV) (requires co-infection with HBV)
	Hepatitis E virus (HEV)
Retroviruses	**Human immunodeficiency virus (HIV) 1 + 2**
	Human T-cell leukaemia virus (HTLV) I + 2
Herpes viruses	**Cytomegalovirus (CMV)**
	Epstein–Barr virus (EBV)
Parvoviruses	Parvovirus B19
Miscellaneous viruses	GBV-C—previously referred to as hepatitis G virus (HGV)
	Transfusion transmitted virus (TTV)
	West Nile virus
	Dengue
	Zika virus
	Lassa fever virus
	Chikungunya virus

Bacteria

Endogenous	***Treponema pallidum* (syphilis)**
	Borrelia burgdorferi (Lyme disease)
	Brucella melitensis (brucellosis)
	Yersinia enterocolitica/Salmonella spp.
Exogenous	Environmental species – staphylococcal spp./*Pseudomonas/Serratia* spp.
Rickettsiae	*Rickettsia rickettsii* (Rocky Mountain spotted fever)
	Coxiella burnettii (Q fever)

Protozoa

	***Plasmodium* spp. (malaria)**
	***Trypanosoma cruzi* (Chagas' disease)**
	Toxoplasma gondii (toxoplasmosis)
	Babesia microti/divergens (babesiosis)
	Leishmania spp. (leishmaniasis)

Prions

	New variant Creuzfeldt–Jacob disease (nvCJD)

The infections depicted in bold type are those for which microbial testing of donor blood is carried out in the UK (see Table 30.2).

Techniques in blood group serology

The most important technique is based on the agglutination of red blood cells. Saline agglutination is important in detecting IgM antibodies, usually at room temperature or at 4°C (e.g. anti-A, anti-B; Fig. 30.4). Addition of colloid to the incubation or proteolytic enzyme treatment of red cells increases the sensitivity of the indirect antiglobulin test (see below), as does low ionic strength saline (LISS). These latter methods can detect a range of IgG antibodies.

The antiglobulin (Coombs') test is a fundamental and widely used test in both blood group serology and general immunology. Antihuman globulin (AHG) is produced in animals following the injection of human globulin, purified complement or specific immunoglobulin (e.g. IgG, IgA or IgM). Monoclonal preparations are also now available. When AHG is added to human red cells coated with immunoglobulin or complement components, agglutination of the red cells indicates a positive test (Fig. 30.5).

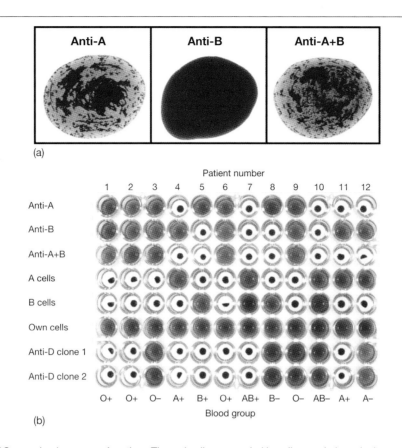

(a)

(b)

Figure 30.4 **(a)** The ABO grouping in a group A patient. The red cells suspended in saline agglutinate in the presence of anti-A or anti-A + B (serum from a group O patient). **(b)** Routine grouping in a 96-well microplate. Positive reactions show as sharp agglutinates; in negative reactions the cells are dispersed. Rows 1–3, patient cells against antisera; rows 4–6, patient sera against known cells; rows 7–8, anti-D against patient cells.

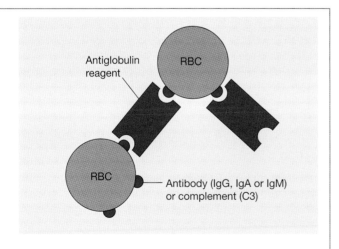

Figure 30.5 The antiglobulin test for antibody or complement on the surface of red blood cells (RBC). The antihuman globulin (Coombs') reagent may be broad spectrum or specific for immunoglobulin G (IgG), IgM, IgA or complement (C3).

The antiglobulin test may be either direct or indirect. The **direct antiglobulin test (DAT)** is used for detecting antibody or complement already on the red cell surface where sensitization has occurred *in vivo*. The AHG reagent is added to washed red cells and agglutination indicates a positive test. A positive test occurs in haemolytic disease of the newborn, autoimmune or drug-induced immune haemolytic anaemia and haemolytic transfusion reactions.

The **indirect antiglobulin test (IAT)** is used to detect antibodies that have coated the red cells *in vitro*. It is a two-stage procedure: the first step involves the incubation of test red cells with serum; in the second step, the red cells are washed and the AHG reagent is added. Agglutination implies that the original serum contained antibody which has coated the red cells *in vitro*. This test is used as part of the routine antibody screening of the recipient's serum prior to transfusion and for detecting blood group antibodies in a pregnant woman.

Most of the above methods were originally developed for tube techniques. These were replaced by 96-well microplates, but most laboratories now use gel-based technology (Fig. 30.6).

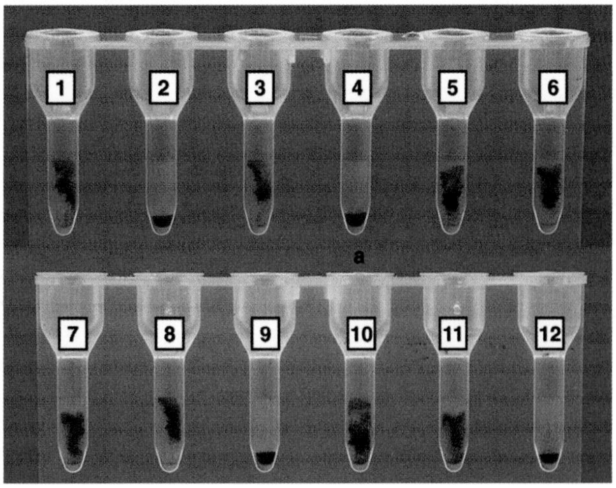

Figure 30.6 Patient antibody screening using the microcolumn (gel) system: 10 tests with two controls (tube 11 is the positive control and tube 12 the negative control) are shown. The patient's serum is tested against screening cells with known red cell phenotype. Tubes 1, 3, 5–8 and 10 show positive results. The patient's serum contained anti-Fyᵃ. Source: Courtesy of Mr G. Hazlehurst.

Table 30.8 Techniques used in compatibility testing. Donor cells tested against recipient serum and agglutination detected visually or microscopically after mixing and incubation at the appropriate temperature.

For detecting clinically significant IgM antibodies
Saline 37°C
For detecting immune antibodies (mainly IgG)
Indirect antiglobulin test at 37°C Low ionic strength saline at 37°C Enzyme-treated red cells at 37°C
Ig, immunoglobulin.

Cross-matching and pre-transfusion tests

A number of steps are taken to ensure that patients receive compatible blood at the time of transfusion. Although group O blood could be given to group A, B or AB recipients since the recipients will not haemolyse the donor red cells, this choice of donor blood should usually be avoided because of the danger of haemolysis of recipient red cells by A and B antibodies in the donor's plasma.

From the patient

1. The ABO and Rh blood group is determined.
2. Serum is screened for important antibodies by an indirect antiglobulin test on a large panel of antigenically-typed group O red cells.

If a red cell alloantibody is discovered in the recipient, donor blood is selected lacking the relative antigen. The most common antibodies are against Rh D, C, c, E, e and K.

From the donor

An appropriate ABO and Rh unit is selected. Donor (blood) testing is described on p. 373.

The cross-match

The techniques that may be used are described in Table 30.8.

Electronic cross-match

In this, a patient has group and antibody screens performed on two separate occasions. If both antibody screens are negative and no blood has been transfused between the test, ABO and Rh compatible blood is issued directly, without further laboratory testing.

Complications of blood transfusion

Haemolytic transfusion reactions

Haemolytic transfusion reactions may be **immediate or delayed** (Table 30.9). Immediate life-threatening reactions associated with massive intravascular haemolysis are the result of complement-activating antibodies of IgM or IgG classes, usually with ABO specificity. Reactions associated with extravascular haemolysis (e.g. immune antibodies of the Rh system which are unable to activate complement) are generally less severe, but may still be life-threatening. The cells become coated with IgG and are removed in the reticuloendothelial system (Fig. 30.7). In mild cases, the only signs of a transfusion reaction may be a progressive unexplained anaemia with or without jaundice. In some cases where the pre-transfusion level of an antibody was too low to be detected in a cross-match, a patient may be reimmunized by transfusion of incompatible red cells, and this will lead to a delayed transfusion reaction with accelerated clearance of the red cells. There may be rapid appearance of anaemia with mild jaundice.

Clinical features of a major haemolytic transfusion reaction

Haemolytic shock phase This may occur after only a few millilitres of blood have been transfused or up to 1–2 hours after the end of the transfusion. Clinical features include urticaria, pain in the lumbar region, flushing, headache, precordial pain, shortness of breath, vomiting, rigors, pyrexia and a fall in blood pressure. If the patient is anaesthetized this shock phase is masked. There is increasing evidence of red cell destruction, and haemoglobinuria, jaundice and disseminated intravascular coagulation (DIC) may all become apparent. Moderate leucocytosis (e.g. 15–20 × 10^9/L) is usual.

Table 30.9 Complications of blood transfusion.

Early (hours)	Late (days or years) Delayed transfusion reaction
Acute haemolytic reaction	Post-transfusion purpura
Reactions caused by infected blood	Immune sensitization, e.g. to red cells, platelets or Rh D antigen
Allergic reactions to white cells, platelets or proteins	Transfusion-associated graft-versus-host disease
Pyrogenic reactions (to plasma proteins or caused by HLA antibodies)	Transfusional iron overload (see Chapter 4)
Circulatory overload	
Hypothermia	
Bacterial contamination (acute sepsis, endotoxin shock)	
Air embolism	
Thrombophlebitis	
Citrate toxicity	
Hyperkalaemia	
Hypocalcaemia (infants, massive transfusion)	
Clotting abnormalities (after massive transfusion)	
Transfusion related acute lung injury (TRALI)	
Anaphylaxis (in IgA-deficient subjects)	

CMV, cytomegalovirus; HIV, human immunodeficiency virus; HLA, human leucocyte antigen; Ig, immunoglobulin.

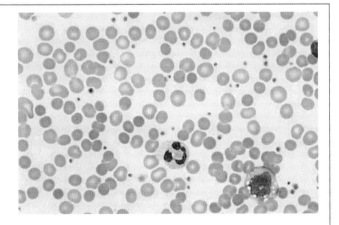

Figure 30.7 Blood transfusion: delayed transfusion reaction. Peripheral blood film showing microspherocytes and polychromasia. *Source:* A.V. Hoffbrand *et al.* (2019) *Color Atlas of Clinical Hematology*, 5th edn. Reproduced by permission of John Wiley & Sons. Courtesy of Dr W Erber.

The oliguric phase In some patients with a haemolytic reaction there is renal tubular necrosis with acute renal failure.

Diuretic phase Fluid and electrolyte imbalance may occur during the recovery from acute renal failure.

Investigation of an immediate transfusion reaction

If a patient develops features suggesting a severe transfusion reaction, the transfusion should be stopped and investigations for blood group incompatibility and bacterial contamination of the blood must be initiated.

1 **Most severe reactions occur because of clerical errors in the handling of donor or recipient blood specimens.** Therefore it must be established that the identity of the recipient (from the patient's wristband) is the same as that on the compatibility label and that this corresponds with the actual unit being transfused.

2 The unit of donor blood and post-transfusion samples of the patient's blood should be sent to the laboratory who will:

   (a) repeat the group on pre- and post-transfusion samples and on the donor blood, and repeat the cross-match;

   (b) perform a direct antiglobulin test on the post-transfusion sample;

   (c) check the plasma for haemoglobinaemia;

   (d) perform tests for DIC; and

   (e) examine the donor sample directly for evidence of gross bacterial contamination and set up blood cultures from it at 20°C and 37°C. If the clinical picture is suggestive of bacterial infection, blood cultures must be taken from the patient and broad-spectrum intravenous antibodies started.

3 A post-transfusion sample of urine must be examined for haemoglobinuria.

4 Further samples of blood are taken 6 hours and/or 24 hours after transfusion for a blood count and bilirubin, free haemoglobin and methaemalbumin (see p. 67) estimations.

5 In the absence of positive findings, the patient's serum is examined 5–10 days later for red cell or white cell antibodies.

Management of patients with major haemolysis

The principal object of initial therapy is to maintain the blood pressure and renal perfusion. Intravenous dextran, plasma or saline and furosemide are sometimes needed. Hydrocortisone 100 mg intravenously and an antihistamine may help to alleviate shock. In the event of severe shock, support with intravenous adrenaline 1 : 10 000 in small incremental doses may be required. Further compatible transfusions may be required in severely affected patients. If acute renal failure occurs this is managed in the usual way, if necessary with dialysis until recovery occurs.

Other transfusion reactions

Hyperhaemolysis syndromes Some patients, particularly with sickle cell anaemia, haemolyse donor blood even though no alloantibodies to red cells can be detected. The haemolysis appears to be due to overactivity of the recipient's macrophages. It is prevented by infusions of gammaglobulin, corticosteroid therapy and eculizumab (see p. 93).

Febrile reactions because of white cell antibodies Human leucocyte antigen (HLA) antibodies (see below and Chapter 23) are usually the result of sensitization by pregnancy or a previous transfusion. They produce rigors, pyrexia and, in severe cases, pulmonary infiltrates. They are minimized by giving leucocyte-depleted (i.e. filtered) packed cells (see below).

Febrile or non-febrile non-haemolytic allergic reactions These are usually caused by hypersensitivity to donor plasma proteins and, if severe, can result in anaphylactic shock. The clinical features are urticaria, pyrexia and, in severe cases, dyspnoea, facial oedema and rigors. Immediate treatment is with antihistamines and hydrocortisone. Adrenaline is also useful. Washed red cells or frozen red cells may be needed for further transfusions if the majority of plasma-removed blood (e.g. saline, adenine, glucose, mannitol (SAGM) blood) causes reactions.

Post-transfusion acute circulatory overload (TACO) The management is that of cardiac failure. These reactions are prevented by a slow transfusion of packed red cells or of the blood component required, accompanied by diuretic therapy.

Transfusion of bacterially contaminated blood This is very rare, but may be serious. It can present with circulatory collapse. It is a particular problem with platelet packs that are stored at 20–24°C.

Graft-versus-host disease (GVHD) This may occur when live lymphocytes are transfused to an immunocompromised patient. It is prevented by irradiation of the blood products for susceptible recipients (Table 30.10). It is uniformly fatal.

Transfusion related acute lung injury (TRALI) This presents within 6 hours of an infusion with cough, breathlessness, fever and rigors, depending on severity. Pulmonary infiltrates are seen on chest X-ray (Figure 30.8). Management is in a high-dependency/intensive care unit with ventilator support if needed. It is caused by transfer of leucoagglutins HLA antibodies in donor plasma or platelets, which cause endothelial and epithelial injury. Most of the donors are multiparous women, so in the UK and USA FFP and plasma to support platelet pools are now from male donors.

Severe anaphylactic reactions This life-threatening reaction in an IgA-deficient subject may result from transfusion of any blood product, most frequently FFP. It is characterized by shock, bronchospasm, laryngeal oedema and widespread skin and mucous membrane angioedema. Intramuscular epinephrine is recommended immediately, followed by parenteral steroids.

Post-transfusion purpura This is a rare problem of severe thrombocytopenia 7–10 days after transfusion of a platelet-containing product, usually red cells. It is caused by an antibody in the recipient (resulting from previous transfusion or pregnancy) which is usually directed against a platelet-specific antigen HPA-Ia (Pl^{A}I). Both the transfused and recipient platelets are destroyed by the immune complexes. It is usually self-limiting, but immunoglobulin or plasma exchange may be needed.

Table 30.10 Indications for irradiated blood products.
Recipients of allogeneic stem cell transplantation
Recipients of autologous stem cell transplantation
Bone marrow or stem cell allogeneic or autologous donors: for 7 days prior to harvest and during harvest
Recipients of solid organ transplants when receiving immune suppressive therapy
Patients with Hodgkin lymphoma
Patients with acute leukaemia
Patients treated with fludarabine, bendamustine, other purine antagonists
Patients treated with anti-CD52
Patients treated with CAR-T cells
Inherited immunodeficiency
Intrauterine and neonatal transfusions

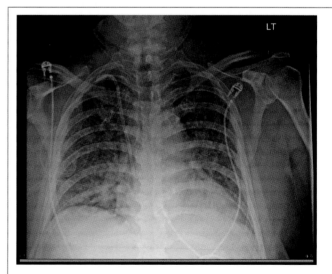

Figure 30.8 Chest X-ray of a 57-year-old man who developed dyspnoea and hypoxia several hours after transfusion of 2 units of red blood cells. Diffuse bilateral airspace infiltrates consistent with transfusion related acute lung injury (TRALI) are present. One of the blood donors was a multiparous woman. Infection and circulatory overload were excluded.

Viral transmission Post-transfusion hepatitis may be caused by one of the hepatitis viruses, although CMV and Epstein–Barr virus (EBV) have also been implicated. Post-transfusion viral hepatitis, HTLV or HIV infection is very rarely seen because of routine screening of all blood donations.

Other infections Toxoplasmosis, malaria and syphilis may be transmitted by blood transfusion. Transfusion-transmitted nvCJD has probably occurred in three cases in the UK.

Post-transfusional iron overload Repeated red cell transfusions over many years, in the absence of blood loss, cause deposition of iron initially in reticuloendothelial tissue at the rate of 200–250 mg/unit of red cells. After 30–50 units in adults, and lesser amounts in children, the liver, myocardium and endocrine glands are damaged, with clinical consequences. This becomes a major problem in thalassaemia major and other severe chronic refractory anaemias (see Chapter 4).

Reduction of blood product use

In the light of transfusion risks and limited resources, appropriate use of blood components is of ever-increasing importance.

Preoperative correction of anaemia (particularly iron deficiency) and cessation of anti-platelet therapies (e.g. aspirin) where possible, together with lower trigger levels for red cell transfusions (haemoglobin 70–80 g/L in most surgical and critical care unit patients), can all help to reduce blood use.

In surgery, the use of alternative fluid replacement, intraoperative or postoperative cell salvage and biological alternatives (e.g. erythropoietin, recombinant clotting factors, recombinant activated clotting factor VII (VIIa) or fibrin glue) all may help.

Blood components

A blood donation is taken by an aseptic technique into plastic bags containing an appropriate amount of anticoagulant, usually citrate, phosphate, dextrose (CPD). The citrate anticoagulates the blood by combining with the blood calcium. Three components are made by initial centrifugation of whole blood: red cells, buffy coat and plasma (Fig. 30.1).

Red cells are stored at 4–6°C for up to 35 days, depending on the preservative. After the first 48 hours there is a slow progressive K+ loss from the red cells into the plasma. In cases where infusion of K+ could be dangerous, fresh blood should be used (e.g. for exchange transfusion in haemolytic disease of the newborn). During red cell storage there is a fall in 2,3-diphosphoglycerate (2,3-DPG), but after transfusion 2,3-DPG levels return to normal within 24 hours. Optimum additive solutions have been developed to increase the shelf-life of plasma-depleted red cells by maintaining both adenosine triphosphate (ATP) and 2,3-DPG levels.

Platelets and plasma may also be collected by apheresis (and centrifuging).

Leucodepletion

In many countries, including the UK and USA, blood products are now routinely filtered to remove the majority of white cells, a process known as leucodepletion. This is usually performed soon after collection and prior to processing, and is more effective than filtration of blood at the bedside (Table 30.1). A blood component is defined as leucocyte-depleted if there are less than 5×10^6/L white cells present.

Leucodepletion reduces the incidence of febrile transfusion reactions and HLA alloimmunization. It is effective at preventing transmission of CMV infection and in addition should reduce the theoretical possibility of transmission of nvCJD in countries where this has been reported.

Red cells

Packed (plasma-depleted) red cells are the treatment of choice for most transfusions (Fig. 30.9a). In older subjects, a diuretic is often given simultaneously and the infusion should be sufficiently slow to avoid circulatory overload. Iron chelation therapy should be considered with patients on a regular transfusion programme to avoid iron overload (see Chapter 4).

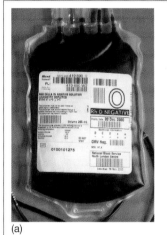
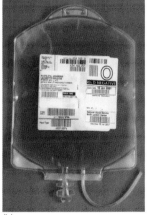
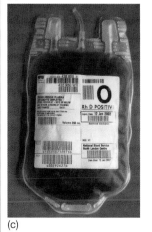

Figure 30.9 Blood components: **(a)** plasma-depleted red cells; **(b)** platelets; and **(c)** fresh frozen plasma.

Recombinant erythropoietin is widely used to reduce transfusion requirements (e.g. in patients with renal failure on dialysis, cancer patients and in myelodysplastic syndromes). Factor VIIa can reduce transfusion need in patients with major haemorrhage (e.g. at surgery or after trauma).

Red cell substitutes are under development, but have not yet proven clinically valuable. These synthetic oxygen-carrying substitutes are often fluorinated hydrocarbons and stromal-free pyridoxylated and polymerized haemoglobin solutions.

Patients with religious objections to red blood cell transfusion such as Jehovah's Witnesses vary in their willingness to receive recombinant erythropoietin and non-red cell blood products such as plasma and platelets.

Autologous donation and transfusion

Anxiety over HIV and other infections has increased the demand for autotransfusion. There are three ways of administering an autologous transfusion:

1 *Predeposit* Blood is taken from the potential recipient in the weeks immediately prior to elective surgery.
2 *Haemodilution* Blood is removed immediately prior to surgery once the patient has been anaesthetized and then reinfused at the end of the operation.
3 *Salvage* Blood lost during the operation is collected during heavy blood loss and then reinfused.

Autotransfusion is the safest form of transfusion with regard to transmission of viral disease, but has a higher risk of bacterial contamination and of clerical errors. The individual involved must be fit enough to donate blood and the predicted operative replacement transfusion should be 2–4 units. Larger replacement transfusions would require blood to be collected over a longer period and red cells stored in the frozen state, which is both labour-intensive and expensive. The high cost of storage and initial restriction of its use to patients undergoing elective surgery means that it can benefit only a minor proportion of the total number of blood recipients. Preoperative autotransfusion is largely reserved for those patients with multiple antibodies for whom it is difficult to identify matching donor blood.

Granulocyte concentrates

These are prepared as buffy coats or on blood cell separators from normal healthy donors or from patients with chronic myeloid leukaemia. They have been used in patients with severe neutropenia (<0.5×10^9/L) and life-threatening infection (e.g., bacterial sepsis or angioinvasive fungus) who are not responding to antibiotic therapy and are expected to eventually recover blood counts. It is not usually possible to give sufficient amounts of granulocytes quickly enough to alter the course of the infection. Granulocytes may transmit CMV infection and must be irradiated to eliminate the risk of causing GVHD.

Platelet concentrates

These are harvested by cell separators or from individual donor units of blood (Fig. 30.9b). They are stored at room temperature. Platelet transfusion is used in patients who are thrombocytopenic, or have disordered platelet function and who are actively bleeding (therapeutic use) or are at serious risk of bleeding (prophylactic use).

For prophylaxis, the platelet count should be kept above 10×10^9/L unless there are additional risk factors such as sepsis, drug use or coagulation disorders for which the threshold should be higher. For invasive procedures (e.g. liver biopsy or lumbar puncture) the platelet count should be raised to above 50×10^9/L. For brain or eye surgery other than cataract removal, the count should be >100×10^9/L.

Therapeutic use is indicated in bleeding associated with platelet disorders. In massive haemorrhage the count should be kept above 50×10^9/L (see Chapter 26).

Platelet transfusions should be avoided in autoimmune thrombocytopenic purpura unless there is serious haemorrhage. They are contraindicated in heparin-induced thrombocytopenia, thrombotic thrombocytopenic purpura and haemolytic uraemic syndrome (see p. 319).

Refractoriness to platelet transfusions is defined by a poor platelet increment post transfusion (less than 7.5×10^9/L per platelet unit transfused at 1 hour or less than 4.5×10^9/L at 24 hours). The causes are either immunological (mostly HLA alloimmunization) or non-immunological (sepsis, hypersplenism, DIC, drugs). Platelets express HLA class I (but not class II) antigens and HLA-matched or cross-match-compatible platelets are needed for patients with HLA antibodies.

The need for platelet transfusions has been reduced with the introduction of direct stimulators of platelet production such as romiplostim or eltrombopag.

Preparations from human plasma

Fresh frozen plasma

Rapidly frozen plasma separated from fresh blood is stored at less than –30°C (Fig. 30.9c). Frozen plasma is usually prepared from single donor units, although pooled products are also available. Its main use is for the replacement of coagulation factors (e.g. when specific concentrates are unavailable) or after massive transfusions, in liver disease and DIC, after cardiopulmonary bypass surgery, to reverse a warfarin effect, and in thrombotic thrombocytopenic purpura (see p. 320). Virally inactivated forms of FFP are now available. Male donors are preferred to reduce the risk of TRALI (see p. 382).

Human albumin solution (4.5%)

This is a useful plasma volume expander when a sustained osmotic effect is required prior to the administration of blood, but it should not be given in excess. It is also used for fluid replacement in patients undergoing plasmapheresis and sometimes for fluid replacement in selected patients with hypoalbuminaemia. For routine volume repletion, there is no benefit from colloidal solutions such as human albumin compared with crystalloid solutions such as normal saline or Lactated Ringer's fluid.

Human albumin solution (20%) (salt-poor albumin)

This may be used in severe hypoalbuminaemia when it is necessary to use a product with minimal electrolyte content. Principal indications for its use are patients with nephrotic syndrome or liver failure.

Cryoprecipitate

This is obtained by thawing FFP at 4°C and contains concentrated factor VIII and fibrinogen and factor XIII. It is stored at less than –30°C or, if lyophilized, at 4–6°C, and was used widely as replacement therapy in haemophilia A and von Willebrand disease before more purified preparations of factor VIII became available. Its main use is in fibrinogen replacement in DIC or massive transfusion or hepatic failure.

Freeze-dried factor VIII concentrates

These are also used for treating haemophilia A or von Willebrand disease. The small volume makes them ideal for children, surgical cases, patients at risk from circulatory overload and for those on home treatment. Their use is declining as recombinant forms of factor VIII become widely available.

Freeze-dried factor IX–prothrombin complex concentrates

A number of preparations are available that contain variable amounts of factors II, VII, IX and X. They are mainly used for treating factor IX deficiency (Christmas disease), but are also used in patients with liver disease or in haemorrhage following overdose with oral anticoagulants or in patients with factor VIII inhibitors. There is a risk of thrombosis.

Immunoglobulin

Pooled immunoglobulin is a valuable source of antibodies against common viruses. It is used in hypogammaglobulinaemia for passive protection against viral and bacterial disease. Repeated doses are needed, for example in the winter months at 3–4-week intervals. It may also be used in immune thrombocytopenia and other acquired immune disorders (e.g. post-transfusion purpura or alloimmune neonatal thrombocytopenia).

Specific immunoglobulin

This may be obtained from donors with high titres of antibody (e.g. anti-RhD, anti-hepatitis B, anti-herpes zoster or anti-rubella).

Acute blood loss and massive haemorrhage

After a single episode of blood loss, there is initial vasoconstriction with a reduction in total blood volume. The plasma volume rapidly expands and the haemoglobin and packed cell volume fall, and there is a rise in neutrophils and platelets. The reticulocyte response begins on the second or third day and lasts 8–10 days. The haemoglobin begins to rise by about the seventh day but, if iron stores have become depleted, the haemoglobin may not subsequently rise to normal. Clinical assessment is needed to gauge whether blood transfusion is needed. This is usually unnecessary in adults at losses less than 500 mL unless haemorrhage is continuing. **The management of massive blood loss with blood, clotting factor and platelet support is described on page 335.**

■ Blood transfusion involves the safe transfer of blood components from a donor to a recipient. Most commonly this is red cells and the red cells must be matched between recipient and donor.
■ Careful donor selection and microbiological testing help to protect both donor and recipient.
■ Red cells contain over 400 antigens. The ABO and Rh systems are most important in transfusion. Subjects lacking an antigen (e.g. group A or B) may develop a naturally occurring antibody to it, usually IgM. These antibodies in a recipient may haemolyse or opsonize donor red cells if these contain the antigen.
■ Antibodies may also develop from exposure to the antigen by a transfusion or pregnancy. Cross-matching of donor red cells with recipient plasma is therefore carried out to ensure they are compatible.
■ Complications of blood transfusion may be acute (within hours) or late (after days or years). They include haemolytic reactions, febrile reactions to white cells or proteins, circulatory overload, shock due to bacterial contamination or anaphylactic reaction, lung injury, transmission of infections, especially viral, transfusion-associated graft-versus-host disease and, in the longer term, iron overload.
■ Blood components other than red cells can also be transfused. These include platelets and protein products including fresh frozen plasma, albumin solutions, coagulation factor concentrates and immunoglobulin.

SUMMARY

Now visit **www.wiley.com/go/essentialhaematology** to test yourself on this chapter.

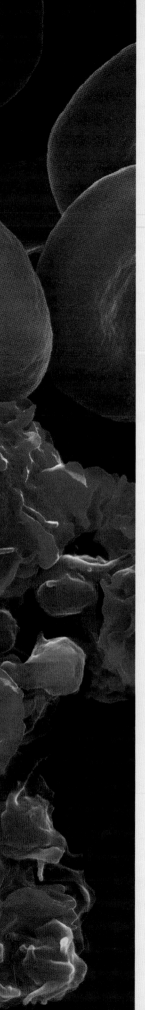

CHAPTER 31
Pregnancy and neonatal haematology

Key topics

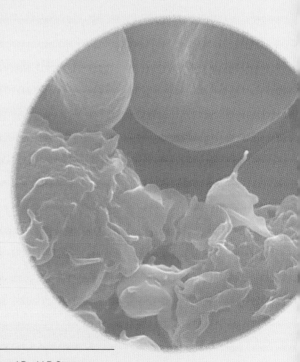

Hoffbrand's Essential Haematology, Eighth Edition. By A. Victor Hoffbrand and David P. Steensma.
© 2020 John Wiley & Sons Ltd. Published 2020 by John Wiley & Sons Ltd.
Companion website: www.wileyessential.com/haematology

Haematology of pregnancy

Pregnancy places extreme stresses on the haematological system and an understanding of the physiological changes that result is obligatory in order to interpret any need for therapeutic intervention.

Definition of anaemia in pregnancy

Physiological anaemia is a term sometimes used to describe the fall in haemoglobin (Hb) concentration that occurs during normal pregnancy (Fig. 31.1), but it is not a true anaemia. Blood plasma volume increases by approximately 1250 mL, or 45%, above normal by the end of gestation and although the red cell mass itself increases by some 25%, this difference still leads to a fall in Hb concentration.

The World Health Organization (WHO) classifies pregnant women with haemoglobin levels of at least 110 g/L as normal; the US Centers for Disease Control (CDC) consider pregnant women with haemoglobin levels of at least 110 g/L in the first and third trimesters and at least 105 g/L in the second trimester as normal. **Values below 100 g/L in the first trimester, 105 g/L in the second and 100 g/L in the third or post-partum are clearly abnormal and require investigation.**

Iron deficiency anaemia

Up to 600 mg iron is required for the mother's increase in red cell mass and a further 300 mg for the fetus and placenta. In addition, a median of 250 mg of iron is lost due to bleeding during delivery. Despite a physiological increase in iron absorption, few women avoid depletion of iron reserves by the end of pregnancy.

In uncomplicated pregnancy, the mean corpuscular volume (MCV) typically rises by approximately 4 fL. A fall in red cell MCV is the earliest sign of iron deficiency. Later, the mean corpuscular haemoglobin (MCH) falls and finally anaemia results. Early iron deficiency is likely if the serum ferritin is below 30 µg/L together with serum iron below 10 mmol/L and should be treated with oral iron supplements. Routine iron supplementation in pregnancy is not carried out in the UK, but is recommended by the CDC in the USA and by the WHO. More than 70% of pregnant patients prescribed oral iron discontinue due to gastrointestinal adverse effects, as pregnant women have decreased bowel motility caused by elevated progesterone, and also have compression of the rectum by the enlarged uterus which can worsen constipation. Intravenous iron infusion is effective (see p. 37) and may be indicated in the second or third trimesters, but is avoided in the first.

Folate and vitamin B₁₂ deficiency

Folate requirements are increased approximately two-fold in pregnancy and serum folate levels fall to approximately half the normal range, with a less dramatic fall in red cell folate. In some parts of the world, megaloblastic anaemia during pregnancy is common because of a combination of poor diet and exaggerated folate requirements. Given the protective effect of folate against neural tube defects (NTDs), folic acid 400 µg/day (5 mg if there has been a previous NTD pregnancy) should be taken periconceptually and throughout pregnancy. Food fortification with folate is now being practised in over 80 countries and has been associated with a fall in incidence of NTDs. Vitamin B₁₂ deficiency has historically been considered rare during pregnancy, but the incidence is increasing in some countries due to

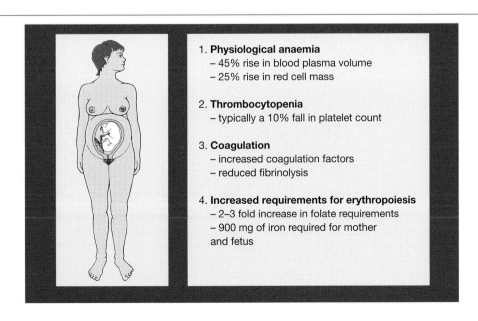

1. **Physiological anaemia**
   – 45% rise in blood plasma volume
   – 25% rise in red cell mass

2. **Thrombocytopenia**
   – typically a 10% fall in platelet count

3. **Coagulation**
   – increased coagulation factors
   – reduced fibrinolysis

4. **Increased requirements for erythropoiesis**
   – 2–3 fold increase in folate requirements
   – 900 mg of iron required for mother and fetus

Figure 31.1 Haematological changes during pregnancy.

the frequency of bariatric surgery. Serum vitamin B$_{12}$ levels fall to below normal in 20–30% of pregnancies and low values are sometimes the cause of diagnostic confusion.

Thrombocytopenia

The platelet count falls by an average of 10% in an uncomplicated pregnancy. The specific cause of this drop is unclear, but there is evidence for both reduced production and increased platelet destruction. In approximately 7% of women this fall is more severe and can result in thrombocytopenia (platelet count less than 140×10^9/L).

In over 75% of cases this is mild and of unknown cause, referred to as **incidental or gestational thrombocytopenia of pregnancy**. Approximately 21% of cases are secondary to a hypertensive disorder and 4% are associated with immune thrombocytopenic purpura (ITP; Fig. 31.2).

Incidental (gestational) thrombocytopenia of pregnancy

This is a diagnosis of exclusion, usually detected at the time of delivery. If the platelet count falls to the range $100–140 \times 10^9$/L, it can confidently be attributed to gestational thrombocytopenia even in the first trimester. It recovers within 6 weeks of delivery. No treatment is needed and the infant is not affected.

Thrombocytopenia of hypertensive disorders

This is variable in severity, with the platelet count usually $<100 \times 10^9$/L. The platelet count rarely falls to below 40×10^9/L except in the setting of severe microangiopathy. It is more severe when associated with pre-eclampsia; the primary treatment is as rapid a delivery as possible. The HELLP syndrome (haemolysis, elevated liver enzymes and low platelets) falls into

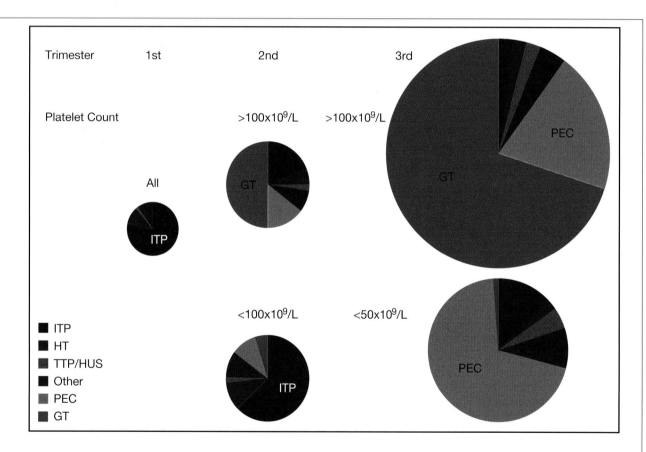

Figure 31.2 Prevalence of causes of thrombocytopenia based on trimester of presentation and platelet count. The size of each circle represents the relative frequency of all causes of thrombocytopenia during each of the three trimesters of pregnancy. All aetiologies and all platelet counts are considered together in the first trimester when thrombocytopenia is uncommon. Distribution of aetiologies during the second and third trimesters is subdivided by platelet count. All results are estimates based on personal experience and review of the literature. 'Other' indicates miscellaneous disorders, including infection, disseminated intravascular coagulation (DIC), type IIB von Willebrand disease, immune and nonimmune drug-induced thrombocytopenia, paroxysmal nocturnal haemoglobinuria, bone marrow failure syndromes (aplastic anaemia, myelodysplasia, myeloproliferative disorders, leukaemia/lymphoma and marrow infiltrative disorders), among others. GT, gestational thrombocytopenia; HUS, haemolytic uraemic syndrome; ITP, immune thrombocytopenia; PEC, pre-eclampsia/HELLP; TTP, thrombotic thrombocytopenic purpura. Source: D.B. Cines *et al*. (2017) *Blood* 130: 144–51. Reproduced with permission of the American Society of Hematology.

this category. It is associated with prolongation of prothrombin time (PT) and activated partial thromboplastin time (APTT).

Immune thrombocytopenic purpura

In pregnancy, ITP (see p. 316) represents a particular problem, both to the mother and to the fetus, as the antibody crosses the placenta and the fetus may become severely thrombocytopenic. Like other adults, pregnant women with ITP and platelet counts higher than 50×10^9/L do not usually need treatment. Treatment is required for women with platelet counts below 10×10^9/L and for those with platelet counts of $10–30 \times 10^9$/L who are in their second or third trimester or who are bleeding. Treatment is with steroids, intravenous immunoglobulin (Ig) G, rituximab or rarely splenectomy as appropriate. Thrombopoietin receptor antagonists are avoided because of potential teratogenetic side-effects.

At delivery, umbilical vein blood sampling or fetal scalp vein sampling to measure the fetal platelet count may be offered, although their exact role is unclear. In general, caesarean section is not indicated when the maternal platelet count is above 50×10^9/L, unless the fetal platelet count is known to be less than 20×10^9/L. Platelet transfusion may be given to mothers in labour with very low platelet counts or who are actively bleeding.

Newborns of mothers with ITP should have a blood count measured for the first 5 days of life, as the platelet count may progressively drop. A count greater than 50×10^9/L is reassuring. Cerebral ultrasonography may be performed to look for intracranial haemorrhage (ICH). In newborns without evidence of ICH, treatment with intravenous IgG is appropriate if the infant's platelet count is less than 20×10^9/L. Neonates with thrombocytopenia and ICH should be treated with steroids and intravenous IgG therapy.

Haemostasis and thrombosis

Pregnancy leads to a hypercoagulable state with consequent increased risks of thromboembolism and disseminated intravascular coagulation (DIC; see p. 333). There is an increase in plasma factors VII, VIII, X and fibrinogen, with shortening of PT and APTT; fibrinolysis is suppressed. These changes last for up to 2 months into the puerperal period and the incidence of thrombosis during this period is increased. There is an association between thrombophilic conditions in the mother and recurrent fetal loss (see p. 344). This is presumed to result from placental thrombosis and infarction.

Treatment of thrombosis

Warfarin has no role in management. It crosses the placenta and in addition is associated with embryopathy, especially between 6 and 12 weeks' gestation. **Low molecular weight heparin is now the treatment of choice**, because it can be given once daily and is less likely than unfractionated heparin to cause osteoporosis.

Neonatal haematology

Haemoglobin and MCV are higher at birth than in adults (Table 31.1). The cord blood Hb varies between approximately 165 and 170 g/L and is influenced by the timing of cord clamping. At birth the haemoglobin ranges from 149 to 23.7 g/L (Table 31.1). The reticulocyte count is initially high (2–6%), but falls to below 0.5% at 1 week as erythropoiesis is suppressed in response to the marked increase in the oxygenation of tissues after birth (Fig. 31.3). This is associated with a progressive fall in Hb to a range of 94–130 g/L at 2 months, from which point it recovers to a mean of 125 g/L at around 6 months. **The lower limit of normal during childhood is 110 g/L.** Preterm infants have a more dramatic fall in Hb to 70–90 g/L at 8 weeks and are more prone to iron and folate deficiency in the first few months of life. Switching of globin types is discussed in Chapter 7.

In the blood film, nucleated red cells will be seen for the first 4 days and for up to 1 week in preterm infants. Numbers are increased in cases of hypoxia, haemorrhage or haemolytic disease of the newborn (HDN).

MCV averages 119 fL at birth (range 100–125 fL), but falls to normal adult values by 2 months (Table 31.1). By 1 year, the MCV has fallen to around 70 fL and rises throughout childhood again to reach adult levels at puberty.

Anaemia in the neonate

This should be considered for Hb below 140 g/L at birth. The clinical significance of anaemia is compounded by the high (70–80%) levels of HbF at birth, as this is less effective than HbA at releasing oxygen to the tissues (see p. 17). Causes include the following (Fig. 31.4):

1. **Haemorrhage** Fetomaternal, twin–twin, cord, internal, placenta.
2. **Increased destruction** Haemolysis (immune or non-immune) or infection.
3. **Decreased production** Congenital red cell aplasia, infection (e.g. parvovirus). Anti-Kell causes alloimmune anaemia of the fetus and newborn with decreased erythropoiesis.

Generally, anaemia at birth is usually secondary to immune haemolysis or haemorrhage; non-immune causes of haemolysis appear within 24 hours. Impaired red cell production is usually not apparent for at least 3 weeks. Haemolysis is often associated with severe jaundice and the causes include HDN, autoimmune haemolytic anaemia (AIHA) in the mother and congenital disorders of the red cell membrane or metabolism.

Red cell transfusion may be needed for symptomatic anaemia with Hb less than 105 g/L, or a higher threshold if there is severe cardiac or respiratory disease.

Anaemia of prematurity

Premature infants have a more marked fall in Hb after birth and this is termed **physiological anaemia of prematurity**. Features include a slowly falling Hb, normal blood film and

Table 31.1 Representative normal haematological values at birth and over the first 2 months of life in term babies.*			
	Birth	**2 weeks**	**2 months**
Hb (g/dL)	14.9–23.7	13.4–19.8	9.4–13
Haematocrit	0.47–75	0.41–0.65	0.28–0.42
MCV (fL)	100–125	88–110	77–98
Reticulocytes (×10⁹/L)	110–450	10–85	35–200
WBC (×10⁹/L)	10–26	6–21	5–15
Neutrophils (×10⁹/L)	2.7–14.4	1.5–5.4	0.7–4.8
Monocytes (×10⁹/L)	0–1.9	0.1–1.7	0.4–1.2
Lymphocytes (×10⁹/L)	2.0–7.3	2.8–9.1	3.3–10.3
Eosinophils (×10⁹/L)	0–0.85	0–0.85	0.05–0.9
Basophils (×10⁹/L)	0–0.1	0–0.1	0.02–0.13
Nucleated RBC (×10⁹/L)	<5	<0.1	<0.1
Platelets (×10⁹/L)	150–450	150–450	150–450

*These data are obtained from a number of sources and have been chosen to represent data most useful for interpreting the significance of haematological results.
Hb, haemoglobin; MCV, mean corpuscular volume; RBC, red blood cells; WBC, white blood cells.
Source: I.A.G. Roberts, N.A. Murray. In J.M. Rennie (ed.) (2011) *Robertson's Textbook of Neonatology*, 4th edn. Philadelphia, PA: Elsevier Churchill Livingstone, pp. 739–72.

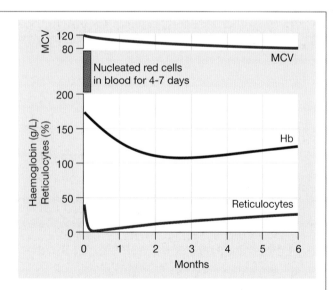

Figure 31.3 Typical profile of the blood count in the neonatal period.

reticulocytopenia. It can be minimized by late (after 1 minute) clamping of the cord and by ensuring adequate iron and folate replacement and limiting phlebotomy. Erythropoiesis-stimulating agents are used in some centres.

Neonatal polycythaemia

This is defined as a venous haematocrit over 0.65 and can occur with twin–twin transfusion, intrauterine growth restriction and maternal hypertension or diabetes. If symptoms are present, it should be treated with partial exchange transfusion using a crystalloid solution.

Neonatal neutropenia

The neutrophil count falls in the first few weeks of life and then rises slowly to adult values by one year. Neutrophil function is also impaired in the first weeks, increasing the risk of infection. From the age of a few weeks, the lymphocyte count is higher than neutrophils throughout childhood.

Fetomaternal alloimmune thrombocytopenia

Fetomaternal alloimmune thrombocytopenia (FMAIT) results from a process similar to that of HDN. Fetal platelets that possess a paternally inherited antigen (HPA-1a in 80%) that is not present on maternal platelets can sensitize the mother to make antibodies which cross the placenta, coat the platelets, which are then destroyed by the reticuloendothelial system, and lead to serious bleeding, including intracranial haemorrhage. Alloimmune thrombocytopenia differs from HDN in that 50% of cases occur in the first pregnancy. Its incidence is approximately 1 in 1000–5000 births.

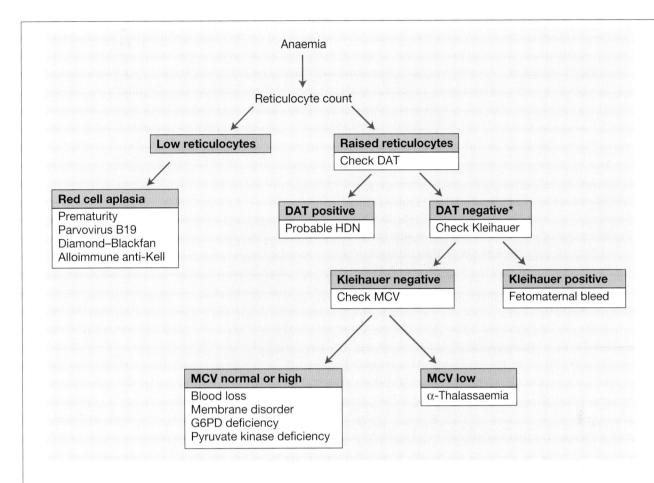

Figure 31.4 The investigation of neonatal anaemia. *The DAT test may be negative in HDN due to ABO incompatibility. DAT, direct antiglobulin test; HDN, haemolytic disease of the newborn; MCV, mean corpuscular volume.

Thrombocytopenia can lead to serious, sometimes fatal, bleeding *in utero* or after birth. Treatment is unsatisfactory. Severe postnatal cases may be treated with a platelet transfusion that is negative for the relevant antigen. Antenatal treatment may be either maternal intravenous immunoglobulin or fetal transfusion with HPA-compatible platelets.

Other causes of neonatal thrombocytopenia include perinatal infection, placental insufficiency and congenital genetic causes.

Coagulation

Standard tests need to be interpreted with caution in the neonate. The APTT and PT are prolonged because of reduced levels of the vitamin K-dependent factors II, VII, IX and X, which become normal at around 6 months. Neonates have an increased risk of thrombosis. This is a result of physiologically low levels of inhibitors of coagulation and the use of in-dwelling vascular catheters. Antithrombin (AT) and protein C levels are approximately 60% of normal for the first 3 months. Homozygous protein C deficiency is associated with fulminant purpura fulminans in early life. Therapeutic protein C concentrates are now available. Homozygous AT deficiency usually presents later in childhood, but arterial and venous thrombosis may also occur in the neonate.

Haemolytic disease of the newborn

HDN is the result of **red cell alloimmunization**, in which IgG antibodies passage from the maternal circulation across the placenta into the circulation of the fetus, where they react with fetal red cells and lead to their destruction. Anti-D antibody is responsible for most cases of severe HDN, although anti-c, anti-E, anti-K and a wide range of other antibodies are found in occasional cases (see Table 30.3). Although antibodies against the ABO blood group system are the most frequent cause of HDN, this is usually mild.

Rh haemolytic disease of the newborn

When an Rh D-negative (p. 376) woman has a pregnancy with an Rh D-positive fetus, Rh D-positive fetal red cells cross into the maternal circulation (especially at parturition and during the third trimester) and sensitize the mother to form anti-D. The mother could also be sensitized by a previous miscarriage, amniocentesis or other trauma to the placenta or by blood transfusion. Anti-D crosses the placenta to the fetus during the next pregnancy, coats Rh D-positive fetal red cells and results in reticuloendothelial destruction of these cells, causing anaemia and jaundice. If the father is heterozygous for D antigen, and mother Rh D negative, there is a 50% probability that the fetus will be D-positive. The fetal Rh D genotype can be established by polymerase chain reaction (PCR) analysis for the presence of Rh D in a maternal blood sample.

The main aim of management is to prevent anti-D antibody formation in Rh D-negative mothers. This can be achieved by the administration of small amounts of anti-D antibody, which 'mop up' and destroy Rh D-positive fetal red cells before they can sensitize the immune system of the mother to produce anti-D.

Prevention of Rh immunization

At the time of booking, all pregnant women should have their ABO and Rh group determined and serum screened for antibodies at least twice during the pregnancy. **All non-sensitized Rh D-negative women should be given at least 500 units (100 µg) of anti-D at 28 and 34 weeks' gestation** to reduce the risk of sensitization from fetomaternal haemorrhage. Fetal Rh D molecular typing from DNA in maternal blood can be used before 28 weeks. If the fetus is Rh D-negative, no further anti-D prophylaxis is needed. In addition, at birth the babies of Rh D-negative women who do not have antibodies must have their cord blood grouped for ABO and Rh. If the baby's blood is Rh D-negative, the mother will require no further treatment. If the baby is Rh D-positive, prophylactic anti-D should be administered to the mother at a minimum dose of 500 units intramuscularly within 72 hours of delivery. A **Kleihauer test** is performed. This uses differential staining to estimate the number of fetal cells in the maternal circulation (Fig. 31.5a). If the Kleihauer is positive, many centres will perform flow cytometry for a more accurate estimate of the volume of feto-maternal haemorrhage (FMH; Fig. 31.5b). The chance of developing antibodies is related to the number of fetal cells found. The dose of anti-D is increased if there is greater than 4 mL transplacental haemorrhage. Anti-D IgG (125 units) is given for each 1 mL of FMH greater than 4 mL.

Sensitizing episodes during pregnancy

Anti-D IgG should be given to Rh D-negative women who have potentially sensitizing episodes during pregnancy: 250 units is given if the event occurs up to week 20 of gestation and 500 units thereafter, followed by a Kleihauer test.

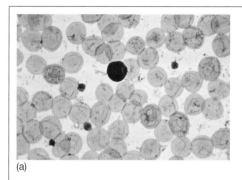

(a)

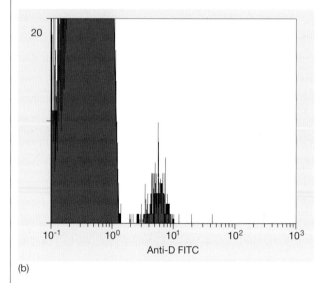

(b)

Figure 31.5 (a) Kleihauer test for fetal red cells; a deeply eosin-staining cell containing fetal haemoglobin is seen at the centre. Haemoglobin has been eluted from the other red cells by an incubation at acid pH and these appear as colourless ghosts. **(b)** Determination by flow cytometry of the number of RhD fetal cells in maternal blood using fluorescent-labelling of antibody to RhD, the mother being RhDd. Source: Courtesy of Dr W Erber.

Potentially sensitizing events as well as delivery are listed in Table 31.2.

Treatment of established anti-D sensitization

If anti-D antibodies are detected during pregnancy, they should be quantified at regular intervals. The clinical severity is related to the strength of anti-D present in maternal serum, but is also affected by such factors as the IgG subclass, rate of rise of antibody and past history. The development of haemolytic disease in the fetus can be assessed by velocimetry of the fetal middle cerebral artery by Doppler ultrasonography, as increased velocities correlate with fetal anaemia (Fig. 31.6). If anaemia is detected, fetal blood sampling and intrauterine transfusion of irradiated Rh D-negative packed red cells may be indicated.

Table 31.2 Potentially sensitizing events in pregnancy (from British Committee for Standards in Haematology (BCSH) Guidelines 2014: https://b-s-h.org.uk/guidelines).

Amniocentesis, chorionic villus biopsy and cordocentesis

Antepartum haemorrhage/per vaginal bleeding in pregnancy

External cephalic version

Fall or abdominal trauma (sharp/blunt, open/closed)

Ectopic pregnancy

Evacuation of molar pregnancy

Intrauterine death and stillbirth

In utero therapeutic interventions (transfusion, surgery, insertion of shunts, laser)

Miscarriage, threatened miscarriage

Therapeutic termination of pregnancy

Delivery – normal, instrumental or caesarean section

Intraoperative cell salvage

Source: S. Allard, M. Contreras. In A.V. Hoffbrand *et al.* (2016) (eds) *Postgraduate Haematology*, 7th edn. Reproduced by permission of John Wiley & Sons.

Clinical features of HDN

1 **Severe disease** Intrauterine death from hydrops fetalis (Fig. 31.7a).
2 **Moderate disease** The baby is born with anaemia and jaundice and may show pallor, tachycardia, oedema and hepatosplenomegaly. If the unconjugated bilirubin is not controlled and reaches levels exceeding 250 μmol/L, bile pigment deposition in the basal ganglia may lead to **kernicterus** – central nervous system damage with generalized spasticity and possible subsequent mental deficiency, deafness and epilepsy. This problem becomes acute after birth as maternal clearance of fetal bilirubin ceases and conjugation of bilirubin by the neonatal liver has not yet reached full activity.
3 **Mild disease** Mild anaemia with or without jaundice.

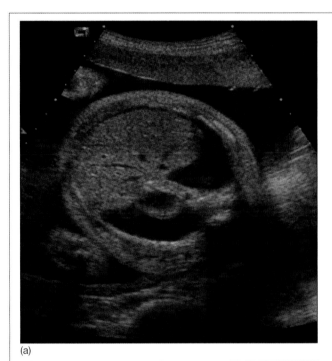

(a)

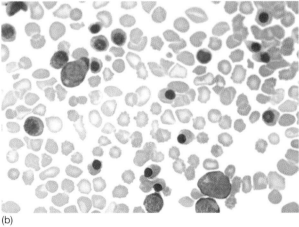

(b)

Figure 31.7 (a) Ultrasound features of hydrops fetalis showing skin oedema, hepatomegaly and ascites. Source: S. Kumar, F. Regan (2005) *BMJ* 330: 1255–58. Reproduced with permission of BMJ. **(b)** Rh haemolytic disease of the newborn (erythroblastosis fetalis): peripheral blood film showing large numbers of erythroblasts, polychromasia and crenated cells.

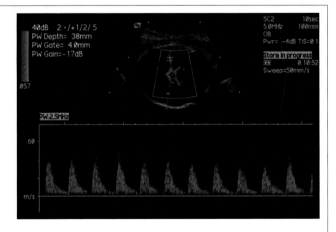

Figure 31.6 Doppler ultrasonography of the circle of Willis in a fetus. The cursor is placed over the middle cerebral artery and an increased blood velocity correlates with anaemia. Source: S. Kumar, F. Regan (2005) *BMJ* 330: 1255–58. Reproduced with permission of BMJ.

Investigations will reveal variable anaemia with a high reticulocyte count; the baby is Rh D-positive, the direct antiglobulin test is positive and the serum bilirubin raised. In moderate and severe cases, many erythroblasts are seen in the blood film (Fig. 31.7b); this is known as **erythroblastosis fetalis**.

Treatment

Exchange transfusion may be necessary; the indications for this include severe anaemia (Hb <100 g/L at birth) and severe or rapidly rising hyperbilirubinaemia. More than one exchange transfusion may be required and 500 mL is usually sufficient for each exchange. The donor blood should be less than 5 days old, CMV negative, irradiated, Rh D-negative and ABO compatible with the baby's and mother's serum. Phototherapy (exposure of the infant to bright light of appropriate wavelength) degrades bilirubin and reduces the likelihood of kernicterus.

ABO haemolytic disease of the newborn

In 20% of births, a mother is ABO incompatible with the fetus. Group A and group B mothers usually have only IgM ABO antibodies (p. 373). **The majority of cases of ABO HDN are caused by 'immune' IgG antibodies in group O mothers.** Although 15% of pregnancies in white people involve a group O mother with a group A or group B fetus, most mothers do not produce IgG anti-A or anti-B and very few babies have severe enough haemolytic disease to require treatment. Exchange transfusions are needed in only 1 in 3000 infants. The mild course of ABO HDN is partly explained by the A and B antigens not being fully developed at birth and by partial neutralization of maternal IgG antibodies by A and B antigens on other cells, in the plasma and tissue fluids.

In contrast to Rh HDN, ABO disease may be found in the first pregnancy and may or may not affect subsequent pregnancies. The direct antiglobulin test on the infant's cells may be negative or only weakly positive. Examination of the blood film shows auto-agglutination spherocytosis, polychromasia and erythroblastosis.

SUMMARY

- Pregnancy results in multiple changes in the haematological systems.
- There is a fall in haemoglobin because of an increased plasma volume that is proportionally greater than a 25% increase in red cell mass.
- Iron deficiency is frequent; folate deficiency is associated with maternal anaemia and also with neural tube defects (NTDs) in the fetus.
- Serum vitamin B$_{12}$ levels fall in pregnancy, but recover post-partum.
- Platelets counts fall on average by 10%. If the count falls below 100×10^9/L other causes than gestational thrombocytopenia are sought, e.g. immune thrombocytopenia, hypertensive disorders.
- Pregnancy is a hypercoagulable state with increased levels of coagulation factors and risk of thrombosis or disseminated intravascular coagulation.

- Neonates have higher haemoglobin levels than adults. Anaemia at birth is usually caused by haemorrhage or immune haemolysis.
- Haemolytic disease of the newborn is brought about by Rh D antibodies made by a Rh D-negative mother crossing the placenta. It may cause death of the fetus (hydrops fetalis) or haemolytic anaemia. It is now rare because of administration of Rh anti-D to Rh D-negative mothers at the time of exposure to Rh D-positive fetal cells or blood products.
- ABO haemolytic disease of the newborn is more frequent. It is usually mild and may occur in the first pregnancy. It is most frequently caused by group O mothers making immune IgG antibodies (which cross the placenta) against a group A or B fetus.

Now visit **www.wileyessential.com/haematology** to test yourself on this chapter.

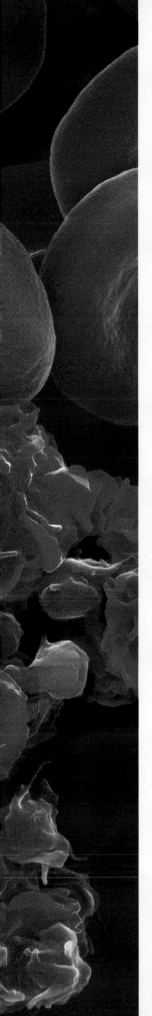

APPENDIX

2016 World Health Organization classification of lymphoid and myeloid neoplasms

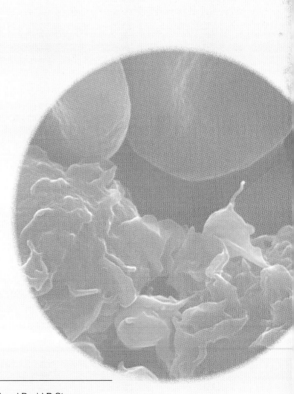

Hoffbrand's Essential Haematology, Eighth Edition. By A. Victor Hoffbrand and David P. Steensma.
© 2020 John Wiley & Sons Ltd. Published 2020 by John Wiley & Sons Ltd.
Companion website: www.wileyessential.com/haematology

Swerdlow SH, et al. *Blood* 2016;127:2375–2390.
Arber DA, et al. *Blood* 2016;127:2391–2405.
Swerdlow SH, et al. eds. WHO *Classification of Tumours of Haematopoietic and Lymphoid Tissues*. International Agency for Research on Cancer, Lyon, 2017.

Myeloproliferative neoplasms

Chronic myeloid leukemia, *BCR-ABL 1*-positive	9875/3
Chronic neutrophilic leukemia	9963/3
Polycythemia vera	9950/3
Primary myelofibrosis	9961/3
Essential thrombocythemia	9962/3
Chronic eosinophilic leukemia, NOS	9964/3
Myeloproliferative neoplasm, unclassifiable	9975/3

Mastocytosis

Cutaneous mastocytosis	9740/1
Indolent systemic mastocytosis	9741/1
Systemic mastocytosis with an associated hematologic neoplasm	9741/3
Aggressive systemic mastocytosis	9741/3
Mast cell leukemia	9742/3
Mast cell sarcoma	9740/3

Myeloid/lymphoid neoplasms with eosinophilia and gene rearrangement

Myeloid/lymphoid neoplasms with *PDGFRA* rearrangement	9965/3
Myeloid/lymphoid neoplasms with *PDGFRB* rearrangement	9966/3
Myeloid/lymphoid neoplasms with *FGFR1* rearrangement	9967/3
Myeloid/lymphoid neoplasms with *PCM1-JAK2*	9968/3[a]

Myelodysplastic/myeloproliferative neoplasms

Chronic myelomonocytic leukemia	9945/3
Atypical chronic myeloid leukemia, *BCR-ABL1*-negative	9876/3
Juvenile myelomonocytic leukemia	9946/3
Myelodysplastic/myeloproliferative neoplasm with ring sideroblasts and thrombocytosis	9982/3
Myelodysplastic/myeloproliferative neoplasm, unclassifiable	9975/3

Myelodysplastic syndromes

Myelodysplastic syndrome with single lineage dysplasia	9980/3
Myelodysplastic syndrome with ring sideroblasts and single lineage dysplasia	9982/3
Myelodysplastic syndrome with ring sideroblasts and multilineage dysplasia	9993/3[a]
Myelodysplastic syndrome with multilineage dysplasia	9985/3
Myelodysplastic syndrome with excess blasts	9983/3
Myelodysplastic syndrome with isolated del(5q)	9986/3
Myelodysplastic syndrome, unclassifiable	9989/3
Refractory cytopenia of childhood	9985/3

Myeloid neoplasms with germline predisposition

Acute myeloid leukemia with germline *CEBPA* mutation	
Myeloid neoplasms with germline *DDX41* mutation	
Myeloid neoplasms with germline *RUNX1* mutation	
Myeloid neoplasms with germline *ANKRD26* mutation	
Myeloid neoplasms with germline *ETV6* mutation	
Myeloid neoplasms with germline *GATA2* mutation	

Acute myeloid leukemia (AML) and related precursor neoplasms

AML with recurrent genetic abnormalities

AML with t(8;21)(q22;q22.1); *RUNX1-RUNX1T1*	9896/3
AML with inv(16)(p13.1q22) or t(16;16) (p13.1;q22); *CBFB-MYH11*	9871/3
Acute promyelocytic leukemia with *PML-RARA*	9866/3
AML with t(9;11)(p21.3;q23.3); *KMT2A-MLLT3*	9897/3
AML with t(6;9)(p23;q34.1); *DEK-NUP214*	9865/3

AML with inv(3)(q21.3q26.2) or t(3;3) (q21.3;q26.2); *GATA2, MECOM* — 9869/3

AML (megakaryoblastic) with t(1;22) (p13.3;q13.1); *RBM15-MKL1* — 9911/3

AML with *BCR-ABL1* — 9912/3[a]

AML with mutated *NPM1* — 9877/3[a]

AML with biallelic mutation of *CEBPA* — 9878/3[a]

AML with mutated RUNX1 — 9879/3[a]

AML with myelodysplasia-related changes — 9895/3
Therapy-related myeloid neoplasms — 9920/3
Acute myeloid leukemia, NOS — 9861/3

AML with minimal differentiation — 9872/3

AML without maturation — 9873/3

AML with maturation — 9874/3

Acute myelomonocytic leukemia — 9867/3

Acute monoblastic and monocytic leukemia — 9891/3

Pure erythroid leukemia — 9840/3

Acute megakaryoblastic leukemia — 9910/3

Acute basophilic leukemia — 9870/3

Acute panmyelosis with myelofibrosis — 9931/3

Myeloid sarcoma — 9930/3
Myeloid proliferations associated with Down syndrome

Transient abnormal myelopoiesis associated with Down syndrome — 9898/1

Myeloid leukemia associated with Down syndrome — 9898/3

Blastic plasmacytoid dendritic cell neoplasm — 9727/3
Acute leukemias of ambiguous lineage

Acute undifferentiated leukemia — 9801/3

Mixed-phenotype acute leukemia with t(9;22) (q34.1;q11.2); *BCR-ABL1* — 9806/3

Mixed-phenotype acute leukemia with t(v; 11q23.3); *KMT2A*-rearranged — 9807/3

Mixed-phenotype acute leukemia, B/myeloid, NOS — 9808/3

Mixed-phenotype acute leukemia, T/myeloid, NOS — 9809/3

Mixed-phenotype acute leukemia, NOS, rare types

Acute leukemias of ambiguous lineage, NOS

Precursor lymphoid neoplasms

B-lymphoblastic leukemia/lymphoma, NOS — 9811/3

B-lymphoblastic leukemia/lymphoma with t(9;22) (q34.1;q11.2); *BCR-ABL 1* — 9812/3

B-lymphoblastic leukemia/lymphoma with t(v;11q23.3); *KMT2A*-rearranged — 9813/3

B-lymphoblastic leukemia/lymphoma with t(12;21) (p13.2;q22.1); *ETV6-RUNX1* — 9814/3

B-lymphoblastic leukemia/lymphoma with hyperdiploidy — 9815/3

B-lymphoblastic leukemia/lymphoma with hypo-diploidy (hypodiploid ALL) — 9816/3

B-lymphoblastic leukemia/lymphoma with t(5;14) (q31.1;q32.1); IGH/IL-3 — 9817/3

B-lymphoblastic leukemia/lymphoma with t(1;19) (q23;p13.3); *TCF3-PBX1* — 9818/3

B-lymphoblastic leukemia/lymphoma, *BCR-ABL 1*-like — 9819/3[a]

B-lymphoblastic leukemia/lymphoma with IAMP21 — 9811/3

T-lymphoblastic leukemia/lymphoma — 9837/3

Early T-cell precursor lymphoblastic leukemia — 9837/3

NK-lymphoblastic leukemia/lymphoma

Mature B-cell neoplasms

Chronic lymphocytic leukemia (CLL)/small lymphocytic lymphoma — 9823/3

Monoclonal B-cell lymphocytosis, CLL-type — 9823/1[a]

Monoclonal B-cell lymphocytosis, non-CLL-type — 9591/1[a]

B-cell prolymphocytic leukemia — 9833/3

Splenic marginal zone lymphoma — 9689/3

Hairy cell leukemia — 9940/3

Splenic B-cell lymphoma/leukemia, unclassifiable — 9591/3

   Splenic diffuse red pulp small B-cell lymphoma — 9591/3

   Hairy cell leukemia variant — 9591/3

Lymphoplasmacytic lymphoma — 9671/3

   Waldenström macroglobulinemia — 9761/3

IgM monoclonal gammopathy of undetermined significance — 9761/1[a]

Heavy chain diseases

   µ Heavy chain disease — 9762/3

   γ Heavy chain disease — 9762/3

   α Heavy chain disease — 9762/3

Plasma cell neoplasms

Non-IgM monoclonal gammopathy of undetermined significance	9765/1
Plasma cell myeloma	9732/3
Solitary plasmacytoma of bone	9731/3
Extraosseous plasmacytoma	9734/3
Monoclonal immunoglobulin deposition diseases	
Primary amyloidosis	9769/1
Light chain and heavy chain deposition diseases	9769/1
Extranodal marginal zone lymphoma of mucosa-associated lymphoid tissue (MALT lymphoma)	9699/3
Nodal marginal zone lymphoma	9699/3
Pediatric nodal marginal zone lymphoma	9699/3
Follicular lymphoma	9690/3
In situ follicular neoplasia	9695/1[a]
Duodenal-type follicular lymphoma	9695/3
Testicular follicular lymphoma	9690/3
Pediatric-type follicular lymphoma	9690/3
Large B-cell lymphoma with IRF4 rearrangement	9698/3
Primary cutaneous follicle center lymphoma	9597/3
Mantle cell lymphoma	9673/3
In situ mantle cell neoplasia	9673/1[a]
Diffuse large B-cell lymphoma (DLBCL), NOS	9680/3
Germinal centre B-cell subtype	9680/3
Activated B-cell subtype	9680/3
T-cell/histiocyte-rich large B-cell lymphoma	9688/3
Primary DLBCL of the CNS	9680/3
Primary cutaneous DLBCL, leg type	9680/3
EBV-positive DLBCL, NOS	9680/3
EBV-positive mucocutaneous ulcer	9680/1[a]
DLBCL associated with chronic inflammation	9680/3
Fibrin-associated diffuse large B-cell lymphoma	
Lymphomatoid granulomatosis, grade 1, 2	9766/1
Lymphomatoid granulomatosis, grade 3	9766/3[a]
Primary mediastinal (thymic) large B-cell lymphoma	9679/3
Intravascular large B-cell lymphoma	9712/3
ALK-positive large B-cell lymphoma	9737/3
Plasmablastic lymphoma	9735/3
Primary effusion lymphoma	9678/3
Multicentric Castleman disease	
HHV8-positive DLBCL, NOS	9738/3
HHV8-positive germinotropic lymphoproliferative disorder	9738/1[a]
Burkitt lymphoma	9687/3

Burkitt-like lymphoma with 11q aberration	9687/3[a]
High-grade B-cell lymphoma	
High-grade B-cell lymphoma with MYC and BCL2 and/or BCL6 rearrangements	9680/3
High-grade B-cell lymphoma, NOS	9680/3
B-cell lymphoma, unclassifiable, with features intermediate between DLBCL and classic	
Hodgkin lymphoma	9596/3

Mature T- and NK-cell neoplasms

T-cell prolymphocytic leukemia	9834/3
T-cell large granular lymphocytic leukemia	9831/3
Chronic Lymphoproliferative disorder of NK cells	9831/3
Aggressive NK-cell leukemia	9948/3
Systemic EBV-positive T-cell lymphoma of childhood	9724/3
Chronic active EBV infection of T- and NK-cell type, systemic form	
Hydroa vacciniforme-like lymphoproliferative disorder	9725/1[a]
Severe mosquito bite allergy	
Adult T-cell leukemia/lymphoma	9827/3
Extranodal NK/T-cell lymphoma, nasal type	9719/3
Enteropathy-associated T-cell lymphoma	9717/3
Monomorphic epitheliotropic intestinal	
Hydroa vacciniforme T-cell lymphoma	9717/3
Intestinal T-cell lymphoma, NOS	9717/3
Indolent T-cell lymphoproliferative disorder of the gastrointestinal tract	9702/1[a]
Hepatosplenic T-cell lymphoma	9716/3
Subcutaneous panniculitis-like T-cell lymphoma	9708/3
Mycosis fungoides	9700/3
Sézary syndrome	9701/3
Primary cutaneous CD30-positive T-cell lymphoproliferative disorders	
Hydroa vacciniforme lymphomatoid papulosis	9718/1[a]
Hydroa vacciniforme primary cutaneous anaplastic large cell lymphoma	9718/3
Primary cutaneous γδT-cell lymphoma	9726/3
Primary cutaneous CD8-positive aggressive epidermotropic cytotoxic T-cell lymphoma	9709/3
Primary cutaneous acral CD8-positive T-cell lymphoma	9709/3[a]
Primary cutaneous CD4-positive small/medium T-cell lymphoproliferative disorder	9709/1
Peripheral T-cell lymphoma, NOS	9702/3

Angioimmunoblastic T-cell lymphoma	9705/3
Follicular T-cell lymphoma	9702/3
Nodal peripheral T-cell lymphoma with T-follicular helper phenotype	9702/3
Anaplastic large cell lymphoma, ALK-positive	9714/3
Anaplastic large cell lymphoma, ALK-negative	9715/3[a]
Breast implant-associated anaplastic large cell lymphoma	9715/3[a]

Hodgkin lymphomas

Nodular lymphocyte predominant Hodgkin lymphoma	9659/3
Classic Hodgkin lymphoma	9650/3
Nodular sclerosis classic Hodgkin lymphoma	9663/3
Lymphocyte-rich classic Hodgkin lymphoma	9651/3
Mixed cellularity classic Hodgkin lymphoma	9652/3
Lymphocyte-depleted classic Hodgkin lymphoma	9653/3

Immunodeficiency-associated lymphoproliferative disorders

Post-transplant lymphoproliferative disorders (PTLD)	
Nondestructive PTLD	

Plasmacytic hyperplasia PTLD	
Infectious mononucleosis PTLD	
Florid follicular hyperplasia	
Polymorphic PTLD	9971/1
Monomorphic PTLD	[b]
Classic Hodgkin lymphoma PTLD	9650/3
Other iatrogenic immunodeficiency-associated lympho-proliferative disorders	

Histiocytic and dendritic cell neoplasms

Histiocytic sarcoma	9755/3
Langerhans cell histiocytosis, NOS	9751/1
Langerhans cell histiocytosis, monostotic	9751/1
Langerhans cell histiocytosis, polystotic	9751/1
Langerhans cell histiocytosis, disseminated	9751/3
Langerhans cell sarcoma	9756/3
Indeterminate dendritic cell tumor	9757/3
Interdigitating dendritic cell sarcoma	9757/3
Follicular dendritic cell sarcoma	9758/3
Fibroblastic reticular cell tumor	9759/3
Disseminated juvenile xanthogranuloma	
Erdheim–Chester disease	9749/3

The morphology codes are from the International Classification of Diseases for Oncology (ICD-O). Behaviour is coded /0 for benign tumors; /1 for unspecified, borderline, or uncertain behavior; /2 for carcinoma in situ and grade III intraepithelial neoplasia; and /3 for malignant tumors. The classification is modified from the previous WHO classification, taking into account changes in our understanding of these lesions.

[a]These new codes were approved by the IARC/WHO Committee for ICD-O.

[b]These lesions are classified according to the lymphoma to which they correspond, and are assigned the respective ICD-O code.

Italics: Provisional tumor entities.

Index

Page locators in **bold** indicate tables. Page locators in *italics* indicate figures. This index uses letter-by-letter alphabetization.

Hoffbrand's Essential Haematology, Eighth Edition. By A. Victor Hoffbrand and David P. Steensma.
© 2020 John Wiley & Sons Ltd. Published 2020 by John Wiley & Sons Ltd.
Companion website: www.wileyessential.com/haematology

BMA LIBRARY
BRITISH MEDICAL ASSOCIATION

WITHDRAWN
FROM LIBRARY